A Textbook of

HOMOEOPATHIC PHARMACY

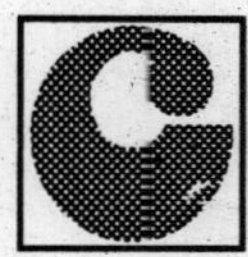

A Textbook of

HOMOEOPATHIC PHARMACY

[For Students of Homoeopathy, Homoeopathic Pharmacists, Practising Homoeopaths and all interested in Homoeopathy]

Dr Biman Mandal BHMS [Gold Medallist]

Foreword by

Dr S K Dubey
DMS [Hons], Gold Medallist, MBS [Hons]
Ex-Principal CHMC
Chairman of Literary Research
Central Council for Research in Homoeopathy [Govt. of India]

Globally Distributed by
New Central Book Agency (P) Ltd
8/1 Chintamoni Das Lane, Kolkata 700 009

NCBA

REGD OFFICE
8/1 Chintamoni Das Lane, Kolkata 700 009, India
email: ncbakolkata@gmail.com

OVERSEAS
NCBA (UK) Ltd, 149 Park Avenue North, Northampton, NN3 2HY, UK
email: ncbauk@yahoo.com

CORPORATE OFFICE
212 Shahpur Jat, New Delhi 110 049
email: delhincba@gmail.com

A TEXTBOOK OF HOMOEOPATHIC PHARMACY • Mandal & Mandal

First Published: 1994
Second Edition: 2004
Reprinted: 2005, 2007, 2009, 2010, 2011
Thoroughly Revised and Enlarged Third Edition: 2012
Fourth Edition: 2022
Thoroughly Revised and Enlarged Fifth Edition: 2024

PUBLISHER
Central Educational Enterprises (P) Ltd
54-B Patuatola Lane, Kolkata 700 009

TYPESETTER • PRINTER
New Central Book Agency (P) Ltd
8/1 Chintamoni Das Lane, Kolkata 700 009

TECHNICAL EDITOR: Dr Mita Sen

PROJECT SUPERVISOR: Meenakshi Bhattacharya, Subas Maitra

PROJECT TEAM: Pradip Baidya and Ashit Ghosh

ISBN: 978 81 7381 743 4

Price ₹ 750.00

NEW SYLLABUS 2015

By Central Council of Homoeopathy

HOMOEOPATHIC PHARMACY

Applicable from the Academic Session 2015-2016

Instructions

Instruction in Homoeopathic Pharmacy shall be so planned as to present-

1. Importance of homoeopathic pharmacy in relation to study of Homoeopathic Materia Medica, Organon of Medicine and National Economy as well as growth of homoeopathic pharmacy and research;
2. Originality and specialty of homoeopathic pharmacy and its relation to pharmacy of other recognised systems of medicine;
3. The areas of teaching shall encompass the entire subject but stress be laid on the fundamental topics that form the basis of homoeopathy.

A. Theory:

I. General concepts and orientation:

1. History of pharmacy with emphasis on emergence of Homoeopathic Pharmacy.
2. Official Homoeopathic Pharmacopoeia (Germany, Britain, U.S.A., India).
3. Important terminologies like scientific names, common names, synonyms.
4. Definitions in Homoeopathic Phamacy.
5. Components of pharmacy.
6. Weights and measures.
7. Nomenclature of homoeopathic drugs with their anomalies.

II Raw material: drugs and vehicles:

1. Sources of drugs (taxonomic classification, with reference to utility).
2. Collection of drugs substances.
3. Vehicles.
4. Homoeopathic Pharmaceutical Instruments and Appliances

III Homoeopathic Pharmaceutics:

1. Mother tincture and its preparation – old and new methods.
2. Various scales used in Homoeopathic Pharmacy.
3. Drug dynamisation or potentisation.
4. External applications (focus on scope of Homoeopathic lotion, glycerol, liniment and ointment).
5. Doctrine of signature.
6. Posology (focus on basic principles related aphorisms of Organon of Medicine).
7. Prescription (Including abbreviations).

8. Concept of Placebo.
9. Pharmaconomy – routes of homoeopathic drug administration.
10. Dispensing of medicines.
11. Basics of adverse drug reactions and Pharmacovigilance.

IV. Pharmacodynamics:

1. Homoeopathic Pharmacodynamics.
2. Drug Proving (related aphorisms 105-145 of Organon of Medicine) and merits and demerits of Drug Proving on Humans and Animals.
3. Pharmacological study of drugs listed in appendix – A

V. Quality Control:

1. Standardisation of homoeopathic medicines, raw materials and finished products.
2. Good Manufacturing Practices (GMPs); Industrial Pharmacy.
3. Homoeopathic Pharmacopoeia Laboratory (HPL) – functions and activities, relating to quality control of drugs.

VI. Legislations pertaining to Pharmacy:

1. The Drugs and Cosmetics Act, 1940 (23 of 1940 ((in relation in Homoeopathy);
2. Drugs and Cosmetics Rules, 1945 (in relation to Homoeopathy);
3. Poisons Act, 1919 (12 of 1919);
4. The Narcotic Drugs and Psychotropic Substance acts, 1985 (61 of 1985);
5. Drugs and Magic Remedies (Objectionable Advertisements) Act, 1954 (21 of 1954);
6. Medicinal and Toilet Preparations (Excise Duties) Act, 1955 (16 of 1955).

B. Practical:

Experiments:

1. Estimation of size of globules.
2. Medication of globules and preparation of doses with sugar of milk and distilled water.
3. Purity test of sugar of milk, distilled water and ethyl alcohol.
4. Determination of specific gravity of distilled water and ethyl alcohol.
5. Preparation of dispensing alcohol and dilute alcohol from strong alcohol.
6. Trituration of one drug each in decimal and centesimal scale.
7. Succussion in decimal scale from Mother Tincture to 6X potency.
8. Succussion in centesimal scale from Mother Tincture to 3C potency.
9. Conversion of Trituration to liquid potency: Decimal scale 6X to 8X potency.
10. Conversion of Trituration to liquid potency: Centesimal scale 3C to 4C potency.
11. Preparation of 0/1 potency (LM scale) of one Drug.
12. Preparation of external applications – lotion, glycerol, liniment, ointment.
13. Laboratory methods – sublimation, distillation, decantation, filtration, crystallisation.
14. Writing of prescription.
15. Dispensing of medicines.
16. Process of taking minims.
17. Identification of drugs (listed in Appendix B):
    (i) Macroscopic and Microscopic characteristic of drug substances - minimum 05 drugs);
    (ii) Microscopic study of trituration of two drugs (up to 3X potency).
18. Estimation of moisture content using water bath.
19. Preparation of mother tincture – maceration and percolation.
20. Collection of 30 drugs for herbarium.
21. Visit to Homoeopathic Pharmacopoeia Laboratory and visit to a large scale manufacturing unit of homoeopathic medicine. (GMP compliant). (Students

shall keep detailed visit reports as per Proforma at Annexure – 'B').

C. Demonstration:

1. General instructions for practical or clinical in pharmacy.
2. Identification and use of homoeopathic pharmaceutical instruments and appliances and their cleaning.
3. Estimation of moisture content using water bath.
4. Preparation of mother tincture – maceration and percolation.

APPENDIX – A

List of drugs included in the syllabus of pharmacy for study of pharmacological action:

1. Aconitum napellus
2. Adonis vernalis
3. Allium cepa
4. Argentum nitricum
5. Arsenicum album
6. Atropa belladonna
7. Cactus grandiflorus
8. Cantharis vesicatoria
9. Cannabis indica
10. Cannabis sativa
11. Cinchona officinalis
12. Coffea cruda
13. Crataegus oxyacantha
14. Crotalus horridus
15. Gelsemium sempervirens
16. Glonoinum
17. Hydrastis canadensis
18. Hyoscyamus niger
19. Kali bichromicum
20. Lachesis
21. Lithium carbonicum
22. Mercurius corrosivus
23. Naja tripudians
24. Nitricum acidum
25. Nux vomica
26. Passiflora incarnata
27. Stannum metallicum
28. Stramonium
29. Symphytum officinale
30. Tabacum

APPENDIX – B

List of drugs for identification

I. Vegetable Kingdom

1. Aegle folia
2. Anacardium orientale
3. Andrographis paniculata
4. Calendula officinalis
5. Cassia sophera
6. Cinchona officinalis
7. Cocculus indicus
8. Coffea cruda
9. Colocynthis
10. Crocus sativa
11. Croton tiglium
12. Cynodon dactylon
13. Ficus religiosa
14. Holarrhena antidysenterica
15. Hydrocotyle asiatica
16. Justicia adhatoda
17. Lobelia inflata
18. Nux vomica
19. Ocimum sanctum
20. Opium
21. Rauwolfia serpentina
22. Rheum
23. Saraca indica
24. Senna
25. Stramonium
26. Vinca minor

II. Chemicals or Minerals

1. Acetium acidum
2. Alumina
3. Argentum metallicum
4. Argentum nitricum
5. Arsenicum album
6. Calcarea carbonica
7. Carbo vegetabilis

8. Graphites
9. Magnesium phosphoricum
10. Natrum muriaticum
11. Sulphur

III. Animal kingdom

1. Apis mellifica
2. Blatta orientalis
3. Formica rufa
4. Sepia
5. Tarentula cubensis

Note:1. Each student shall maintain practical or clinical record or journal and herbarium file separately.

2. College authority shall facilitate the students in maintaining record as per Appendix– C.

D. Examination:

1. Theory

1.1 Number of Paper – 01

1.2 Marks: 100

2. Practical including viva voice or oral

2.1 Marks: 100

2.2	Distribution of marks:	Marks
2.2.1	Experiments	15
2.2.2	Spotting	20
2.2.3	Maintenance of practical records or journal	10
2.2.4	Maintenance of herbarium record	05
2.2.5	Viva voice (oral)	50
	Total	100

Contents

Foreword

I have gone through "A Textbook of Homoeopathic Pharmacy" by Dr Partha Pratim Mandal and Dr Biman Mandal. I am pleased to note that the treatise is very competent and up-to-date, and will be useful not only to the students but also to the profession at large.

Within the short compass of Homoeopathic Pharmacy, the authors have endeavoured to incorporate all the important matters in a systematic, logical, and schematic manner with due consideration to the long-felt need of the students and busy practitioners.

The book seeks to make everything as up-to-date as can be in this fast-moving world. It will certainly be a trusty companion to the practising physicians and pharmcists.

The chapters which deserve special mention deal with sources of Homoeopathic drugs, different scales of preparation of drugs, methods of preparing Homoeopathic drugs, potentisation, and list of drugs with their common name, family, distribution, and parts used.

The authors, as I well know, are brilliant students of Homoeopathy with genuine research and scientific aptitude. They have earned well-deserved reputation in practising Homoeopathy. I am sure that they will be able to offer more excellent works in future for the students and the profession.

Dr S K Dubey

12 Blank

Preface to the Fourth Edition

The fourth edition of this classic text has been fully updated to reflect the latest research and development in Homoeopathic Pharmacy.

This thoroughly revised edition includes new chapters in 'Contribution of Homoeopathic Stalwarts in the field of Pharmacy', 'Pharmacovigilance', 'Artificial Intelligence in the Homoeopathy', and 'Abbreviations used in Homoeopathic Pharmacy'.

In this edition some important additions have been made in the text of original chapters such as 'Pharmacopoeia and Pharmacy', 'Methods of preparing Homoeopathic Drugs' (Old method), 'Pharmacology', 'Identification of some Homoeopathic Drugs', 'Drug action: Characteristics of some important Drug Substances', 'Weights and Measures', 'Doctrine of Signature', 'Recent advances in Homoeopathic Pharmacy'.

I hope this edition will be invaluable to degree and post-graduate students, Pharmacist's in the Homoeopathic Medicine Industry, Clinical Researchers and Physicians.

Hearty congratulations to Dr. Sumit Pramanik and Dr. Debasish Mandal for thier kind cooperation in writing this edition.

I express my gratitude to the publisher and the entire production unit of New Central Book Agency Pvt. Ltd. whose tireless efforts have made it possible to publish this edition.

Ratha Jatra
7th July 2024

Dr Biman Mandal

Preface to the First Edition

There are undeniably some literature which embraces the subject of Homoeopathy Pharmacy. But from our student life in B.H.M.S. of Calcutta University, we felt the necessity of a complete and standard Textbook on Homoeopathy Pharmacy which can give students the factual profile and conceptual perception.

Keeping such a need in view, **the book has been planned and written in accordance with the syllabi of BHMS and DHMS courses of all Indian Universities.** And also for those who are interested in the subject. Endeavour has been made in this book not only to portray the factual profiles with their interpretations but also, as far as possible, to dovetail the concept developed with practices that existed in different pharmacopoeias.

The subject matter, both as regards the arrangements of chapters as well as the contents of each chapter, has been so graded that the students may follow the course with ease and inte-rest. From that point of view, the book may claim its specialities for schematic presentation, diagram, and biochemical analysis.

It is meant not only for Students but also useful for practising Physicians and for the Laboratory Technicians in this field. We feel indebted to the great scholars in the sphere of Pharmacy, our teachers, and our colleagues from whom we received help in any form.

We take this opportunity to gratefully acknowledge the guidance of our teacher and mentor Dr S K Dubey, Ex-Principal, Calcutta Homoeopathic Medical College and the Chairman, Central Council for Research in Homoeopathy.

We convey our gratefulness to Dr C R Paithankar of Calcutta, Dr Madhusudan Dutta and Dr Sujit Mandal of Bankura, Dr Prabir Mukherjee of Durgapur, Dr Pradip Saha of Krishnanagar, and Dr Chandan Sarkar of Balurghat.

We are happy to record our thanks to friends and well-wishers like Sri Asim Chatterjee, Sri Bidyut Gorai, Sri Sukomal Ghosh, Sri Tushar Kanti Ghosh, and Sri Kamal Das of Bankura. Prof. Siddhartha Bhattacharya of Bankura Sammilani College deserves our deep gratitude for his constant help and cooperation in publishing such a book.

Sri Amitabha Sen, Director of New Central Book Agency (P) Ltd, and his colleagues deserve high praise for undertaking the publication of the book in a highly commendable and elegant form.

We would like to place on record our gratitude for the assistance and encouragement from Miss Soma Maiti.

First edition might have some errors of omission and commission and we will always be grateful to our readers for any advice that may help us to improve the next edition of this work.

Dr Partha Pratim Mandal
Dr Biman Mandal

Chapter 01

Pharmacopoeia and Pharmacy

PHARMACOPOEIA

Etymology

The word 'pharmacopoeia' is derived from two Greek words—*'pharmakon'* meaning 'a drug' and *'poiein'* meaning 'to make'.

Definition

It is the supreme (standard) authoritative book, published by the authority of government of any country, which deals with the scientific facts and logical attitude of the rules and regulations of standardisation of drug substances, containing directions for collecting drug materials from different sources, for preparing, preserving, compounding and combining of various drugs.

Besides, it contains—external applications, prescription writing, posology and monograph of drugs. It is officially published by the authority of government of any country or any/medical or pharmaceutical society, either constituted or authorised by government.

Pharmacopoeia is the theoretical part of pharmacy.

Types of Pharmacopoeia

Two types of pharmacopoeia are present:

(a) *Official pharmacopoeia*: The official (Lat. *officium,* authority) pharmacopoeia is published by the government or any authority of the government of a country.

(b) *Unofficial pharmacopoeia*: It is published by any person or pharmaceutical company other than the government.

First Recognised Pharmacopoeia

Perhaps the first widely recognised pharmacopoeia was the Dispensatorium of Valerius Cordus (1515-1544) (First edition 1546*). This contain many old formulae derived from traditional sources including Galen, Avicenna, Mesue and Rhazes, but also contained a number of unique references to medicines, including the first accurate description of Nux vomica and many preparations of essential oils.

The Dispensatorium of Valerius Cordus, was adopted by the Senate of Nuremberg, which gave rise to the work being known later as the 'Nuremberg Pharmacopoeia'. It was well known in England in the sixteenth century, along with other similar works such as The Grete Herball, an

English translation of Le Grant Herbier en Francoys (1516-1520), which was itself sourced from the first herbal compiled in French, Arbolayre (c. 1485).

In the dispensatorium the herbs, minerals and other crude drugs were arranged in alphabetical order and information was given about their identification, sources, preparation and uses, together with some detail of pathology and therapeutics.

Father of Homoeopathic Pharmacopoeia

Dr. Carl W. Caspari (1798-1828) of Leipzig, Germany.

The first homoeopathic pharmacopoeia was published by him in 1825. He published '*Homöopathisches Dispensatorium für Aerzte und Apotheker*' thereby giving the first idea of homoeopathic pharmacopoeias for physicians and pharmacists.

Previously, medicines were prepared by extemporaneous pharmacy till 1825.

History and Development of Homoeopathic Pharmacopoeia

Hahnemann was not only the inventor of homoeopathy, at the same time he was the pioneer of 'Experimental Pharmacology'. He was the first to ascertain the positive effects of drugs on healthy human beings. The fruits of his labour in the field of pharmacology or pharmacodynamics are preserved in—

(a) Materia Medica Pura

(b) Organon of Medicine

(c) The Chronic Diseases, Their Peculiar Nature and Their Homoeopathic Cure.

Though he never wrote any separate book on, 'Pharmacopoeia' his scattered records regarding the basic principles of homoeopathic preparation of drugs and medicines, served as the basis of homeopathic pharmacopoeia in future.

1805: In 1805, Hahnemann announced his new method of pharmacological process in the treatise, '*Fragmenta de Viribus Medicamentorum Positivis Sive in Sano Corpore Humano Observatis*', which included the first repertory of homoeopathic materia medica. Between 1811 and 1833 were published his 'Materia Medica Pura' and 'Chronic Diseases'.

1825: Firstly, the homoeopathic pharmacopoeia was written by Dr. Carl W. Caspari of Leipzig, Germany, in 1825. He published a, 'Homöopathisches Dispensatorium für Aerzte und Apotheker'. Dr. Caspari was a member of Samuel Hahnemann's provers Union and wrote the Homoeopathic Domestic Physician which included a chapter on mesmerism.

1829: Hartmann: Pharmacopoeia Homoeopathica.

1834: Frederick Hervey Foster Quin (1799-1878), the president of British Homoeopathic Society, edited, 'The Pharmacopoeia Homoeopathica' in Latin, published in 1834 in London, dedicated to Leopold I, king of the Belgians. This pharmacopoeia contains 188 medicines.

1840: Joseph Benedict Buchner published Homoeopathische Arzneibereitungs lehre to which Jahr refers.

1842: New Homoeopathic Pharmacopoeia and Posology, or The Preparation of Homoeopathic medicines and The Administration of Doses, by Gottlieb Heinrich Georg Jahr, appeared in Germany, and was translated into English by James Kitchen, M. D. and published in Philadelphia, New York, in 1842. First independent U.S. publication.

1845: Carl Ernest Gruner's Homoopathische Pharmacopoe, compiled and published in 1845.

1850: New Homoeopathic Pharmacopoeia and Posology, or the mode of preparing homoeopathic medicines and the administration of doses compiled and translated from the German works of Buchner and Gruner and the French work of Jahr, with original contributions by Chas. J. Hempel, M.D. This work contains 304 medicines.

1852: Buchner's 2nd and enlarged edition of his Homoopathische Arzneibereitungslehre published in 1852.

1855: An authorised English edition of Gruner's Homöopathische Pharmacopoe, published in Leipzig, London and New York, in 1855.

1870: British Homoeopathic Pharmacopoeia published by British Homoeopathic Society, Great Ormond Street, London, W.C. First edition.

1872: Von Willmar Schwabe's, '*Pharmacopoeia Homoeopathica Polyglotta*' published in 1872.

1876: British Homoeopathic Pharmacopoeia, published by the British Homoeopathic Society, Second edition.

1882: In 1882 the first edition of 'The American Homoeopathic Pharmacopoeia' edited by Joseph T. O'connor and published by Boericke and Tafel in Philadelphia. The description of drugs were taken largely from the United States Dispensatory, the United States Pharmacopoeia, and the National Dispensatory: the rules for preparation were taken from the "*Pharmacopoeia Homoeopathica Polyglotta*". It was therefore essentially a reprint of Schwabe's pharmacopoeia.

1882: British Homoeopathic Pharmacopoeia published by the British Homoeopathic Society, Third edition. This edition of B.H.P. contains a total of 510 medicines (of which 268 are in the text of the book and 242 in the Appendix).

1884: Theodore D. Williams '*The American Homoeopathic Dispensatory*' published in 1884. It contains 871 medicines.

1892: In India, M. Bhattacharya and Co. published '*Pharmaceutics Manual*' in 1892.

1897: '*Pharmacopoeia of the American Institute of Homoeopathy*' was published in June, 1897, by the American Institute of Homoeopathy, with thd help of Otis Clapp and Son, Agents, Boston, USA. First edition.

1898: Pharmacopie Homoeopathique Francaise (PHF).

1901: After revision, 2nd edition of the *Pharmacopoeia of the American Institute of Homoeopathy* was published and its title was changed to the more comprehensive "*Homoeopathic Pharmacopoeia of the United States (HPUS)*". It thus became the official guide for the pharmacists and physicians, and they should conform their methods to its requirements.

1938: The FDA regulates the manufacture and sale of homoeopathic medicines. The Homoeopathic Pharmacopoeia of the US was written into federal law in 1938.

1945: N. Nundie's, 'A short sketch of States Homoeopathic Pharmacopoeia of USA' published in 1945. It contains 713 medicines.

1962: The Government of India constituted the Homoeopathic pharmacopoeia committee in September, 1962. Dr. B. K. Sarkar was the first chairman of Homoeopathic pharmacopoeia committee.

1975: Homoeopathic pharmacopoeia Laboratory, Ghaziabad (HPL) was set up in September, 1975 as a sub-ordinate organisation of the Department. It is recognised by the Department of Science and Technology, as Scientific, Technological and Research Institution.

Types of Homoeopathic Pharmacopoeias

Homoeopathic pharmacopoeias may be official and un-official.

- Official Homoeopathic Pharmacopoeias:
  1. German Homoeopathic Pharmacopoeia (GHP).
  2. British Homoeopathic Pharmacopoeia (BHP).
  3. Homoeopathic Pharmacopoeia of United States (HPUS).
  4. Homoeopathic Pharmacopoeia of India (HPI).
  5. French Homoeopathic Pharmacopoeia (FHP).

  The homoeopathic pharmacopoeias was gradually made official throughout the world. It appeared:

  in 1938 in the United States

  in 1965 in France

  in 1971 in India

  in 1978 in Germany

- Unofficial Homoeopathic Pharmacopoeias:
  1. M. Bhattacharya and Co's Homoeopathic Pharmacopoeia.
  2. Encyclopaedia Homoeopathic Pharmacopoeia by P. N. Verma and Indu Vaid.

3. Brazilian Homoeopathic Pharmacopoeia.
4. Pakistan Homoeopathic Pharmacopoeia.
5. Mexican Homoeopathic Pharmacopoeia.

Pharmacopoeias Recognised World-wide

While a number of countries may not have their own homoeopathic pharmacopoeias, they do recognise the French, German (HAB), American (HPUS) and European Pharmacopoeias. This is notably the case in Australia, Tunisia, Morocco, Lebanon and Ukraine. Russra also recognises these pharmacopoeias, in addition to its own.

German Homoeopathic Pharmacopoeia (G.H.P.)–1825

The first homoeopathic pharmacopoeia was published by Dr. Carl W. Caspari of Leipzig, Germany. He published a '*Homöopathisches Dispensatorium fur Aerzte ünd Apotheker*', thereby giving the first ideä of homoeopathic pharmacopoeias for physicians and pharmacists.

Every new edition of G.H.P. contains new developments. In the 1979 edition, there was inclusion of new direction methods such as spectral analysis. Hahnemann's work has been so accurate that, except for technical changes, the G.H.P. still follows his directions.

Dr. Willmar Schwabe of Leipzig founded the Homoeopathic Central Pharmacy to manufacture and sell homoeopathic medicines in 1866. He created precise standards for homoeopathic pharmaceutical production which was published in 1872 as, '*Pharmacopoeia Homoeopathica Polyglotta*'. In 1880, the first English edition of this work was published. In 1929 the second English edition was published. This was later revised and is known today as 'Dr. Willmar Schwabe Homoeopathisches Arzneibuch' which was subsequently accepted as the official German Homoeopathic Pharmacopoeia (GHP) or. Homoeopathisches Arzneibuch (HAB). Today HAB serves as an international reference standard for homoeopathic medicines.

G.H.P. Supplement 2005, edited by Stephen Benyunes and published in Dec. 03, 2005.

G.H.P. 2nd Supplement, edited by Stephen Benyunes and published in January 17, 2006.

British Homoeopathic Pharmacopoeia (B.H.P.)–1870

The first edition of the B.H.P. was published for the British Homoeopathic Society in 1870 by J. E. Altard and followed by the publication of the second and third editions in 1876 by W. J. Johnson and 1882 by E. Gould, respectively, and Son of London. It then went out of print for over a century. New editions of the B.H.P. were published by the British Association of Homoeopathic Manufacturers (B.A.H.M.) in 1993 and 1999.

The book is in a clear loose-leaf format and reflects many of the current practices developed by British Manufacturers by adopting German methods. It is designed to be used in conjunction with the G.H.P.

The B.H.P. has no official status, having not been adopted as a national standard by the M.H.R.A. (Medicines and Health care products Regulatory Agency).

The *first part* of the book contains background information to the manufacture of homoeopathic preparations, including abbreviations, analytical methods, reagents and general regulations for the manufacture of homoeopathic medicines. Cross-reference is made to the G.H.P. and other pharmacopoeias. At the start of the section on manufacturing methods there is an index to all the methods of preparation, referencing the source of the method concerned.

The monographs are set out in the *second part.*

Note: Companion to the, British and American Homoeopathic Pharmacopoeias—arranged in the form of dictionary, was compiled by Lawrence T. Ashwell, London, in 1881. Its 2nd, 3rd and 4th editions have been published in July 1883, May 1884, Sept. 1890, respectively. These compilations had been accepted by the physicians.

Homoeopathic Pharmacopoeia of USA (H.P.U.S.)–1897

It was published in June 1897, by Otis Clapp and Son, Agents under the direction of '*Committee on American Institute of Homoeopathy*' named as '*Pharmacopoeia of the American Institute of Homoeopathy*'.

Its 2nd edition was published in 1901, under the direction of *'Committee on American Institute of Homoeopathy'* and its title was changed to the more comprehensive one – *'Homoeopathic Pharmacopoeia of United States'*, in short 'H.P.U.S'.

Further, the 6th edition was published in 1941 which introduced the *'New Method of Mother Tincture Preparation'* keeping the water content of the drug substance in mind.

The 7th edition was published in 1964 and 8th edition Volume 1 was published in 1979 with an addendum, *'Compendium of Homoeotherapeutics'*.

In June 1938, 'Food, Drug and Cosmetic Act' (commonly known as the Pure Food Law) was passed and the HPUS became the official pharmacopoeia of USA. for the preparation of all remedies used in homoeopathic practice.

In December 1980, the *'Homoeopathic Pharmacopoeia Convention of the United States'*(H.P.C.U.S) was incorporated as an independent body assumed responsibility for future publication. The H.P.C.U.S. published Supplement 'A' of the H.P.U.S. 8th edition in 1982.

In reality, the H.P.U.S. comprises of three different books: (i) Compendium of Homoeotherapeutics (1974) (ii) 7th edition Volume 1 (1978) and (iii) Supplement 'A' of the H.P.U.S. 8th edition (1982). This system of three texts caused information to be difficult to access.

To eliminate the difficulties *'Homoeopathic Pharmacopoeia Convention of the United States'* (H.P.C.U.S.) decided to republish these texts into one compilation to be known as the *'Homoeopathic Pharmacopoeia of United States/Revision Service'* (H.P.R.S).

Editions of Homoeopathic Pharmacopoeia of United States

An H.P.U.S. time line: Phase One 1841-1897

The H.P.U.S. has been in continuous publication since 1897.

Roots:

1841 Jahr's *'New Homoeopathic Pharmacopoeia and Posology'*, which appeared in Germany, and was translated into English by James Kitchen and published in Philadelphia in 1842. First independent US publication.

1868 *'American Institute of Homoeopathy'* (A.I.H) formed its committee to prepare a dispensatory, chaired by Carroll Dunham.

1882 *'The American Homeopathic Pharmacopoeia'*, written by Boericke and Tafel, was first published in 1882.

An H.P.U.S. time line: Phase Two 1897-1980

Publication by the American Institute of Homoeopathy (A.I.H.)

1897 *'Pharmacopoeia of the American Institute of Homoeopathy'* was published in June 1897 by Otis Clapp and Son, Agents under the direction of *'Committee on American Institute of Homoeopathy'*. First edition.

1901 2nd Edition (Mohr/Clapp)

1914 3rd Edition (TH Carmichael/Clapp)

1936 4th Edition (TH Carmichael)

1938 'Food, Drug and Cosmetic Act' was passed and the HPUS became the official pharmacopoeia of USA. for the preparation of all remedies used in homoeopathic practice.

Editions	Name of Pharmacopoeia	Published under the direction of
1st edition (1897)	Pharmacopoeia of the American Institute of Homoeopathy (A.I.H)	Committee on American Institute of Homoeopathy (A.I.H)
2nd to 7th edition	Title changed to Homoeopathic Pharmacopoeia of United States (H.P.U.S)	Committee on American Institute of Homoeopathy (A.I.H)
8th edition	Homoeopathic Pharmacopoeia of the United States (H.P.U.S)	Homoeopathic Pharmacopoeia Convention of the United States (H.P.C.U.S)

1938:5th Edition (TH Carmichael)

1941:6th Edition (TH Carmichael)

1964:7th Edition (Roger Schmidt)

1974:Compendium of Homoeotherapeutics (Baker)

1978:7th Edition, Vol. 1 (Rogers/Baker).

An H.P.U.S. time line: Phase Three 1980–present

Publication by the independent Homoeopathic Pharmacopoeia Convention of the United States (H.P.C.U.S).

1980:In December 1980, the *'Homoeopathic Pharmacopoeia Convention of the United States'* (H.P.C.U.S) was incorporated as an independent body with a focus to update and continue publication of the H.P.U.S.

1982:The H.P.C.U.S published Supplement 'A' of the H.P.U.S 8th edition.

1983-1988: Development of *Compliance Policy Guide,* 7132-15 (Borneman).

1988:Homoeopathic Pharmacopoeia of United States/Revision Service (H.P.R.S). It is the official guide in homoeopathy. It contains information and manufacturing standards for over 1,300 official homoeopathic substances.

1990:Compliance Policy Guide (C.P.Gs), 713.15 becomes effective.

1992:H.P.R.C. (Homoeopathic Pharmacopoeia of United States/Revision Committee) is complete semiannual updates, supersedes compendium and Supplement 'A' as the official compendium.

1992-2004: Monographs, General Pharmacy. Standards and Controls updated semi-annually.

2004:H.P.U.S. online begins, immediate/real-time updates. Today, the H.P.U.S is published online and continuously updated by multiple working committees of the H.P.C.U.S.

Homoeopathic Pharmacopoeia of India (H.P.I.)–1971

H.P.I, is the official pharmacopoeia of India. Worked out standards of drugs are released by the Ministry of HealtK and Family Welfare in the form of Homoeopathic Pharmacopoeia of India (H.P.I.). Ten volumes consisting of standard for drugs have already been published by the Government of India (Ministry of Health), compiled by the 'Homoeopathic Pharmacopoeia Committee', appointed by the Central Government of India, in Sept. 1962 under the Chairmanship of Dr. B. K. Sarkar.

Several experts have contributed from time to time for the publications of Ist – Xth Volume of Homoeopathic Pharmacopoeia of India (HPI) that comprises monographs of 1111 drugs. The details are as under:

Volume	Year	New	Revised	Total
Volume I	1971	180	---	180
Volume II	1974	99	---	99
Volume III	1978	105	---	105
Volume IV	1984	104	02	106
Volume V	1987	109	01	110
Volume VI	1990	103	01	104
Volume VII	1999	77	28	105
Volume VIII	2000	74	27	101
Volume IX	2006	73	27	100
Volume X	2013	101	---	101
Total	1025	86	1111	

There are total 1,111 monographs has been published in ten volumes by the Council till date and out of which, 1,025 monographs are new and 86 monographs are revised.

Latest Research on H.P.I under C.C.R.H.

1. **Homoeopathic Pharmacopoeia of India (HPI) revision and updating work (Volume I to X):** About 60 monographs from plants and chemicals have been updated so far as advance analytical method in H.P.L.

2. **Preparation of monographs for H.P.I Volume XI:** About 11 monographs from plants and chemicals have been incorporated in H.P.I Volume XI from Dr D. P. Rastogi Central Research Institute for Homoeopathy (D.D.P.R.C.R.I.H), Noida. The publication work of H.P.I Volume XI is under progress.

3. **H.P.I-H.P.U.S Harmonisation Work:** 50 monographs of both pharmacopoeias have been harmonise so far in order to duplication of work.

The functions of the Homoeopathic Pharmacopoeia Committee (H.P.C.) were—

(a) **To prepare a pharmacopoeia of Homoeopathic drugs, whose therapeutic usefulness has been proved on the lines of the American, German, and British Pharmacopoeias.**

(b) **To lay down principles and standards for the preparation of homoeopathic drugs.**

(c) **To lay down tests for identity, quality, and purity.**

(d) **Such other matters as are incidental and necessary for the preparation of a homoeopathic pharmacopoeia.**

In the course of compiling the H.P.I., the Indian Pharmacopoeia (I.P.), the American Homoeopathic Pharmacopoeia (A.H.P.), the Homoeopathic Pharmacopoeia of United States (H.P.U.S.), British Homoeopathic Pharmacopoeia (B.H.P.) and the German Homoeopathic Pharmacopoeia (G.H.P.) are consulted.

The H.P.C. has been assigned the above work; besides, it also had to prepare a Homoeopathic Pharmaceutical Codex.

The H.P.C. was constituted in Sept, 1962, on the recommendation of the Homoeopathic Advisory Committee and Homoeopathic Subcommittee of the Drug Technical Advisory Board, on the question of control of homoeopathic drugs under The Drugs and Cosmetics Act., 1940, and Rules 1945. The homoeopathic drugs are prepared mainly from plants, animals, and minerals. For this purpose, the committee has experts from Chemistry, Botany and Pharmacology branches besides manufacturers of medicines and homoeopathic practitioners as well as officials who are concerned with the work of testing and research in drugs. H.P.I, is included in the second Schedule of 'Drugs and Cosmetic Act—1940'.

We in India used to follow the H.P.U.S. upto 1971 because there was no separate book of our own.

French Homoeopathic Pharmacopoeia (F.H.P.)–1898

F.H.P. is named as *Pharmacopie Homoeopathiaue Francaise* firstly published in 1898.

The homoeopathic system is highly accepted in France and medicines are available in almost all homoeopathic pharmacies. The F.H.P. is somewhat different from pharmacopoeias of other countries.

The F.H.P. gives valuable information on nosodes, sarcodes and introduced many new drugs on gemmotherapie (extraction on glycerine), organotherapie (parts of the body—similar to sarcodes); lithotherapie (from crude materials).

F.H.P. is not recognised in India, but the physicians believe in the new drugs introduced in France and they tend to use the product when available.

F.H.P. has the following features:

1. Categories of products:
   (i) Mother tincture TM (of plants, animals and chemicals).
   (ii) Potencies—decimal (D, DH, X or XH) and centesimal (C or CH).
   (iii) Combination of the above.
2. Material source:
   (i) Vegetables (or botanicals)
   (ii) Animals
   (iii) Minerals and inorganic chemicals
   (iv) Organic substances and chemicals
   (v) Biological and microbiologicals.
3. Therapeuticals forms:
   (i) Drops and combination of monodilutions or tinctures
   (ii) Triturations
   (iii) Granules or globules (impregnated)
   (iv) Tablets and capsules
   (v) Ampoules
   (vi) Suppositories
   (vii) Pommades.
4. Permitted vehicles:
   (i) Purified water
   (ii) Alcohols of different strengths
   (iii) Glycerol
   (iv) Sugar of milk (or Lactose)
   (v) Sucrose

(vi) Gelatin

(vii) Lanoline

5. Alcohol %: Mostly Hahnemannian principles are adopted.
   (i) Mother tincture contains 40-90% alcohol.
   (ii) Dilution contains 70% alcohol for impregnation and 40% for oral use.
6. Precautions: Proper precautions have been taken for the purity of basic material, procedural precautions and technique of preparation of tincture or triturations; the controls on the alcohol percentage, Chromatography (T.L.C.) and drug content, etc.

M. Bhattacharya and Co.'s Homoeopathic Pharmacopoeia—1892

In India, the first homoeopathic pharmacopoeia was published by M. Bhattacharya and Co. Private Ltd., Kolkata, in 1892 named *'Pharmaceutics Manual'*. Since then it has run into several editions.

The tenth edition was published in 1944, incorporated and contained about 70 of the important Indian drugs. This edition contains 1,193 entries but there are many double entries.

A thoroughly revised and enlarged twelfth edition was published in July, 1962, on behalf of M. Bhattacharya and Co. Private Ltd., Kolkata, under the name and style of, "M. Bhattacharya and Co.'s Homoeopathic Pharmacopoeia".

The thirteenth edition was published in 1970 and fourteenth edition published in 1980. These two editions are only the reprints of the twelfth edition.

This pharmacopoeia is considered as a valuable work but it is not officially recognised by the Govt. of India.

Encyclopaedia of Homoeopathic Pharmacopoeia (E.H.P.)—1997

This pharmacopoeia comprises three volumes containing about 1860 monographs of homoeopathic drugs in alphabetical order, based on H.P.I. It is edited by Dr. P. N. Varma and Dr. Mrs. Indu Vaid, published by M/s. B. Jain Pvt. Ltd., India.

It is the useful compilation based on H.P.I., H.P.U.S., H.A.B., F.H.P. and other authoritative homoeopathic literatures:

Vol. I: Contained 697 drugs, which are frequently used by homoeopaths of India, Pakistan and Malaysia.

Vol. II: Contained 713 lesser known drugs and much data in this volume was abstracted from H.P.U.S.

Vol. III: Contained 450 new drugs.

This pharmacopoeia serves as a 'reference book' for standards not covered by H.P.I. The annexures of alcohol contents as recommended by the H.P.I., H.P.U.S., H.A.B., the lowest limit of prescribing of toxic medicines, the glossary of botanical and medical terms have all enhanced the value of the book.

Note: This textbook is the main source of drugs used in Malaysia by Prof. Dr. Nik Omar from the Faculty of Homoeopathy, Malaysia, Pasir Mas, Kelantan.

Brazilian Homoeopathic Pharmacopoeia—1976

The homoeopathic pharmacopoeia of Brazil was first published in 1976.

The second edition, part 1 was published in 1997. The pharmacopoeia may be called as Farmacopoeia Homeopathis Brasileira (FHB). Its 3rd edition was published in 2011.

Pakistan Homoeopathic Pharmacopoeia

The Homoeopathic Pharmacopoeia of Pakistan was published in Lahore, by the Board of Homoeopathic System of Medicine, in 1978, 1st edition. Its second edition was published in 1997.

Mexican Homoeopathic Pharmacopoeia

First edition of homoeopathic pharmacopoeia in Mexico was published in 1998, in Spanish. It is named as Farmacopea Homeopatica Mexicana. Its 2nd edition was published in 2007.

MONOGRAPHS

The general plan of pharmacopoeias is to lay down the direction for the selection and preparation of drugs that are thoroughly adapted to the purpose of homoeopathic prescribing. These directions and specifications for each drug are called 'monograph'.

Features

(i) The standards and strengths are stated in the monographs of the pharmacopoeia and are applied to articles that are intended for medicinal use, but not necessarily to articles that may be sold under the same name for other purposes.

(ii) All statements contained in the monographs constitute standards for the official substances.

(iii) There is no set framed to provide against all possible impurities.

General pattern of a monograph

The general pattern of monographs has the following features—

(a) Plant:
1. Name with abbreviation
2. Botanical name
3. Family
4. Common names
5. Description
6. Part used
7. Macroscopical
8. Microscopical
9. Identification tests
10. Distribution
11. History and authority
12. Preparation
13. Storage
14. Caution

(b) Animal:
1. Name with abbreviation
2. Zoological name
3. Family
4. Common name
5. Description
6. Part used
7. Microscopical
8. Distribution
9. History and authority
10. Preparation
11. Storage
12. Caution.

(c) Chemical:
1. Name with abbreviation
2. Symbol
3. Molecular weight
4. English name
5. Description
6. Identification
7. Reaction
8. Limit tests
9. Assay
10. History and authority
11. Preparation
12. Storage
13. Caution.

(d) Nosode:
1. Name with abbreviation
2. Microbiological name
3. History and authority
4. Biological distribution
5. Source of preparation
6. Description/Morphology of the organism
7. Cultural characteristics
8. Resistance and metabolism
9. Biochemical reactions
10. Preparation
11. Storage
12. Caution.

Object of Homoeopathic Pharmacopoeia

The object of homoeopathic pharmacopoeia is to list of remedies used in homoeopathic treatment and give proper instructions as to their identity and preparations aiming to give preference to preparation of the drugs similar to those used in the original proving.

Pharmacopoeia also describes the standard methods and gives the standards of purity that has to be followed when preparing the medicines.

If the drug proving appears to be adequate and demand for the medicine by pharmacists sufficient to warrant the manufacture and stocking of the medicines, it may be listed in the homoeopathic pharmacopoeia.

PHARMACY

Definition

It is an art and science of identifying, selecting, collecting, combining, preparing, preserving and standardization of drugs and medicines either from natural and synthetic sources. It also embraces knowledge of medicine, art of compounding and dispensing them.

Dr. William Boericke, in his, "A Compend of the Principles of Homoeopathy" defines pharmacy as "the art of preparing drugs for use and dispensing them as medicines".

According to Chambers Dictionary—"Pharmacy is the art, practice or science of collecting, preparing, preserving, and dispensing of medicines".

History of Pharmacy

The history of pharmacy is nothing but the history of medicine. It is very difficult to begin or point out the beginning of pharmacy. There are no such documentary proof or evidence in respect of historical development of pharmacology.

Fighting against the diseases with drugs is a timeless struggle. Its beginning echoed out in early ages when mankind lived in jungle. Man's survival and enjoyment for better health has depended partly upon the success of pharmacy.

There are significant events in the history of this part of the specific science which led to the development of pharmacy as a separate and distinct discipline. This can be explained according to the countrywise and century-wise parameter.

A. Primitive Period

The disease was considered as a displeasure of God or the priests were considered to be the only personnel who are capable of driving out the disease process and they used to prescribe some folk-medicine.

B. Period before 13th Century

This period includes (i) Egyptian and Babylonian medicine, (ii) Mohammedan and Jewish medicine, (iii) Ancient Hindu medicine, (iv) Greek and Roman medicines.

During these periods there are certain notable facts:

(a) The medicine box of Egyptian queen of 11th Dynasty containing dried drugs and roots, spoons, vases are the important findings in support of pharmacological thoughts.

(b) Charak whose Charak Samhita is the first authentic pharmacopoeia in India. Susruta (5th century B.C.): Hindu medicines were very rich in drug. Susruta mentioned 760 medicinal plants and their use, some ointments, sneezing powders and inhalations. These were the part of Ayurveda (about 700 B.C.).

(c) Ibn Sinna or Avicenna (980-1037 A.D.): He was called Prince of Physicians in Mohammedan period. He wrote a treatise known as "Canon", where he described the preparation of alcohol and sulphuric acid.

(d) Abu Mansur: His book on Materia Medica was an important work on pharmacology. Their disciplines of Materia Medica and preparation of drugs became standard authority throughout the Middle Ages.

(e) Shen Nung: A Chinese emperor who lived about 3000 B.C., wrote a book known as "Pen Tsoas" (Chinese Materia Medica). This book contains description of thousands of drugs. Different vegetable substances (e.g. Opium, Rhubarb, Aconite, Croton), inorganic substances (e.g. Iron, Arsenic, Sulphur) are mentioned in this book.

C. Period after 13th Century

(a) Paracelsus (1493-1541): He was the precursor of chemical pharmacology and therapeutics of the 16th century. He was contemporary of Columbus, Martin Luther and Michelangelo.

(b) In 1630: The use of Peruvian bark for the treatment of malaria was discovered. After two centuries, two French pharmaceutical chemists—Caventor and Pelletier—isolated the alkaloid of quinine.

(c) In 1760: Louis Cadet, a French chemist, made Cacodyl oxide by heating together Potassium acetate and Arsenious oxide.

(d) In 1790: Dr. Hahnemann discovered homoeopathy from the experiment with Preuvian bark (Cinchona).

(e) Alexander Wood of Edinburg developed hypodermic needle, which created a great advancement on drug administration. Before 1853, drugs were administered orally, rectally, or by inhalation.

(f) In 1865: Dr. Count Ceaser Mattei, an Italian herbalist, discovered Electro-homoeopathy, having full pharmacological details.

By the end of 19th century, the need for the science of pharmacology was well recognized throughout the world and thus the studies in experimental pharmacodynamics were being carried out in the different laboratories of Biological Chemistry and Physiology.

Homoeopathic Pharmacy

It is an art and science, by means of which we can acquire a sound knowledge about the art of identifying and collecting medicinal substances from the different sources of nature, preparing, preserving them in the laboratory, combining and compounding according to the rules and regulations of homoeopathic pharmacopoeia and dispensing them according to the physician's prescription. It also embraces the legal and professional aspects as also regulates the proper distribution of drugs and medicines.

H.P.I says "Homoeopathic Pharmacy is concerned with collection, identification, preparation, standardization and preservation of the drugs used in homoeopathic practice."

Basis of homoeopathic pharmacy: Homoeopathic pharmacy is based on monopharmacy, pharmacodynamics, and potentisation.

Contributions: Homoeopathic pharmacy is contributed by Dr. Aegidi, Dr. Carl W. Caspari of Leipzig, Germany, Dr. C. Hering, Dr. Von Boenninghausen and different pharmaceutical organisations.

'Pharmacy is an art and science'—Explain

Science: A department of systematised knowledge as an object of study; knowledge of covering general truths or the operation of general laws, especially as obtained and tested through scientific methods.

Art: Systemic application of knowledge of skill in effecting a desired result.

Pharmacy is the study of the cardinal principles of a subject. The scientific process is adopted in the nature. The principles are applied successfully for the attainment of higher purposes of the healing art. Therefore, pharmacy is a science as well as art.

Sources of Homoeopathic Pharmacy

The main sources are Hahnemann's writings, especially—

1. Materia Medica Pura, Part I to Part VI (1811 to 1821).
2. Organon of Medicine 1st to 6th edition (1810 to 1921).
3. Chronic diseases, their nature and homoeopathic treatment, Part to Part IV (1828 to 1830).
4. Lesser writings of Hahnemann:

   (a) Essay on a New Principle for Ascertaining the Curative Powers of Drugs, and some Examinations of the Previous Principles.

   (b) On the Value of Speculative Systems of Medicine, Especially in connection with the Various Systems of Practice (1808)—appeared in Allegemine Anzeiger der Deutschen.

   (c) On the Preparation and Dispensing of Medicines of Homoeopathic Physicians (1820).

These form the basis of all subsequent instructions given by his followers.

Homoeopathic Pharmacy Includes

1. *Collecting*—How to collect the drug or medicinal substances in crude natural form.
2. *Identifying*—How to identify (macroscopically, microscopically and chemically) the drug substance—before using for preparation. For proper identification, help of a qualified and experienced botanist (for vegetable substance), zoologist (for animal substance) and chemist (for chemicals) is necessary.
3. *Quality inspecting*—Not only identification but also quality of drugs or characteristic features of a drug must be ascertained by physical and analytical process with the help of instruments and chemicals, respectively.
4. *Preserving*—How to preserve the drug materials, mother tinctures and potentised medicines.
5. *Standardising*—Drugs or medicines so prepared must be made to conform to some standards, prescribed by 'Appropriate authority' or official homoeopathic pharmacopoeia and the process is known as 'Standardising'.
6. *Combining*—It means joining two or more things together. Scientifically, the product of a combination is called 'Mechanical mixture'.
7. *Compounding*—It means uniting two or more different elements or constituents together so as to form an altogether new product. This new product will have new properties different from those of its constituents. e.g. Cal. phos; Cal. carb; Mag. sulph; Nat. carb, etc.

Criticism: There is some criticism about the definition of pharmacy. So far identification, collection, preparation, preservation and dispensing is concerned it is all right; but confusion arises in case of compounding and combining. The 2nd homoeopathic cardinal principle is 'Law of Simplex' (Law of Similia being the 1st law) which means that a single and simple substance is to be administered to the patient at a time. So there is no question of compounding and combining in homoeopathy. But while making homoeopathic medicines, one neither combines nor compounds, he only applies the method of trituration and succussion of the entity as a whole.

As such, when combining and compounding precede the preparing of homoeopathic medicines—then it can be definitely said that the homoeopathic cardinal principle, 'the Law of Simplex', is not contraindicated. Therefore, it is suggested that 'compounding' and 'combining' should be mentioned before 'preparing' is mentioned.

Thus the better definition of homoeopathic pharmacy is: "Pharmacy is the art of collecting, compounding, combining, preparing, preserving and dispensing of medicines according to the prescriptions of the physician".

8. *Preparing*—It includes preparations of mother tincture, mother solution and mother substance from different crude drugs. Further 'attenuations' are made from mother preparations. All the preparations are made according to 'old Hahnemannian method', or the 'New method of homoeopathic pharmacopoeia of U.S.A.'
9. *Quality control*—The quality of all finished medicinal preparations must be carefully controlled.
10. *Dispensing*—It means preparing and serving the medicinal preparation in proper form (solid or liquid) as per direction of a physician.

SPECIALITY AND ORIGINALITY OF HOMOEOPATHIC PHARMACY

Homoeopathic Pharmacy has a philosophical background and a scientific application. Homoeopathic Pharmacy deals with a specialised system of therapeutical art and science, having specificity in its mode of preparation, administration and modus operandi. Homoeopathy is based on holistic and individualistic approach of disease. It treats the patient as a whole and not the disease. Hahnemann says: "There is no disease but sick people". But other systems of medicine treat the disease and not the patient.

1. Theory of Potentisation

Homoeopathic dynamisations are processes by which the medicinal properties that are latent in crude substances become aroused and enabled to act in an almost spiritual manner in our life. This discovery that the subdivision of crude substances and their diffusion, through an inert vehicle, developed in them new and previously unappreciated curative powers, when properly administered, is a feature that is a signature of homoeopathy. Homoeopathic pharmacy demonstrates the power or capacity of an infinitesimal small dose.

2. Homoeopathic Pathogenetic Trial (H.P.T)

(i) Each and every drug gets its entry in homoeopathy after "complete proving". Homoeopathic drugs are tested on healthy persons (Sec.108), in both males and females (Sec. 127) in different ages and different constitutions.

(ii) In H.P.T, the subjective symptoms are noted with great importance.

(iii) Drugs are proved in their natural form, though attempts are being made to prove alkaloids or artificial chemical substances.

(iv) In H.P.T, doses used are from minute infinitesimal potencies to the crude drug.

3. Single, Simple Remedy

The conventional (allopathic) system uses complex mixtures in medicines, containing several ingredients. But the homoeopathic system has no such compound prescriptions, and in all cases of illness one single simple medicinal substance is prescribed at one time.

4. Rich Source of Curative Drugs

In homoeopathic pharmacy, there are varied sources of substances which are taken into consideration as medicines, thus, it provides a wide range of curative drugs. Apart from the plant, animal and chemical kingdoms, introduction of nosodes, sarcodes, imponderabilia and synthetically prepared compounds as a source of drug is a specific aspect of homoeopathic pharmacy.

5. New Introduction

Introduction of 'Allersodes' and 'Isodes' as a source of drug is also peculiar to homoeopathic pharmacy.

6. Purity and Totality of the Drug Source

Homoeopathy accepts a drug with its entity and totality, without attempting to separate a drug into its specific chemical constituents. However, specific constituents of certain substances may also used as drugs in homoeopathy.

7. In-process Quality Control

The "in-process" quality control includes 'every step of the preparation' from raw materials to finished products. It is critical in ensuring the purity and safety of homoeopathic medicines. The system of quality control is even more vital in the manufacturing process than with their allopathic counterparts. In case of highly diluted and potentised medicines, care should be taken in every step of manufacture to maintain the quality and reliability of the final product.

Freshness of materials used is also an important feature in homoeopathy.

8. Simple to Dispense and easy to Administer

Homoeopathy employs no complex methods and compound formulations in preparing medicines. The methods of dispensing homoeopathic medicines are very simple, guided solely by convenience and ease to the physician, and, at the same time, easy to administer to the sick, thus ensuring a good compliance.

9. Drug Action

Homoeopathic medicine acts on dynamic plane. Pharmacodynamics specialises in studying individual drug actions, in addition to its general (i.e physical and chemical) actions.

10. Cost Effective

Manufacturing cost of homoeopathic medicines is comparatively cheaper than other systems of medicine. These are economically viable for every aspect of life.

11. Long Shelf Life

The official life of a homoeopathic medicine is five years after its manufacturing. But it has been observed that a dose of potentised homoeopathic remedy in its paper envelope in the desk is said to retain its medicinal virtue for years. In homoeopathy, mother tinctures certainly have expiry dates. But these expiry dates vary from mother tincture to mother tincture based on the type of ingredient and method of preparation.

Mother tincture will expire after 5 years, 10 years or more but they will definitely expire depending upon the environment. It is a common observation that fresh mother tinctures gave better and prompt results as compared to the old mother tinctures. The reason is the same—with the passage of time these mother tinctures will lose strength. Generally mother tinctures will lose their strength and medicinal power after ten to twenty years in case of juicy plants like Calendula prepared in alcohol—depending upon the density in the surroundings. While those prepared in distilled water will expire earlier like Acid phos.

SCOPE OF HOMOEOPATHIC PHARMACY

A. During Study and Practice of Homoeopathy

1. **Posology**: At bedside of a patient, after selecting the proper medicine, the physician may be confused with the 'doses' of medicines, because dose or potency depends upon many factors. But if the physician has thorough knowledge about the posology, i.e. doctrine of doses—he will never be confused with the doses. So a detailed knowledge of pharmacy helps us in this context.
2. **Preparation of Medicines**: Pharmacy gives us the practical knowledge about the preparation of mother tincture, mother solution and mother substances.
3. **External Application:** We get the knowledge of drug for external application from the study of pharmacy.
4. **Prescription Writing:** Pharmacy helps us to write the prescriptions in proper order.

B. As a Career

Due to increased pharmaceutical needs all over the world, career opportunities for pharmacists are expected to grow in different circles:

1. **Government Services**: Pharmacist may be appointed in health departments of the government as commissioned and non-commissioned officers. Foods and Drug Administration (FDA) and Indian Health Services (IHS) also appoint homoeopathic pharmacists. Presently, some state governments recruit homoeopathic pharmacists in homoeopathic hospitals and health centres.
2. **Industrial (Institutional) Pharmacy:** Homoeopathic pharmaceutical companies appoint qualified homoeopathic pharmacists for marketing and administration. Some pharmacists work as medical representative who visits homoeopathic physicians and educate them with their products.
3. **Health System Pharmacy**: The pharmacist may work in private physicians' clinic, private or government hospitals, nursing homes and health maintenance organisations. The pharmacist dispenses medicines and advises patients about the use of drugs.
4. **Community Pharmacy**: The Community Pharmacists are needed in community dispensing pharmaceuticals, to answer for the prescriptions and over the counter (OTC) drugs. They give advices about home health care supplies and durable medical equipments.
5. **Pharmacy Courses**: Presently, some State Governments started homoeopathic pharmacy courses (Diploma) to make qualified pharmacists. This will enrich different homoeopathic pharmacy.
6. **Publication of Pharmaceutical Journal:** Some homoeopathic pharmaceutical companies are regularly publishing journals to promote their products. Presently, it is conducted by the expert homoeopaths but, with the gradual development of pharmacy, the involvement of pharmacists will be required in near future.

BRANCHES OF HOMOEOPATHIC PHARMACY

Homoeopathic Pharmacy has mainly two branches:

A. Pharmacy Proper

It consists of

1. Official Pharmacy: Consists of the preparation of drugs according to the processes prescribed in official pharmacopoeias (e.g., HPI, HPUS. GHP/HAB, BHP).

2. Extemporaneous Pharmacy: Consists of the preparation and distribution of medicine according to the prescription of physician. Previously, medicines were prepared by this pharmacy till 1825.

B. Galenical Pharmacy

It was Galen, a Greek pharmacist of Rome (131-200 AD) who described various methods of extracting the crude drugs for the first time and, hence, the branch dealing with the extraction of plant and animals drug is known as Galenical Pharmacy and the product as Galenicals.

Galenicals are pharmaceutical preparations obtained by macerating or percolating drugs with alcohol of appropriate strength, or some menstrum carefully selected to remove as thoroughly the desired principle and to leave the inert and other undesirable constituents of the plant undissolved.

The preparations include under the Galenicals are infusions, decoctions, fluid extracts and fluid glycerites, vinegars, and tinctures.

Other Branches

1. **Hospital (Institutional) Pharmacy**: Hospital pharmacy may be defined as the practice of pharmacy in hospitals, health maintenance organisations and nursing homes.

   Hospital pharmacy is a discipline concerned with the objects of planning, organising, directing, motivating, communicating and controlling all aspects related to drugs with a view to contributing to the overall objectives of the homoeopathic hospital as an organisation of health care.

   Its scope ranges from drug procurement to drug administration. A hospital pharmacy is a drug procurement, processing and dispensing, a storage, distribution and administration centre, depending upon the size and nature of the hospital in which it is set up.

2. **Clinical Pharmacy**: It is that branch of pharmacy where pharmacists provide patient care that optimises the use of medication and promotes health, wellness and disease prevention.

3. **Theoretical Pharmacy**: It is that branch of pharmacy which deals with the teaching of pharmacy in homoeopathic institutions and is theoretical in nature.

4. **Operative Pharmacy**: This branch of pharmacy is related to different aspects of standardisations, manufacturing retail and also includes administrative and hospital pharmacy.

5. **Wholesale Pharmacy**: This pharmacy maintains a linkage between the homoeopathic manufacturer, hospital (institutional) pharmacist and community pharmacist. It helps to maintain the supply of the medicines up to end level. In India, anyone can get license for trading homoeopathic wholesale pharmacy. For this purpose only trading knowledge is sufficient and no pharmaceutical knowledge is required.

6. **Retail Pharmacy**: This pharmacy deals with the selling of homoeopathic medicines in retail. For retail selling of medicines in India the dealing person should have an official license of pharmacy.

SPAGYRIC PHARMACY

The term 'Spagyria' has been used by the 16th century Swiss physician Paracelsus (1493-1541), in his book 'Liber Paragranum', deriving from the Greek words 'spao' (separate) and 'ageiro' (combine), the essential meaning of which is to 'separate and to combine'.

In its original use, the word spagyric was commonly used synonymously with the word alchemy; however, in more recent times it has often been adopted by alternative medicine theorists and various techniques of holistic medicine. The spagyrism represents a form of homoeopathy in which both vital healing energy and active substances are extracted from medicinal plants, creating powerful mother tinctures that can be further potentised.

The spagyric remedies were originally created by fermenting parts of wild herbs. This process produced concentrated aromatic solutions that were extracted and separated from the bulk plant matter. After fermentation was completed, the plant material was distilled in a special device, and the remainder dried and burned. The ashes were extracted and purified via distillation, then recombined with the concentrated solution. As a result, the finished spagyric essence contained the mineral constituent parts of the plant.

Paracelsus pointed out that the vital energy of an herb is more important than the plant material itself. Combining the ideas of Paracelsus with modern manufacturing techniques, **Pekana** (Naturheilmittel GmbH of Kisslegg, Germany) founded in 1974 the preparation technique of spagyric remedies using four key steps: separation, purification, incineration and reunification:

1. **Separation**: Using only the specific parts of either fresh or dried herbs as prescribed in the Homeopathic Pharmacopoeia, **Pekana** adds special yeast, sucrose and pharmaceutical grade water to initiate fermentation. This three-week process produces a natural alcohol intrinsic to the particular plant, resulting in a high quality mother tincture solution that contains vital energy specific to that herb.
2. **Purification**: Next, Pekana repeatedly filters the tincture solution until it is completely free of impurities. Similar to producing a fine wine, this process requires time and precision because new particles created by the plant tincture during the various filtering phases must be removed to achieve an absolutely pure liquid solution. Unlike other manufacturers, Pekana never distills its spagyric tinctures to ensure that biocatalysts (enzymes), vitamins and other vital substances remain active.
3. **Incineration**: In step three, the original plant material used to produce the mother tincture solution is dried, caked and burned at very high temperatures, creating an ash. After **Pekana's** advanced processing technique removes all impurities from the ash, only the remaining pure plant minerals are extracted.
4. **Reunification**: Finally, the pure plant crystals that stimulate metabolic processes in the body are combined with the mother tincture solution. Until this final step, the tincture is odourless. However, at the precise moment **Pekana** adds the minerals to the solution, a dramatic colour change takes place and the specific aroma distinctive to the plant flows from the fluid creating the "miracle" of spagyrics.

Importantly, practitioners are able to experience the excellent efficacy of these homoeopathic-spagyric medications through the fast, lasting results produced in patients.

If the excretion process is not stimulated, and the internal terrain not improved, then the ill body may be forced to store toxins in the connective tissues, or aid excretion by other means such as fever, diarrhea, and excessive sweating. This can be avoided by using Pekana remedies.

Lists of Spagyric Remedies

Delima (Pomegranate seed high grade oil), Habifac, AILGENO, AKUTUR spag. Drops, Alfalfa, apo-Dolor, apo-Haem, apo-Hepat, apo-Infekt, apo-Oedem, apo-Pulm, apo-Rheum, apo-Stom, apo-Strum, apo-Tuss, Bronchi-Pertu, Cangust, Cardinorma, Citriplus, Clauparest, Corocalm, Dalektro, Defaeton, Dercut, Fattex, Ferrodonna, Fluofin, Formiplus, Glautarakt, Helmin, Inflamyar, Inflamyar ointment, Itires, Lactic Plus, Lassitul, Mucan, Muliton, Mundipur 250 mls tonic, Neocard, Neu Regen, Neu Regen tonic, Okoubaka, Opsonat, Oss-regen, Otidolo, Plevent, Pollon, Proaller, Proscenat, Psystabil, Radinex, Renelix, Ricura, Sedicelo, Septonsil, Somcupin, Specichol, Supren, Thuja, Toxex.

ASPECTS OF PHARMACY

The pharmacy has different aspects. But from the homoeopathic point of view pharmacy has two important aspects:

1. Conceptual (Doctrinal) aspects, and
2. Technological (Technical or mechanical) aspects.

1. Conceptual (Doctrinal) Aspects

(i) It deals with the basic laws and principles of pharmaceutical process.

(ii) The knowledge about the conceptual aspect of pharmacy depends on the principles and physiology, which guides the practice of any particular system.

(iii) The conceptual aspect of pharmaceutics vary considerably in different system of treatment.

(iv) It is the basis on which the technological aspect works.

(v) It decides whether a substance will be used as medicine or not.

(vi) It decides the individuality or distinction of any particular school of therapeutics.

In Ayurvedic and Unani: The conceptual aspect of pharmacy is based on books of Materia Medica and Practice of Medicine where the concept of drugs and diseases are described respectively.

In Homoeopathy: The basic laws and principles are laid down in Organon of Medicine and other philosophy.

In Allopathy: This system has no separate book on principles or philosophy. Its principles of drug application depends on concepts of pathology and practice of medicine.

Examples

(i) The characteristics of a vehicle.

(ii) The ratio between the drug substance and vehicle

(iii) Quantity of dose.

(iv) Route of administration of medicines.

(v) The principles of preparation of drugs.

(vi) Method of dispensing of medicine.

(vii) Precautions before, during, and after administration of medicines.

2. Technological (Technical or Mechanical) Aspects

(i) It deals with the manual, physical, chemical and mechanical processes involved in pharmaceutical methods.

(ii) Allopathic and homoeopathic pharmacies are closely related in the technological aspect and homoeopathy takes the help of allopathy.

(iii) The knowledge of the technological aspect depends on the sciences of botany, zoology, chemistry, physiology, pathology, practice of medicine etc.

(iv) The sources of pharmaceutical knowledge have a common technological aspect and all the systems of medicine have the same common source with minor exceptions.

(v) If the conceptual aspect is the vital force, then technological aspect is its body. The former is formless without the latter and the latter is lifeless without the former.

In all system of medicine, the technological aspect of pharmacy follows the same fundamental processes and do not manifest remarkable differences. The homoeopathic pharmacy is closely related to pharmaceutical methods of other schools of treatment regarding the technological aspect of identifying, collecting, combining, compounding, filtration, sublimation, decantation, maceration, percolation, grinding etc.

Examples

(i) Processes of identifying, cultivating, collecting, cleansing, processing, preparing, preserving, labeling, dispensing, administration of medicine.

(ii) The mechanical process of cutting, grinding, triturating and the chemical process of sublimation, percolation, maceration etc.

Relationship of the two Aspects of Pharmacy

1. Recognition of a Substance as a Drug

The conceptual aspect of pharmacy decides whether a substance can be used as medicine or not. In homoeopathic system many substances are used as medicines which are not used in other systems of medicine e.g., *Bacillinum*, *Medorrhinum*, *Syphillinum* etc. On the other hand, in allopathy, many substances are used as medicines which are not used in homoeopathy and other systems of medicine.

2. Identification and Collection

The conceptual aspect decides which part of the plants, animals, minerals, nosodes and sarcodes will be used for preparation of a particular medicine. On the other hand technological aspect informs about the habitat or distribution of the plant, time of blossoming or maturity, the test for proper identification of the drug substance and the method of collection.

3. Compounding

The conceptual aspect decides the applicability, acceptance and/or rejection of a compound. Compounding is a chemical process. The preparation of compounds from more than one element is guided by the rules of chemistry and related to technological aspect.

4. Combining

The conceptual aspect decides the quantity of medicine and vehicle required for combining. The process of combining is a chemical process like compounding and related to technological aspect.

5. Preparing

The conceptual aspect decides the ratio between the vehicle and the drug substance, the kind of processing before preparation, the part of substance to be used, the nature and kind of vehicle, the time to be spent on making a mixture or trituration, the time allotted for grinding, the quantity of vehicle to be mixed with drugs, the days allotted for keeping the mixture before filtration, the principles of physico-mechanical processes etc.

The processing, cleansing, making a pulp or powder, weighing etc. are all physical and mechanical process and done before preparing the drugs into medicines.

All schools of pharmacy use the technological processes of heating, grinding, filtration, percolation etc. in the preparation of their medicines.

6. Preserving

The site and process of preservation (e.g., in cool dark place, refrigerator or cold storage) will depend on the conceptual aspect.

Labelling and storing of medicines are technological processes, so related to technological aspects.

7. Dispensing

The conceptual aspect decides the quantity of dose, the art of dispensing, the vehicle used in dispensing.

The technological aspect deals with the mechanical processes of mixture during dispensing.

8. Administration

The conceptual aspect decides the routes and the methods of administration of medicines. The very processes of administration of medicine or injection are technological processes, so are related to technological aspects.

Relationship of Homoeopathic Pharmacy and Allopathic Pharmacy

1. Naming

Both the systems of treatment—allopathy and homoeopathy consist of two Greek words. Both the terms allopathy and homoeopathy were coined by Dr. Samuel Hahnemann.

Allopathy: The word allopathy is derived from Greek words 'Alloeos' means 'dissimilar, heterogeneous' and 'pathos' means 'suffering, disease.' This system has no fixed principles between the drug and disease. The term allopathy was used by Samuel Hahnemann and other early homoeopathic doctors to highlight the difference they perceived between homoeopathy, a pseudoscience, and the conventional medicine of that era. This system is based on the principles of the ancient Greeks such as Hippocrates.

Homoeopathy: The word homoeopathy is derived from Greek words 'Homoeos' means 'similar, alike' and 'pathos' means 'suffering, disease.' This system has a fixed principle between the drug and disease. It is based on 'Similia Similibus Curantur' which means 'likes cure likes'.

2. Origins

Both the systems have their roots in Ancient Medicine of Greece and gradually flourished in Europe.

Allopathy: Practitioners of alternative medicine have used the term "allopathic medicine" to refer to the practice of conventional medicine in both Europe and United States since the 19th century.

Homoeopathy: Homoeopathy was founded by Samuel Hahnemann (1755–1843) of Germany in 1796.

3. Therapeutic Approach

Allopathy

(i) Being guided by the materialistic view of disease, allopathy attempts to kill or remove the bacteria and parasites in order to cure diseases. Hence they treat the results of disease, though the interior of man remains disea-sed as before, sometimes worse than before.

(ii) They use material doses for killing bacteria, and also in the treatment of several diseases.

(iii) Being guided by the concept of local diseases they try to remove the local symptoms, ignoring the whole. Hence they become organo-specialist.

Homoeopathy

(i) Being guided by the dynamic concept of disease, Homoeopathy treats the deranged vital force to restore back the previous healthy state. Hence, homoeopathy treats the diseased, not the disease.

(ii) Very minute amount of medicine is administered in this system.

(iii) Homoeopathy treats the patient as a whole, not the lung, not the kidney, not the particular parts of the body.

4. Sources of Drugs

Both the systems acquires drug substances from plants, animals and chemicals.

Allopathy: Source of drugs is largely synthetic and chemicals.

Homoeopathy: The medicines are prepared from different sources such as vegetables, animals, minerals, nosodes, sarcodes, imponderabilia, allersodes, isodes and synthetics.

5. Nomenclature of Drugs

Both the systems use Latin and Greek names of the plants and animals, with some exceptions where common names of regional language are used. In case of minerals, nosodes and sarcodes the principles of nomenclature are same. These names have been accepted by the international bodies. In allopathy, proprietary names (i.e. known by their commercial or trade names) are mostly used whereas, in homoeopathy, non-proprietary names (i.e. official names) are used.

6. Identification

The methods and techniques of identification of drug substance is more or less same in both systems. Knowledge of allied sciences (botany for plants, zoology for animals and chemistry for minerals) which bears the description of drugs, is helpful. Nowadays botanists, zoologists and chemists perform their functions for identification of drug substances.

7. Collection

The process and time of collection is same in both the systems. There are some separate instructions for collection of some drugs which are used exclusively either in allopathy or homoeopathy.

8. Combining

Both the systems follow common methods of combining, mixing, dissolving etc. The process of combination is guided by fixed principles which differ in allopathy and homoeopathy. The choice of medicine in mixture, ratio of combination and duration of combining period are different.

9. Compounding

Both the systems follow same chemical processes in making compounds from elements.

Allopathy: Compounding of two separately prepared medicines are done by the employees of the physician who dispenses medicines for the patient.

Homoeopathy: Compounding of two separately prepared medicines are against the principles of homoeopathy.

10. Preparation

(a) Process used

Both the systems follow some common processes of preparation of drugs such as mother tinctures, aqueous solutions, macerations, percolations and triturations.

Allopathy: There are some processes which are only used in allopathy, but not in homoeopathy—decoctions, granulations, fusions, scaling etc.

Homoeopathy: There are some processes which are only used in homoeopathy, but not in allopathy—potentisation etc.

(b) Vehicles

Some vehicles are common in both the systems e.g., sugar of milk, tablets, purified water, different varieties of alcohol, olive oil, glycerine, white petroleum jelly etc.

There are many vehicles which are only used in allopathy, but not in homoeopathy such as ether, chloroform, dilute acetic acid, acetone etc.

(c) Forms of Preparation

Both the systems prepare medicines in the form of tinctures, tablets, lotions etc.

Allopathy: There are some preparations which are only used in allopathy such as mixtures, suppositories, injections, capsules, elixirs etc.

Homoeopathy: There are some preparations which are only used in homoeopathy such as medicated globules, back potencies, different potencies as per different scales.

(d) Ratios between the Drugs and Vehicles

Allopathy: Mother tinctures are prepared by various methods and different vehicles are used for extracting the active principles and preparing drugs. The quantity of vehicle varies with each individual drug. Further preparations are done according to the individual drug and they are prepared in the form of mixtures, suppositories, injections, capsules, tablets, elixirs etc.

Homoeopathy: Mother tinctures, solutions and substances (as per old method) are prepared by using vehicles of different types such as strong alcohol, purified water, sugar of milk, and glycerine. The ratio between the drug substance and vehicle varies with the different classes. Further preparations are made under three scales, viz., decimal (1: 9), centesimal (1: 99) and 50-millesimal (1: 50,000).

11. Doses (Posology)

Allopathy: Allopathy uses relatively large doses of unnatural drugs, synthesised in chemical laboratories, tested in vitro in test tubes and in vivo in animals or sick persons. These chemical drugs derange the innate physiological mechanisms by removing symptoms, often in small groups which are conceptually aggregated into alleged disease entities.

Homoeopathy: Homoeopathy employs infinitesimal potentised doses of natural drugs derived from vegetable, animal and mineral kingdom. These natural substances have been previously tested on healthy volunteers (proving), whose aggregate symptom totality (drug pictures) very precisely matches the symptom totality of each individual patient in all its rich and diverse idiosyncrasy, excluding nothing and involving no false demarcation of the patient totality into arbitrarily conceived fragments or diseases.

12. Dispensing of Medicines

Allopathy: Allopathic medicines are available in the form of tablets, capsules, syrups etc. and administered in large doses.

Homoeopathy: Homoeopathic medicines are dispensed in sugar of milk (Sac lac), globules and purified water in most cases. The dispensing process is simple. As minimum doses are sufficient, the patient is not allowed to purchase a whole phial (esp. dilution) from the shop.

13. Administration of Medicine (Pharmaconomy)

In both systems, medicines are administered in oral route (through mouth) and inhalation.

Allopathy: Allopathy mostly depends on injections (like intramuscular, subcutaneous, intro-venous. This system also admits external applications (ointments, creams, lotions etc.).

Homoeopathy: Homoeopathy mostly depends on oral administration of medicines.

The external applications are against the principles of homoeopathy. However, different external preparations are manufactured and used.

14. Preservations

The general rules for preservation of drugs and medicines are more or less the same, but the methods differ in both systems.

Allopathy: Some of the allopathic medicines require very elaborate process of preservation like keeping in a refrigerator etc. Things like scent, smell etc. do not matter much with the finished products of allopathic pharmaceuticals.

Homoeopathy: Homoeopathic medicines should not be kept in refrigerator. The wooden chest, *neutral glass bottles*, velvet cork and paper packs generally used for preserving potentised homoeopathic medicines are all known as highly resistive to heat. A dose of homoeopathic potentised medicine in its paper envelop in the desk is said to retain its medicinal virtue for years. Homoeopathic medicines are also advised to kept protected from sunlight and even body heat. Homoeopathic medicines—esp. in the form of globules—has a longevity of as many as 19/20 years according to Hahnemann.

15. New Drugs Development

Allopathy: In allopathy, any manufacturing company may prepare a medicine and market it. Medicine will be accepted by the physician and will be prescribed. The manufacturing industries guide the physician in accepting or rejecting a drug.

Homoeopathy: In homoeopathy, a medicine has to be proved on healthy human beings, its symptoms are recorded and verified by HPL.

16. Conceptual Allegiances

Allopathy: The primary conceptual allegiance of allopathy is not really to Nature but to a theory of how life is: to a preconceived and fragmented view of the patient as a mere collection of parts, never conceived as a whole.

Homoeopathy: The primary conceptual allegiance of homoeopathy is an empirical one to Nature, a faithfulness in compiling a natural, an accurate and complete image of the sick persons in all their aspects—mind, body, modalities, generalities, sleep and dreams, preferences etc.

Relation of Homoeopathic Pharmaceutics with Allied Sciences

The term pharmaceutics means the science or art of preparing medicines. The science of pharmacy is that branch of medical science which relates to the use of medicinal drugs.

On the other hand, allied sciences means botany (i.e., plant biology), zoology, chemistry, biochemistry, physiology as well as physics.

The relation between these allied sciences and pharmaceutics is necessary in every step for nomenclature, identification, collection, cultivation, preservation, preparation, separation of active principles of drugs from plants, separation of healthy parts from diseased parts of a plant or animals etc.

Each allied science is well known in their separate scientific disciplines in relation to pharmaceutics such as pharmaceutical botany, pharmaceutical zoology, pharmaceutical chemistry, clinical chemistry etc.

Botany

The term 'botany' comes from Greek Botany, meaning 'pasture, grass, fodder'.

Botany (or plant biology) is a branch of biology that involves the scientific study of plant life. Botany covers a wide range of scientific disciplines concerned with the study of plants, algae and fungi, including structure, growth, reproduction, metabolism, development, diseases, chemical properties, and evolutionary relationships among taxonomic groups. It has many specialised branches such as:

1. Plant systematics (Taxonomy): Classification and nomenclature for identification of plants.
2. Plant ecology: Role of plants in the environment.
3. Plant geography: Distribution of plants in different regions.
4. Agronomy (Agriculture): Application of plant science to crop production.
5. Horticulture: Cultivated plants.
6. Forestry: Forest management and related studies.
7. Phytopathology—Plant diseases.
8. Pharmaceutical or medical botany (Pharmacognosy): Pharmacy related to botany or botany related to pharmacy.

Botany is closely related to pharmaceutics and is one of the important pillars of technological (Technical or Mechanical) aspects of pharmacy.

In homoeopathic system, about 75% of the medicines are derived from plant sources (Exotic—60% and Indigenous—40%).

The knowledge of botany is essential for pharmacy and pharmaceutics due to the following reasons:

1. **Largest source**: The vegetable kingdom is the largest source of drugs in homoeopathic system for preparation of medicines. Whole plants or its parts (e.g. roots, stems, leaves, fruits, flowers and barks), fungi, algae are used for this purpose.
2. **Identification**: The identification of particular species of plants, containing active principles is done with the help of knowledge and experience based on botany. The books of botany contains the description of plants, which are helpful for identification.
3. **Collection**: The collection of drug substances should be done by an experienced and qualified botanist having a special knowledge of Taxonomy and Systemic Botany. He should also possess the basic knowledge of homoeopathic pharmaceutics.
4. **Cultivation and Preservation**: Knowledge of botany is essential for cultivation and preservation of drugs.
5. **Nomenclature**: The International Codes of Botanical Nomenclature are followed for the medicines prepared from the vegetable kingdom.
6. **Plant Pathology**: Most of the homoeopathic medicines of vegetable kingdom are prepared from healthy plants but some are prepared from diseased plants (e.g., Secale cornutum, Ustilago maydis, Nectrianinum). Plant pathology helps in differentiating healthy plants from diseased plants. It also helps in determination of the nature and extent of plant diseases.

Zoology

The term zoology is derived from ancient Greek, 'zoon' means 'animal' and 'logos' means 'knowledge'.

It is the branch of biology which relates to the animal kingdom, including the structure, embryology, evolution, classification, habits, and distribution of all animals, both living and extinct.

In homoeopathic system, animal sources are the second largest group, accounting for about 20% of the medicines.

In the field of homoeopathy animal models are used both for testing the principle of dilution/ potentisation and for studying the possible mechanism of action of homoeopathic medicines in a thorough and repeatable manner, as well as for discovering medicines to be used in the veterinary context. The animal models are selected from the thorough knowledge of zoology.

1. **Identification**: Both healthy and diseased animals are used for preparation of medicines. The proper knowledge of zoology is essential for the distribution (i.e., habitat), characteristic points for identification, for the functions and importance of the organs, the secretions, discharges etc.
2. **Nomenclature**: The International Codes of Zoological Nomenclature are followed for the medicines prepared from the animal kingdom.
3. **Preparation of Nosodes**: The knowledge of zoology is helpful for preparing medicines from diseased animals, diseased tissue and clinical materials (secretions, discharges etc.). These are included under the name of Nosodes.
4. **Preparation of Sercodes**: The knowledge of zoology is helpful for preparing medicines from healthy endocrine glands as a whole, healthy secretions from endocrine glands, normal secretion of animals, product (or extract) of animal glands and tissues, healthy organs of animals. These are included under the name of Sarcodes.

Chemistry

Pharmaceutical chemistry is a discipline at the intersection of chemistry, pharmacology, and biology involved with designing, synthesising and developing pharmaceutical drugs. Pharmaceutical chemistry involves the identification, synthesis and development of new chemical entities suitable for therapeutic use. It also includes the study of existing drugs, their biological properties, and their quantitative structure-activity relationships (QSAR). Pharmaceutical chemistry is focused on quality aspects of medicines and aims to assure fitness for the purpose of medicinal products. With the advancements of chemistry and biochemistry, the homoeopathic pharmacy gives emphasis on chemicals.

Chemistry is closely related to pharmaceutics and is one of the important pillar of technological (Technical or Mechanical) aspects of pharmacy.

The knowledge of chemistry is essential in homoeopathic pharmaceutics. The role of chemistry for pharmacy and pharmaceutics are:

1. **Identification**: The identification of constituents of drugs done by crystallography, melting point determination and chemical test (colour reaction test). These are learnt from the knowledge of chemistry.
2. **Isolation**:
   (a) Knowledge of chemistry helps in isolation of different components of a crude drug substance. It isolates the non-medicinal from the medicinal component of a drug substance.
   (b) Knowledge of chemistry also helps in isolation of active principles of drugs from vegetable source.
3. **Nomenclature**: The International Codes of Nomenclature of Chemical substances, are followed for the medicines prepared from the mineral kingdom.
4. **Detection of impurities**: Thorough knowledge of chemistry helps in detection of impurities in medicines or vehicles by different chemical tests.
5. **Standardisation and quality control**: The quality control of raw materials, finished products, and vehicles is a vital problem where knowledge of chemistry is helpful.
6. **Laboratory methods**: Different laboratory methods, techniques and processes such as sedimentation, decantation, filtration, evaporation, distillation, sublimation, crystalisation, precipitation, maceration, percolation, etc. used in the preparation of homoeopathic drugs are learnt from the knowledge of chemistry.
7. **Preservation**: The techniques of preservation and the knowledge of preservatives is known through the knowledge of chemistry.

Biochemistry

It is the study of the chemical processes and transformations in living organisms, including the structure and function of cellular components (such as proteins, carbohydrates, lipids, nucleic acids, and other biomolecules) and various aspects of cellular and intercellular changes.

The modern biochemistry has two aspects—descriptive and dynamic. The descriptive biochemistry deals with the chemical nature of cell components and dynamic biochemistry deals with various aspects of metabolism, chemical regulation, as well as cellular and intercellular changes.

It gives information about the biochemical actions of substances. The knowledge derived from biochemical study about the curative power of a drug deals with the sphere of action of drugs on one or two systems and organs.

Physiology

The word physiology is from Ancient Greek: '*physis*' means 'nature, origin' and '*logos*', means 'study of'.

Physiology is that branch of science which deals with the normal functions of the cells, tissues, organs, and systems. The study of physiological action of drugs in vegetable and chemical kingdom is helpful for their inclusion or exclusion. On the basis of importance in physiological functions of healthy and diseased individuals some substances such as vitamins (Vitamin A, Vitamin B, Vitamin E), hormones (e.g., Insulin, Adrenocorticotropin) and enzymes (e.g., Pepsinum, ATP, AMP) are used as homoeopathic medicines. Most of the vitamins are available as potentised homoeopathic medicines prepared according to the law of symptom similarity.

PHARMACIST

Definition

A Pharmacist is a person who is skilled or engaged in pharmacy, one who prepares or dispenses medicines, one who is legally qualified to sell drugs.

Features

(i) A pharmacist should hold the health and safety of the patient at first consideration.

(ii) A pharmacist should never condone the dispensing, promoting or distributing of drugs or assist therein, which are not of good quality, which do not meet the standards required by law or which lack therapeutic value for the patient.

(iii) He should not engage in any illegal or unethical conduct in the profession.

(iv) A pharmacist should seek at all times only fair and reasonable remuneration for his services. He should never agree to or participate in transactions with practitioners of other health professions or any other person under which fees are divided or which may cause financial or other exploitation in connection with the rendering of his professional services.

(v) No attempt should be made to capture the business of a contemporary by cut-throat competition, by offering prizes or gifts or allurement to physicians.

(vi) A pharmacist should strive to provide information to the patient regarding professional services truthfully, accurately and fully and should avoid misleading the patient regarding the nature, cost or value of the professional services.

Qualities

The pharmacist should possess the following qualities:

1. Knowledge of pharmacy, regarding collection of drug substances, preparation of medicines, preservation, handling and dispensing.
2. Perfect perception in different homoeopathic pharmacopoeias such as HPI, HPUS, GHP/HAB and BHP.
3. Qualified, honest, humanitarian, trustworthy and must be fully aware of his/her responsibilities.
4. Profound love and sympathy for the sick.
5. Proper skill in performance.
6. The pharmacist must exercise painstaking care and accuracy in every step of preparation, handling and dispensing.

Since the Homoeopathic physician has to depend almost entirely on infinitesimal doses, it is essential that the homoeopathic medicinal preparation must be absolutely accurate and dependable. So the homoeopathic pharmacist must know the proper way of preparation of various drugs. He must have knowledge of collection of drug substances, because the first job of a pharmacist is to procure or collect drug substance. So, great care should be taken in selecting the drug materials. As there are no available tests to see if the medicines obtained are genuine, one has to depend completely on the pharmacist.

PHARMACIST'S OATH

1. I Swear by the code of Ethics of Pharmacy Council of India in relation to the community and shall act as an integral part of health care team.
2. I shall uphold the laws and standards governing my profession.
3. I shall strive to perfect and enlarge my knowledge to contribute to the advancement of pharmacy and public health.
4. I shall follow the system which I consider best for pharmaceutical care and counseling of patients.
5. I shall endeavour to discover and manufacture drugs of quality to alleviate sufferings of humanity.
6. I shall hold in confidence the knowledge gained about the patients in connection with professional practice and never divulge unless compelled to do so by the law.
7. I shall associate with organisations having their objectives for betterment of the profession of Pharmacy and make contribution to carry out the work of those organisations.
8. While I continue to keep this Oath unviolated, may it be granted to me to enjoy life and the practice of pharmacy respected by all, at all times!
9. Should I trespass and violate this oath, may the reverse be my lot!

Chapter 02

Sources of Homoeopathic Drugs

The different sources of homoeopathic drugs are:

1. Vegetable kingdom
2. Animal kingdom

Sub-sources

(a) Ophidia—This specific source of snake venoms was first suggested by E. A. Farrington in his *Clinical Materia Medica.*

(b) Lacs—The milk and milk products of several animals. Even human milk is employed as a homoeopathic drug.

3. Mineral kingdom
4. Nosodes
5. Sarcodes
6. Imponderabilia
7. Synthetic source.
8. Allersodes
9. Isodes.

VEGETABLE KINGDOM

It includes whole plants, roots (fresh and dried), stems, leaves, herbs, flowers, fruits, seeds, barks, algae, fungi etc. The different plants and parts thereof are used for the preparation of mother tincture and mother substances.

1. **Whole Plants**

(a) INCLUDING ROOTS

Acalypha indica
Aconitum napellus
Adonis vernalis
Aethusa cynapium
Anagallis arvensis
Andrographis paniculata
Anthoxanthum odoratum
Arnica montana
Asarum europaeum
Belladonna
Bellis perennis
Boerhaavia diffusa
Branca ursina
Caladium seguinum
Caltha palustris
Chamomilla
Chelidonium majus
Chelone glabra
Chenopodium anthelminticum
Chimaphila umbellata
Cineraria maritima
Cistus canadensis
Conium maculatum
Convallaria majalis
Cynodon dactylon
Damiana
Drosera rotundifolia
Dulcamara
Echinacea angustifolia
Epiphegus virginiana
Equisetum hyemale
Erigeron canadense
Eupatorium purpureum
Euphrasia officinalis
Fagopyrum esculentum
Gnaphalium polycephalum
Gratiola officinalis
Hydrocotyle asiatica
Hyoscyamus niger
Hypericum perforatum

Lachnanthes tinctoria
Ledum palustre
Lemna minor
Lilium tigrinum
Lobelia cardinalis
Lycopersicum esculentum
Lycopus virginicus
Menyanthes trifoliata
Mercurialis perennis
Millefolium
Paris quadrifolia
Petroselinum sativum
Plantago major
Pulsatilla nigricans
Ranunculus bulbosus
Ranunculus acris
Rheum
Ruta graveolens
Sarracenia purpurea
Senecio aureus
Solanum carolinense
Spigelia marylandica
Stramonium
Teucrium marum varum
Thlaspi bursa pastoris
Tribulus terrestris
Tussilago farfara
Tussilago petasites
Urtica urens
Verbascum thapsus
Vinca minor
Viola odorata
Viola tricolor.

(b) EXCLUDING ROOTS

Achyranthes aspera; Alfalfa; Blumea odorata; Lobelia inflata; Mentha piperita; Myrtus communis; Ocimum sanctum, Ranunculus sceleratus.

2. **Roots (Radices)**

(a) FRESH: Abroma augusta radix; Actaea spicata; Apocynum cannabinum; Aralia racemosa; Aristolochia clematitis; Artemisia vulgaris; Arum dracontium; Arum triphyllum; Bryonia alba; Cicuta virosa; Cyclamen europaeum; Eryngium aquaticum; Euphorbia corollata; Gentiana cruciata; Jalapa; Nymphaea odorata; Oenanthe crocata; Paeonia officinalis; Paullina pinnata; Phytolacca decandra; Raphanus sativus; Withania somnifera.

(b) DRIED: Calotropis gigantia; Ipecacuanha; Ratanhia; Geranium maculatum; Rauwalfia serpentina; Senega; Sumbul; Tamus communis.

(c) HANGING AERIAL ROOTS: Ficus indica.

(d) ROOT AND RHIZOME: Asarum canadense; Aletris farinosa.

3. **Stems (Stipities)**

(a) ONLY STEM: Cactus grandiflorus; Tinospora cordifolia.

(b) STEM WITH LEAVES: Clematis erecta; Rhus venenata; Sabina.

(c) MODIFIED UNDERGROUND STEM:

(i) Rhizome (Thick, fleshy, underground stem with distant nodes and internodes, growing horrizontally—sometimes more or less vertically—beneath the surface of the body): Caulophyllum thalictroides; Cimicifuga racemosa; Collinsonia canadensis; Curcuma longa; Cypripedium pubescens; Dioscorea villosa; Filix mas; Gelsemium sempervirens; Helleborous niger; Hydrastis canadensis; Iris versicolor; Juncus effusus; Podophyllum peltatum; Rumex crispus; Sanguinaria canadensis; Valeriana officinalis; Veratrum album; Veratrum viride.

(ii) Stem-tuber (It is the swollen tip of an underground creeping branch which arises from the axil of a leaf on the main stem).

(iii) Corm (It is an elongated, more or less round solid vertical fleshy underground stem with few nodes and internodes, very often internodes are reduced to one): Colchicum autumnale; Crocus sativus.

(iv) Bulb (It is a small modified disc-like underground stem. The stem is extremely reduced and takes the shape of a disc): Allium cepa; Allium sativum.

4. **Leaves (Folia),**

(a) FRESH: Aegle folia; Ceanothus americanus; Cephalendra indica; Digitalis purpurea; Duboisia myoporoides; Ficus religiosa; Gaultheria procumbens; Jaborandi; Justicia adhatoda; Kalmia latifolia; Laurocerasus; Rhus toxicodendron; Thea sinensis.

(b) DRIED: Barosma crenata; Coca; Eucalyptus globulus; Gymnema sylvestre; Tabacum.

5. **Young Shoots**

Asparagus officinalis; Pinus sylvestris.

6. **Flowers (Flores)**

(a) FLOWERING HEADS: Cannabis sativa; Cina; Helianthus annus; Melilotus alba; Solidago; Trifolium pratense.

(b) FLOWERING HEADS AND LEAVES: Calendula officinalis; Eupatorium perfoliatum.

(c) STIGMA (Dried): Crocus sativus.

(d) FLOWER BUD: Prunus spinosa.

7. Fruits (Fructus)

(a) FLESHY FRUITS

(i) BERRY OR BACCA (It is usually a many-seeded fleshy fruit, develops from monocarpellary or polycarpellary, superior or inferior ovary): Agnus castus; Juniperus communis; Crataegus oxyacantha; Rhamnus cathartica; Sabal serrulata; Symphoricarpus racemosus.

(ii) FRESH LEAVES AND BERRIES: Viscum album.

(iii) WHOLE PLANT WITH BERRIES INCLUDING ROOTS: Solanum nigrum.

(b) DRIED FRUITS

(i) NUTS (Dry, one-celled and one seeded fruit which develops from a superior bi- or poly-carpellary ovary, having a hard and woody polycarp): Aesculus glabra; Sterculia accuminata.

(ii) PODS OR LEGUMES: Dolichos pruriens.

(iii) OTHERS: Embelia ribes; Capsicum annum; Phellandrium aquaticum; Terminalia chebula.

(c) PULPS: Carica papaya; Colocynthis.

8. Seeds (Semina)

(a) FRESH: Avena sativa; Cucurbita pepo; Ignatia amara; Lolium temulentum; Physostigma venenosum; Strophanthus hispidus; Syzygium Jambolanum.

(b) DRIED: Carduus marianus; Cedron; Cocculus indicus; Coffea cruda; Iberis amara; Jatropha curcas; Lathyrus sativus; Nux moschata; Nux vomica; Psoralea corylifolia; Sabadilla; Staphysagria.

9. Bark or Cortices (Bark as a mass of dead tissues lying in the peripheral region of the plant body as a hard dry covering):

(a) OUTER BARK OR RHYTIDOME (All the cork layers together with cortical and dry phloem tissues external to the innermost phellogen are called outer bark):

(i) FRESH: Abies canadensis; Ptelea trifoliata; Salix nigra; Viburnum opulus; Viburnum prunifolium.

(ii) DRIED: Alstonia scholaris; Cascara sagrada; Condurango; Cinchona officinalis; Mezereum.

(b) INNER BARK (All the tissues external to vascular cambium): Cinnamomum; Fraxinus americana; Populus tremuloides; Prunus virginiana.

(c) BARK OF THE ROOT

(i) FRESH: Baptisia tinctoria; Berberis vulgaris; Hamamelis virginica; Juglans cinerea; Myrica cerifera.

(ii) DRIED: Gossypium herbaceum.

(d) BARK OF YOUNG BRANCHES: Daphne indica.

(e) BARK OF ROOT AND STEM: Robinia pseudocacia.

(f) BARK OF THE TREES: Azadhirachta indica; Jonosia asoka; Terminalia arjuna.

(g) BARK and LEAF: Comocladia dentata; Prunus padus.

(h) LEAF, BARK and FRUIT: Mancinella.

(i) BARK and YOUNG TWIG: Ampelopsis quinquefolia.

10. Wood (Ligna)

Ostrya virginica (heart-wood)

Santalum album (dried-wood).

11. Extractions

(a) JUICES: Aloe socotrina (Inspissated juice of leaves); Anacardium occidentale (black oily juice of the shell); Anacardium orientale (Resinous fluid of seed); Elaterium (Sediment from the juice of the fruit); Opium (Gummy juice of Poppy).

(b) RESINS: Abies nigra; Guaiacum officinale.

(c) GUM-RESINS: Asafoetida.

(d) BALSAMS: Balsamum peruvianum, Balsamum tolutanum.

(e) OILS:

(i) FIXED or FATTY OIL:

Oleum chaulmoogra (seeds)
" crotonis (seeds)
" ricini (seeds)
" sesame (seeds)

(ii) VOLATILE or ESSENTIAL OIL:

Oleum cajuputi (leaves)
" caryophyllum (dried ovary of flower)
" chenopodium (fresh flowering and fruiting plants, excluding roots)
" cinnamomum (leaves and twigs)
" eucalyptus (dried leaves)
Oleum gaultheria (leaves)
" lavender (flowers)
" myristica (dried kernel of the seeds)
" santali (sandal wood)
" terebinth (various species of pinus).

12. Cryptogamia

(a) THALLOPHYTA:

(i) ALGAE: Fucus vesiculosus

(ii) FUNGI:

Agaricus emeticus
" muscarius
" phalloides
Boletus laricis
" satanas
" luridus
Bovista
Phallus impudicus
Polyporus pinicola
Russula
Secale cornutum (Claviceps purpurea)
Ustilago maydis

(iii) LICHENS:

Cetraria islandica
Sticta pulmonaria
Usnea barbata

(b) BRYOPHYTA: Polytrichum juniperinum

(c) PTERIDOPHYTA: Lycopodium clavatum (spores)
Filix mas
Equisetum hyemale.

13. Alkaloids

Name of Alkaloids	*Source*
Aconitine ($C_{34}H_{45}NO_{11}$)	Aconitum napellus (Root)
Apomorphia and its salt Apomorphinum muriaticum ($C_{17}H_{17}O_2N, HCl, \frac{1}{2}H_2O$)	Morphine
Areolin hydrobrom	Areca
Aspidospermine and its salt A. hydrochlor	Aspidosperma
Atropine or Atropinum ($C_{17}H_{23}NO_3$) and its salt A. sulphuricum [$(C_{17}H_{23}NO_3)_2H_2SO_4H_2O$]	Belladonna
Berberine and its salt B. sulph [$C_{20}H_{18}O_4N(HSO_4)$]	Berberis vulgaris
Brucine ($C_{23}H_{26}N_2O_4$) and its salt B. nitric	Nux vomica
Caffeinum and theine ($C_8H_{10}N_4O_2, H_2O$) and its salts C. bromicum, C. citrate ($C_8H_{10}N_4O_2C_6H_8O_7$), C. hydrobrom	Coffea; Ilex opaca; Thea sinensis
Quinidine ($C_{20}H_{24}N_2O_2$) and its different salts, C. arsenicum [$(C_{20}H_{24}N_2O_2)_3H_3ASO_3.4H_2O$], C. bisulphuricum ($C_{20}H_{24}O_2N_2H_2SO_4, 7H_2$), C. bromicum, C. ferrocyanicum, C. hydrocyanicum, C. hypophosphoricum, C. Iodatum, C. muriaticum($C_{20}H_{24}O_2N_2, HCl, 2H_2O$), C. phosphoricum, C. salicylicum, C. sulphuricum [$(C_{20}H_{24}O_2N_2)_2H_2SO_4, 2H_2O$], C. sulph. carb., C. valerianicum.	Cinchona officinalis
Colchicine ($C_{22}H_{25}O_6N$)	Colchicum autumnale
Conine ($C_8H_{17}N$) and its salts C. bromatum, C. mur	Conium maculatum

Name of Alkaloids	*Source*
Cocainum mur ($C_{17}H_{21}NO_4$, HCl)	Coca
Codeine ($C_{18}H_{21}NO_3$, H_2O) and its salts C. hydrochlor, C. phos ($C_{18}H_{21}NO_3H_3PO_4$, $2H_2O$)	Opium
Duboisine and its salt D. sulphate	Duboisia myoporoides
Emetine hydrochloride (salt of an alkaloid emetine, $C_{29}H_{40}O_4N_2$, 2HCl, $7H_2O$)	Ipecacuanha
Ephedrine ($C_{10}H_{15}ON$)	Ephedra vulgaris
Ergotin ($C_{35}H_{41}O_6N_5$)	Secale cornutum
Eserine and its salt E. sulph, ($C_{15}H_{21}$, $N_3O_2)_2$, H_2SO_4	Physostigma venenosum
Gelsemin	Gelsemium sempervirens
Hyoscyaminum ($C_{17}H_{23}NO_3.½H_2SO_4$) and its salt, H. hydrobromicum ($C_{17}H_{21}NO_4$, Hbr, $3H_2O$), H. sulph, [($C_{17}H_{23}NO_3)_2H_2SO_4$, $2H_2O$]	Hyoscyamus niger
Hydrastine ($C_{21}H_{21}NO_6$) and its salts H. hydrobrom, H. sulph	Hydrastis canadensis
Lobeline	Lobelia inflata
Morphine ($C_{17}H_{19}O_3N$) and its salt Morphinum aceticum ($C_{17}H_{19}NO_3$, $C_2H_4O_2$, $3H_2O$), Morphinum muriaticum ($C_{17}H_{19}O_3N$, HCl, $3H_2O$), Morphinum sulphuricum [($C_{17}H_{19}O_3N)_2$, H_2SO_4, $5H_2O$]	Opium
Muscarinum and its salt Muscarinum sulphuricum	Agaricus muscarius
Narceinum ($C_{23}H_{27}NO_8 3H_2O$)	Opium
Nicotinum ($C_{10}H_{14}N_2$)	Tabacum
Narcotinum ($C_{22}H_{23}NO_7$)	Opium
Pilocarpinum and its salt Pilocarpinum muriaticum ($C_{11}H_{16}N_2O_2$,HCl)	Pilocarpus microphyllus
Piperine ($C_{17}H_{19}O_3N$)	Piper methysticum
Sanguinarin and its salt Sanguinarina nitrica, S. sulphurica, S. tartaricum	Sanguinaria
Senecin	Senecio aureus
Spartein sulphuricum (salt of an alkaloid spartein)	Spartium scoparium
Strychninum ($C_{21}H_{22}N_2O_2$) and its salts Strychninum arsenicum, S. nitricum ($C_{21}H_{22}O_2N_2$, HNO_3) S. hydrochlor ($C_{21}H_{22}O_2N_2$, HCl, $2H_2O$), S. phosphoricum ($C_{21}H_{22}N_2O_2.H_3PO_4.2H_2O$) S. sulphuricum ($(C_{21}H_{22}N_2O_2)_2H_2SO_2.5H_2O$), S. valerianum	Nux vomica
Veratrinum	Sabadilla

14. Resinoids

Name of Resinoids	*Source*
Aletrin	Aletris farinosa
Ampelopsin	Ampelopsis quinquefolia
Apocynin	Apocynum cannabinum
Asclepin	Asclepias tuberosa
Baptisin	Baptisia tinctoria
Caulophyllin	Caulophyllum thalictroides
Cerasin	Cerasus virginiana
Collinsonin	Collinsonia canadensis
Cornin	Cornus florida
Corydalin	Corydalis formosa
Cypripedin	Cypripedium pubescens
Dioscorin	Dioscorea villosa
Euphorbin	Euphorbia villosa
Geranin	Geranium maculatum
Gossypin	Gossypium herbaceum
Irisin	Iris versicolor
Jugulandin	Juglans cinerea
Leptandrin	Leptandra virginica
Macrotin	Cimicifuga racemosa
Podophyllin	Podophyllum peltatum
Scutellarin	Scutellaria lateriflora
Senecin	Senecio aureus
Stillingin	Stillingia silvatica
Xanthoxylin	Xanthoxylum fraxineum

15. Glycosides

Name of Glycosides	Source
Adonidin	Adonis vernalis
Aloin	Aloe socotrina
Arbutin	Uva ursi
Colocynthin	Colocynthis
Digitalin	Digitalis
Phloridzin	Bark of the root of the apple and other trees
Sanguinarin	Sanguinaria canadensis
Saponinum	Quillaya saponaria
Viburnin	Viburnum opulus
Picrotoxinum($C_{30}H_{34}O_{13}$)	Anamirta paniculata (seed).

ANIMAL KINGDOM

The drugs prepared from living or dried whole animals, different parts, secretions etc. and also from the venoms of poisonous animals as well as milk and milk products.

(a) Whole Living Animals

Name of animal or drug	*Common name*	*Class*	*Phyllum*
Apis mellifica	Hive bee (throughout world)	Insecta	Arthropoda
Bombyx chrysorrhoea	Brown tailed Moth (Europe)	"	"
Bombyx processionae	Procession Moth (Europe)	"	"
Chenopodium glauci	Plant-lice from Chenopodium	"	"
Cimex acanthia	Bed bug (India)	"	"
Coccinella septempuncata	Lady bug (India)	"	"
Culex musca	Mosquito—culex	"	"
Doryphora decemlineata	Colorado potato-bug	"	"
Formica rufa	Crushed live ants (Europe)	"	"
Vespa crabro	Common wasp (Europe)	Insecta	Arthropoda
Pulex irritans	Common flea	"	"
Pediculus capitis	Head louse	"	"
Millepedes (Oniscus asellus)	Wood louse or saw bug (Europe)	Crustacea	"
Astacus fluviatilis	River crab; cray fish (Pacific slope; Europe; Asia; England)	Crustacea	"
Spider group			
Aranea avicularis	Mygale avicularis (Middle Europe)	Arachnida	
Aranea diadema	Papal cross spider; garden spider (Europe; America)	"	"
Aranea scinencia	Grey spider (Kentucky, on old walls)	"	"
Latrodectus hasselti	Large black spider (New South Wales)	"	"
Latrodectus katipo	Poison spider (New Zealand & California)	"	"
Latrodectus mactans	Black widow spider (South Europe; New Zealand)	"	"
Mygale lasiodora	Black cuban spider (Island of Cuba; Texas ; South America)	"	"
Tarentula cubensis	Large, dark brown & hairy spider (Cuba; Mexico)	"	"
Tarentula hispanica	Spanish spider (Spain; South Europe; South America)	"	"
Theridion curassavicum	Orange spider (West Indies)	"	"

Contd.

Name of animal or drug	Common name	Class	Phyllum
Scorpion Group			
Scorpio europus	Bichchu (Europe)	Arachnida	Arthropoda
Aurelia medusa	Jelly-fish (Entire Atlantic coast & Pacific coast)	Scyphozoa	Coelentereta
Physalia	Portugese man-of-war	Hydrozoa	"
Sanguisuga officinalis	The leech	Hirudinea	Annlida
Helix tosta	Snail; shamuk (paleoarctic region; poorly represented in America)	Gastropoda	Mollusca
Asterias rubens	Common starfish (Europe; America; India)	Asteroidea	Echinodermata
Pyrara	River fish (South America; Brazil)	Osteichthyes	Chordata
(b) **Whole Dried Animals**			
Blatta americana	Great American cockroach (America)	Insecta	Arthropoda
Blatta orientalis	Indian cockroach (India)	"	"
Cantharis vesicatoria	Spanish fly (Middle and Southern Europe)	"	
Coccus cacti	Grana fine cochineal insect (Mexico; America; Peru; Spain)	Insecta	Arthropoda
Armadillo officinarum	Ant-eater (South America)	Crustacea	"
Lacerta agilis	Green lizard	Reptila	Chordata
(c) **Different Parts, Secretions of Animals**			
1. *Skeletons:*			
Spongia tosta	Roasted sponge (Syria; Greece)	Calcarea or Calcispongiae	Porifera
Badiaga (Spongilla fluviatilis)	Fresh water sponge (Atlantic; European and American waters)	"	"
Corallium rubrum	Red coral or prabala	Arthozoa	Colenterata
2. *Acarus:*			
Trombidium	Red acarus of the fly (Philadelphia	Arachnida	Arthropoda
3. *Blood:*			
Limulus or Xiphosura americana	The king-crab or horse foot (Asia, North America)	"	"
4. *Juices:*			
Araneinum	Juice of greasy spider, Aranea scinencia	"	"
Mephitis mephitica	Skunk—poison; Fluid secretion of the anal gland of wild cat (U.S.A.)	Mammalia	Chordata
Murex purpurea	Purple fish (Syrian coast, Greece, Italy, India, West Indies and U.S.A.)	Gastropoda	Mollusca
Sepia succus	Cuttle fish (India, Europe)	Cephalopoda	"
5. *Shells:*			
Calcarea calcinata	Calcineed oyster shell	Bivalvia	"
Pecten	Scallop (India and U.S.A.)	"	"
Calcarea ovorum	Toasted egg-shell of hen	Aves	Chordata
Ovi gallinae pellicula	Membrane of egg-shell	"	"

Contd.

Name of animal or drug	*Common name*	*Class*	*Phyllum*
6. *Backbone:*			
Gadus lata	Cod-fish spp.	Osteichthyes	Chordata
7. *First cervical vertebra:*			
Gadus morrhua	Cod-fish spp.	"	"
8. *Thumb-nail:*			
Castor equi	A red substance growing on the inside of the legs of the horse (Rudimentary thumbnail of the horse)	Mammalia	"
9. *Prickles:*			
Sphingurus maritini	Large rodent (Brazil)	"	"
10. *Hide:*			
Carbo animalis	Animal charcoal	Insecta	Arthropoda
Cervus braziliens	Hide of Brazilium stag with hair on (Brazil)	"	"
11. Gizzard:			
Ingluvin	Gizzard of a fowl	"	"
12. *Extracts:*			
Orchitinum	Testicular extract of man	"	"
Oophorinum	Ovarian extract of cow or sheep	"	"
Hippomanes	Meconium deposit from newborn horse or calf	"	"
Moschus moschiferus	Dried secretion of preputial follicles of male musk-deer (East Asia)	"	"
Castoreum	Extract from the preputial sacs of the beaver	"	"
13. *Animal brain:*			
Lecithin	Phosphorus containing complex organic body	"	"
14. *Gall-bladder:*			
Fel piscinum	Fresh gall of dog	"	"
Fel tauri	Fresh gall of horse	"	"
Vulpis fel	Fresh gall of ox	"	"
15. *Liver:*			
Vulpis hepar	Fresh liver of fox	"	"
16. *Small intestine:*			
Typho-febrinum	Large rodent (porcupine), having spines or sharp quills in its horny coat (Sajarur Kutilantra)	"	"
17. *Lung:*			
Vulpis pulmo or pulmo vulpis	Fresh lung of wolf or fox	"	"
18. *Digestive fluid:*			
Homarus	Digestive fluid of live lobster	Crustacea	Arthropoda
19. Serum:			
Serum anguillae ichthyotoxin	Eel serum (Serum of the eel)	Pisces	Chordata

Contd.

Name of animal or drug	*Common name*	*Class*	*Phyllum*
20. *Oil:*			
Oleum animale	Dippel's animal oil or bone oil (It is the secretion of the mare i.e. female horse)	Mammalia	Chordata
Oleum jecoris aselli	Fresh liver of the cod, *Gadus morrhua*	Osteichthyes	"
(d) VENOMS			
1. *Snake Poison (Ophidia):*			
Ancistrodon contortrix or Cenchris contortrix	Pit-viper, Copper head snake (Hilly region in North and Eastern parts of India and Asia)	Reptila	Chordata
Bungarus fasciatus	Banded krait (South East Asia; All over India and Malayasia)	Reptila	Arthropoda
Chelone	Snake head (Indian, Pacific and Atlantic Oceans and coasts of the United States)	"	"
Crotalus horridus	Rattle snake (North America; Europe)	Reptila	Chordata
Elaps corallinus	Coral snake (Brazil)	"	"
Lachesis lanceolatus or Bothrops lanceolatus	Yellow viper	"	"
Hydrophis cyanocynatus	Sea snake	"	"
Lachesis trigonocephalus	Surukuku snake (South America)	"	"
Naja tripudians	Indian headed snake, Gokshura (India)	"	"
Toxicophis	Moccasin snake	"	"
Vipera berus	Common viper	"	"
2. *Lizard Poison:*			
Amphisboena vermicularis	Glass snake; Snail-like Lizard (South America)	"	"
Heloderma horridus	Gill-monster or Hella monster (Deserts of Mexico and U.S.A.)	"	"
3. *Scorpion Poison:*			
Centruroides elegans	Scorpion (Mexico)	Arachnida	Arthropoda
4. *Spider Poison:*			
Latrodectus mactans	Black widow spider; Hour glass spider (South Europe; Southern United States; New Zealand)	"	"
5. *Insect Poison:*			
Apium virus	Poison of honey bee	Insecta	"
6. *Poison of Aqueous Animal:*			
Bufo rana	Toad	Amphibia	Chordata
(e) MILK AND MILK PRODUCTS (LACS)			
Lac. caninum	Dog's milk	Mammalia	"
Lac. felinum	Cat's milk	"	"
Lac. vaccinum	Cow's milk	"	"
Lac. defloratum	Skimmed cow milk	"	"
Lac. vaccinum coagulatum	Curd	"	"
Lac. vaccini floc	Cream	"	"
Koumyss	Fermentation from ass's milk	"	"

MINERAL KINGDOM AND CHEMICALS

A. **Acids** (Acids are compounds containing hydrogen in which the hydrogen can be replaced by metals)

(a) *Organic Acids*

1. Alliphatic monobasic acids—Acidum aceticum (CH_3COOH); Acidum formicum ($HCOOH$); Acidum butyricum ($CH_3CH_2CH_2COOH$).
2. Substituted fatty acids—Acidum lacticum [$CH_3\ CH(OH)COOH$]; Acidum sarcolacticum ($CH_3CH\ OHCOOH$).
3. Cyanogen compounds—Acidum hydrocyanicum (HCN).
4. Saturated di-carboxylic acids—Acidum oxalicum ($HOOC—COOH$); Acidum succinicum ($HOOCCH_2\ CH_2COOH$).
5. Hydroxy polybasic acids—Acidum tartaricum ($C_4H_6O_6$); Acidum citricum ($C_6H_8O_7$).
6. Phenol—Acidum carbolicum or Acidum phenic (C_6H_5OH); Acidum picricum or Tri-nitrophenol [$C_6H_2(NO_2)_3OH$].
7. Aromatic carboxylic acids—Acidum benzoicum (C_6H_5COOH); Acidum hippuricum ($C_6H_5—CONHCH_2COOH$); Acidum gallicum [$C_6H_2(OH)_3\ COOH$]; Acidum salicylicum ($HO—C_6H_4COOH$); Acidum acetyl salicylicum or Aspirin ($CH_3COO — C_6H_4—COOH$).
8. Derivatives of carbonic acid—Acidum uricum ($C_5H_4O_3N_4$).

(b) *Inorganic Acids*

Acidum arsenicosum or Arsenicum album (AS_2O_3); A. boracicum (H_3BO_3); A. bromicum ($HbrO_3$); A. chromicum ($HCrO_3$); A. hydrofluoricum (HFl); A. muriaticum (HCl); A. nitricum (HNO_3); A. phosphoricum (H_3PO_4); A. sulphuricum (H_2SO_4).

B. **Elements** (Elements are defined as a homogeneous substance which cannot be decomposed or disintegrated further to get substances of different characteristics)

(a) *Metals:* Aluminium met (Al); Argentum met. (Ag); Aurum met (Au.); Beryllium met (Be.); Bismuthum met (Bi); Cadmium met (Cd.); Cobaltum met (Co.); Cuprum met (Cu.); Ferrum met (Fe); Indium met (In); Iridum met (Ir); Manganum met (Mn); Magnesia met (Mg); Merc. vivus (Hg); Niccolum met (Ni); Osmium met (Os); Palladium met (Pd); Platinum met (Pt); Plumbum met (Pb); Rhodium met (Rh); Stannum met (Sn); Tellurium met (Te); Thallium met (Tl); Titanium met (Ti); Uranium met (U); Vanadium met (V); Zincum met (Zn.)

(b) *Non-metals:* Bromium (Br); Chlorinum or Chlorum (Cl_{12}); Iodum (I); Selenium (Se); Phosphorus (P); Sulphur (S).

(c) *Metalloids* (The elements which exhibit more or less the properties of both metals and non-metals—they are referred to as metalloids): Arsenic (As); Antimony (Sb.)

C. **Compounds** (are defined as homogeneous substances which are formed through chemical combination of two or more elements in definite proportion and, hence, they can be broken down, either by chemical or physical method, into simpler ingredients, viz. the elements.)

(a) *Inorganic compounds:*

1. Aluminium group—Aluminium acetate [$Al(CH_3\ COO)_3$]; A. chloridum ($AlCl_3$); Alumina or Oxide of Aluminium or Argilla (Al_2O_3); A. phosphorica ($Al\ PO_4$); A. silicata or Kaolin or China-clay or Bolus alba (Al_2O_3, $2SiO_2$); Alumen (Common potash alum) K_2SO_4, $Al_2(SO_4)_3.24H_2O$.
2. Ammonia group—Ammonium aceticum or Acetate of ammonia ($CH_3COO\ NH_4$); A. arsenicum [$(NH_4)_3AsS_4$]; A. benzoicum or Benzoite of Ammonia or Sal volatile (NH_4HCO_3, $NH_4NH_2CO_2$); A. causticum or Hydrate of ammonia, ammonia water (NH_4OH); A. fluoricum or Fluoride of Ammonia (NH_4F); A. formaldehyde or cystogen or urotropine ($(CH_2)_6N_4$; A. iodatum or Iodide of Ammonia (NH_4I); A. muriaticum or Sal ammoniac (NH_4Cl);

A. nitricum (NH_4NO_3); A. phosphoricum or Phosphate of ammonia [$(NH_4)_2HPO_4$]; A. picricum or Picrate of ammonia ($C_6H_6N_4O_7$); A. sulphuricum [$(NH_4)_2SO_4$]; A. tartaricum ($(CHOH.COONH_4)_2$; A. valerianicum or valerianate of ammonia ($NH_4C_5H_9O_2$); A. vanadiate (NH_4VO_3).

3. Antimony group—Antimonium arsenium or Arsenite of antimony ($SbAsO_4$); A. chloridum or Butter of antimony ($SbCl_3$); A. crudum or Antimony trisulphide (Sb_2S_3); A. iodatum (Sb_2I_3); A. oxydatum (Sb_2O_3); A. sulphuratum aureum or Golden sulphuret of antimony (Sb_2S_5); A. tartaricum or Emetic tartar or Double tartarate of antimony and potash {$2[K(SbO)C_4H_5O_6]H_2O$}.

4. Silver group—Argentum cyanatum (AgCN); A. iodatum (AgI); A. muriaticum (AgCl); A. nitricum ($AgNO_3$); A. oxydatum (Ag_2O); A. phosphoricum (Ag_3PO_4).

5. Arsenic group—Arsenicum bromatum or Bromide of arsenic ($AsBr_3$); A. hydrogenisatum or Arseniuretted hydrogen (AsH_3); A. iodatum or Iodide of Arsenic (AsI_3); A. sulphuratum flavum or Arsenic trisulph (AS_2S_3); A. sulphuratum rubrum (AS_2S_2).

6. Gold group—Aurum bromatum ($AuBr_3$); A. iodatum (AuI_3); A. muriaticum ($AuCl_3$); A. muriaticum natronatum ($NaAuCl_4$, $2H_2O$); A. sulphuratum or Gold trisulphate (Au_2SO_3).

7. Barium group—Baryta acetica (CH_3COOBa); B. carbonica ($BaCO_3$); B. caustica [$Ba(OH)_2$]; B. iodata (BaI_2); B. muriatica ($BaCl_2$, $2H_2O$); B. nitrica [$Ba(NO_3)_2$]; B. sulph ($BaSO_4$);

8. Bismuth group—Bismuthum nitricum [$Bi(NO_3)_3$. $5H_2O$]; B. sub. nitricum ($6Bi_2O_35N_2O_5$, $9H_2O$).

9. Cadmium group—Cadmium brom ($CdBr_2$); C. carb ($CdCO_3$); C. fluor (CdF_2); C. iodatum (CdI_2); C. oxide (CdO); C. phos ($CdPO_4$); C. sulphuricum (Cd $SO_4.8H_2O$).

10. Calcium group—Calcarea acetica or Acetate of lime [$(CH_3COO)_2Cu_2$]; C. arsenicosa or Arsenite of lime [$Ca_3(ASO_3)_2$]; C. bromata ($CaBr_2$); C. carbonica or Carbonate of lime ($CaCO_3$); C. caustica or Slaked lime [$Ca(OH)_2$]; C. fluorica or Fluoride of lime (CaF_2); C. formata [$Ca(HCOO)_2$]; C. hypophosphorosa [$Ca(PH_2O_2]_2$)]; C. iodata or iodide of lime ($CaI_2.6H_2O$); C. lactic [$(CH_3CXHOHCOO)_2C_8$]; C. muriatica or C. chloratum ($CaCl_2$); C. nitrica [$Ca(NO_3)_2$]; C. oxalica (CaC_2O_4. H_2O); C. phosphorica [$Ca_3(PO_4)_2$]; C. silicata or Silicate of lime ($Ca.SiO_3$); C. sulphurica ($CaSO_4$); Hepar sulphurica (CaS).

11. Chromium group—Chromium oxydatum (Cr_2O_3); C. sulphate ($CrSO_4$, $7H_2O$); Chromico kali sulphuricum or chrome alum [K_2SO_4, $Cr_2(SO_4)_3$, $24H_2O$].

12. Cobalt group—Cobaltum nitricum or cobaltous nitrate [$CO(NO_3)_2$, $6H_2O$].

13. Copper group—Cuprum aceticum (CH_3COOCu); C. ammonio—sulphuricum [$Cu(NH_3)_4]SO_4$; C. arsenicum or Arsenite of copper or scheele's green [$Cu_3(ASO_3)_2.2H_2O$]; C. carbonicum [$CuCO_2$ + $Cu(OH)_2$]; C. cyanatum (CuCN); C. nitricum [$Cu(NO_3)_2.3H_2O$]; C. oxydatum (CuO); C. sulphuricum ($CuSO_4.5H_2O$).

14. Iron group—Ferrum aceticum [$(CH_3COO)_3Fe$]; F. arsenicum [$Fe_3(ASO_4)_2$]; F. bromatum ($FeBr_2$); F. carbonicum ($FeCO_3$); F. citricum [$Fe_3(C_6H_5O_7)_2$]; F. iodatum (FeI_2); F. lacticum [$(CH_3CHOHCOO)_2$ Fe]; F. magneticum or Load-stone (Fe_3O_4); F. muriaticum ($FeCl_3$. $6H_2O$); F. phosphoricum [$Fe_3(PO_4)_2$. $8H_2O$]; F. sulphuricum ($FeSO_4$. $7H_2O$); F. tartaricum [$CH(OH)COOFe]_2$.

15. Potash group—Causticum or Hahnemann's tintura acris sine kali; K. aceticum (CH_3COOK); Kali arsenicosum or Fowler's solution ($KASO_2$ + H_3ASO_3); K. benzoicum ($KC_7H_5O_2$); K. bi-carb ($KHCO_3$); K. bichromicum

($K_2Cr_2O_7$); K. bromatum (KBr); K. carbonicum (K_2CO_3); K. causticum (KOH); K. chloricum ($KClO_3$); K. chromicum (K_2CrO_4); K. citricum ($K_3C_6H_5O_7.H_2O$); K. cyanatum (KCN); K. ferrocyanatum or prussian blue [$K_4Fe(CN)_6$] $3H_2O$; K. iodatum or hydroiodatum (KIO_3); K. muriaticum (KCl); K. nitricum (KNO_3); K. oxalicum (KOOC—COOK, H_2O); K. permanganum ($KMnO_4$); K. phosphoricum (K_2HPO_4); K. picricum (C_6H_2 KN_3O_7); K. salicylate ($KC_7H_5O_3$); K. sulphuricum (K_2SO_4); K. sulphchrom (Alum of Chrom) [K_2SO_4,$Cr_2(SO_4)_3$, $24H_2O$]; K. tartaricum ($K_2C_4H_5O_6$. H_2O); K. telluricum (K_2TeO_4);

16. Lithium group—Lithium benzoicum ($LiC_7H_5O_2$); L. bromicum (LiBr); L. carbonicum (Li_2CO_3); L. citricum [$C_3H_4OH(COOLi)_3.4H_2O$]; L. lacticum [$(CH_3CH\ OH.COO)_2Li$] L. phosphate (Li_3PO_4).

17. Magnesium group—Magnesia acetica (CH_3COO Mg); M. carbonica [$(MgCO_3)_4.Mg(OH)_2.5.H_2O$]; M. iodata ($MgI_2.8H_2O$); M. muriatica ($MgCl_2.6H_2O$); M. phosphorica ($MgHPO_4.7H_2O$); M. sulphurica or Epsom salt ($MgSO_4.7H_2O$).

18. Manganese group—Manganum aceticum [$Mn(CH_3.\ COO)_2.4H_2O$]; Manganum bin-oxydatum (MnO_2); M. carbonicum ($MnCO_3$); M. muriaticum ($MnCl_2$. $4H_2O$); M. phos. ($MnPO_4$. H_2O); M. sulphuricum [$Mn_2(SO_4)_3$].

19. Mercury group—Mercurius aceticus (CH_3COOHg); M. biniodatus or M. iodatus ruber (HgI_2); M. bromatus (Hg_2Br_2); M. corrosivus or corrosive sublimate ($HgCl_2$); M. cyanatus [$Hg(CN)_2$]; M. dulcis or Calomel (HgCl); M. et. kali iodatus ($HgI_2 2KI$); M. nitricus [$Hg(NO_3)_2$]; M. praecipitatus albus [NH_2 HgCl]; M. precipitatus ruber (HgO); M. proto iodatus or M. iodatus flavus (HgI); M. sulphuricus ($HgSO_4$).

20. Soda group—Borax veneta or bi-borate of soda ($Na_2B_4O_7.10H_2O$); N. aceticum (CH_3COONa); N. arsenicum (Na_2HASO_4. $7H_2O$); N. benzoicum ($NaC_7H_5O_2$); N. bi-carbonicum ($NaHCO_3$); N. bromatum (NaBr); N. cacodylas or cacodylate of Soda [$(CH_3)_2$.ASOOH]; N. carbonicum ($Na_2CO_3.10H_2O$); N. chloratum or Labarraque's solution ($NaClO_3$); N. caust (NaOH); N. hypochloricum (NaOCl); N. hypophosphoricum ($NaPH_2O_2$); N. iodatum (NaI); N. lacticum [$CH_3.CHOH.COO)_2.Na$]; N. nitrosum ($NaNO_2$); N. phosphoricum (Na_2HPO_4. $12H_2O$); N. salicylicum ($NaC_7H_5O_3$); N. selenicum (Na_2SeO_4); N. silicatum ($Na_2SiO_5.H_2O$); N. succinate ($(CH_2COONa)_2$; N. sulphocarbolicum (C_6H_5 SO_3Na); N. sulphuricum or glauber's salt (Na_2SO_4. $10H_2O$); N. sulphurosum ($Na_2SO_3.7H_2O$); N. telluricum (Na_2TeO_4).

21. Nickel group—Niccolum bromatum ($NiBr_2$); N. carbonicum [$NiCO_3$. $2Ni(OH)_2.4H_2O$]; N. sulphuricum ($NiSO_4.7H_2O$).

22. Platinum group—Platinum muriaticum (H_2PtCl_6. $6H_2O$).

23. Plumbum group—Plumbum aceticum [$Pb(CH_3\ COO)_2.3H_2O$]; P. carbonicum ($PbCO_3$); P. chromi cum ($PbCrO_4$); P. iodatum (PbI_2).

24. Radium group—Radium bromide ($RaBr_2$); R. chloride ($RaCl_2$).

25. Stannum group—Stannum iodatum (SnI_2); S. muriaticum ($SnCl_2$).

26. Strontium group—Strontiana carbonica or Strontium carbonate ($SrCO_3$).

27. Thallium group—Thallium acetate (CH_3COOTt).

28. Uranium group—Uranium aceticum (CH_3COOU); Uranium nitricum [$UO_2(BO_2)_2.6H_2O$].

29. Zinc group—Zincum aceticum [$Zn(CH_3COO)_2$. $2H_2O$]; Z. arsenicum [$Zn_3(ASO_2)_2$]; Z. bromatum ($ZnBr_2$);

Z. carbonicum ($ZnCO_3$); Z. oxydatum (ZnO); Z. phosphoratum (Zn_3P_2); Z. sulphuricum ($ZnSO_4.7H_2O$); Z. valerianicum [$Zn(C_5H_9O_2).2H_2O$].

(b) *Organic compounds:*

1. Acetanilidum (C_8H_9NO) or Antifebrinum, Phenyl acetamide.
2. Allyl sulphide [$(CH_2{=}CH{-}CH_2)_2S$]: It is the main component of oil of garlic (allium, garlic).
3. Amyl nitrosum or Amyl nitrite ($C_5H_{11}O.NO$): It consists chiefly of iso-amyl nitrite but also contains other nitrites of the homologous series.
4. Anilinum or Aminobenzene or Phenyl amine: ($C_6H_5NH_2$): Aromatic amino compound; a coal tar product.
5. Antipyrine or phenazone ($C_{11}H_{12}N_2O$): A coal tar derivative.
6. Benzinum or Benzol (C_6H_6): A mixture of homologous hydrocarbons obtained from light coal-tar oil. It contains about 70% of benzene and 20–30% toluene.
7. Benzinum di-nitricum or dinitrobenzene [$C_6H_4(NO_2)_2$]: It is prepared by heating Nitrobenzene with a mixture of conc. H_2SO_4 and fuming HNO_3.
8. Benzinum nitricum or nitrobenzene ($C_6H_5NO_2$): It is the simplest aromatic nitro-compound.
9. Benzoinum or Benzoin ($C_{14}H_{12}O_2$): A balsamic resin obtained from the incised stem of Styrax benzoin, known as sumatra benzoin.
10. Camphora ($C_{10}H_{16}O$), Karpur.
11. Chloralum or Chloral hydrate [$CCl_3.CH.(OH)_2$]: Ethylic alcohol is saturated with dry chlorine and thus chloral is formed. It is purified and water is added to form a hydrate.
12. Chloroformum or chloroform ($CHCl_3$) or trichloromethane.
13. Chrysorobinum.
14. Eosin (Tetra bromo fluorscein): Results on brominating at room temp., fluorscein in acetic acid.
15. Ethylic ether or Ethyl oxide ($C_4H_{10}O$) or Etherum.
16. Ethylum nitricum ($C_2H_5NO_3$).
17. Eupionum: A product of wood-tar distillation.
18. Formalin (CH_2O): Aqueous solution (35%) of formaldehyde gas.
19. Glonoinum or Nitroglycerine ($C_3H_5N_3O_9$).
20. Glycerinum [$C_3H_5(OH)_3$], Glycerin or Glycerol.
21. Guaiacol ($C_7H_8O_2$): A product obtained by fractional distillation of beech tar kreosote.
22. Ichthyolum [$C_{28}H_{36}S_5O_6(NH_4)_2$]: A combination of sulphonated hydrocarbon; a fossil product of complex structure found in Tyrol, supposed to be fish deposits, contains 10% sulphur.
23. Indigo ($C_{16}H_{10}O_2N_2$): Dye-stuff.
24. Indol (A crystalline compound derivable from indigo, but also a product of putrefaction of proteins).
25. Iodoform (CHI_3): It is prepared by reacting acetone or ethyl alcohol with iodine and alkali.
26. Kreosotum: A product of beech-tar distillation. It consists of a mixture of guaiacol ($C_7H_8O_2$), cresol ($C_8H_{10}O_2$) and less of other phenols.
27. Menthol ($C_{10}H_{20}OH$): It is a saturated secondary alcohol. It is the main constituent of peppermint oil (Mentha piperata) which is obtained from the plant by steam distillation.
28. Methylene blue ($C_{16}H_{18}N_3ClS, 3H_2O$): One of the aniline dyes.
29. Naphthalinum ($C_{10}H_8$): A chemical compound from coal tar distillation; tar camphor.
30. Petroleum: Crude rock-oil.
31. Phenacetin ($C_{10}H_{13}N_2O$) or P-aceta-

minophenetole: Is obtained from P-nitrophenol by ethylation, reduction and acetylation.

32. Pix liquida: A bituminous liquid obtained from the wood pinus sylvestris and other species of pinus by wood tar distillation.
33. Propylamine (C_3H_9N): Distilled-Hering-brine.
34. Resorcinum or meta di-hydroxy benzene [$C_6H_4(OH)_2$].
35. Sulphonal ($C_7H_6S_2O_4$): Product of coal tar distillation.
36. Thiosinaminum ($NH_2CSNHCH_2CH_2CH_2$): A chemical derived from oil of Mustard seed.
37. Tri-nitro-toluene [CH_3—$C_6H_2(NO_2)_3$].

D. Minerals (Mineral is a term by which is meant a naturally occurring substance which contains essentially one of the chemical elements of interest):

1. Adamas.
2. Aethiops mercurialis mineralis (Black sulphide of Mercury).
3. Aethiops antimonalis (Hydrar-gyrum stibiato sulfuratum).
4. Anthracite.
5. Anthrakokali (Anthracite coal derived in caustic potash).
6. Benzoaris-Lapis (Gorochana).
7. Fluorspar (Fluorite, CaF_2).
8. Graphites (Plumbago; Black lead).
9. Hekla-lava (Lava scoriae from Mt. Hekla).
10. Kaolin or Alumina silicata.
11. Mica [$KH_2Al_3(SiO_4)_3$], Abhra.
12. Sal marinum (Sea salt).
13. Silicea or Silicon di-oxide or Silica or pure flint.
14. Tetradymitum (Bi_2Te_3)—Crystals from Georgia and North Carolina containing Bismuth, Tellurium and Sulphur.

E. Mineral-Spring Water (Mineral water, impregnated with minerals)

Aqua calcarea (lime-water); Aqua petra; Aqua marina (Isotonic plasma); Aqua regia (Acidum nitro-muriaticum); Aqua sanicula; Carlsbad salz (The waters of the Sprudel springs); Equx bonnes; Lapis albus (Silicofluoride of Calcium; Gastein rock); Levico water (containing Ars., Iron, and Copper of South Tyrol); Vichy; Wiesbaden; Skookum chuck (salts from water of 'medical lake' near Spokane, Wash.)

Notes:

1. **Carlsbad:** Bohemia, altitude 1,214 feet (370 metres). April to October. One of the largest bathing stations in Europe.—Hot mineral, purgative, diuretic, and resolvent waters, catarrhs of mucous membranes, congestions of liver, urinary calculus, gravel, chronic gout, diabetes, obesity etc. are the features.
2. **Vichy:** 228 miles (365 kms) from Paris—May to October, Alkaline springs, with or without iron. Dyspepsia, hepatic and renal disorders, gout, diabetes, catarrhs and malarial cachexia etc. treated by it.
3. **Wiesbaden:** Alkaline saline waters of a muddy brown hue. Is one of the most popular spas in Prussia of Germany. The treatment is both internal and external—gout, catarrh, diabetes etc. In fact, the baths and waters are stated to cure almost everything that is curable.
4. **Levico:** Situated in south Iyrol, on the confines of Italy, Levico has for many years been a favourite sanatorium of the Italian medical profession for their nervous and skin patients. Of late years, Levico water has also been increasingly recognised by the German and Austrian faculty, among whom Baberger, Billroth, Hebra, Nussbaum, and others testify to the extraordinary remedial activity of the waters, favouring assimilation, increasing nutrition, and in chronic and dyscratic skin diseases functioning as antiseptic or astringent.

NOSODES OR BIOTHERAPEUTIC PREPARATIONS

Definition

The word 'Nosode' is derived from '*Nosos*' (Gr.) means 'Disease' and '*Cidos*' means 'appearance'. It may also be compared with '*Noxa*' (L), which means 'noxious or damage'.

Willium Lux, who is considered to be the founder of Isopathy, used the discharges of human and animals to treat the people. Dr. Hering used it after proving it on humans as homoeopathic remedies.

The name nosodes has given way to a new term—'Biotherapeutics' which seems to be more appropriate. This includes disease products, disease-causing organisms and disease-preventing vaccines and toxins.

The term 'Nosode' has no legal existence in France and Germany and has been replaced by the term 'biotherapy'.

1. Dewey—"The homoeopathic designation from the morbid product of disease, when employed as remedies'.
2. Pierre Schmidt—'an isopathic remedy'. According to him, "If it is applied after having been tested on a healthy man, it becomes a nosode".
3. H.P.I. (Vol. IV)—'Homoeopathic preparation from pure microbial culture obtained from diseased tissue and clinical materials (secretions, discharges etc.)'.
4. Rene Allendy—'The nosode is characterised by a pathological substance used as the medicine prepared in advance and according to the homoeopathic method of dilution.'
5. Stedman's Medical Dictionary—'An agent administered in minute doses in the treatment of the disease, it causes; an isopathic term, signifying a bacterine or bacterial vaccine.'
6. H.P.C.U.S.—According to the Homoeopathic Pharmacopoeia Convention of the United States, 'Nosodes are homoeopathic attenuations of pathological organs or tissues; causative agents such as bacteria, fungi, parasites, virus particles, and yeast; disease products; excretions or secretions.'
7. Others—Remedies which are prepared from diseased products of human beings, lower animals and diseased plant products are called nosodes.

Classification of Nosodes

The nosodes are classified in the following types:

1. Basic nosodes: Psorinum, Tuberculinum, Bacillinum, Syphillinum, Medorrhinum, Carcinosinum
2. Exanthem (= a widespread rash): Morbillinum, Parotidinum, Vaccininum, Variolinum, Influenzinum, Diphtherinum, Pertussinum, Anthracinum, Malandrinum.
3. Isopathic nosodes: Streptococcinum, Staphylococcinum, Pneumococcinum, Malaria officinalis, Pyrogeninum.
4. Intestinal nosodes: Proteus, Dysentery co., Morgan, Gaertner bacillus etc.
5. Autogenous: Nosodes prepared from discharges or secretions from the pathological tissues or organs of the patient himself for treatment of that very diseased state (tautopathy).
6. Lesser used: Ambra grisea, E. coli, Microfilaria, Histaminum, Eosinophillinum.

Depending upon the nature of materials used, nosodes are divided into four catagories (HPI—Vol IV). They are denoted by NI, NII, NIII and NIV:

- NI: Nosodes prepared from lysates of micro-organisms capable of producing bacterial endotoxins, e.g., Typhoidinum, Paratyphoidinum, E. coli., Staphylococcinum.
- NII: Nosodes prepared from microorganisms capable of producing exotoxins, e.g., Diphtherinum.
- NIII: Nosodes prepared from purified toxins.
- NIV: Nosodes prepared from microorganisms/viruses/clinical materials from human convalescence or diseased subjects. e.g., Psorinum, Syphillinum, Morbillinum, Influenzinum, Variolinum etc.

Examples

	Name of the Drug	*Source*
A.	**Diseased products of Human beings**	
	Aids nosode	Prepared from the blood of a man suffering from AIDS.
	Bacillinum Burrett	Sputum of tuberculosis patients containing the bacteria.
	Bacillinum testinum	Prepared from the testicle of tuberculosis patient.
	Carcinosinum (= Carcinosin)	Prepared from tissues of liver metastasis.
	Coqueluchinum or Pertussin	Lysate from expectoration of patient suffering from whooping cough.

Name of the Drug	*Source*
Diphtherinum	From diphtheritic membrane of a patient; diphtheria toxin.
Epihysterinum	From the tissues of uterine fibroid patient, possibly with malignant elements.
Influenzinum	Stock prepared by Pasteur Institute, Paris, esp. for homoeopathic use.
Medorrhinum or Glinicum	From purulent urethral discharge in patient suffering from acute gonorrhoea with *Neisseria gonorrhoeae*.
Melitagrinum	From the discharge of eczema capitis.
Morbillinum	From exudate of mouth and pharynx of measles affected patients.
Parotidinum	Lysate from the saliva of a patient suffering from mumps.
Osteo arthritic nosode (O.A.N.)	From synovial fluid of articulations esp. knee and hip of osteo arthritic patient.
Psorinum	From exudate in patients suffering from itch eruptions.
Rheumatoid arthritic nosode (R.A.N.)	From synovial fluid of knee affected with rheumatoid arthritis.
Scarlatininum	Lysate from scabs of a patient suffering from scarlatina.
Syphillinum or Lueticum	Prepared from the serosity of *Treponema pallidum* of a patient in primary (hard chancre) or early secondary stage.
Tuberculinum	From culture of *Mycobacterium tuberculosis.*
Toxoplasma gondi	From Lysate of *Toxoplasma gondi.*
Variolinum	Lysate obtained from serosity of small pox pustules.

B. Diseased Products of Aniamals

Anthracinum	Lysate obtained without addition of antiseptic from the liver of rabbit suffering from Anthrax.
Anti-coli bacillary	Purified form of stock serum anti-coli bacillary of caprine origin, made from goats immunised with *E. coli*.
Botulinum	*Clostridium botulinum* toxin (exotoxin) made from putrefied pork.
Ambra grisea	Morbid secretion from the liver of Spermaceti whale (Physeter macrocephalus). It is extracted from the rectum of the whale, found floating on the sea along the coasts of Madagascar and Sumatra.
Hippozaenium	Lysate from the 'glanders' in horses.
Hydrophobinum or Lyssin	From the saliva of rabid dog.
Malandrinum	Lysates from exudates of the horse malandra; discharge of eczema in the fold of the knee of horse.
Malaria officinalis	From mire taken during dryness of a malarial marsh.
Oscillococcinum	Autolysate filtered from liver and heart of a duck.
Pyrara	Lard of pyrarara, a fish of the Amazon river.

Name of the Drug	Source
Pyrogenum	Prepared originally from decomposition of meat of beef.
Sanguisuga	Prepared from leech.
Serum of Yersin	From the anti-pest serum obtained from animals that have been immunised by means of live or killed cultures of Yersinia pestis.
Vaccininum	From the lymph of cowpox pustules.

C. Diseased Plant Products

Agaricus muscarius	From entire fresh fungus, found in dry pine-woods.
Boletus laricus	From the dried fungus purging agaric/tarch boletus.
Candida albicans	Lysate of culture of *Monilia albicans.*
Mucor mucido	Lysate obtained by isolating and transplanting the mushroom mucor mucido from the culture media.
Nectrianinum	Nosode of cancer of trees (*Nectria ditissima*).
Secale cornutum	Prepared from the fungus *Claviceps purpura,* growing upon the seed of the secale cereal and other grains.
Ustilago maydis	Prepared from the fungus, growing on the stem, grains of Indian corn.
Usnea barbata	Prepared from lichen infecting soft maple.

D. Other Nosodes

Brucella melintensis	A filtrate of a 21-day old culture of the microbe of undulating fever.
D.T., T.A.B.	Mixed vaccine of anti-diphtheric, antitetanic and antitypho-paratyphoid.
Eberthinum	Prepared from culture of mixture of many stocks of *Salmonella typhi.*
Entero coccinum	Stocks of Streptococcus faecalis.
Flavus	Prepared from *Neisseria pharingis.*
Gonotoxinum	Prepared from anti-gonococcal vaccine.
Leptospira	Lysate of *Leptospira icterohaemarrhagie.*
Meningococcinum	Prepared from stocks of *Neisseria meningitidis.*
Pneumococcinum	*Diplococcus pneumoniae* found in saliva.
Staphylococcinum	Lysate of culture of many stocks of *Staphylococcus aureus.*
Staphylotoxinum	Antitoxin of *Staphylococcus aureus.*
Streptococcinum	Lysate of culture of stocks of *Streptococcus β-haemolyticus.*
Strepto-enterococcinum	Lysate of culture of *Streptoenterococcus.*
Tetanotoxinum	Dilution of tetanic toxin.

E. Bowel Nosodes

Bacillus No. 7 (Paterson)	Morgan-pure (Paterson)
Bacillus No. 10 (Paterson)	Mutabile (Bach)
Dysentery co. (Bach)	Proteus (Bach)
Faecalis (Bach)	Sycotic co. (Bach)
Gaertner (Bach)	
Morgan (Bach)	
Morgan-Gaertner (Paterson)	

Carcinosinum Group of Nosodes

Epitheliomine	Extract of epithelioma
Carcinosin	Prepared from tissues of liver metastasis.

Carcinosin adeno-vesica	Papillary adenocarcinome of bladder.
Carcinosin pulmonale	Pulmonary caseous.
Schirrinum	Carcinoma Schirrus (Stomach).

Tuberculinum Group of Nosodes

Tuberculinum avis	Prepared from mycobacterium tuberculosis of chicken.
Tuberculinum bovinum	Prepared from the pus of tuberculous abscess in animal.
Tuberculinum (Koch)	Prepared from culture of *Mycobacterium tuberculosis.*
Tuberculinum Marmoreck	Obtained from horses vaccinated by the filtrates of young cultures of *Mycobacterium tuberculosis.*
Bacillinum Burnett	From sputum of tuberculosis patients containing the bacteria.
Bacillinum testinum	From the testicle of tuberculosis patient.

SARCODES

Meaning

'Sarcode' means 'fleshy' (Greek, *sarkos* = flesh and *eidos* = form or resemblance). It can be termed protoplasm of animals.

Sarcodes belong to the branch of homoeopathy called organotherapy—developed in France. They have been in use for generations and even the highly esteemed C. Hering advocated their use as early as 1834.

Description

In fact, sarcodes may be considered to belong to the animal kingdom. Secretions of poisonous animals and venoms are not included in this group. Most of the sarcodes, however, have not been proved and are prescribed clinically rather than homoeopathically, but there are some exceptions.

Sarcodes are prepared from:

1. Healthy endocrine glands as a whole.
2. Healthy secretions from endocrine glands.
3. Normal secretions of animals.
4. Product (or extract) of animal glands and tissues.
5. Healthy organs of animals.

Sarcodes are derived from healthy glands, organs or tissues of animals, usually slaughtered animals such as pigs, sheep, or cattle. Besides these, oxes, foxes, insects, spiders, and snakes may be used for preparation of sarcodes.

Utility

A sarcode homoeopathically restores targeted glands or organs by producing the healthy template of the tissue from which the body can rebuild, restore, and restimulate.

"Healthy organ extracts or organ secretions prepared according to the general rules of homoeopathic remedies, which will help to slow down the natural and pathological deterioration of the organ."—Michel M. Bouko Levy.

Examples

Name of the Drug	*Source*
A. From healthy endocrine glands as a whole	
1. Parathyroidinum	From the parathyroid gland of ox.
2. Pituitaria glandula (Pituitrin)	From the entire pituitary gland.
3. Pituitaria anterior	From the anterior lobe of pituitary gland.
4. Pituitaria posterior	From the posterior lobe of pituitary gland of sheep.
5. Thyroidinum	From healthy thyroid tissue of sheep or calf.
6. Hypothalamus	From hypothalamus of ox.
7. Thymus	From thymus gland of animal.
8. Pinealis	From the pineal gland.

Name of the Drug	Source
B. From healthy secretions of endocrine glands	
1. Adrenocorticotropinum (A.C.T.H.)	From anterior pituitary gland of pig.
2. Adrenalinum	From internal secretion of adrenal medulla.
3. Castoreum	From dried Graffian follicles of ovary.
4. Corpus luteum	From the ovaries of pregnant animals.
5. Cortisone	From adrenal cortex of man.
6. Folliculinum	From oestrone, an oestrogenic hormone, secreted by Graffian follicles of ovaries.
7. Insulin	From β-cells of Islets of Langerhans of Pancreas.
8. Oophorinum	From the ovarian extract (expressed juice) of sheep and cow.
9. Orchitinum	From the testicular extract of sheep.
10. Pancreatinum	From pancreatic extract of beef, ox and sheep.
11. Secretinum	A hormone secreted from gut.
12. Thymi glandula extractum	From the extract of thymus gland.
13. Thyreostimuline	From internal secretion of anterior lobe of pituitary gland.
C. From normal secretions of animals or humans	
1. Colostrum	From mother's milk after recent birth of a baby.
2. Lac caninum	From dog's milk.
3. Lac felinum	From cat's milk.
4. Lac vaccinum	From cow's milk.
5. Lac humanum	From human breast milk.
6. Liquor amni	From amniotic fluid in pregnant women.
7. Meconium	From the stool in new-born baby, passed within first three or four days.
8. Pepsinum	From an enzyme, secreted from peptic cells of stomach of sheep or calf.
9. Placenta humana	From human placental fluid.
10. Placenta suis	From placenta of pigs.
11. Serotoninum (5-HT)	From a neurotransmitter, secreted from the gut.
D. From product of animal glands and tissues	
1. Adeps suis	From pig's fat.
2. Cholesterinum	From epithelial lining of gall-bladder and bile duct.
3. Fel tauri	From fresh bile of ox.
4. Fel vulpis	From fresh gall of fox.
E. From healthy organs of animals	
1. Bulbinum	From medula oblongata of brain.
2. Cartilago suis	From cartilage of pigs.
3. Cerebellum	From cerebellar part of brain.
4. Cerebrinum	From cerebrum part of brain.
5. Colon mucosa	From healthy colonic mucus membrane.
6. Duodenum	From duodenum part.
7. Embryo suis	From embryo of pigs.
8. Gastric mucosa	From inner lining of stomach.
9. Kidney (Nephrino)	From entire kidney tissue of animal.
10. Liver (Hepatine)	From healthy liver tissues.
11. Mammal (Glandula mammalis)	From mammary gland of cow and sheep.

Name of the Drug	*Source*
12. Medula ossis suis	From bone marrow of pigs.
13. Medula spinalis	From spinal cord.
14. Mucosa nasalis	From mucous membrane of human nose.
15. Myocardium	From middle (myocardial) layer of heart.
16. Nervous auditorius	From auditory (VIIIth cranial) nerve.
17. Pancreas suis	From pig's pancreas.
18. Prostate	From prostate.
19. Pulmine (Lung)	From lung tissues.
20. Neurinum	From neurone (nerve cell).
21. Retina	From nerve layer of eyeball.
22. Spleen (Splenine)	From healthy spleen of animal.
F. Others	
1. Aorta	From the aorta, arising from heart.
2. Arteria (artery wall)	From the artery.
3. Conjunctiva	From the conjunctiva.
4. Diaphragma	From the diaphragm.
5. Discus intervertebralis	From intervertebral disc.
6. D.N.A.	From thymus and latiance of fishes.
7. Fibrinum	From the fibrin.
8. Haemoglobinum	From the haemoglobin.
9. Labyrinthinum	From labyrinth of internal ear.
10. Lymphaticus	From lymph vessel.
11. R.N.A.	From yeast sources.
12. Veinous wall	From the vein.

IMPONDERABILIA

(Direct physical energy medicines)

The word imponderabilia has came from, 'imponderable' that means which is not weighable, i.e., the substances which have no perceptible weights.

Imponderabilia medicines can also be termed as direct physical energy medicines as these medicines utilise energy directly, available from natural and physical reactions.

Different forms of energy are potent sources of imponderabilia medicines. They are electromagnetic, electrical, magnetic, nuclear, gravitational, thermal, electrostatic and cosmic energy.

Presently available imponderabilia medicines belong to magnetic, electromagnetic, electrical, nuclear and cosmic category of energies.

Different authors mentaining about Imponderabilia

1. Hahnemann (F.N. Sec. 280)—'Even imponderable agencies can produce most violent medicinal effects upon man'.
2. H. C. Allen describes their mode of preparation and symptoms in 'Materia Medica of Nosodes'.
3. Elizabeth Wright mentions in her book 'A Brief Study Course in Homoeopathy' the imponderabilia, which include positive and negative magnetic forces, electricity, sun-force etc.
4. P. Sankaran also mentions this source in his book 'Elements of Homoeopathic Pharmacy.'
5. Carl W. Caspari, Gottlieb Heinrich Georg Jahr, J. H. Clarke, Swan etc. have described their symptoms.

Examples

A. Natural source

1. Magnetis poli ambo	From both pole of a magnet.
2. Magnetis polus Arcticus	From north pole of a magnet.
3. Magnetis polus Australis	From south pole of a magnet.
4. Luna	From light rays of full moon.
5. Sol	From sunrays (i.e., sunlight).

B. **Artificial source**

1.	Magnetis artificialis	From artificial magnet.
2.	X-ray	From X-rays.
3.	Radium bromide	From radioactivity of element.
4.	Electricitus	From atmospheric and artificial (Electric current) electricity.
5.	Mobile Phone Radiation	From radiation of mobile phone.

TAUTOPATHIC OR SYNTHETIC SOURCES

Fautopathy (*Tauto* means 'same') is a method of curing or removing bad or side-effects of drugs by iso-intoxication, i.e., curing by means of the identical harmful agent in potentised form.

This form the source of those medicines which are taken from the synthetic and chemical products.

Tautopathic drugs can be proved according to homoeopathic proving and can be assimilated in homoeopathic materia medica and can be given to antidote the bad effects of crude or offending and harmful identical agents. Tautopathy cannot cure all types of drug diseases but it can help to cure many and varied diseases.

Tautopathy is indirect homoeopathy. It is homoeopathy minus actual proving of the drugs on healthy prover. It is used on the basis of:

(i) Causative factor (abuse of the corresponding drug) and (ii) The symptoms produced as side-effects of the abused drug.

As per J. N. Kanjilal

"Tautopathic drugs have nothing to do with allopathy on the following grounds:

(i) they are used on the basis of symptoms produced by the crude drug on diseased person (unhealthy provers);

(ii) they are prepared strictly in the process of homoeopathic pharmaceutical discipline":

Examples

- Acetazolamide ($C_4H_6N_4O_3S_2$)
- Acetohexamide ($C_{15}H_{20}N_2O_4S$)
- Allopurinol ($C_5H_4N_4O$)
- Alloxan ($C_4H_2N_2O_4$)
- Alphaprodine ($C_{16}H_{23}NO_2$)
- Alprajolum ($C_{17}H_{13}ClN_4$)
- Aminopyrine ($C_{13}H_{17}N_3O$)
- Aminophylline ($C_{16}H_{24}N_{10}O_4$)
- Amoxycillin ($C_{16}H_{19}N_3O_5S$)
- Amphetamine sulphate ($C_9H_{13}NH_2SO_4$)
- Anti rabies vaccine
- Aspirin, Acidum Acetyl Salicylicum ($C_9H_8O_4$)
- Aureomycin ($C_{22}H_{23}ClN_2O_8$)
- Benadryl or Diphenhydramine ($C_{17}H_{21}NO$)
- Butazolidin ($C_{19}H_{20}N_2O_2$)
- B.C.G. (Bacillus Calmette-Guerin)
- Carbamazepine ($C_{15}H_{12}N_2O$)
- Carbimazole ($C_7H_{10}N_2O_2S$)
- Cephalexin ($C_{16}H_{17}N_3O_4S.H_2O$)
- Cephradine ($C_{16}H_{19}N_3O_4S$)

Table 2.1: Imponderabilia medicines in relation to energy and miasm

	Medicines	Energy	Miasm
1.	Magnetis poli ambo	Magnetic energy	Syphilitic
2.	Magnetis polus Australis	"	"
3.	Magnetis polus Arcticus	"	"
4.	Magnetis artificialis	Electromagnetic energy	
5.	Luna	Light energy	
6.	Sol	Heat and light energy	
7.	X-ray	Electromagnetic radiation energy	Mixed miasmatic state
8.	Radium bromide	"	"
9.	Electricitus	Electrical energy	

Chloramphenicol, Chloromycetin or Synthomycetine and Kemicetine ($C_{11}H_{12}Cl_2N_2O_5$)

Chloroquine ($C_{18}H_{26}ClN_3$)

Chlorothiazide ($C_7H_6ClN_3O_4S_2$)

Chlorpromazinum hydrochloride (Largactil) ($C_{17}H_{19}ClN_2S$. HCl)

Chlorpropamide ($C_{10}H_{13}ClN_2O_3S$)

Chlortetracycline hydrochloride (Ledermycin) ($C_{22}H_{23}ClN_2O_8$· HCl)

Chlorthalidone ($C_{14}H_{11}ClN_2O_4S$)

Cimetidine ($C_{10}H_{16}N_6S$)

Clotrimazole ($C_{22}H_{17}ClN_2$)

Corticotrophin, Adreno corticotrophic hormone (ACTH)

Cortisone (17, Hydroxy corticosterone and 11, dehydroxy 17, hydroxy corticosterone) ($C_{21}H_{28}O_5$)

Deriphylline ($C_{11}H_{10}N_2O_2$)

Diazepam ($C_{16}H_{13}ClN_2O$)

Dichloral phenazone ($C_{15}H_{18}C_{16}N_2O_5$)

Diphenytoin or Dilantin ($C_{15}H_{12}N_2O_2$)

Diprophylline ($C_{10}H_{14}N_4O_4$)

Dopamine ($C_8H_{11}NO_2$)

Durabolin ($C_{28}H_{44}O_3$)

Emitine hydrochloride ($C_{29}H_{40}N_2O_4$, 2HCl)

Ephidrine ($C_{10}H_{15}NO$)

Erythromycin ($C_{37}H_{67}NO_{13}$)

Ethambutol hydrochloride ($C_{10}H_{24}N_2O_2$, $2H_2O$)

Furosemide ($C_{12}H_{11}ClN_2O_5S$)

Furazolidone ($C_8H_7N_3O_5$)

Gammexane ($C_6H_6Cl_6$)

Gentamycin ($C_{21}H_{43}N_5O_7$)

Hetrazan or Diethylcarbamazine ($C_{10}H_{21}N_3O$)

Histaminum hydrochloride ($C_5H_{11}C_{12}N_3$)

Ibuprofen ($C_{13}H_{18}O_2$)

Isoniazid ($C_6H_7N_3O$)

Kanamycin ($C_{18}H_3N_4O_{11}$)

Levodopa ($C_9H_{11}NO_4$)

Mannitol ($C_6H_{14}O_6$)

Methionine ($C_5H_{11}NO_2S$)

Metronidazole ($C_6H_9O_3N_3$)

Mytomycin ($C_{15}H_{18}N_4O_5$)

Neomycin ($C_{23}H_{46}N_6O_{13}$)

Natamycin ($C_{33}H_{47}NO_{13}$)

Oxytetracycline hydrochloride, terramycin ($C_{22}H_{24}O_9N_2$, HCl)

Paracetamol or Acetaminophen ($C_8H_9NO_2$)

Penicillin (Benzyl penicillin sodium, $C_{16}H_{17}N_2O_4$, SNA)

Prednisolone ($C_{21}H_{28}O_5$)

Rastinon ($C_{12}H_{18}N_2O_3S$)

Rifampicin ($C_{43}H_{58}N_4O_{12}$)

Salbutamol ($C_{13}H_{21}NO_3$)

Streptomycin ($C_{21}H_{39}N_7O_{12}$)

Sulpha guanidine ($C_7H_{10}N_4O_2S$)

Sulphnilamidum (Sulphanilamid), P-Amino benzene sulphonamide (P.A.B.S.), Protonsil album, Streptocide ($C_6H_8O_2N_2S$).

Sulphonamides ($C_{10}H_{10}N_4O_2S$)

Tetracycline hydrochloride (Achromycin) ($C_{22}H_{24}N_2O_8$·HCl)

Theophylline ($C_7H_8N_4O_2$)

Thymolum or Isopropyl metacresol ($C_{10}H_{14}O$)

Tobramycin ($C_{18}H_{37}N_5O_9$)

ALLERSODES

Allersodes are homoeopathic attenuations of antigen, i.e., substances which, under suitable conditions, can stimulate the formation of antibodies.

Antigens include toxins, ferments, precipitonogens, agglutinogens, opsonogens, lysogens, venins, agglutinins, complements, opsonins, amboceptors, precipitins, and most native proteins.

Technically, allersodes are a sub-set of isopathic remedies.

They are prepared from routine allergens whose presence in the environment or in the food chain cause problems to people. They are prepared according to homoeopathic specifications, provided the basic substance is not altered and the final product is not adulterated by any pathogen or other deleterious substances.

The administration of this type of remedy is designed to reduce the sensitivity of people to a particular allergen. Examples would be grass, pollen, dairy products, house dust mites or animal hair which are usually presented as a homochord, a mixture of potencies.

Allersodes may not be dispensed in attenuations below 6X, 3CH, or 3CK.

ISODES

These are homoeopathic medicines prepared from plant, animal or chemical substances, including drugs, excipients or binders, which have been ingested or otherwise absorbed by the body and are believed to have produced a disease or disorder which interferes with homeostasis. They may be called detoxodes. These also contains the preparations made from commonly used allopathic medicines. They are prepared as per HPI. They are prepared generally at physician/prescriber level. Generally isodes are not used below 6x potency. Awareness of side-effects of these drugs and their lower attenuations up to 3x is essential.

Chapter 03

Collection of Drug Substances

Hahnemann does not mention directly the process of collection of drug-substances in his 'Organon of Medicine' (5th edition)—which helps in the collection of drug-substances:

Aphor. 264: 'The true physician must be provided with genuine medicine of unimpaired strength, so that he may be able, himself, to judge of their genuineness.'

Aphor. 266: 'Substances belonging to the animal and vegetable kingdoms possesses their medicinal qualities most perfectly in their crude state.'

VEGETABLE KINGDOM

The collection of drug substances should be done by an experienced and qualified botanist having a special knowledge of Taxonomy and Systemic Botany. He should also possess the basic knowledge of homoeopathic pharmacy.

A. General rules of collection

(a) Regarding character of plants:

1. Medicinal plants should be gathered in localities to which they are indigenous.
2. Wild plants are more effective and possess more medicinal virtue than those cultivated in gardens. Cultivated plants should never be used if the wild ones can be procured. Plants cultivated in botanical gardens should not be used for medicinal purposes.
3. Only healthy, well-developed, fresh (except substances which have to be imported from outside), perfect and vigorous plants are to be used which are regularly formed and free from—(i) all kinds of dust, (ii) worms, insects and caterpillar's nest, (iii) worm eaten things and things which are spoilt by dirt and mud, (iv) discolouration, abnormal odour or any sign of detorioration.
4. Plants that through old age have acquired a woody consistence ought not to be used. All sickly-looking, partially withered, or decayed plants or roots should be discarded.
5. Plants which have the greatest degree of medicinal activity are those found in their natural places of growth and are perfect plants.

(b) Regarding time of collection:

1. They should be collected: (i) In fine, sunny, dry weather, (ii) Early morning, (iii) Just after disappearance of morning dew, (iv) When their medicinal virtue is greatest.
2. They should not be collected: (i) During early morning dew, (ii) After heavy rainfall, (iii) During excessive heat of the day.

(c) Regarding cleansing of drug materials, after collection: Cleansing should be done carefully so that no part of it is eroded. Large amount of water should not be used for washing; if unavoidable, only too little water may be used for washing.

B. Particular rules of collection

As regards the plants, the parts which are used for preparation of mother tincture (Q) and mother substance (O) are to be collected at the specified time.

The directions are given, with the few exceptions:

Name of the different parts	Proper time and method of collection
1. Whole plant:	In flowering season, partly in flower and partly in bud during sunny weather. They should be carefully cleansed by shaking, brushing or gentle rubbing. Washing with profuse water should be avoided.
2. Roots (radices):	(a) Annuals—early in Autumn, as they die, after ripening of the seeds. (b) Biennials—in the spring of the 2nd year. (c) Perennials—in the 2nd or 3rd year, before they develop woody fibres. Roots are to be collected by cutting just under the stem. Roots should be cleaned without using much water. They should be free from moulds and woody appearances. After the collection of fresh material they should be processed as early as possible to avoid deterioration.
3. Stems (stipites):	After development of leaves.
4. (a) Leaves (folia):	Before, during and early part of flowering time.
(b) Leaves of biennial plants	In spring of 2nd year, as soon as the flowering stems begin to shoot.
5. Young shoots:	In spring, when the whole plant is in full vigour.
6. Herbs (herba):	When they are fully developed, should be cut just above root-leaves.
7. Twigs:	Of present year's growth only.
8. Flowers (flores):	Partly in bud and partly in blossom; in the dry weather.
9. Fruits (fructus), seeds (semina) berries (baccae):	When they are fully ripe. Succulent fruits, seeds or berries should be used while fresh. Only dried fruits, seeds or berries may be stored in well-closed glass-containers.
10. Bulbs:	As soon as they mature, when the leaves begin to decay.
11. Woods (ligna):	In early spring or late in autumn before the juices are not exhausted and also from mature young trees or tree-like shrubs.
12. Barks (cortices)	
(a) Resinous:	In early spring, i.e. at or about the time of development of leaves and blossoms.
(b) Non-resinous:	Late in autumn from young vigorous trees.
13. Narcotic plants:	While in bloom and just before—or when coming into—bloom.

Notes:

1. Exotic drug substances should never be imported in powder form and without proper identification of their genuineness (Aphor. 268). They are to be obtained from reputed firm but preferably in their natural form or state and proper identification should be carried out before using them in the preparation of mother tincture.
2. For exporting vegetable products to the foreign countries, they should be tied in loose bundles and then hanging in the shade away from direct sunlight, rain etc.—when they will be perfectly dried they should be packed well and sent.

ANIMAL KINGDOM

A. General rules

1. They must be thoroughly identified and collected by a zoologist.
2. Selection of animals must be perfect.
3. Animals must be healthy and hygienic, coming from good stock.
4. Animal substances must be genuine. They must not be spoilt by dirt. Decomposed and worm-eaten substances must not be used.
5. Secretions and excretions should be collected from healthy animals, which must be examined by animal doctors, i.e., veterinary physicians.
6. When the animal substances are not available nearby, they may be taken from reliable sources but never in the form of powder.
7. If the specimens are to be stored before use, they should be protected from light, heat, moisture and other contaminations.

B. Particular rules

	Mode of collection	*Name of the animals*
1.	Gathered by fishing	1. Star fish (Ast. rub.) 2. River fish (Pyrara) 3. Cuttle fish (Sepia) 4. Purple fish (Murex) 5. Alive jelly-fish (Aurelia medusa) 6. Cray-fish (Astacus fluviatilis) 7. Cod-fishes (Godus lota; Godus morrhua; Oleum. jac. aselli)
2.	Caught by different processes	1. Toads (Bufo rana) 2. Spiders (Aranea avicularis, Aranea diadema, Aranea scinencia; Latrodectus hasseti, Latrodectus kalpio, Latrodectus mactans; Mygale lasiodora; Tarentula cubensis; Tarentula hispanica; Theridion) 3. Lizards (Lacerta agilis)
3.	Wild animals collected by hunting	1. Sperm-whale (Ambra grisea) 2. Musk-deer (Moschus) 3. Beaver (Castoreum)
4.	From wild or cultivated in scientific way	1. Honey-bee (Apis mel) 2. Cantharides (Cantharis) 3. Cochineal (Coccus cacti) 4. Cockroach (Blatta americana; Blatta orientalis). 5. Bugs (Cimex; Coccinella; Doryphora). 6. Ants (Formica rufa). 7. Moth (Bombyx chrysorhoea).
5.	Snake venoms collected from wild snakes or cultivated ones from snake firm	1. Coral snake (Elaps) 2. Rattle snake (Crotalus) 3. Surukuku snake (Lachesis)

		4. Gokshura or Cobra (Naja)
6.	From domestic animals	Lacs (Lac. can; Lac. def; Lac. fel; Lac vac).

Collection of Snake Venoms

1. Elaps corallinus: The venom collected by pressing a butter-plate against the fangs or by letting the snake bite through a cloth covering a wide-mouth bottle. Only experts in handling snake attempt to collect the venom.
2. Vipera and Crotalus horridus: The venom collected by compressing the gland, when the serpent is either pinioned in a frame or under the influence of chloroform ($CHCl_3$) (H.P.I.).
3. Lachesis: The venom is obtained from living snake by stunning it with a blow and then collecting the poison on sugar of milk by pressing the fangs upwards against the 'poison sac.'
4. Naja: The venom is obtained by a special device by compressing the glands of the serpent when it is either pinioned in a frame or under the influence of chloroform (H.P.I.).

Note: Different types of venoms may be obtained from serological laboratory and they are quickly dry freezed and preserved.

Collection of Poisons of Toad (Bufo rana)

The live toad is fastended to a slab of cork by four strong pins struck through the webs of the feets. Then the poles of an 'induction apparatus' in action are slowly drawn over the back of the animal, where upon the poison exudes from the dorsal glands of the toad, which is removed with a small horn-made knife.

MINERAL KINGDOM

1. They should be collected very carefully from reliable sources and should be thoroughly tested (if necessary) in analytical laboratory (according to the rules of chemistry and mineralogy)—before they are used for homoeopathic purposes.
2. They should not be obtained in finely powdered form.

NOSODES

1. They should be collected after proper diagnosis of disease.
2. They should be obtained from standard serological laboratory who deal with the manufacture of the cultures of these organisms.
3. They are collected as per rules laid down in the following authoritative books:
   (i) Swan's Materia Medica of Nosodes.
   (ii) 'The Materia Medica of the Nosodes'—by H. C. Allen.
   (iii) The North American Journal of Homoeopathy—Volume 1, Page 366.
   (iv) 'Dictionary of Practical Materia Medica'—by J. H. Clarke.

SARCODES

1. The animals must be perfectly healthy.
2. The animals should be kept under observation on restricted food before the drug substances are collected from them.
3. The products or parts that are to be used must be treated first.
4. These should be collected from standard serological laboratory who deal with the manufacture of the culture of these organisms.
5. The 'endocrine' products and few 'enzymes' may be collected from cattle, sheep etc. from the slaughter houses.

IMPONDERABILIA

1. The rules for collecting and of preparing of medicine is given in pharmacopoeia.
2. The respective magnet can be had from some physical laboratory.
3. In case of 'Luna', 'full-moon' is suggested to be considered.
4. For X-ray purpose the respective chemical testing laboratory may be contacted.
5. Potentisation of imponderabilia should be done very carefully.

Chapter 04

Homoeopathic Pharmaceutical Instruments and Appliances

List of the instruments and appliances in a standard homoeopathic laboratory

1. Mortar and pestle
2. Spatula
3. Presses
4. Sieves
5. Chopping board
6. Chopping knife
7. Bottles (glass-stoppered)
8. Cork
9. Spoon
10. Scale
11. Funnel
12. Beaker
13. Measuring cylinder
14. Volumetric flask
15. Burettes
16. Pipettes
17. Graduated dropping pipette
18. Graduated conical testing glasses
19. Stirrer
20. Spirit lamp
21. Hydrometer
22. Lactometer
23. Desiccator
24. Water bath
25. Hot air oven
26. Thermometer
27. Test tube
28. Crucible
29. Porcelain basin
30. Tripod stand
31. Wire-gauze
32. Burner
33. Glass-retort
34. Watch glasses
35. Wash bottles
36. Specific gravity bottle (pyknometer)
37. Cork borer set
38. Balance
39. Microscope
40. Percolator.

Mortar and Pestle

1. Shape—Mortars are available in diverse shapes. Generally, the shape is hemispherical.
2. Varieties according to the material used—Different kinds of mortar have specific utility in preparing and grinding different materials. These are made up of Iron, Porcelain, Agate, Glass and Wedgewood.
   (a) Iron or steel mortar and pestle—They should be always kept clean. These must be lightly polished and keep them perfectly free from rust, as rust decomposes many vegetable juices at once.
   (b) Porcelain mortar and pestle—The inside of the mortar and the face of the pestle should be ground and unglazed. If not, make unglazed by rubbing wet sand upon their surfaces.
   (c) Glass mortar and pestle—They are made up of glass.

The pharmacist must keep at least three mortars: (i) One of porcelain for trituration of drugs having strong smell, (ii) Second one made of glass for mercurial prepa-

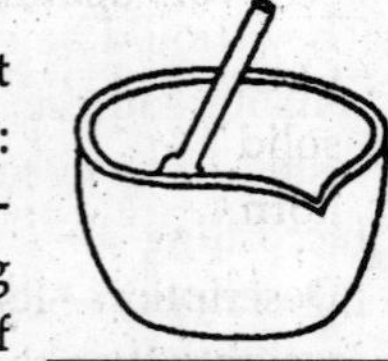
Mortar and Pestle

rations, and (iii) The third one for the rest of the remedies.

Pestle is made of same material as that of mortar. The handle of pestle is made up of wood, which are screwed into the head of the pestles. The cementing material is used to fix the handle to the head of the pestle. This material should be of superior quality, otherwise, due to wear and tear, handle tends to come out from the head. Pestle entirely made up of porcelain matter is not suitable as they are easily broken.

3. Uses—The different kinds of mortar and pestle have different use:
   (a) Iron or steel mortar and pestle—For pulverising very hard substances, e.g. hard seeds of Nux vomica, Sabal serrulata etc.
   (b) Porcelain mortar and pestle—For triturating purposes of soft substances, e.g., charcoal, fresh vegetable materials.
   (c) Glass mortar and pestle—For mercurial preparations.
4. Precautions in using mortar and pestle:
   (a) Mortar and pestle should not be interchanged.
   (b) If only one mortar is kept for all medicines, it should be washed immediately after every use.
   (c) Maximum contact between the surfaces of the head of the pestle and the interior of the mortar should be maintained.

Spatula

1. Varieties—It may be: (i) Stainless steel rather of iron spatula, (ii) Solid hard rubber spatula, (iii) Horn spatula, (iv) Bone spatula, (v) Porcelain spatula, (vi) Ivory spatula.

   Generally stainless steel spatula, solid hard rubber spatula, and horn spatula are used.

Spatula

2. Description—Its handle is more weighty than the blade. So when it is kept on the table, the blade does not touch the surface of the table. The spatula should be free from rust.
3. Uses:

Name of Spatula	*Uses*
(i) Stainless steel spatula (Modern powder spatula)	(i) During the process of trituration—to loosen the powdered material as it becomes packed on the inner sides of the mortar. Due to increased pressure exerted by pestle many substances are packed in inner side of mortar. So unless the compacted mass is loosened with the help of spatula—trituration process is hampered.
	(ii) Used in weighing the powder.
	(iii) Used in the preparation of ointments.
(ii) Solid hard rubber spatula or horn spatula	Used when corrosive substances capable of reacting with steel are handled.

Presses

1. **Description**
   (a) It is constructed in such a way that it can easily separate its several parts and cleansed thoroughly.
   (b) The press is made up of wood or iron.
   (c) Wooden press—Each press has two wooden parts each of which consists of one handle. These two parts are connected to each other by two hinges. One part has deep concave coning at the centre, whereas the other has an elevated rounded convex part, so that each of them is fitted with another when pressed.
2. **Uses**
   (a) For squeezing juices from the medicinal plants, herbs, leaves, seeds etc.
   (b) They are also used as 'filter' after the 'maceration' and 'percolation' process of

preparing mother tincture (Q). After the filtering of mother tincture the sediments or magma may retain with them a part of the tincture. This is also pressed out by using the press.

3. **Process:** The materials (such as plants, seeds or magma) to be pressed are enclosed in a new well-cleansed linen bag (free from starch or bleaching materials) and then subjected to the action of screw press; the juice runs into a suitable vessel below. The one and the same bag should never be used for two distinct drugs. The container of the press is double chambered. The drug will be inside the inner chamber which has got several holes to let out the juices.

4. **Precaution**

(a) Presses should be properly cleansed before as well as after use. They should be separated and cleansed.

(b) Linen clothes should be reserved for one and the same drug only, the other drug material should be prepared in separate linen clothes.

Sieves

These are vessels with meshed or perforated bottom for separating fine powders from coarser substances. The sieves that are used today are made up of silk, hair or stainless steel wire. But A.H.P. advises the use of hair or silk sieves only.

Varieties and uses

Varieties	*Uses*
1. Silk sieve	In making trituration: (i) For very fine powder (≠ 80) 80 meshes sieve in a sq. inch (all the potencies will pass through a No. 80 sieve) (ii) For fine powder (≠ 60) 60 meshes sieve in a sq. inch (all of the particles will pass through a No. 60 sieve and not more than 40% through a No. 100 sieve). *Note:* Never use the sieves for sugar of milk to shift other substances.
2. Hair or stainless steel wire sieve	In making tinctures: (i) For moderately coarse powder (≠ 40) 40 meshes sieve in a sq. inch (all of the particles will pass through a No. 40 sieve and not more than 40% through a No. 80 sieve). (ii) For coarse powder (≠ 20) 20 meshes sieve in a sq. inch (all of the particles will pass through a No. 20 sieve and not more than 40% through a No. 60 sieve). *Note:* When acid substances are to be shifted, horse-hair sieve may be used.

Chopping Board

Description—They should be made of sound, strong wood free from any holes and knots. It may be either circular or oval shaped. Centrally, it is concave with prominent margin. Marble or glazing porcelain slabs may serve better as they are easy to be cleansed.

Cleansing—It should be cleaned thoroughly after using and dried well before the next use.

Uses—They are used as the base for cutting fresh medicinal plants, herbs, roots, barks and flowers into small pieces.

Chopping Knife (Chopper)

Description—The chopping knife should be made of very good steel. They should always be well-polished and free from rust, as rust decomposes many vegetable juices at once. One side of the blade is sharp for chopping the soft substances. Iron-made chopping knife should never be used, as it may form rust.

Uses—Soft vegetable substances are chopped by the knife placing it over the concave surface of the chopping board.

Corks

1. It should be of best velvet quality, smooth, well-polished and without any holes or discolouration.
2. As soon as they shrink or become soft, they should be replaced by new ones.
3. Never use any used cork that has ever been in contact with any medicine.
4. For every fresh bottle, a fresh cork should always be used.

Spoons

These are made up of ivory, horn, bone, porcelain or stainless steel.

Uses—Spoon is used to transfer liquid or semi-liquid substances from one container to another and also for handling sugar of milk, and some other purposes.

Scale

It is an instrument for measuring length. It is a thin plate made up of wood, steel or plastic. It is one or half metre in length and 2½ to 4 centimetres in breadth. Its one side is graduated in centimetre and millimetre, other side in inches. The scale is sometimes graduated only in centimetre and millimetre. This scale is known as metre scale. Here, each centimetre is divided into 10 millimetres. The centimetre marks are longer than the millimetre marks. (1 mm = 0.1 cm).

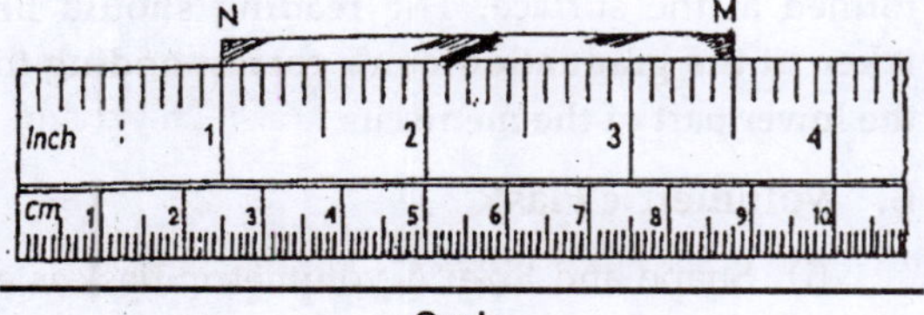

Scale

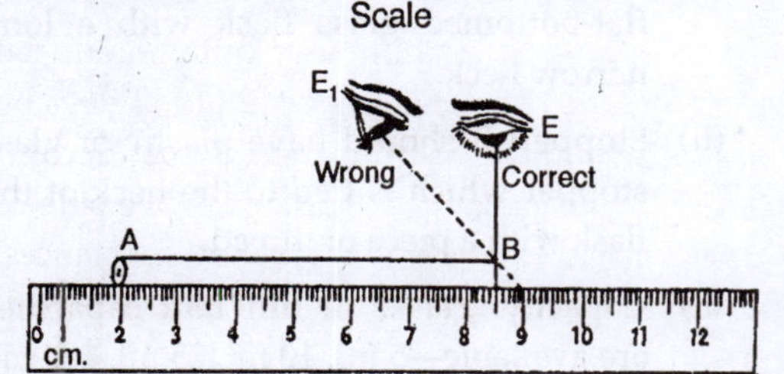

Measurement with the help of Scale

Sometimes, the scale only graduated in inches and one-tenth division of an inch. This scale is known as foot-rule. Its smallest division = 0.1 inch.

Say, with the help of scale, the length of AB (shown in figure) is to be measured. The pencil is placed by the side of the scale in such a way that the one end of AB coincide with any full number (in figure 1 cm). Now, reading is taken where other end (B) touches the scale. It is seen in the figure that it touches the 7.5 graduation. So length of AB = 7.5 – 1 = 6.5 cm = 6 cm 5 mm.

Notes:

(i) Do not place the zero end of the scale in contact with one end of the distance to be measured. Sometimes zero end of a scale is worn out by use. So the exact position of the zero becomes uncertain.

(ii) Look perpendicular to the scale while taking a reading. Otherwise you get a wrong value. This is called error of parallax.

Uses—It is used for measuring globules (scale in mm is used) and for measuring in different pharmaceutical works.

Funnel

It is made of either glass, high polythene or porcelain. It has an expanded upper conical part. Its lower part is a narrow pipe-like structure.

Uses—The chief utility is in trituration, sublimation and transfer of liquid.

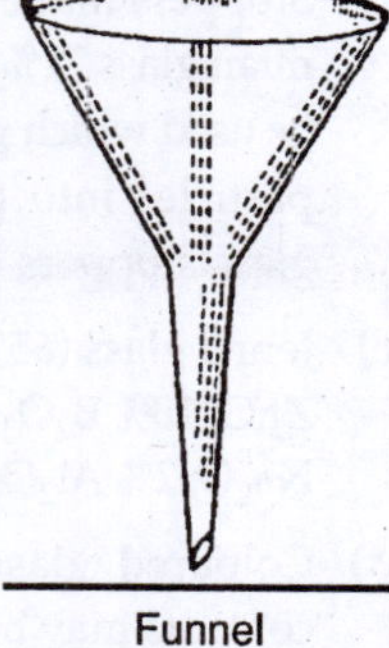
Funnel

Container, Bottles and Glasses

(a) New well-cleansed bottles which should be (i) Colourless (white) and (ii) Made of neutral flint glasses. [Flint glass: It contains 53% SiO_2; 14% K_2O and 33% PbO and has high density and refractive index. It is very soft].

Neutral flint glasses are essential because cheap glasses may have excess of free alkali in them. This can be tested chemically and selected accordingly. Especially bottles in which potentisation is done should be completely neutral. Otherwise, the potentised medicines will be a mixture of free alkali and the drug potentised together.

Neutral glass bottles are more superior than made up by polymers for preserving and dispensing homoeopathic medicines.

(b) For substances easily decomposed by sunlight—Yellow (colouring agent: cadmium sulphide and uranium oxide) or amber coloured (colouring agent: carbonaceous material with sulphur or iron sulphide) phials or white phials covered with a solution of asphaltum or black varnish are to be used.

Note: Burt advises to avoid blue-coloured (colouring agent: cobalt oxide, cupric oxide) bottles, as blue has certain dynamic effects injurious to remedies.

(c) Bottles made of gutta-purcha are requisitioned for keeping fluoric acid.

Bottles (Glass-stoppered)

(a) These should be used for substances which corrode cork (as acids, chlorine, bromine and iodine preparations, chloroform, kreosote etc. in their 1X or 2X potencies).

(b) Stoppers made of glass (potash glass or Bohemian glass 71% SiO_2; 18% K_2; 11% CaO) should be used which prevent the introduction of glass particles into the drugs from friction of the glass-stoppers in opening and shutting them.

(c) Jenna glass (65% SiO_2; 8% Na_2; 5% Al_2O_3; 12% ZnO; 10% B_2O_3) and pyrex glass (81% SiO_2; 5% Na_2O; 2% Al_2O_3; 12% B_2O_3) are also preferable.

(d) Coloured glass bottles are used where the contents may be affected by light.

Uses—All homoeopathic mother tincture and solution (excepting a few) should be stored in glass-stoppered bottles. But in certain cases of acids, e.g., Fluoric acid, glass-stoppered bottles prove insufficient in as much as the acid will eat away the glass—however strong it may be.

Gutta-purcha bottle or other kinds of containers serve useful purposes in this respect.

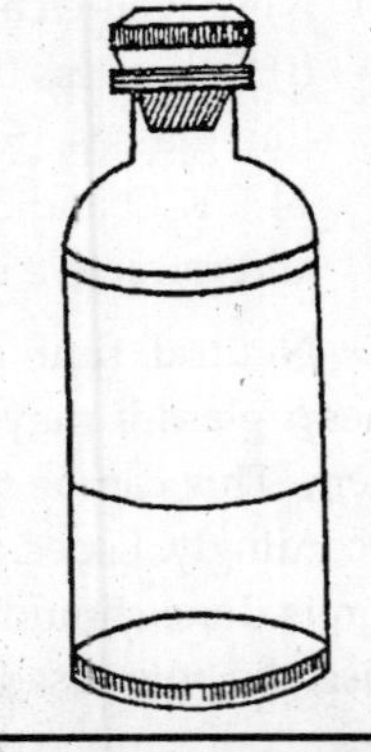

Glass-stoppered Bottle

INSTRUMENTS FOR MEASURING VOLUME

A. Measuring Cylinder

These are the long cylinders of glass by which various volumes can be measured but without great accuracy.

The measuring cylinder is to be used with a capacity close to the volume required. e.g.,

(i) 50 ml capacity used to measure 45 ml

(ii) 100 ml capacity used to measure 95 ml

(iii) 150 ml capacity used to measure 140 ml

(iv) 200 ml capacity used to measure 180 ml

(v) 250 ml capacity used to measure 230 ml.

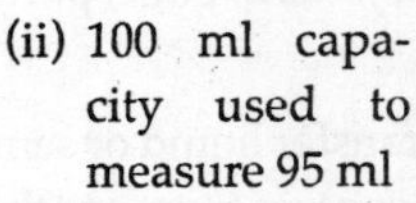

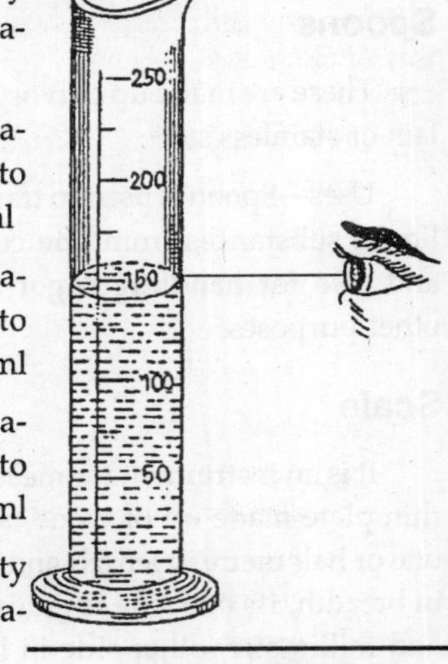

Measuring Cylinder

How will you take the reading?

The measuring cylinder is allowed to stand on a table. Then the eye-level is adjusted to the surface of liquid. It will be seen that a concave meniscus is formed at the surface. **The reading should be taken at the graduation mark corresponding to the lower part of the meniscus.**

B. Volumetric Flask

(i) Shape and Size: A volumetric flask is a flat-bottomed glass flask with a long narrow neck.

(ii) Stopper: It should have plastic or glass stopper which is tied to the neck of the flask with a piece of thread.

(iii) Capacity: Flasks of different capacities are available—5 ml, 10 ml, 25 ml, 100 ml, 250 ml, 500 ml, 1,000 ml, 2,000 ml.

The capacity of a flask at a paticular temperature is usually engraved on its wall. The

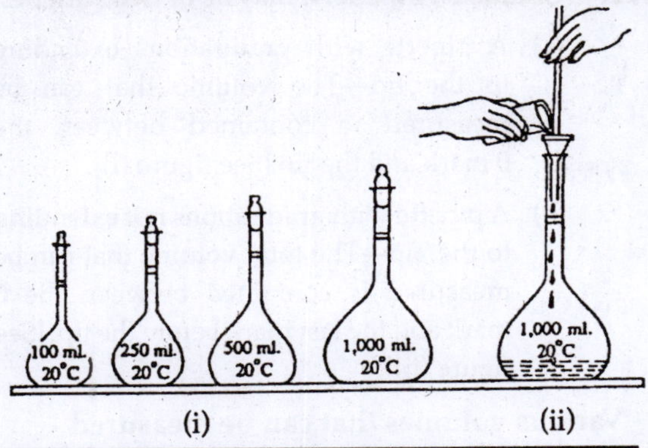

(i) A few volumetric flasks of different sizes, and (ii) The way of filling up a volumetri flask during preparatin of solution

neck carries a thin circular mark etched glass, which indicates the capacity of the flask.

(iv) Temperature of the liquid: The temperature at which liquids should be measured is etched on the flask (after the capacity figure). Example—1,000 ml : 20°C.

(v) Uses of volumetric flasks: It is generally used for the preparation of reagents and also for storing standard solutions. Before use, the volumetric flasks must be cleansed properly to remove dirt and grease.

C. Burette

(a) Description of Apparatus: A burette is a long glass tube of uniform bore (10–15 mm diam.) throughout its length and is graduated in fractions of cubic centimetres. One end (upper) of the tube is open and the other (lower) end is drawn to a jet and is fitted with a glass stopcock about 5–6 cms above the lowest jet point. The graduation begins from a few centimetres below the upper end and goes downwards to a few centimetres above the stopcock, the uppermost graduation being marked 'zero', the lowermost graduation being marked according to the capacity of

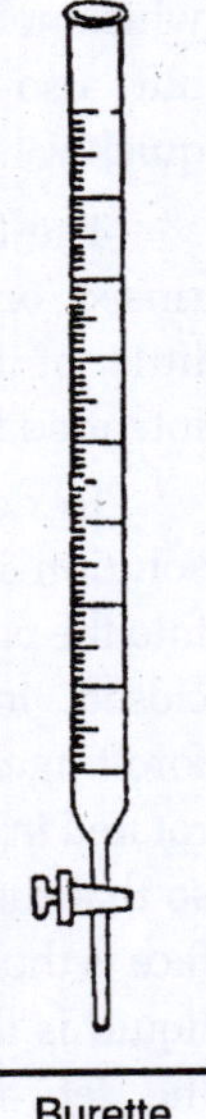

Burette

23 24 25 26 27 28

Correct measurement of volume of liquid (or soln.) in a burette

the burette. A burette may be of different capacities—25 ml, 50 ml, 100 ml, etc. of which a burette of 50 ml capacity is generally used. The burettes are filled from the top with the liquid to be measured.

(b) The use of a burette: A burette is a very suitable apparatus for delivering variable exact volumes of a liquid contained in it and the rate of delivery can be controlled by means of the stopcock. It is, therefore, generally used for various types of triturations, in analytical laboratory, for the analysis of drug substances.

(c) Cleansing and rinsing: The burette must be cleaned and made grease-free before use, which may be done in the same way as described for the cleansing of a pipette.

The clean burette is rinsed twice with the liquid with which the burette is to be filled, in the same way as the rinsing of a pipette.

(d) Measurement of the volume of a liquid by a burette: The burette is filled up with the solution (generally acid solutions are taken in burette) to a little above the zero mark. The burette is held vertically and the liquid is allowed to flow out slowly by opening the stopcock slightly, until the lowest point of the liquid meniscus just coincides with the zero graduation. The position of the meniscus is read by placing the eye at the same horizontal level as the lowest point of the concave meniscus in order to avoid errors due to parallax.

The burette is now clamped vertically to a stand at a convenient height on the table. Particular care must be taken so that no air-bubble remains inside the jet or the burette. In such case, the stopcock is fully opened and the liquid is allowed to run out with a force till the air-bubbles are expelled. The liquid is then poured in the burette to fill up to the zero mark again.

Micro-Burette: For finer measuring which measure 1 ml in fraction.

D. Pipette

The pipettes that are used in the pharmaceutical laboratory may be graduated or volumetric type:

1. Volumetric pipette: These are used to measure precise volume with a high degree accuracy. The volumetric pipette may be of two types:
   (a) A pipette with single graduation mark—A pipette is a glass tube with a cylindrical bulb in the middle, one end of the tube being drawn into a jet, while the other stem carries a thin circular mark etched on it. This mark indicates the volume of the liquid to be measured out by the pipette. This volume, i.e., the capacity of the pipette at a particular temperature, is usually engraved on the bulb. Pipettes of different capacities (2 ml, 5 ml, 10 ml, 25 ml, or 50 ml etc.) are available.
   (b) A pipette with two graduation marks—It is applicable by the well-experienced person for more accuracy. It is not reliable by the beginners as it is easy to overrun the lower graduation when discharging.

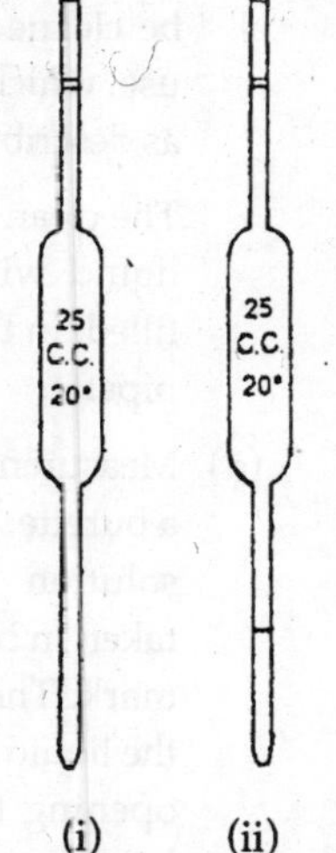

Volumetric Pipette
(i) A pipette with a single graduation mark.
(ii) A pipette with two graduation marks.

2. Graduated Pipette: It may be of two varieties:
   (a) A pipette with graduations extending to the tip—The volume that can be measured is contained between the 0 mark and the tip [See figure (i)].
   (b) A pipette with graduations not extending to the Tip—The total volume that can be measured is contained between the 0 mark and the last mark before the tip. [See figure (ii)].

Various volumes that can be measured

1 ml pipette to measure 0.8 ml

2 ml pipette to measure 1.8 ml

5 ml pipette to measure 3.5 ml

10 ml pipette to measure 8.5 ml can be used.

The use of a Pipette

Pipettes are employed for withdrawing a measured volume of a liquid accurately from a vessel and to transfer it to another.

Cleansing and rinsing of a Pipette

The pipette must be clean and free from grease before use. For this purpose, the pipette is washed first with sodium carbonate solution, then with dilute hydrochloric acid. It is then washed thoroughly with purified water and, finally, with absolute alcohol or acetone, which not only removes grease but also helps in drying it quickly.

The clean pipette is then rinsed once or twice with a little of the liquid which is intended to be measured.

To do this, a little of the solution is sucked by mouth into the pipette, the open end is closed immediatley by the fore-finger. The pipette is now rotated in a horizontal position so that the whole internal surface is thoroughly washed. The liquid is then run out through the jet and discarded. The

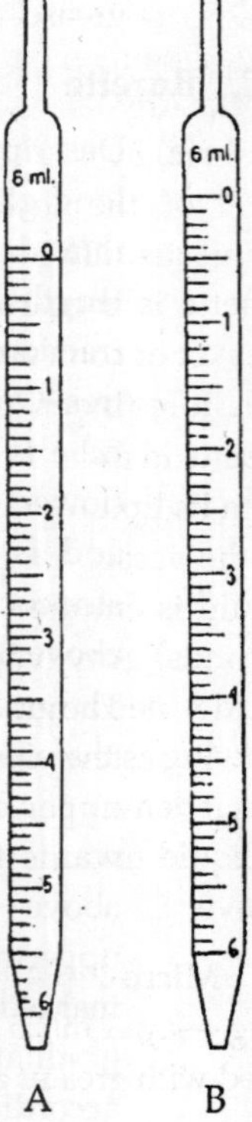

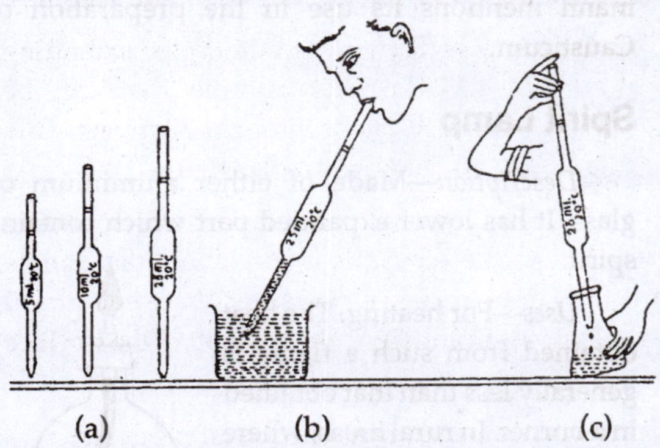

(a) pipette of different size, (b) sucking of liquid (or soln.) with the help of a pipette, (c) the method of transferring liquid (or soln.) from a pipette to a vessel

process is repeated again to ensure complete removal of any water that might have adhered inside the pipette.

Measurement by a Pipette

The given solution, of which a definite aliquot is to be measured out, is sucked by mouth into the pipette, until it rises a little above the mark. The open end is closed very quickly by the dry fore-finger. The pipette is now held in a vertical position and the liquid is allowed to run out slowly by slightly relaxing the pressure at the finger until the lowest point of the meniscus just coincides with the mark. Any error due to parallax is avoided by keeping the eye at the level of the **lowest point of the meniscus.** The liquid inside the pipette is then run out in a vessel (beaker or conical flask), by releasing the fore-finger and holding the pipette in a slightly inclined position with its tip touching against the wall of the vessel, until the whole of the liquid is emptied (it takes about 15 seconds). Any liquid, still remaining inside, need not be forced out by blowing as the pipette is so calibrated that it delivers the measured quantity of liquid under the conditions stated above.

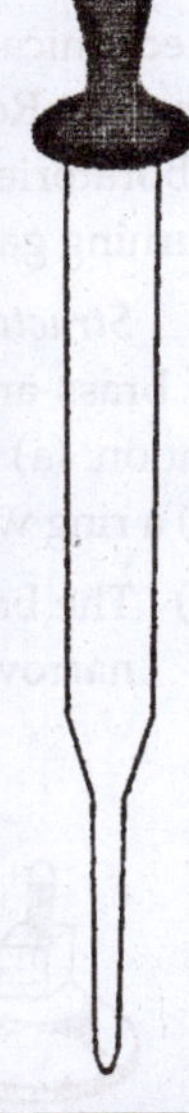

Dropping Pipette

Micro-Pipette: For finer measuring—say, .1 ml, .5 ml, 1 ml—these are used with greater accuracy.

E. Calibrated Dropping Pipettes

Calibrated dropping pipettes generally deliver divider 20 drops per ml of purified water. So 1 drop = 0.05 ml.

To measure the drops dropping pipette should be held in absolutely vertical position.

Calibration of Dropping Pipette:

(i) 1 ml of water is measured by volumetric pipette and taken in a small test tube.

(ii) Water is drawn into the dropping pipette to be calibrated.

(iii) No. of drops that are delivered from the ml of water, counted.

The process is repeated at least three times to check the accuracy.

F. Graduated Conical Testing Glasses

These are not accurate for measuring. It is better to avoid using them for laboratory tests only.

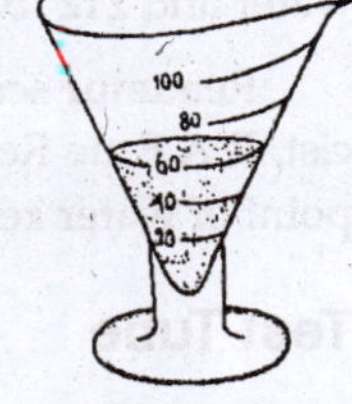

Graduated Conical Glass

Beaker

It is generally made up of glass. Different sizes of beaker are available. The mouth of the beaker is generally circular but in some beakers there is a lip or spout in the mouth for better discharging. It is used to store the liquid substances.

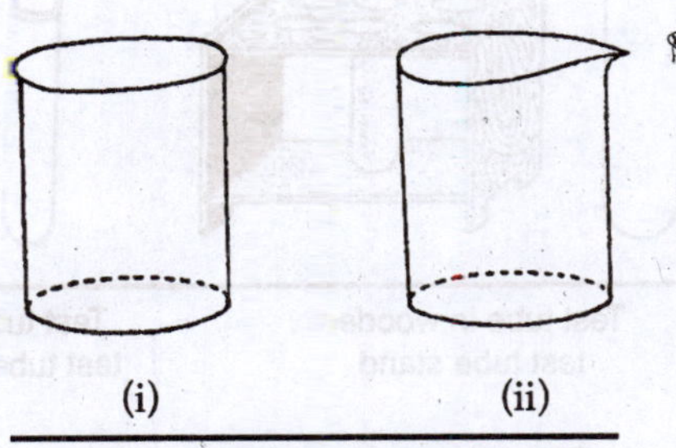

Beakers: (i) without lip, (ii) with lip

Thermometer

The simplest and commonly used instrument for measuring temperature in homoeopathic pharmaceutical laboratory is 'Liquid Thermometer'. But the most accurate ones are 'Gas Thermometer', which work on the principle of the relation of pressure and temp. However, this cannot be used because of difficulty in using the glass apparatus that are used in pharmacy laboratory. The liquid thermometer is used for analytical purposes. They are made up of glass tubes having the capillary bores, and mercury is the most common liquid used in thermometer.

There are three scales viz. Celsius, Fahrenheit and Reaumur:

Celsius Scale—Constructed by Swedish astronomer, Anders Celsius (1701–44)—scale divided into 100 degrees (centigrade), zero degree is freezing point of water and 100° boiling point.

Fahrenheit Scale—Invented by German physicist Gabriel Daniel Fahrenhiet (1686–1736)—scale divided into 180 degrees, 32° is freezing point of water and 212° boiling point.

Reaumur scale—Introduced by French physicist, R.A.F. de Reaumur (1683–1757) with freezing point of water zero and boiling point 80°R.

Test Tube

The apparatus which is always and most essential in a pharmacy laboratory is test tube. It is a thin glass tube whose one end is closed. Wooden test tube stand is used to place the test tube. During heating, the test tube is held with test tube holder.

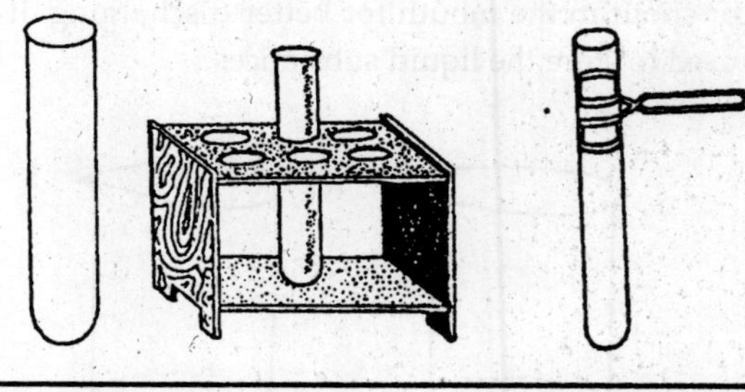

Test tube in wooden test tube stand — Test tube with test tube holder

Glass Retort

It is a flask-like round-bottomed apparatus and its one side is bent and looks like a tube.

It is generally used in pharmacy laboratory as distilling flask. Hahnemann mentions its use in the preparation of Causticum.

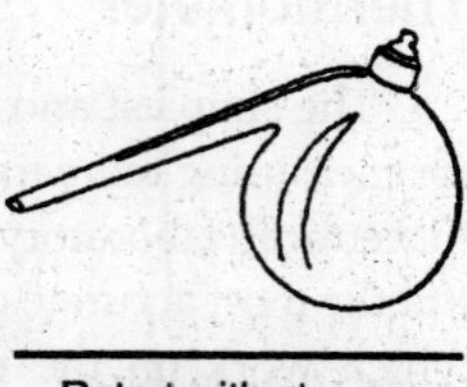

Retort with stopper

Spirit Lamp

Description—Made of either aluminium or glass. It has lower expanded part which contains spirit.

Uses—For heating. The heat obtained from such a flame is generally less than that obtained in a burner. In rural areas, where gas production is not available, spirit lamp is used in pharmaceutical laboratory, instead of burner.

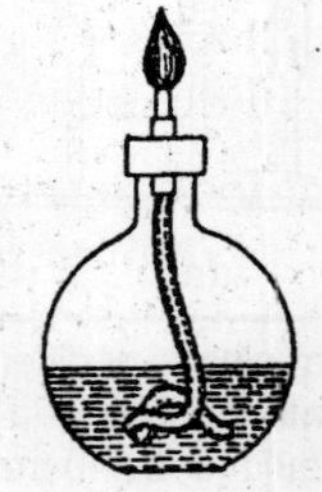

Spirit Lamp

BURNERS

To perform some chemical tests or to carry out some experiments involving chemical reactions, application of heat is necessary. Gaseous fuels are very suitable for laboratories. But, for burning gaseous fuels, some special mechanical devices are required which would allow the gas to burn without causing disturbance or danger. Such devices are called burners.

Bunsen Burner

Definition—A bunsen burner is a simple mechanical device, discovered by the German scientist Robert Bunsen (1811-99) in 1855, used in laboratories for producing heat and flame by burning gaseous fuel (commonly coal gas).

Structure—A bunsen burner is generally made of brass and iron and has three parts in combination: (a) a base, (b) a burner tube or barrel, and (c) a ring with a hole.

(a) The base (made of cast iron) is fitted with a narrow nozzle (jet) at the centre and an inlet

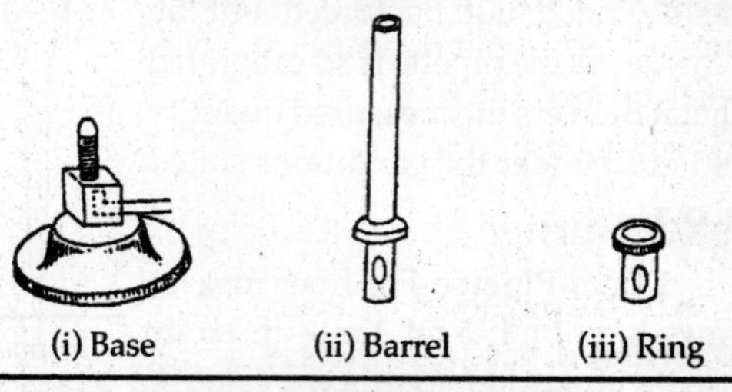

Three main parts of a Bunsen burner

tube at one side (both made of brass), which are in communication with each other through the body of the base. The nozzle is provided with screw thread on its outer surface to which the burner tube is fitted. The inlet tube allows coal gas to flow in and its speed is increased by passing through the narrow nozzle which throws the gas in a fine jet upwards through the burner tube.

(b) The burner tube (also called barrel) is a narrow cylindrical pipe (made of brass) of varying length depending upon the overall size of the burner. It has, at its lower end, an air-hole, either on one side or on both diametrically opposite sides, linearly with the tip of the inlet jet.

(c) The ring, also called the air-regulator or collar, is an annular ring (made of brass) fitted over the burner tube at the junction of its lower end and the base. The ring has holes corresponding to the number of air-holes in the barrel. The ring is so placed round the barrel that its holes exactly align themselves with those of the barrel. The ring can be rotated round the burner tube and the air-holes can be made fully-open, partially open or fully closed by rotating the air-regulator and thereby regulating the access of air into the burner.

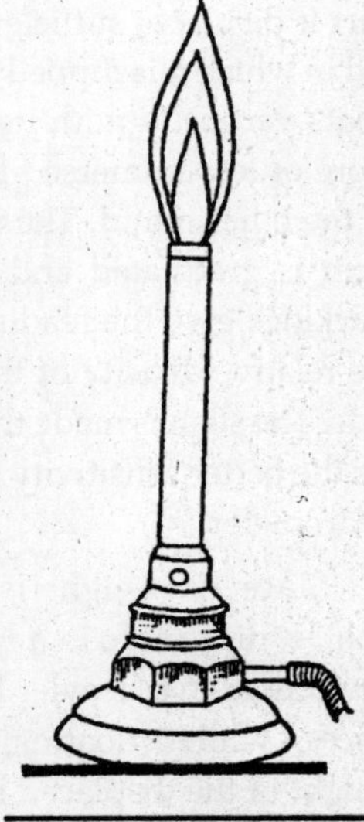

A Bunsen Burner with all parts duly fitted together

Other types of burners—Some types of burners, other than the bunsen burner, which are in common use in pharmaceutical laboratory are: (i) Meker burner, (ii) Teclu burner, (iii) Ring burner, (iv) Fish-tail burner.

Meker Burner

It is so designed that it can make use of higher proportion of air with the gas, which cannot be done with a Bunsen burner due to the danger of

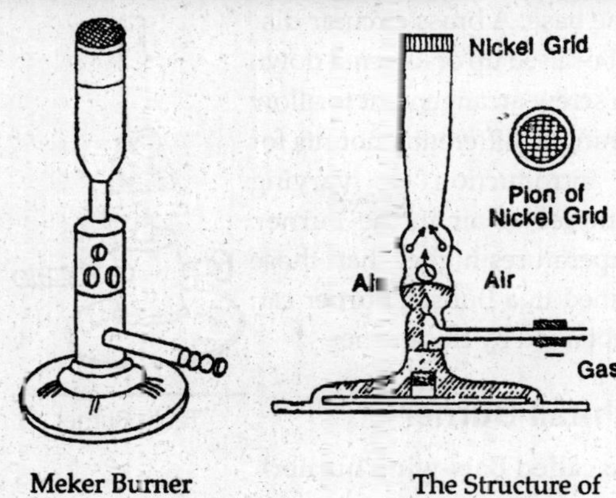

Meker Burner

The Structure of Meker Burner

'Striking back'. For complete combustion of coal gas, a proportion of 6 volumes of air to one volume of the gas is required, while the proportion of air and gas producing normal Bunsen flame is about 2.5 volumes to 1 volume. So, the Bunsen burner cannot make use of the total heating capacity of the fuel gas, and also it is not without the danger of 'Striking back'. These two difficulties are overcome in a Meker burner which are provided with larger air-holes which supply air required for complete combustion of the fuel gas and it is provided with a wider barrel with a nickel or copper grid (or wire-gauge) placed at top which prevents the flame from striking back. Thus, in a Meker burner, a temperature of 1,100°–1,200°C can be ordinarily attained without danger.

Ring Burner

May be considered as made up of a series of small Bunsen burners placed in a circle with a cast iron setting. It is widely used in laboratories, where large vessels are to be heated more or less rapidly and uniformly.

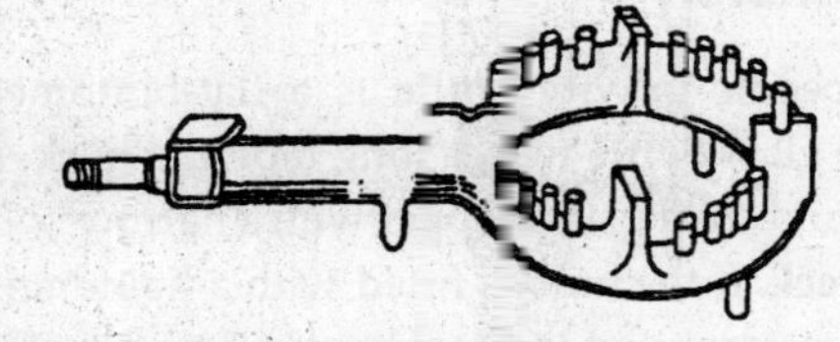

Ring Burner

Teclu Burner

It is a modified type of an ordinary Bunsen burner. Its barrel is of the shape of a conical drum at the base. A brass circular disc can be raised up or lowered down by a screw arrangement to allow opening of different amounts for the introduction of varying quantities of air in the burner. Temperatures higher than those attained in a Bunsen burner can be obtained by this burner.

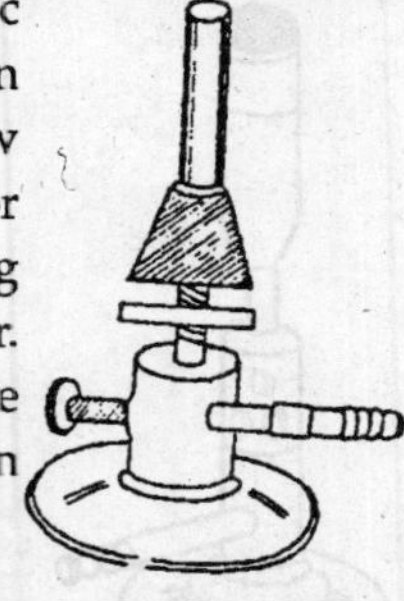
Teclu Burner

Fish-tail Burner

(also called Bats-wing burner)

It is so named because of the very shape of its flame which resembles the tail of a fish (or the wings of a bat). The burner has no air-hole or air-regulator and the top of the burner tube is fitted with a special cap provided with a thin narrow slit-opening which is responsible for producing the flame of a fish-tail shape.

This burner produces a luminous flame which is thin and widened and, as such, it is best suitable for bending glass tubes, because it can heat uniformly a large area of the tube.

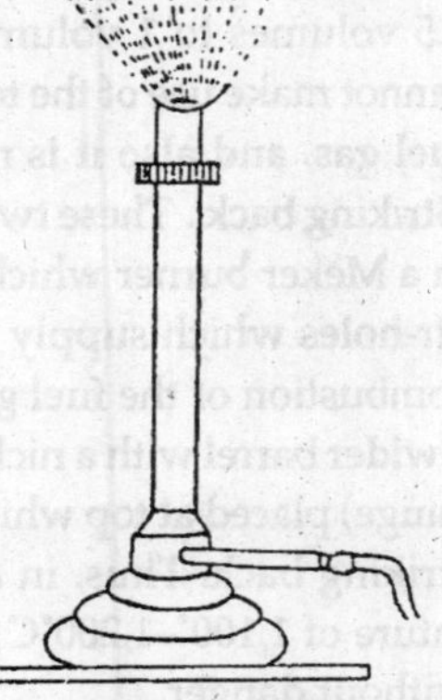
Fish-tail Burner

Stirrer

Description—It is generally made of glass or steel. It is a rod having a long handle and a small rounded tip.

Uses—It is used to stir and mix the liquid.

Specific Gravity Bottle (Pyknometer)

A specific gravity bottle is a flat-bottomed bulb-like glass bottle with a long tapering neck. A well-ground solid glass stopper with a narrow bore fits the neck. If the bulb is fitted with a liquid and the stopper dropped in place, some liquid comes out through the bore and the bottle contains a fixed volume of the liquid. The internal volume of the bottle is often 20, 25 or 50 cm^3.

In a standard bottle the volume and the temperature at which the volume is exact are marked on the bottle. But a beginner may not get a standard bottle for use because it is costly.

Since volume changes with temperature, a specific gravity bottle should always be held by the neck and never by the bulb. The bottle is particularly suitable for measuring the Sp. Gr. of liquids and of granular solids.

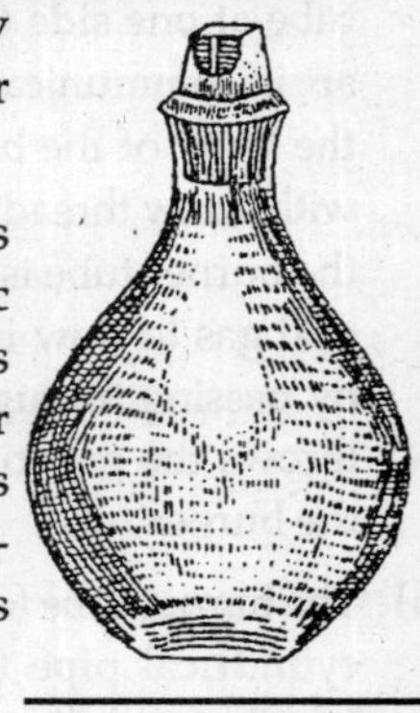
Specific Gravity Bottle

Hydrometer

A common hydrometer consist of three parts—a long narrow graduated stem (B), a tubular bulb (A), and a round bulb (C) as shown in the figure.

The round bulb (C) contains lead shots or mercury, making the apparatus heavy at the bottom.

Due to the tubular hollow part it displaces sufficient liquid in which it is dipped and it floats vertically with its stem more or less immersed in one or the other liquid. The upper stem is graduated and these markings give the readings of the relative density of the liquids. The stem is made thinner for the better sensitivity of the hydrometer.

Since its weight is constant, it dips more in a lighter liquid than in a heavier liquid since, while floating, the weight of the displaced liquid must be equal to its weight in every case.

Uses—It is used for rapid and easy measurement of the 'relative density' or 'specific gravity' of different liquids.

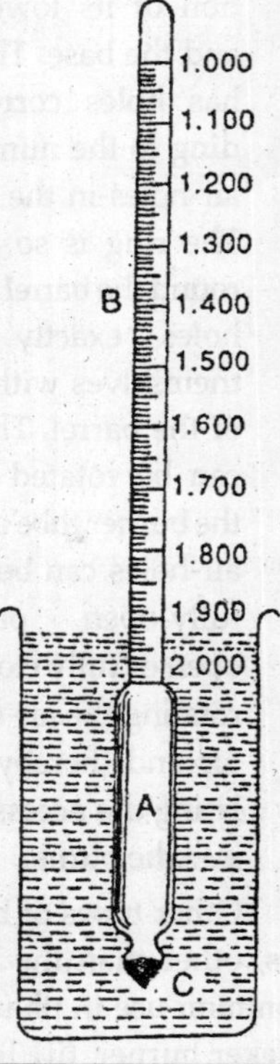

Common Hydrometer

Lactometer

It is a glass-tube with a buldge in the middle part. The bottom is a 'bulb' with a few spots. The top portion is a tube closed at the end and graduated. The markings gives the readings of Sp. Gr.

This instrument registers Sp. Gr. from 1015–1040. The first two digits are omitted. Only 15 is written in place of 1015. Lactometer is graduated for a definite temperature, especially 60°F. When lactometer is used for other temperatures add 0.1 to the reading of every degree above 60°F or subtract 0.1 from the reading of every degree below 60°F.

Uses—It is used for testing milk.

Porcelain Basin

It is made up of porcelain. It is used for evaporation of liquids at high temperature.

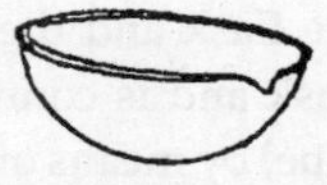

Porcelain Basin

Crucible

It is made up of porcelain. It is used for drying the hard substances in small amounts at a high temperature. For drying at very high temperature, the crucible is made by silica.

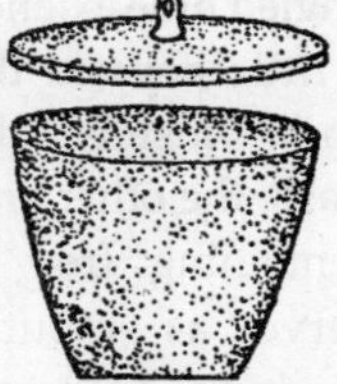

Porcelain Basin

Water Bath

Description—Round or pan-shaped vessel, generally made up of copper. It is fitted with two handles on either side of the vessel—for easy handling. The vessel is covered with concentric reducible flat ring-like lids which are made up of copper. Porcelain covers are also used. The lids are arranged one above another. All the lids are perforated except which is placed above. The vessel is partially filled with water and is placed on a tripod stand and heated from below by a bunsen burner, gas, or spirit lamp.

Uses—(i) To calculate the moisture content of drug substances. (ii) For indirect heating at low temperature, (iii) For sublimation.

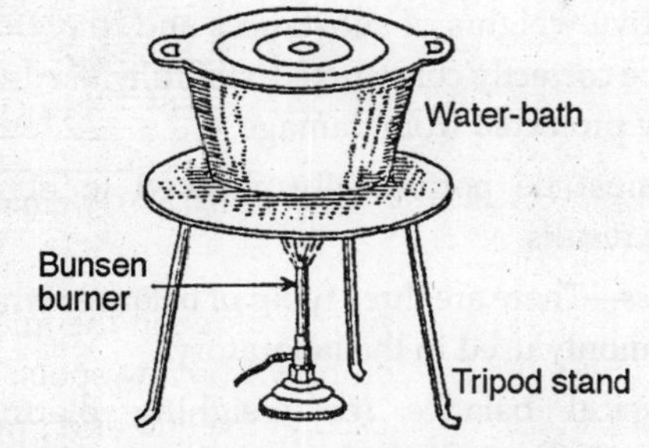

Water Bath

Desiccator

It is an air-tight thick-walled hard glass vessel provided with a lid fitting perfectly on the upper ground rim of the desiccator, which is greased. The desiccator is contracted at the middle—a circular perforated zinc-sheet placed on a shelf above the constriction separates the upper from the lower half. The air inside the desiccator is kept always dry by placing some drying agents, e.g., concentrated sulphuric acid, fused calcium chloride etc. The substances to be dried are kept on a porcelain basin in the upper half.

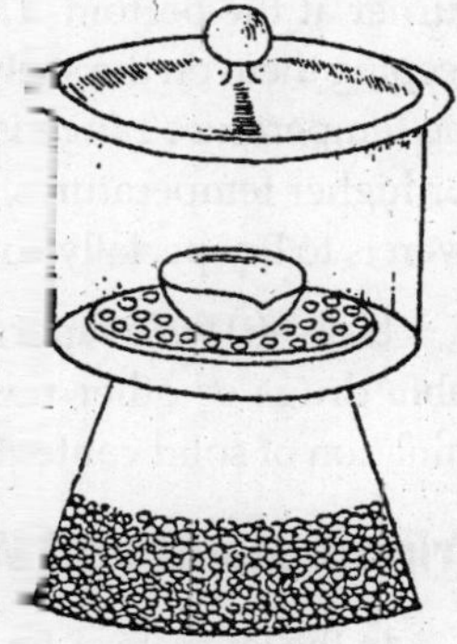

Desiccator (ordinary)

For quick drying, a vacuum desiccator is used, the vacuum is created through an adjustable opening at the top of the desiccator—being connected with a vacuum pump.

Uses—It is used for desiccation, i.e. removing moisture completely from substances for keeping 'hygroscopic' materials, i.e., those which absorb moisture from atmosphere.

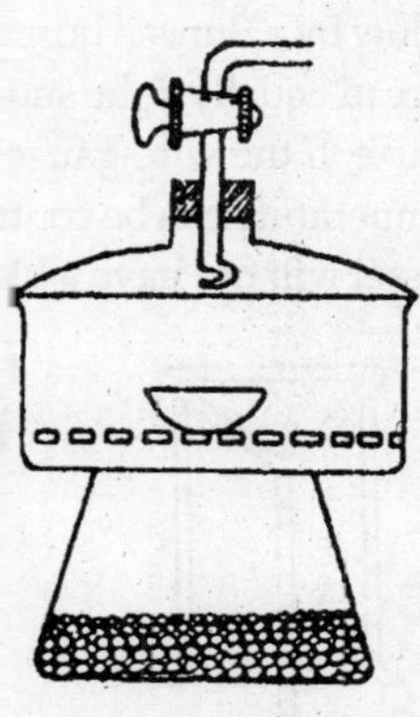

Desiccator (vacuum)

Hot-air Oven

Description—The air is ignited in a closed chamber known as hot air oven. It is a small almirah-like chamber, made of aluminium or stainless steel (for higher temperatures), formerly made of copper. Two or more perforated and

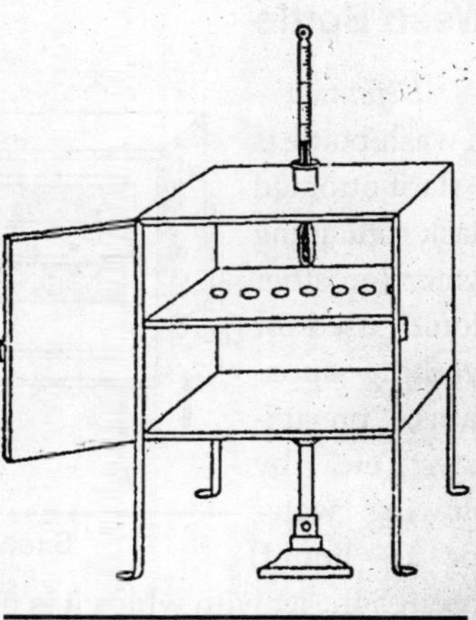

Hot-air Oven

movable racks are provided within the chamber, having a hinged door, so that the oven can be opened or closed, as required. At the top of the chamber there is a hole, where a thermometer is inserted for recording temperatures of the air inside. The oven is heated electrically or by gas-burner at the bottom. The materials are dried by keeping them on the shelves of the oven. Generally, the temperature range is from 50°C to 250°C; but for higher temperatures, viz., 450°C or higher, the oven is to be specially constructed.

Uses—(i) For evaporating the moisture of vegetable drugs or other raw materials. (ii) In determination of solid contents of mother tinctures.

Tripod Stand and Wire-gauze

In the laboratory, for the purpose of heating of any substance, it is placed over the wire-gauze. This wire-gauze is kept on a three-legged stand i.e., Tripod stand, and the substance is heated from below by a Bunsen burner. The Bunsen flame will be spread equally if the substance is kept over the wire-gauze. If the wire-gauze is coated with asbestos the temperature can be controlled and the surface of the vessel will not have a blackish discolouration.

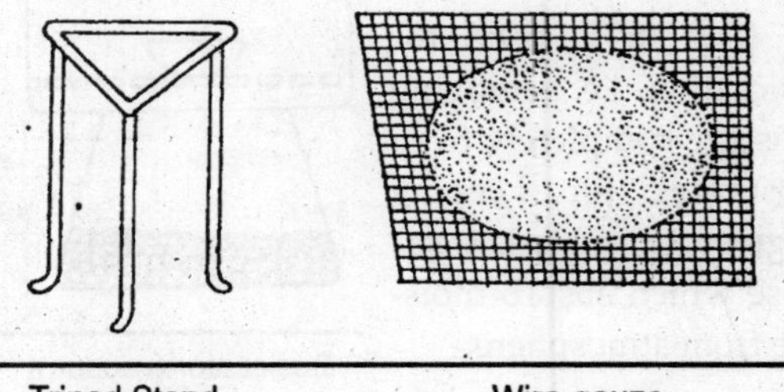

Tripod Stand Wire-gauze

Wash Bottle

Definition—A wash-bottle is a flat-bottomed flask containing water (or other liquid) used for washing apparatus, precipitates etc. by blowing water (or liquid) through the jet with which it is fitted.

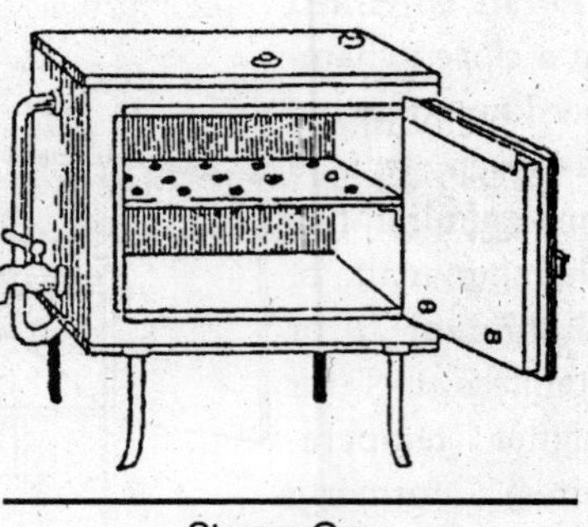

Stream Oven

Description of a Wash-bottle—It is a flat-bottomed flask of 500 ml (or 1 litre) capacity, fitted with an air-tight cork having two holes, through which pass two glass-tubes, one long and bent at an acute angle near one of its ends, and the other short and bent at an obtuse angle in the middle. The two angles of the two tubes are so made as to form about 180° together. The cork, along with the tubes inserted through it, is carefully fitted to the flask to make air-tight joints. The longer arm of the acute-angled tube reaches almost to the bottom of the flask and the other arm remains outside the flask and is connected with a jet (made of glass tube) by means of a piece of rubber-tubing. On the other hand, one arm of the obtuse-angled tube extends a little beyond the cork inside the flask, the other arm remaining free to serve as mouth-piece for blowing. About three-fourth of the flask is filled with purified water.

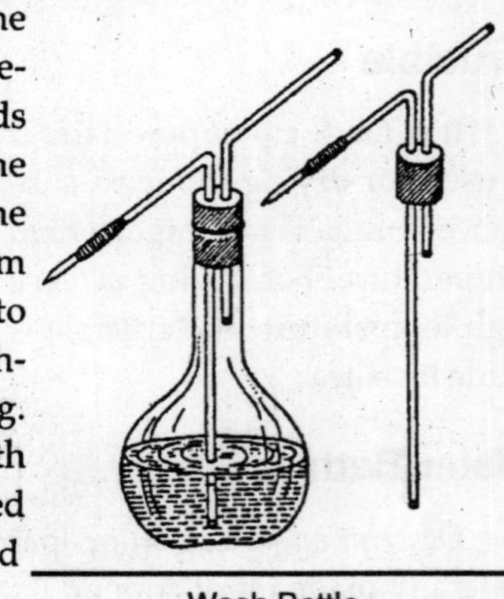

Wash Bottle

Uses—It is used for washing purposes and for transfering precipitates adhering to the vessel to a filter.

Balances

Introduction—Successful performance of many of the operations in pharmacy depend upon a thorough knowledge of the principle of the balance and a correct understanding of its care and use, and weighing is nearly always the first step in any compounding.

Balance is an instrument devised to determine the relative weights of substances and, therefore, should be correctly constructed, skillfully used and carefully protected from damage.

It must be periodically checked to obtain accurate results.

Types—There are three types of balances which are commonly used in the laboratory:

(a) Physical balance (or weighing platform balance, also called a beam balance): Physical balance of three varieties of scales are used for ordinary weighing.

Uses—It is used in weighing larger quantities which do not need finer sensitivity.

(i) Scales with brass-pan—for serving prescription.

(ii) Scales with glass-pan—for hygroscopic and caustic substances.

(iii) Scales with horn-pan—for poisonous substances and sugar of milk.

(b) Chemical balance: It is used for minute quantities where fine degree of sensitivity is needed.

(c) Single pan balance: It is of recent origin. There is only one pan where the substance to be weighed is kept and adjusted by turning the knobs and its weight will be directly read on the scale.

Uses—It is used where putting in and putting out of weights is not required.

Open Two-pan Balance

This balance has two pans, supported by shafts. It may be designed for separate weights or incorporate a graduated arm with a sliding weight (Harvard Trip balance).

Uses—To weigh large amounts (up to several kilograms) when a high degree of accuracy is not required, e.g., 25.5 gm, 40 gm, 8.5 gm etc. sensitivity: 0.5 g (500 mg).

Set of Weights for use:

500 gms	1	10 gms	1
200 gms	2	5 gms	1
100 gms	1	2 gms	2
20 gms	2	1 gm	1

Dispensary Balance

This balance also has two suspended pans but it has no glass case and no rests. Sensitivity: 5–10 mg.

The dispensary balance is more accurate than the open two-pan balance, but can weigh only up to 50 gm.

Sensitivity of Balance

This corresponds to the smallest mass that makes the pointer move over one division on the scale, e.g., if the sensitivity of a balance is 1 mg this means that a mass of at least 1 mg is needed to move the pointer.

Chemical Balance

Uses—

(i) To weigh small quantities (up to 20 or 200 gm, depending on the model), (ii) When great accuracy is required: e.g., 3.85 gm, 0.110 gm, 7.530 gm Sensitivity: 0.5 mg. to 0.1 mg depending on the model.

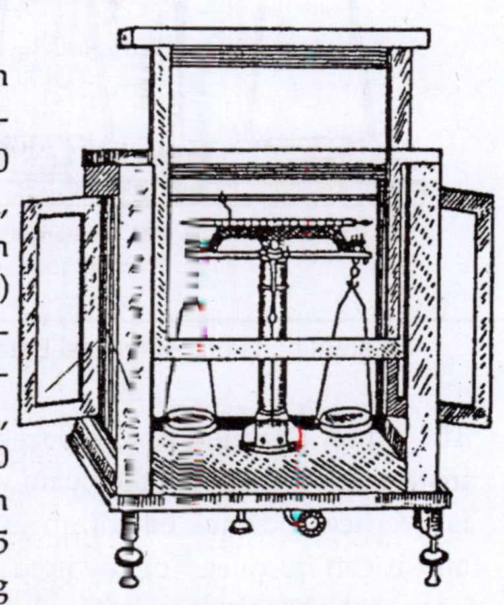

Chemical Balance

Components of the Balance

The essential parts of a common chemical balance are:

1. The Balance beam—It is a horizontal metal or alloy casting, generally of the form of a thin bar, which is capable of turning freely about a sharp steel or agate knife-edge at the middle, which is called the fulcrum. The sharp end of the knife-edge rests on a small plate of steel or agate to minimise friction. At the ends of the beam, two similar agate knife-edges are attached with their sharp edges upwards.
2. The Stirrups or pan supporters—These rest on the terminal knife-edges. In the better type of balances, these are provided with agate pieces attached at the lower surfaces of their upper arms. These are furnished with hooks at the lower end, from which the pans are suspended. The distances from the fulcrum to the centre of gravity of the stirrups are called the arms of the balance, which are equal in length.
3. The scale pans, on which standard weights and bodies to be weighed are placed.

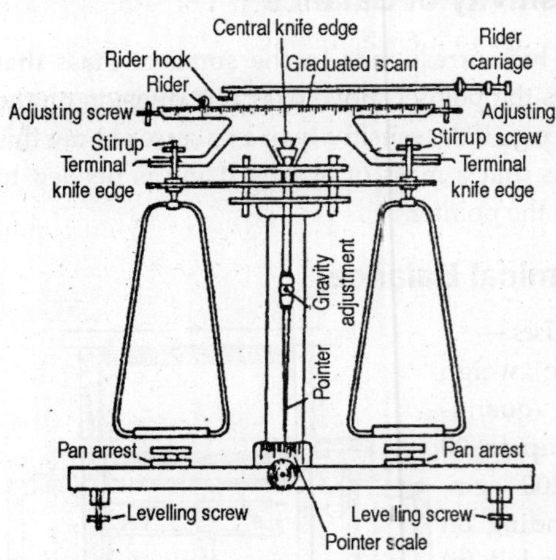

Different parts of a Chemical Balance

4. The pillar, attached to the base-plate of the instrument to support the beam when at rest, is a vertical rod encased within an outer cover, and it can be raised or lowered by a key or knob at the base, when required. The pillar has an agate at the top, upon which the central knife-edge of the beam rests.
5. The pointer—This is attached at its upper end to the middle part of the beam and the lower end can move freely over a graduated scale attached to the bottom of the pillar. When the beam is horizontal, the pointer should be vertical and its lower end should point to the zero mark of the scale.
6. The Arresting arrangement—When the balance is not in use, the pillar supporting the beam is lowered so that the beam rests on another support attached to the outer casing of the pillar as horizontal projections, and the under-surfaces of the pans just touch the pan-rests on the base-board. Thus the knife-edge at the centre of the beam does not always rest on the agate plate and so its sharpness is preserved.
7. The Adjusting nuts—At each end of the beam there is a nut working in a screw. By displacing the position of the nuts, the effective weight on each side can be altered through a small range, and thus weighing accuracy of the balance can be adjusted.
8. The plumb-line and the levelling screws—The base of the instrument is provided with levelling screws by whose adjustment the pillar is made vertical, so that the balance-beam becomes horizontal; the correct adjustment is indicated by the exactly vertical position of the plumb-line attached to the instrument.

The whole instrument is placed in a glass-casing to protect it from dust (and fumes) and to avoid air-convection during weighing.

The Rider

The rider is a small piece of wire weighing 10 mgs, made of platinum, gold, stainless steel etc. and bent twice at about 90°, with a loop at the middle. A chemical balance is provided with such a rider for taking fractional weights less than 10 mgs. For this purpose, the whole of the balance beam is divided by serrated marks (like a saw-blade) into 100 equal parts and marked accordingly.

The use of rider during weighing in a chemical balance—while weighing, if it is found that weights less than 10 mgs (which are not provided with in the weight box) are required for correct balancing, the rider is moved by the rider carriage and placed by trial and error method on a suitable position on the beam. From the position of the rider on the scale engraved on the beam, the extra weight is calculated and added to the 'weights' placed on the pan. Each smallest sub-division on the beam of the sartorius balance corresponds to 0.2 mg and, in the Bunge type, it is 0.1 mg. Sartorius type of balances are commonly used in chemical laboratories.

The Weight Box

It is a wooden box with hinged lid. The standard weights are kept in the grooves cut in the box. The standard weights are generally made of brass, plated with nickel or chromium (Stainless steel weights are also available). Standard set generally comprises the following weights:

100 gms	1	500 mgs	1
50 gms	1	200 mgs	2
20 gms	2	100 mgs	1
10 gms	1	50 mgs	1
5 gms	1	20 mgs	2
2 gms	2	10 mgs	1
1 gm	1		

The heavier weights (up to 1 gm) are more or less cylindrical solid metal blocks with a knob at the top, while the fractional weights are generally rectangular or triangular metal plates. The value of each weight is inscribed or embossed on it. The weights are arranged in the box in a regular way and fractional weights are generally covered by a glass plate. A pair of forceps is also provided in the box for handling the weights.

Instructions for use: Points to be followed before, during, and after the weighing in a chemical balance:

1. The balance should be kept on a strong table so that it is not affected by vibration. It should be placed in a room free from dust and fumes.
2. The balance may not be properly levelled. This is easily detected by looking at the plumb line, which should not be exactly vertical under such conditions. This defect should be corrected by adjusting the levelling screws provided at the base of the instrument, till the plumb line is exactly vertical.
3. The beam of the balance may not be perfectly horizontal when freed, i.e., one side is heavier than the other side. This can be adjusted by screwing in or out the nuts provided at the ends of the beam of the balance.
4. The stirrups may be displaced. This should be properly placed on the beam before weighings are made.
5. The pans may not be cleaned. It should be properly cleaned by a camel-hair brush before using the balance.
6. A hot body must not be weighed in a chemical balance.
7. The weights should not be lifted with fingers.

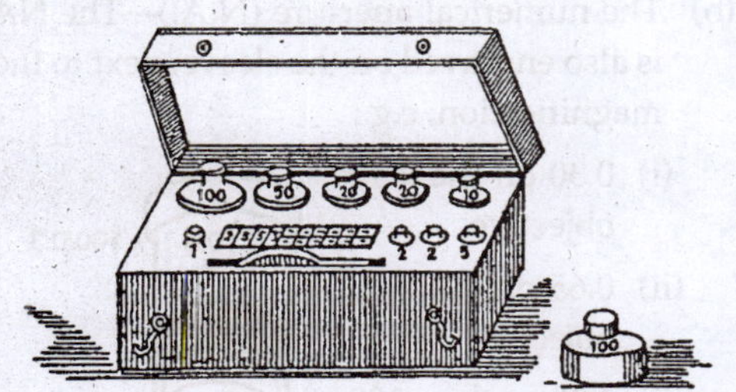

A weight box used with a chemical balance

They should be handled with forceps provided in the weight box.

MICROSCOPE

In homoeopathic laboratory, a microscope is highly essential for the purpose of identification and physical examination of vegetable drugs.

Types:

A. **Light Microscope**

When artificial light or sunlight is used to see the object. It may be: (i) Simple, and (ii) Compound.

B. **Electron Microscope**

Electron microscope totally modernised the concept of structure at cellular and molecular levels and now—instead of structure—it is ultrastructure which has become the most fashionable study. It is the electron microscope through which human eye can see and measure the ultramicroscopic particles.

Principles

(i) A beam of electrons is used instead of a beam of light.

(ii) Electromagnetic fields used instead of glass lenses.

(iii) The resolving power (0.6–0.7 nm) is much greater than that of the light microscope.

(iv) Magnification: Up to 10 lakh or 1 million (1,000,000) times i.e., 10^6.

Disadvantages

(i) Only very small fragments of tissue can be examined. Ultra-thin sections are cut on a specially designed microtome with glass or diamond knives. The ultra-thin section is placed on a very thin 150A membrane made from colloidion (nitrocellulose), formvar (poly-vinyl fermol) carbon, aluminium, or beryllium.

(ii) Since the electrons travel long distances in a vacuum the instrument must be completely enclosed in a vacuum. So living cells cannot be used.

(iii) To prevent damage to the tissues, the material to be studied is fixed in osmium tetraoxide and formaldehyde.

Light Microscope

A. **Components of Light Microscope**

(a) The support system

(b) The magnification system

(c) The illumination system

(d) The adjustment system.

(a) The Support System

This consists of:

1. The foot—It is the lowest part.
2. The limb—The limb carries the main part of the mechanism and is mounted on a strong, elliptical or horse-shoe shaped metallic base, called the foot. The limb carries, towards the lower region, a flat horizontally placed plate, the stage and the sub-stage attachments, and towards the upper region, the body and the body tube, which is sometimes referred to as a draw tube. The body contains the focussing mechanism that consists of two components:

   (i) A pair of large milled heads, working on the principle of 'rack and pinion' mechanism, operate the coarse focussing by moving the body tube up and down, and

   (ii) A pair of smaller milled heads, working in the same manner, operate the fine focussing. They are also known as the coarse or crude-adjusting or focussing-knobs and fine adjusting or focussing-knobs, respectively.

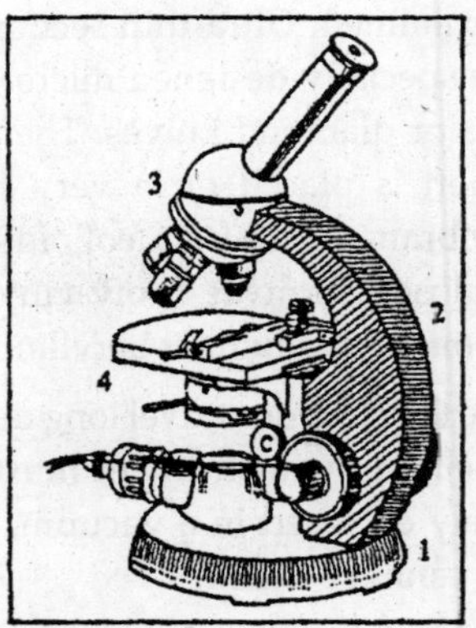

Light Microscope:1. The Foot, 2. The Limb, 3. Objectives, 4. Mechanical stages.

3. The revolving-nose piece—It is placed almost at right angles to and at the base of the body-tube, carries a set of two or three objective lenses which are designed to 'click home' when they are properly positioned. The top end of the body-tube carries the eye-piece through which the image formed by the objective is viewed.

(b) The Magnification System

This system consists of two groups of lenses situated in both the ends of the body tube:

1. The objectives: This group of lenses is at the bottom of the tube, just above the object.
2. The eye-piece: This group of lenses is at the top of the tube, where the microscopist applies his/her eyes.

I. **The Objectives**

(a) Magnification—The magnifying power of each objective is shown by a figure on the sleeve of the lens:

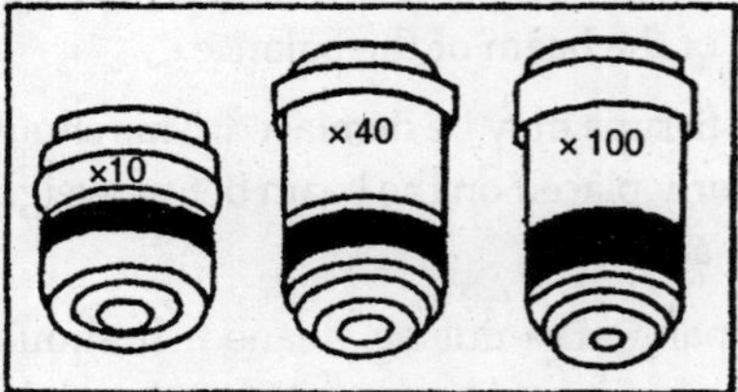

(i) The × 10 objective magnifies 10 times.

(ii) The × 40 objective magnifies 40 times.

(iii) The × 100 objective magnifies 100 times.

(b) The numerical aperture (N.A.)—The NA is also engraved on the sleeve, next to the magnification, e.g.:

(i) 0.30 on the × 10 objective

(ii) 0.65 on the × 40 objective

(iii) 1.30 on the × 100 objective

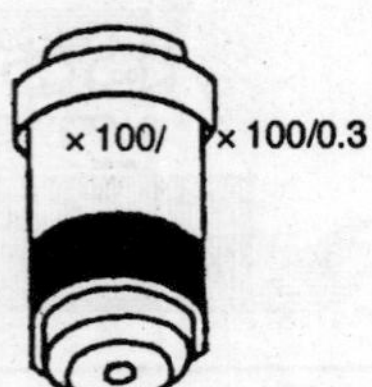

N.A. is directly proportional to resolving power (R.P.)—N.A. ∝ R.P.

(c) Other figures:

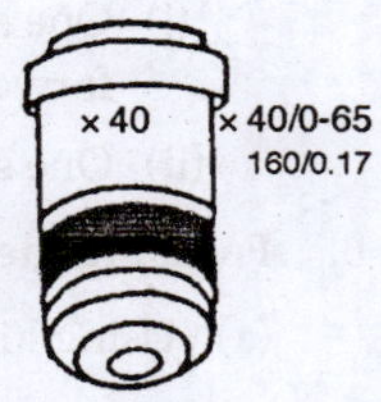

(i) Recommended length of body tube (between the objective and eye-piece) = 160 mm.

(ii) Recommended thickness of cover-slip to cover the object slide = 0.17 mm.

(d) Working distance of an objective—(distance between front lens of objective and object slide when the image is in focus).

Magnifying power of objective is inversely proportional to working distance i.e., Magnifying power ∝1 / working distance:

(i) × 10 objective: working distance = 5–6 mm.

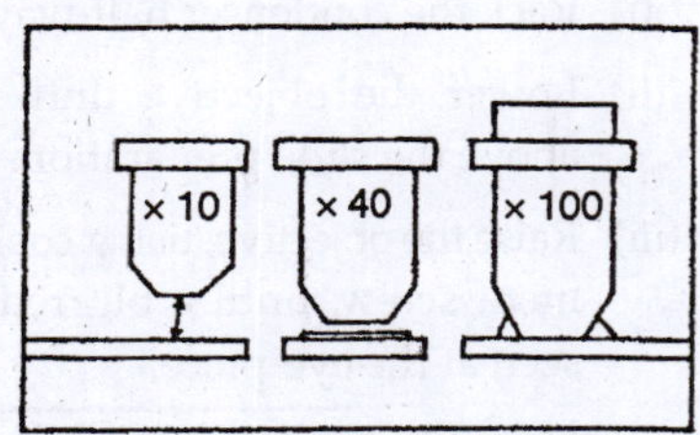

(ii) × 40 objective: working distance = 0.5–1.5 mm.

(iii) × 100 objective: working distance = 0.15–0.20 mm.

(e) Resolving power—It is the ability to distinguish between two adjacent point sources of light.

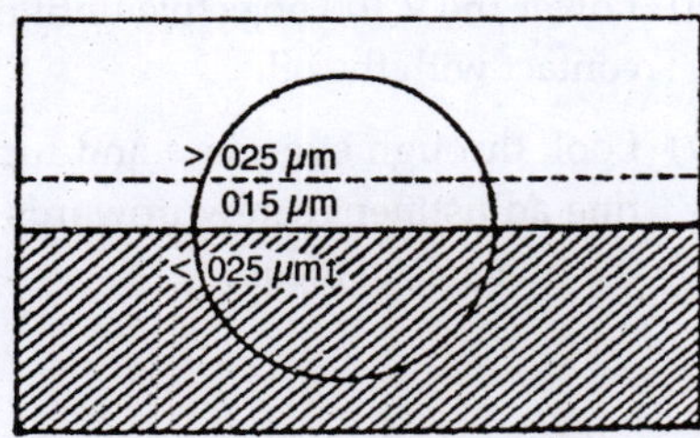

In other words, it is the minimum distance separating two point sources of light, at which they are distinctly seen as two images.

Measurement: R.P. = ½ of the wave length of the light used. R.P. of light microscope: with average light → 0.25 μm (average).

II. The Eyepiece: Magnification—

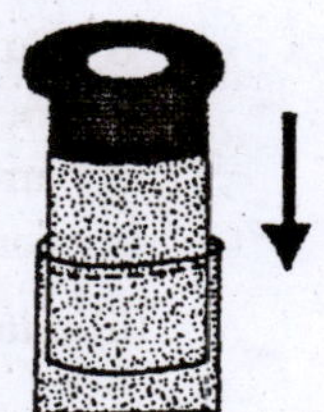

(i) The × 4 eyepiece magnifies 4 times.

(ii) The × 6 eyepiece magnifies 6 times.

(iii) The × 10 eyepiece magnifies 10 times.

If the object is magnified 40 times by the × 40 objective, then 6 times by × 6 eyepiece, the total magnification = 40 × 6 = 240.

Calculation of total magnification = Magnifying power of objective × magnifying power of eyepiece.

(c) The Illumination System

1. **The source of light:** Electric light is preferable. It is provided with lamp built beneath the mechanical stage. Otherwise, daylight can be used.

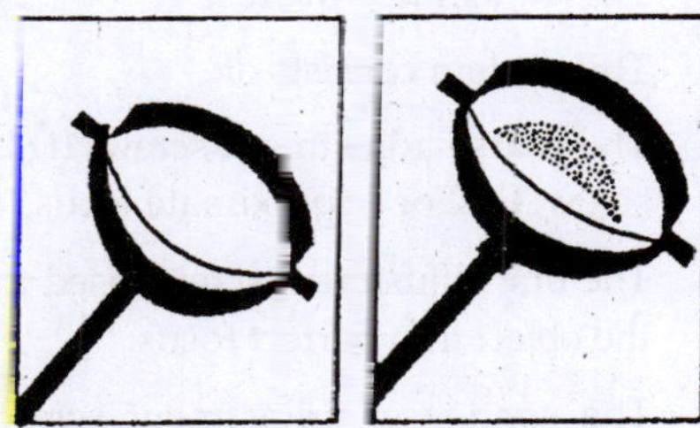

2. **The mirror:** It reflects rays from the light source on the object.

(i) Concave mirror: for low and high power objective.

(ii) Plane mirror: for oil immersion objective.

3. **The condenser**

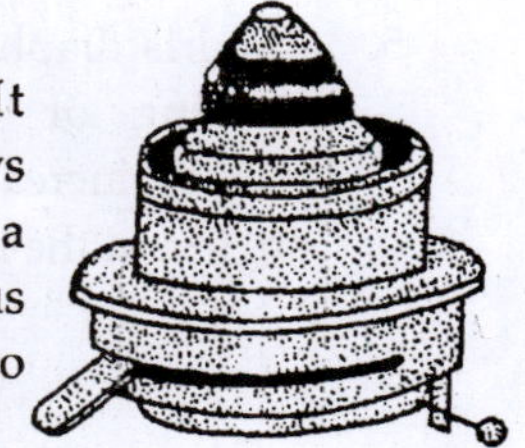

(i) Function—It brings the rays of light to a common focus on the object to be examined.

(ii) Situation—Between the mirror and mechanical stage.

(iii) Adjustment—(a) Low and high power objective: condenser low, and

(b) Oil immersion objective: condenser up.

4. **The diaphragm**

(i) Function—It is used to reduce or increase the angle and, therefore, also the amount of light that passes into the condenser.

(ii) Situation—Within the condenser.

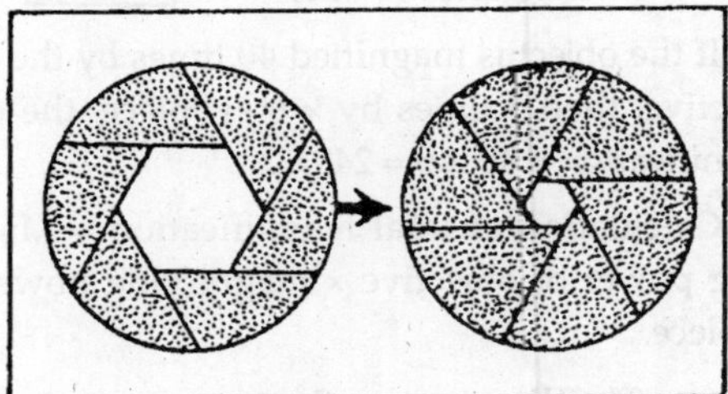

5. **Filters:** In some microscopes, coloured filters (especially blue filters) are fitted below the condenser.

(d) The Adjustment System

This system consists of:

1. The coarse adjustment screw: (i) Largest screw; (ii) For approximate focus.
2. The fine adjustment screw: used to bring the object into perfect focus.
3. The condenser adjustment screw: It is used to raise for maximum illumination and lowered for minimum illumination.
4. Condenser centering screws: There may be three screws around the condenser—One in front, one on the left and one on the right. They are used to centre the condenser exactly in relation to the objective.
5. The iris diaphragm lever: It is used for opening or closing the diaphragm, thereby increasing or reducing both the angle and the intensity of light.
6. Mechanical stage controls: used to move the object slide on the stage.

(i) One screw: to move it backwards and forwards.

(ii) One screw: to move it to left or right.

B. **Focusing the Object**

(a) Using low power objective (× 5 or × 10)

(i) Rack the condenser down to the bottom.

(ii) Lower the objective until it is just above the slide preparation.

(iii) Raise the objective, using coarse adjustment screw, until a clear image is seen in the eyepiece.

(iv) Rack the condenser up slightly if there is insufficient illumination.

(b) Using a high-power objective (× 40)

(i) Rack the condenser half-way down.

(ii) Lower the objective until it is just above the slide preparation.

(iii) Raise the objective, using coarse adjustment screw, until a blurred image is seen at the eye-piece.

(iv) Using fine adjustment screw, bring into focus. Raise the condenser to obtain sufficient illumination.

(c) Using the oil-immersion objective (× 100)

(i) Place a drop of ciderwood oil on the part to be examined.

(ii) Rack the condenser up as far as it will go and open the iris diaphragm fully.

(iii) Lower the × 100 objective until it is in contact with the oil.

(iv) Look through eye-piece and turn the fine adjustment screw upwards until the image is in focus.

Chapter 05

Cleansing of Utensils

General Rules or Instructions

1. Utensils should be thoroughly washed even when used for first time and should be again washed immediately after use.
2. HCl, HNO_3, Aqua regia or a concentrated solution of Potassium bichromate ($K_2Cr_2O_7$) in conc. H_2SO_4 may be beneficial, to remove dirt and other stains from glass vessels.
3. Ordinary cleaning can be done with soda and hot water.
4. To remove greasy or oily materials, methylated spirit, ether, chloroform ($CHCl_3$) or benzene (C_6H_6) can be used.
5. Vessels made up of metals should never be washed with acids.

Particular Rules or Instructions

1. **Mortar and Pestles**

(a) Glass mortar and pestles

(i) Firstly, the glass mortar and pestles are washed with hot water.

(ii) Then with the help of hard brush and cold water they are cleaned properly.

(iii) Then by using soft brush, mortar and pestles are rubbed and washed under tap water.

(iv) Then they are dried at high temperature.

(v) Mortar and pestles are then further dried by pouring small quantity of strong alcohol inside the mortar and burning it. But precaution should be taken with handle of pestles.

SCHEMATIC REPRESENTATION

Hot water wash

↓

Hard brush and cold water application

↓

Rubbing by soft brush

↓

Washed under tap water

↓

Dried at high temperature

↓

Small quantity of strong alcohol is burnt inside the mortar

(b) Porcelain mortar and pestles

(i) Firstly, they are washed with cold water.

(ii) Then scraped with brush and cleaned by using boiling water.

(iii) By using fine sand they are rubbed and rinsed with purified water.

(iv) Then thoroughly dried up at high temperature.

Note: After mercurial preparations the porcelain mortar and pestle should be washed with HNO_3 to neutralise residue.

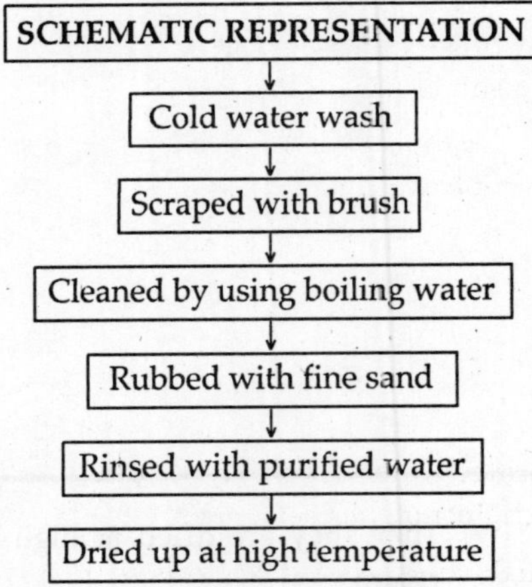

(c) Iron (or steel) mortar and pestles

(i) Firstly, they are washed by running tap-water.

(ii) Then scraped with hard brush and cleaned by using boiling water.

(iii) Again, rubbed with soft brush and washed with purified water.

(iv) Lastly, dried with clean cloth and alcohol to prevent rusting.

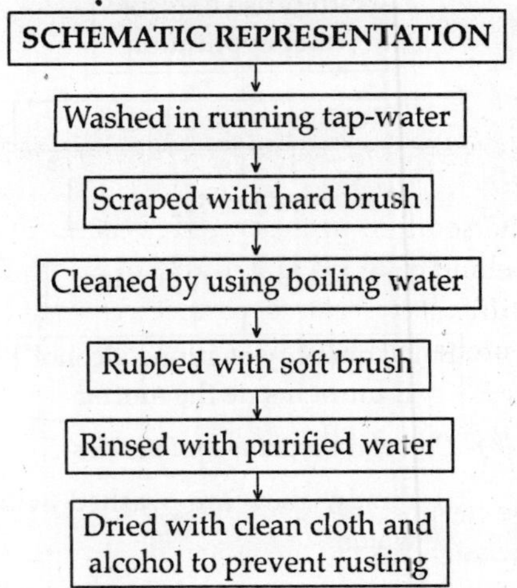

2. Spatula

Horn-made spatulas are usually used in homoeopathic pharmaceutical laboratory:

(i) Horn spatula is at first cleaned with a soft cloth.

(ii) Then it is washed by running tap-water. It is kept for hours immersed in the water.

(iii) Finally alcohol is used to wash it carefully and then it is wiped dry with a clean cloth.

Caution: Horn-made spatula should never be washed with hot water or boiled in water.

Comments of Hahnemann

Hahnemann in his "Organon of Medicine" in *Sec. 270* (6th edition) states: "Mortar, pestle and spatula must be cleaned well before they are used for another medicine. Washed first with warm water and dried. Both mortar and pestle, as well as spatula are then put in a kettle of boiling water for half an hour."

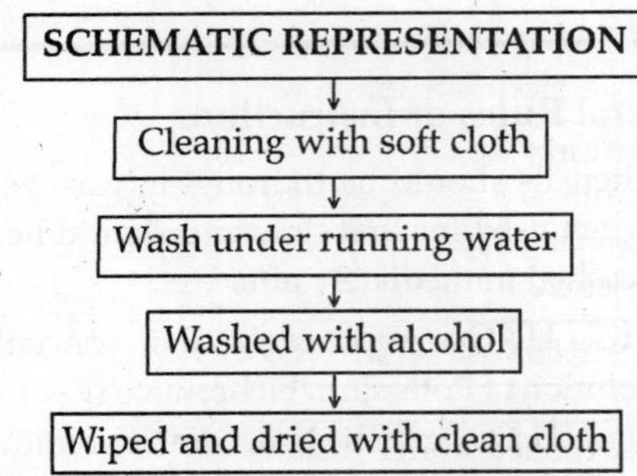

3. Bottles

(i) The bottles are kept in the cold or rain water for 6-7 hours. By using hard brush they are washed several times by shaking and brushing consecutively to remove stains, precipitates or dirt.

(ii) Then they are washed with moderately warm water and rubbed with soft brush.

(iii) Then they are washed with purified water.

(iv) Lastly some amount of strong alcohol is poured inside the bottles to wash them properly.

(v) Then the bottles are exposed to sun for drying purpose.

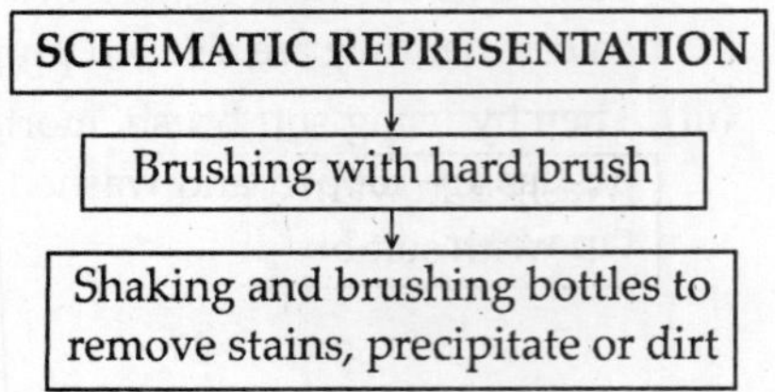

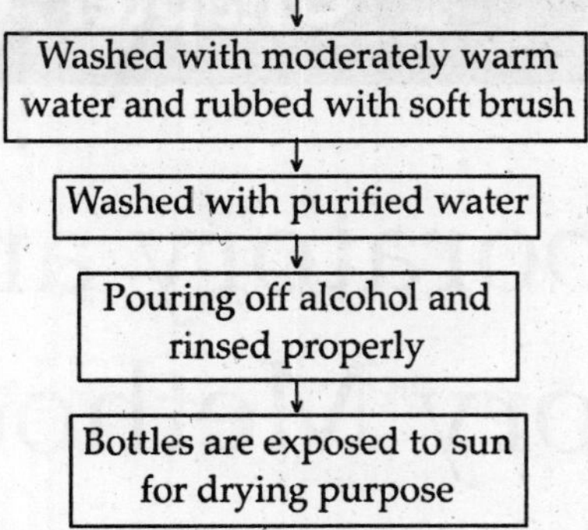

4. **Corks**

(i) The corks are firstly rubbed under running tap-water and then with purified water in a hair-sieve.

(ii) Then they are kept to dry and, after drying, again rinsed with dilute alcohol.

(iii) Afterwards, they are dried thoroughly at a moderate temperature under sunrays.

Note: The corks should never be treated with hot water or steam as it gives them irregular shape and dingy colour. As soon as they shrink, they should be rejected.

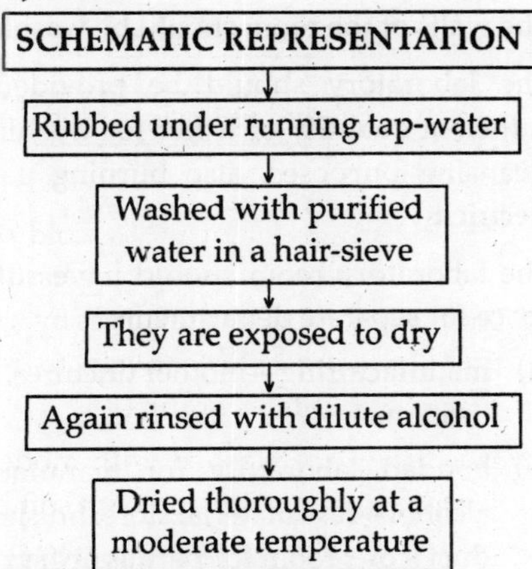

5. **Wooden Instruments**

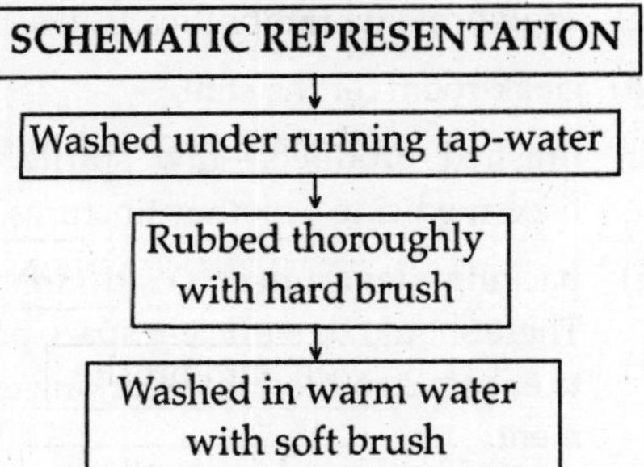

Final wash by purified water

↓

Dried thoroughly at a moderate temperature

(i) Wooden instrument is washed under running tap-water and rubbed thoroughly with hard brush.

(ii) It is then washed with warm water with soft brush.

(iii) Lastly, purified water is used to give it a final wash.

(iv) It is then kept under sunlight for drying.

6. **Tincture Press:** The press is separated into its component parts. Then the parts are washed carefully with cold and hot water, next with purified water. Then they are dried well, after each tincture has been made.

7. **Phials and glasses:** The dust is removed by shaking. Then they are washed several times with hot water, using phial brush. Then rinsed with alcohol. After that, dried at moderate temperature.

8. **Knife:** It should always be wiped off after washing and kept dry to avoid rusting.

9. **Percolator:** It is cleaned after each preparation throughout the filter-bed and washing by the same method as the process adopted in cleaning bottle and phials. The velvet cork which is used earlier is to be thrown away.

10. **Burette:** The burette should be carefully washed free from grease. If it contains grease, the solution in the burette will leave a tail behind when it is run out of it, making it difficult to take a correct reading of the burette. In such a case, the burette should be cleaned with sodium carbonate, using burette brush and then washed with purified water. If the burette still contains grease, it should be cleaned with a little chromic acid solution or a mixture of alcohol and ether, and then with purified water. The burette should not contain any adhering grease.

Chapter 06

General Laboratory and Laboratory Methods

HOMOEOPATHIC LABORATORY

Location and Surroundings

1. Laboratory should never be situated adjacent to any factory which produces noxious vapours, fumes, dusts etc.
2. It should not be situated in a place close to open sewage, public lavatory or unsanitary filthy surroundings.
3. General environment should be non-polluting.

Room

1. "The room where homoeopathic remedies are prepared, including the cutting, pounding and triturating, should be protected from the rays of the sun, but should be light, airy and dry; all emanations that might vitiate the air of the room, as dust, smoke, dampness, and foetid smells, must be rigidly excluded". (WM. H. Burt).
2. The room temperature should be moderately comfortable. There should be constant circulation of fresh air and good arrangement for exhaust.
3. The entry of bright light—artificial or natural—in room should be avoided.
4. The room should be air-conditioned if possible.
5. The walls of the room should be washable.
6. The laboratory should be provided with sufficient quantity of water for washing and cleansing purposes, also burning gas, and electricity.
7. The laboratory room should have sufficient space for separate departments:
   (a) manufacturing—mother tinctures, potentisation,
   (b) bonded laboratory for manufacturing alcohol—raw material store; finished product store; room for permissible products by Govt. Excise Department,
   (c) analytical laboratory,
   (d) cloak-room for the staff,
   (e) finished products—raw spirits, potentised medicines, mother-tinctures,
   (f) packing department(s) administration. There should be sufficient space provided to ensure a comfortable working environment.

Furniture

1. The laboratory should be furnished moderately.
2. They should be of seasoned wood, well-polished, kept clean and be well-cared.
3. Newly polished furniture should be dried first and then washed.
4. Drawers should be so made that medicines can be kept separate from each other and not jumbled up together.
5. All tables should be provided with marble or sunmica tops.

Arrangements

1. The raw materials and finished products (e.g., mother tinctures, potentised medicines and triturations) should be kept separately.
2. The working room as well as store room for raw material and finished products should be separate.
3. Each raw material should be kept properly and each finished product should be well-stoppered and properly labelled.
4. Storage of all drugs should be in closed cupboards away from direct sunlight. Each drug must be well-stoppered and labelled.
5. Strong odorous drugs should be always kept away from the other drugs.

Workers

1. They must have a cloak-room to change their clothings and shoes.
2. They must be free from any contagious or obnoxious disease.
3. They should be provided with clean dresses and wear masks or clean clothes on the face, covering mouth and nose. They should also be provided with head-wears and washable shoes.
4. All dresses should be sterilised before use.
5. Workers should wash their hands and feet using some disinfectant soaps.

Laboratory Equipments

All manufacturing laboratories of homoeopathic medicines should have an attached analytical laboratory with various scientific apparatus, instruments and appliances for identifying and testing for purity and quality control of homoeopathic drugs and medicines.

(a) For manufacturing: Mortar and pestle; spatula; sieves; presses; bottles; corks; chopping board; chopping knife; balance; spoon; funnel; water bath; measuring cylinder; volumetric flasks; burettes; pipettes; graduated dropping pipettes; graduated conical testing glasses; percolator etc.

(b) For analytical laboratory: Analytical balance; rough balance; hot air oven; water bath; microscope; vacuum pump; hydrometer; thermometer; various glass apparatus.

Functions

The important function of this homoeopathic laboratory is to identify and to test for purity of homoeopathic drugs. This is a very important factor. For the sake of experimentation it becomes necessary even to prepare the drug from the raw material. Such experimentation can further determine the standards for the drugs. This experimentations later on can be utilised on the larger scale to prepare commercial quantity of drugs.

LABORATORY METHODS

1. Solution

(a) *Definition of true solution:* The true solution is a perfectly homogeneous mixture of two or more substances, of which the relative quantities may be varied up to a certain limit.

(b) *Characteristics of a true solution:*

(i) are not distinguishable by their surfaces of separation.

(ii) are not separable by filtration or such forces as gravity.

(iii) can be obtained back in the pure form by such methods as crystallisation, evaporation etc.

(iv) retain their characteristic properties within the mixture to reveal their existence, although they may not be exactly identical with the properties when they exist separately.

(c) *Solute and Solvent:* Any solution consists of two components, viz. the dissolved substances, called the solutes, and the medium in which the solutes are uniformly dispersed through dissolution, known as the solvent. It should be mentioned here that in a solution it is not always very easy to determine which of the substances is the solvent and which is the solute. Usually, the component which is the pure form has the same physical state as the solution itself, is considered as the solvent. Solution = Solute + Solvent.

(d) *Concentration of Solution: Saturated, Unsaturated and Supersaturated solution*—The concentration of a solution is the quantity of the solute contained in a definite weight or in a definite volume of the solution. Solutions with high solute-contents are called concentrated solutions and those with low solute contents are called dilute solutions:

(i) Saturated Solution: Concentration of a solution may be varied from a very low to a sufficiently high value by dissolving more and more quantities of the solute in a given quantity of the solvent. But, during this act of dissolving, it is found that, at a given temperature, as the amount of solute is increased, the rate of dissolution decreases and more vigorous stirring for a longer time is required for the dissolution. After that, a state is reached when the medium refuses to dissolve any further quantity of the solute which, if added, is precipitated, if the temperature is kept constant. This is known as saturation and such a solution is called a saturated solution. Thus, when a certain quantity of a solvent has dissolved as much of a solute as is possible for it to dissolve at a particular temperature, the resultant solution is said to be saturated at that particular temperature.

Saturated solution = Solvent + Excessive solute.

(ii) Unsaturated Solution: If a solution contains less amount of the solute than what is necessary for preparing its saturated solution in the given volume of the solvent and at the given temperature, then such a solution is called an unsaturated solution.

Unsaturated solution = Solvent + less amount of solute.

(iii) Supersaturated Solution: Under certain conditions, e.g., by applying heat, sometimes it is possible to prepare a solution which contains more amount of the solute in a given volume of the solvent than is necessary to make a saturated solution at a given temperature. Such a solution is called a supersaturated solution. Supersaturated solution = Saturated solution + solute.

(e) *Tests of Saturated, Unsaturated and Supersaturated Solution:* If a solution, for example of sugar in water, is to be tested as to whether it is saturated, unsaturated or supersaturated at particular temperatures, a small lump of sugar is to be introduced into the given solution and the following observations are made:

(i) If the lump of sugar does not dissolve or does not change in size or shape, the solution is saturated.

(ii) If the lump of sugar dissolves either wholly or partially (and the concentration of solution is consequently increased), then the solution is unsaturated.

(iii) If the lump of sugar does not dissolve but grows in size (and the concentration of solution consequently diminishes), then the solution is supersaturated.

2. Dilution

(a) *Definition:* Dilution means act of diluting i.e. simply mixing of a liquid with water or any other liquid such as alcohol. As a result, physico-chemical property is reduced but the material quantity is greatly increased.

(b) *Examples:* Nitric acid in crude state when touched with finger, burns it, but when a diluent, say purified water, in good proportion is added to it, it loses its irritating or burning power. The more it is diluted with purified water the more it loses its inner strength, whereas it is increased in quantity more it is diluted.

3. General Laboratory Methods for Purification in Homoeopathic Pharmacy:

e.g., Sedimentation; Decantation; Filtration; Evaporation; Distillation; Sublimation; Crystallisation; Precipitation etc.

Sedimentation

This is the simplest method of separating an insoluble solid from a liquid. When an insoluble solid remains suspended in a liquid (e.g., suspension of clay in water), the solid particles tend to settle down at the bottom of the vessel, if such a mixture is allowed to stand undisturbed for some time (the rate of settling depends mainly on the size and weight of the suspended particles). This process of settling is known as sedimentation and the solid that settles at the bottom of the vessel is called the sediment.

Decantation

It is a process of slowly and carefully pouring out liquids (or solution or tincture) from one vessel to another without disturbing the sediments that have been accumulated at the bottom of the liquid.

It is a rather crude method of separating a liquid (or solution or tincture) from its insoluble solid contents, which settle down at the bottom.

Application: This method is applied in cases of mother tincture or solutions or other liquid preparations, for making them bright by removing their insoluble solid contents.

Filtration

(a) *Definition:* It is an efficient physical process of separation of a liquid—a pure solvent or a solution containing dissolved substances—from the substance(s) insoluble in that liquid with the help of a filter paper (or other filtering medium), through which only the liquid (solvent or solution) can pass but not the other substances insoluble in that liquid.

(b) *Principle:* The process of decantation takes longer time to purify the liquid. Besides, if the particles are too minute—then, after filtration, it is seen that particles remain floating on the surface. For this proper purification of water or other liquid—filtration is necessary.

It involves dissolution of the substance (i.e. the soluble component of the mixture) in water (or the solvent in which it is soluble, while others are not) followed by separation of the solution through a filter paper properly folded and fitted in a filtering funnel, when the insoluble substances will be retained by the filter paper (called the residue) and the solution will pass through the filter paper and collect in a receiver placed beneath the funnel (called the filtrate)

(c) *Apparatus:* (i) 2 beakers (ii) A glass rod (iii) A glass funnel (iv) Filter paper (v) Ring clamped in stand.

(d) *Experiment:*

(i) Say, 10 ml of water is taken in a beaker and one spoonful of sand is poured and thoroughly mixed.

(ii) A piece of filter-paper is folded into halves and then into quadrants. It is then unfolded with three-quadrants on one side and one quadrant on the others, so that a cone is formed. This is fitted to the funnel and is fixed to it by moistening with a little water.

(iii) The funnel with the filter paper is placed on a ring clamped to a stand.

(iv) An empty clean beaker is placed under the funnel in such a position that the

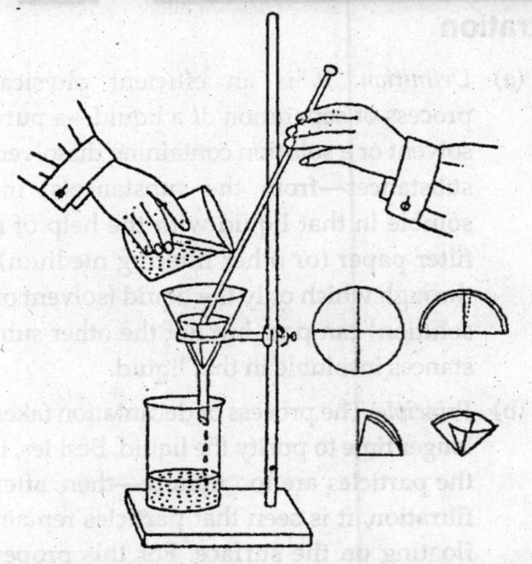
Filtration

stem of the funnel touches the inner side of the beaker.

(v) Now, the solution from the first beaker is poured on the thicker side of the filter cone down the glass rod held against the spout of the beaker.

(vi) The sand is arrested by the filter paper and the purified liquid passes through and is collected in the beaker below.

Special Process of Filtration

A. Rapid Filtration (filtration under reduced pressure)

The ordinary filtration process works slowly and hence the process is time-consuming. The operation can be hastened by adopting rapid filtration process:

Apparatus: (1) A special type of funnel (called Buchner funnel) fitted with a porous plate acting as the filtering medium. (2) A conical flask with a side-tube. The funnel is fitted (air-tight) to the mouth of the flask with the help of a rubber stopper and the side-tube is connected to a water-pump by means of a pressure tube.

Procedure: The mixture to be filtered is poured into the funnel after covering the filtering bed with a piece of filter paper cut exactly according to the shape and size of the porous plate. On running the pump, filtration is performed rapidly.

B. Hot Filtration

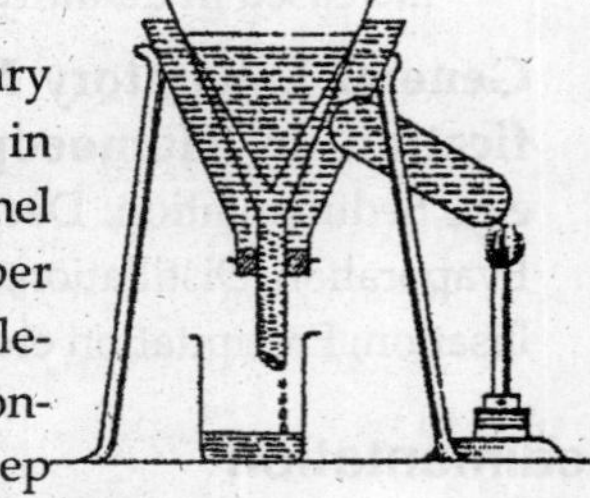

When it is necessary to filter the mixture in that condition, the funnel with the filter paper is placed in a double-walled copper-cone, containing hot water to keep the mixture hot during filtration.

This type of filtration is required where one of the components of the mixture is soluble in hot water but is insoluble in the cold, since the solution made at higher temperature will get cooled and the substances precipitated during ordinary filtration.

"Decantation prior to filtration"—Explain it.

Decantation prior to filtration is necessary, because by decantation only the clear supernatant

Table 6.1: Differences between Decantation and Filtration

Decantation	Filtration
1. In decantation, floating solid substances are sedimented.	1. In filtration, floating solid substance remains as a residue in filter paper.
2. As the weight of solid substance is greater than that of the liquid, the solids are sedimented.	2. Filtration never depends upon the weight of solid substance.
3. It is difficult and time-consuming for complete separation of minute floating substances in the process of decantation.	3. The minute floating solid substances can be separated easily, in short time.
4. The floating substances cannot be separated from colloidal solution by decantation.	4. The floating substances cannot be separated from colloidal solution by simple filter paper. Special membrane is necessary for this purpose.

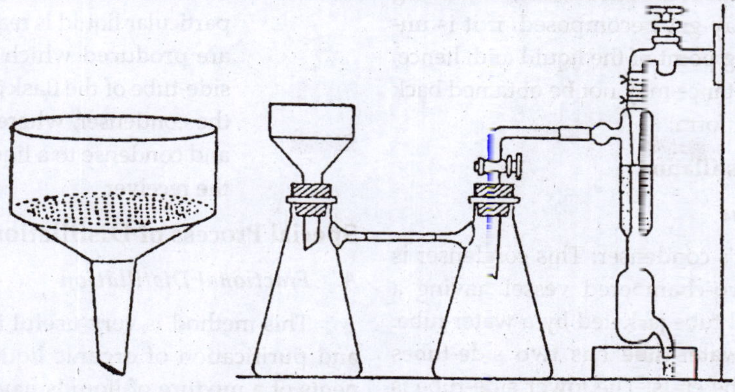

Rapid Filtration

fluid is allowed to pour in another vessel and the solid or semi-solid residues left behind.

If filtration is carried out without decantation, the filter-paper through which the filtration is performed will be choked up with the solid or semi-solid matters and the fluid substance will not be able to pass through the filter paper and there will be a considerable loss by evaporation on account of delay.

Evaporation

It is the simple process of evaporating a liquid (solvent) slowly from the solution, when the solid (solute) is left behind as the residue.

If the liquid is low-boiling i.e., easily volatile (e.g., alcohol, chloroform, ether etc), the solution is taken in a basin and kept exposed to air when the liquid slowly evaporates leaving the solid as the residue.

In other cases, the solution is taken in a water-bath and is slowly warmed or slowly heated by placing it on a suitable heat-bath, which is choosen according to the boiling point of the liquid and the nature of the solid.

Distillation

1. **Definition:** Distillation is a process of purification of liquid substances (i) firstly by converting it at its boiling point into its vapour state by the application of heat or by reduction of pressure—this is known as vapourisation, and (ii) then converting the solid vapour into the former liquid state by cooling, which is known as condensation and the liquid collected in receiver—called distillate.

It is a rapid process and it has the advantage over evaporation (or vapourisation) in that the liquid (solvent) can be recovered. But its main

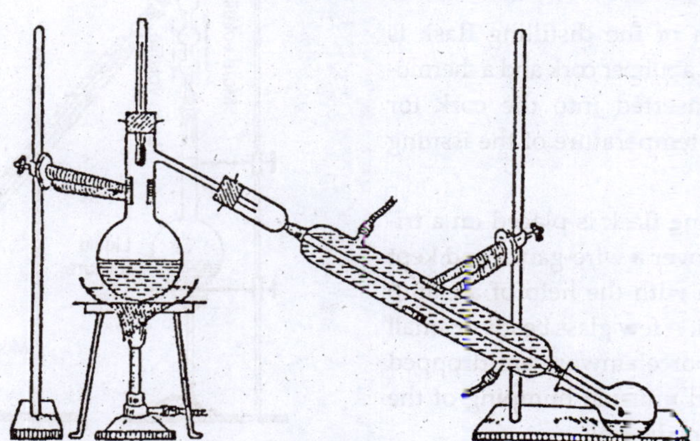

Distillation

disadvantage is that some substances, remaining dissolved in it, may get decomposed, if it is unstable at the boiling point of the liquid and, hence, the dissolved substance may not be obtained back in its pure original form.

2. **Process of Distillation**

(a) *Apparatus*

(i) Liebig's condenser: This condenser is the two-chambered vessel having a central tube jacketed by a water-tube. This water-tube has two side-tubes near the ends. The lower side-tube is attached with a water-tap by means of a rubber tube. When the tap is opened, water enters into the jacket-tube, cools the central tube and comes out through the second side tube at the upper side.

(ii) Flasks: 2 in number: one distilling flask and one receiving flask (to collect the distillate).

(iii) Bunsen burner.

(iv) Tripod stand and wire-gauze.

(b) *Procedure*

(i) The substance to be distilled is taken in a round-bottomed distilling flask. This distilling flask has a side-tube at the top. This side tube is connected by means of a board cork to one end of the Liebig's condenser, the other end of the condenser is inserted into a vessel, called the receiver, to collect the distillate.

(ii) The mouth of the distilling flask is closed with a rubber cork and a thermometer is inserted into the cork for noting the temperature of the issuing vapour.

(iii) The distilling flask is placed on a tripod stand over a wire-gauze and kept in position with the help of a clamp and a stand. A few glass beads or small pieces of porcelainware are dropped in, to avoid unusual bumping of the liquid during boiling.

(iv) The liquid in the distilling flask is heated. When the boiling point of a particular liquid is reached, its vapours are produced which come out of the side-tube of the flask and pass through the condenser, where they cool down and condense to a liquid and collect in the receiver.

Special Process of Distillation

A. *Fractional Distillation*

This method is very useful in the separation and purification of organic liquids. The components of a mixture of liquids having different but somewhat close boiling points may be separated from one another more or less completely by this process. To achieve such separations, a condenser along with a fractionating column is used instead of a single straight condenser. The fractionating columns are so designed that the vapours of the higher boiling liquid (less volatile) are preferentially condensed and return to the distilling flask, where the vapours of the low-boiling liquid (more volatile) are allowed to pass on and condense to liquid in the condenser and, in this way, separation of liquids is made possible.

So long as a particular liquid is distilled off, the temperature, as recorded by the thermometer (inserted in the distilling flask or in the fractionating column), remains unaltered and the liquid is collected in a receiver. As soon as the next higher boiling liquid begins to distil over, the temperature

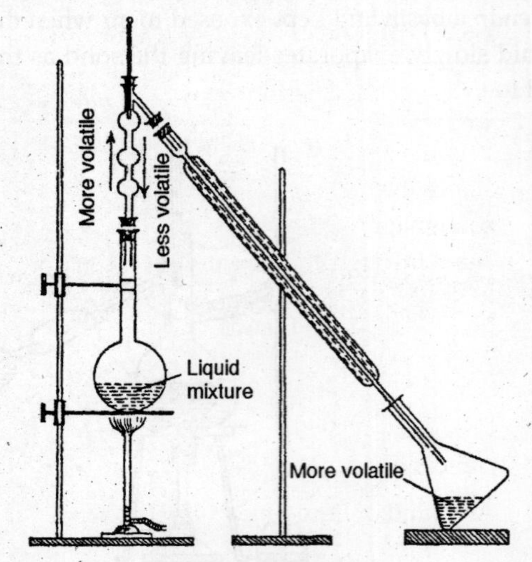

Fractional Distillation

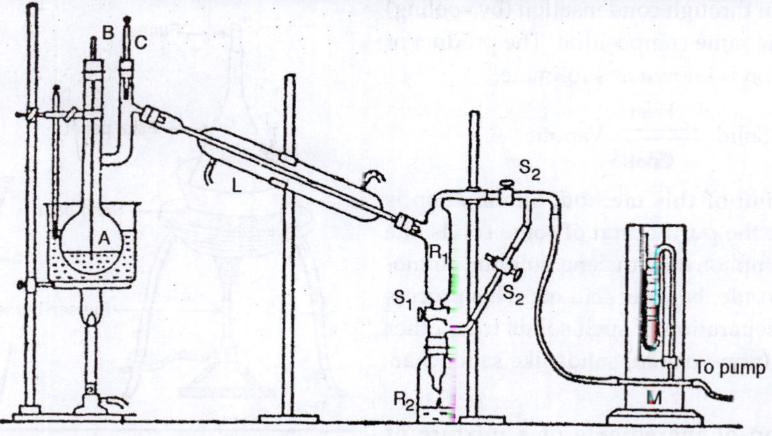

Claisen's Distilling Flask: A. Stops overflow of liquid due to bumping, B. A capillary tube, helps uniform boiling, C. It is a thermometer; L. A Liebig condenser. S_1, S_2 and S_3 are stop-cocks which keep the vacuum of the system intact. R_2. the receiver, can be changed. M is a manometer

changes and the receiver is also then changed. In this way, pure liquids are collected separately.

B. ***Distillation under Reduced Pressure (Vacuum Distillation)***

Distillation of a liquid is affected by atmospheric pressure, since its boiling point depends upon the prevailing atmospheric pressure. If the pressure over a liquid is lowered by some means, its boiling point is also found to be lowered down. Liquids which are susceptible to decomposition at their normal boiling points are distilled at reduced pressures, when they boil at lower temperatures.

This can be done by connecting the distilling flask, through the condenser and the receiver, to a suction-pump (either a water-pump or an oil-pump—depending on the extent of vacuum to be created). The remaining steps are similar to simple or fractional distillations.

Particular occasions where distillation is employed:

Distillation method is employed for the purification of (i) Water, (ii) Alcohol.

Sublimation

1. **Definition:** It is the process of converting a solid substance directly into vapour on heating without being converted to the liquid state and reconversion of the vapour to the solid

Table 6.2: Differences between Distillation and Sublimation

Distillation	Sublimation
1. It is the process of converting a liquid substance directly into vapour on heating and reconversion of the vapour to the liquid state again through condensation (by cooling): $\text{Liquid} \underset{\text{Cool}}{\overset{\text{Heat}}{\rightleftharpoons}} \text{Vapour}$	1. It is the process of converting the solid substance directly into vapour on heating without being converted to the liquid state and reconversion of the vapour to the solid state again through condensation (by cooling): $\text{Solid} \underset{\text{Cool}}{\overset{\text{Heat}}{\rightleftharpoons}} \text{Vapour}$
2. Generally, distillation is possible in liquid substances.	2. Iodine, camphor-like solid substances may undergo sublimation.
3. Any kind of liquid may undergo distillation.	3. Sublimation is not possible for all kinds of solids.
4. Boiling point of the solution is constant.	4. Boiling point of the solution is not constant.

state again through condensation (by cooling) having the same composition. The product of sublimation is known as sublimate.

$$\text{Solid} \underset{\text{Cool}}{\overset{\text{Heat}}{\rightleftharpoons}} \text{Vapour}$$

2. **Application of this method:** Sublimation is useful for the purification of some solids like iodine, camphor, naphthalene, sulphur, ammonium chloride, benzoic acid etc. This process helps in separation of such solids from other common (non-volatile) solids like sand, charcoal etc.

3. **Separation of ingredients of a mixture of Sand and Iodine (or camphor) through sublimation**

(a) *Principle of separation*: Of the two ingredients of the mixture, only iodine (or camphor) can be sublimed, but not the sand. Therefore, it is possible to separate sand from iodine (or camphor) by the process of sublimation.

(b) *Apparatus:* (i) An evaporating porcelain basin, (ii) A funnel with a long stem and wide mouth, (iii) A few pieces of filter paper, (iv) A mortar and a pestle, (v) A tripod stand, (vi) Sand-bath, (vii) Bunsen burner.

(c) *Procedure*

(i) The given mixture of sand and iodine (or camphor) is taken in the mortar and thoroughly mixed with the help of the pestle.

(ii) The mixture is then transferred to the evaporating basin which is placed on the sand-bath over the tripod stand.

(iii) The mixture in the basin is covered by the funnel placed in inverted position, the outer surfaces and the stem of which are wrapped with filter-paper soaked in water.

(iv) Now, the basin with the mixture is warmed slowly by heating the sand-bath with Bunsen burner below the bath.

(v) Iodine (or camphor) will sublime and collect on the cooled inner surfaces of the funnel in the form of small violet crystals (or white crystals in the case of camphor).

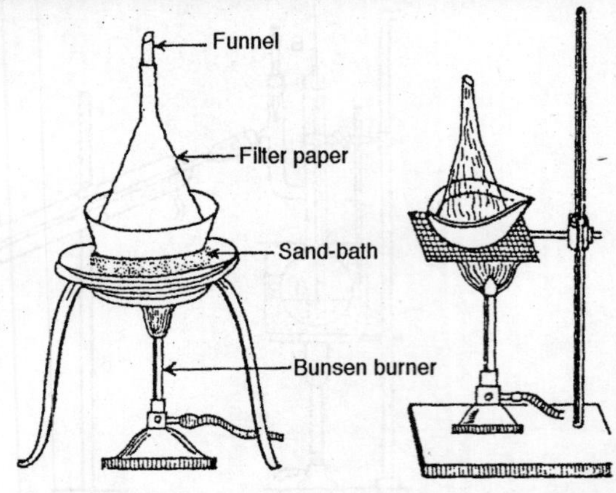

Sublimation Sublimate

(vi) After some time, when sublimation is supposed to be complete, the burner is put off, the basin is taken out of the sand-bath and allowed to cool.

(vii) The funnel is then taken out and the iodine (or camphor) is collected by scraping the inner surfaces of the funnel.

Crystal and Crystallisation

1. **Definition:** When the solution of a solid substance in a liquid, saturated at a higher temperature, is allowed to cool down it is usually found that a quantity of the solid held in solution is deposited at the bottom spontaneously in the form of particles with regular geometric shapes. These particles are called crystals and the process of formation of crystals is known as crystallisation.

Crystals are homogeneous solids with definite geometric shapes and bounded by definite number of plane faces meeting in sharp edges, which they spontaneously acquire during their formation.

2. **Examples:** Each solid has got its own crystalline form. Crystal of common salt (Natrum mur–NaCl) is cubic, of Alum (Alumen) is double-pyramid.

If a perfect crystal is broken, then it breaks in smaller crystals—all of which are similar as the

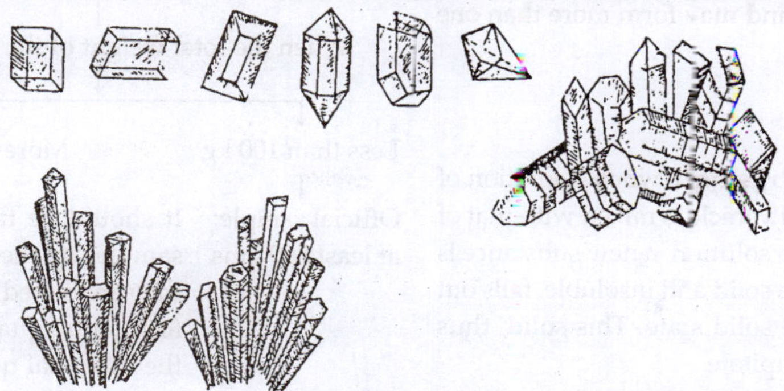

Different shapes of Crystals

bigger mother crystal. The solids which have no crystalline shape are known as amorphous solid, e.g., carbon, sulphur etc.

3. **Principle of Crystallisation:** It is done by cooling saturated solution of solid in a liquid when crystals with definite geometric shape come out gradually from the solution and collect at the bottom.

4. **Different Methods of Crystallisation:** Following methods may be adopted to get solids in their crystalline form:

   (a) Evaporating a saturated solution of a solid in liquid.

   (b) By sublimation and then condensation of substances which have no liquid state, and

   (c) By solidification of a melted substance.

5. **Experiment**

   (a) *First experiment:*

   (i) In a large beaker water is taken and sugar is mixed. Then the mixture is heated to boiling.

   The sugar is added to the beaker until no solid particles are left behind on heating.

   (ii) Then the mixture in hot state is filtered with a filter paper and filtrate is heated with a Bunsen burner until the solution becomes concentrated by evaporating the watery portion of the solution.

   (iii) Concentrated solution is kept in a beaker in cold environment. After one day it is seen that the crystals of sugar deposited at the bottom of the beaker.

   (iv) Then the liquid portion of beaker decanted off and the crystals are dried by blotting paper.

   (b) *Second experiment:* Increase in size of crystals:

   (i) A solution of $CuSO_4$ is made in a beaker and concentrated on heating.

   (ii) A crystal of $CuSO_4$, after tied with a string, suspended in the solution of $CuSO_4$ with the help of a stand.

   (iii) When the solution becomes cold, it will be seen that the $CuSO_4$ of the solution deposited by the side of the suspended $CuSO_4$ crystal and, as a result, size of the crystal become increased.

Application of Crystallisation Method

The crystallisation method is applicable especially in purification of sugar of milk in Stapf's process.

Water of Crystallisation

When crystallised out from saturated solutions, many compounds separate in combination with one or more molecules of water. These water molecules are called water of crystallisation. The number of molecules of water, thus associated with a compound, depends upon the temperature at which crystallisation takes place

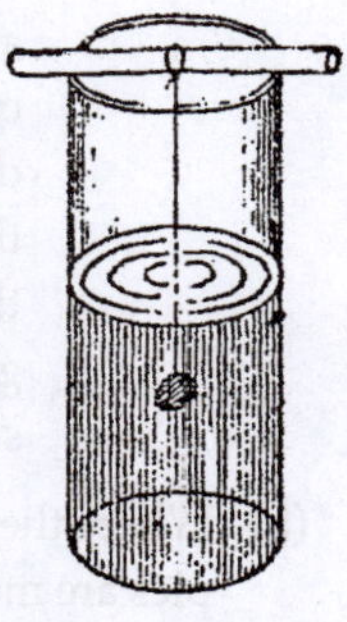

Method of Crystallisation

and the same compound may form more than one hydrate.

Precipitation

This is a process by which, when a solution of a substance in a liquid vehicle is mixed with that of another substance in a solution, a new substance is formed which, being a solid and insoluble, falls out of the solution in the solid state. This solid, thus formed, is called precipitate.

METHOD OF SAMPLING FOR ANALYSIS

A. Process

Official sample of vegetable and animal drugs:

(a) Where the component parts of gross samples are less than 1 cm or less in any dimension, and all powdered or ground drugs.

↓

Taken with the help of sampler which removes a core from the top to the bottom of the container, not more than two cores being taken in opposite directions.

↓

When the total weight of the drug sample:

↓

Less than 100 kg (200 lb)	More than 100 kg
↓	↓
Official sample: at least 250 gms	It should be taken in repeated samples by the same way. Next, they are mixed and divided into four equal quarters. Reject 2 of the diagonal quarters, combine and carefully mix the remaining quarters and again subject the drug to a quartering process in the same manner until two of the quarters weigh at least 250 gms. These latter quarters constitute an official sample.

(b) Where the component parts of gross samples are more than 1 cm in any dimension:

↓

Collect them by hand

↓

When the total weight of the drug sample

↓

Less than 100 kg	More than 100 kg
↓	↓
Official sample: at least 500 gms	It should be taken in repeated samples by the same way. Next, they are mixed and divided into four equal quarters. Reject 2 of the diagonal quarters, combine and carefully mix the remaining quarters and again subject the drug to a quartering process in the same manner until 2 of the quarters weigh at least 500 gm. These latter quarters constitute an official sample.

(c) Where the total weight of the drug sample less than 10 kg:

↓

Same process is to be followed but somewhat smaller quantities be collected

↓

Official sample: at least 125 gms.

B. Preparation of Vegetable or Animal Drugs for Analysis

Following methods is to be used where there is no specific directions given in the text:

Collect official sample by the quartering process as described—as much as may be necessary

↓

In case of unground and unpowdered drugs—grind the collected sample so that it will pass through No. 20 standard mesh sieve.

If the sample cannot be ground, reduce it to as fine a state as possible

↓

Mix it by rolling on paper or sampling cloth

↓

Spread it out in a thin layer and collect the portion for analysis.

C. Determination of the followings

1. Foreign organic matter, 2. Total ash, 3. Acid insoluble ash, 4. Water soluble ash, 5. Sulphated ash, 6. Moisture content, 7. Total solids, 8. Alcohol soluble extractives, 9. Water soluble extractives,

10. Alcohol content, 11. Weight per millimeter, 12. Specific gravity, 13. Boiling range, 14. Melting range, 15. Congealing temperature, 16. Refractive index, 17. Optical rotation and specific rotation, 18. pH value, 19. Acid value, 20. Saponification value, 21. Ester value, 22. Iodine value, 23. Chromatographic analysis.

Determination of Foreign Organic Matter

25–500 gm of the official sample is weighed

↓

Spreadout in a thin layer

↓

The foreign organic matter is separated by hand as completely as possible

↓

Then weight is taken

Then the percentage of foreign organic matter is determined being calculated from the weight of the drugs taken.

For coarse or bulky drug the maximum quantity of the sample is taken.

Determination of Total Ash

About 2–3 gm of powdered drug is taken in a tared platinum or silica dish.

Incinerate at a temperature not exceeding 45.0°C until free from carbon. Then cooled and weighed.

If a carbon free ash cannot be obtained in this way:

Exhaust the charred mass with hot water and residue is collected on an ashless filter paper. Incinerate residue plus filter paper, filter, evaporate filtrate to dryness and heat at a temperature not exceeding 450°C.

Then cooled and weighed.

Then percentage of total ash is calculated with reference to air-dried drug powder.

Determination of Acid Insoluble Ash

The total ash (as obtained in the above method) is boiled with 25 ml dilute alcohol for 5 minutes.

The insoluble matter is collected on an ashless filter-paper or a tared Gooch crucible.

Washed with hot water.

Ignited at a low temperature to constant weight.

Percentage of acid-insoluble ash is calculated from the weight of the air-dried drug taken.

Determination of Water-soluble Ash

The total ash (as obtained in the above method) is boiled with 25 ml of water for 5 minutes.

The insoluble matter is collected on an tared Gooch crucible or on an ashless filter-paper. Washed with hot water.

Ignited it at low temperature to constant weight.

From the weight of total ash, subtract the weight of insoluble matter obtained, and this difference of weight represents the weight of water soluble ash. Percentage of water soluble ash is calculated from the weight of the air-dried drug taken.

Determination of Sulphated Ash

2–3 gm (approx.) accurately weighed air-dried drug is taken in a silica dish.

Moistened with concentrated H_2SO_4.

Ignited gently.

Again, moistened with concentrated H_2SO_4 and reignited.

Next, cooled and weighed.

The percentage of sulphated ash is calculated with reference to the air-dried drug.

Determination of Moisture Content

Following three classes are to be considered to determine the volatile matter (i.e., moisture or water), present in vegetable drug substances and proceed accordingly:

1. When water is the only volatile constituent in the substance—about 10 gm of fresh drug material is taken after accurate weighing, having previously cut into smallest possible pieces.
2. If the drugs are unground or unpowdered, about 10 gm of official sample is prepared by cutting and spreading, so that the parts are about 3 mm in thickness. These are placed in tared evaporating dish.

3. Seeds and fruits larger than 3 mm should be cracked to render them about 3 mm in thickness. High speed mills are avoided in preparing the sample.

Following three methods are employed for the determination of moisture content:

A. *Gravimetric method (as per U.S.P.):* 10 gm (approx.) of the drug, prepared as directed and accurately weighed, is placed on a tared evaporating dish

↓

Dried on a water-bath, until the residue is apperently dry

↓

Transferred to an oven and dried at 105°C for 5 hours, and weighed

↓

Continued the drying and weighing at 1 hour intervals until the difference between two successive weighings corresponds to not more than 0.25%.

B. *Volumetric method (Toluene distillation method):* With the help of Toluene moisture apparatus water may be determined by volume measurement.

The sample and the Toluene ($C_6H_5CH_3$) is placed in flask (A) and the mixture is distilled. Toluene and water form an azeotropic mixture (a mixture of organic liquids with different boiling temperatures but distilling at a constant temperature) and redistill into the condenser (C) and the cooled vapour, after condensation, fall back into receiver (R). Water, being of greater density than toluene, falls to the graduated portion E and the volume read directly. Care must be taken to ensure that any water droplets adhering to 'R' or 'C' are washed into E.

C. *Titrimetric method (Karl Fischer method):*

This method depends upon the fact that a solution of SO_2 and iodine in pyridine and methanol reacts with water quantitatively. The entire operation requires rigid exclusion of atmospheric moisture.

In colourless solution: the end-point of titration may be determined electrometrically or visually by a change from a canary yellow to an amber colour.

In coloured solution: the end-point is obscured and is best determined electrometrically.

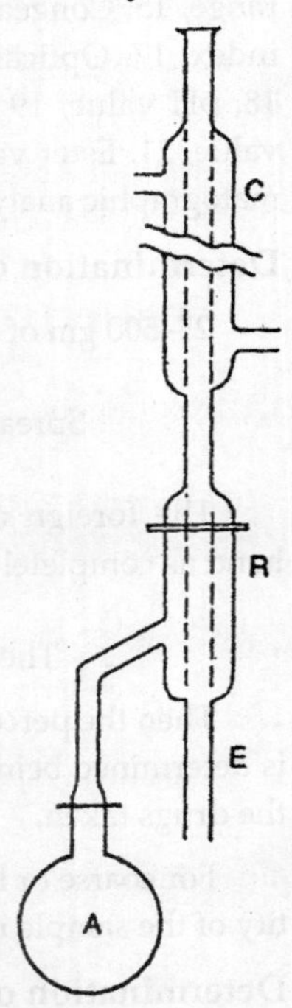

Toluene Distillation Method

Apparatus: The required apparatus embodies a simple electrical circuit which serves to pass 5–10 microamperes (1 ampere = 100 microamperes) or direct current at a 1.5 volt potential between two platinum electrodes immersed in the solution to be titrated. At the end point of titration a slight excess of the reagent increases the flow of current to between 50 and 150 microamperes for 30 seconds or longer—depending upon the solution being titrated. The time is shortest for substances which react with the reagent.

Commercially available apparatus generally comprises a closed system consisting of one or two automatic burettes and tightly covered titration vessel fitted with the necessary electrodes and a magnetic stirrer. The air in the system is kept dry with a drying agent such as P_2O_5, anhydrous granular $CaCl_2$, or silica gel.

Procedure: 25 ml (approx.) of CH_3OH is added to the titration flask and titrate to the end-point with the Karl Fischer reagent, disregarding the volume consumed, since it does not enter into the calculations. Sufficient amount of sample is weighed or measured which contain about 10–50 mg of water and quickly transferred to titration flask. Stirred vigorously and titrated again with Karl Fischer reagent.

The water-content of the sample, in mg, is given by the formula, S × F, where, S = volume of reagent used to titrate the sample and F = water equivalence factor.

Determination of Total Solids

The 'Total Solids' (e.g. chloride, calcium sulphate, heavy metals) means 'residue' obtained when the prescribed amount of the preparation is dried to constant weight under the conditions specified next.

Apparatus: Shallow, flat-bottomed flanged dishes, about 75 mm in diameter and 25 mm deep, made of nickel or other suitable metal of high heat conductivity and which is not affected by boiling water.

Method: An exactly weighed quantity of the preparation is taken in a tared dish

↓

Dried with the help of water-bath

↓

Kept in hot air oven at 105° C for 30 minutes.

↓

The dried dish is again kept in a desiccator

↓

The weight is found out as quickly as possible when cool.

Determination of Alcohol-soluble Extractive

The drug is coarsely powdered and the 5 grams of the powder is macerated with 100 ml of alcohol of specified strength in a closed flask for 24 hours

↓

The flask is shaken frequently

↓

The liquid is filtered

↓

25 ml of the filtrate is dried in a tared-bottomed dish at about 105° C to a constant weight

↓

The weight of the extractive matter will be equivalent to that of 1 gm of the drug. Multiply the same with 100, to give the percentage.

Determination of Water-soluble Extractive

Process 1

Same as determination of alcohol soluble extractive. Chloroform water is used instead of alcohol.

Process 2

5 gm of the sample drug is added to 50 ml of water at 88° C in stoppered flask

↓

Well shaken and allowed to stand for 10 minutes

↓

Cool to 15° C and 2 gm of kieselguhr is added and then filtered.

5 ml of the filtrate is transferred to a tared evaporating basin whose diameter is 7.5 cm

Evaporate the solvent on a water-bath

Continue the drying for 15 minutes and finally dry in steam oven for 2 hours and the residue is weighed.

Percentage of water soluble extractive is calculated from the air-dried drug taken.

Determination of Alcohol Content

Definite amount of test liquid is measured in a round-bottomed 200 to 250 ml flask.

Amount of test-liquid to be taken depends upon the percentage of alcohol present in it.

Take 75 ml for 20% alcohol,

50 ml for 20–50% alcohol,

25 ml for 50% to more alcohol.

(a) *If the test-liquid contains volatile matter (volatile acids or bases):*

(i) For volatile acids—neutralise them with alkali solution.

(ii) For volatile bases—neutralise them with H_3PO_4 and H_2SO_4.

(b) *If test liquid contains free iodine:*

It is treated with small amount of Zn-powder or dry sodium thiosulphate ($Na_2S_2O_3$), the liquids are decolourised. To bind the volatile sulphurous compounds, few drops of NaOH is added.

(c) *If the test liquid contains ether ($C_2H_5-O-C_2H_5$), chloroform ($CHCl_3$), essential oils, camphor etc.:*

Equal volume of saturated NaCl solution and of petroleum ether (boiling point = 30° C to 70° C) is added to the treated sample in a separating funnel. The mixture is shaken for 5 minutes, and wait until two layers separated out within 15–20 minutes.

Run the aqueous alcohol layer into another separating funnel and the same test liquid is treated twice more with half the quantity of petroleum ether.

Run the aqueous alcohol layer into the distilling flask and shake the combined petroleum ether liquids with half the quantity of saturated NaCl solution which is then added to the aqueous alcohol liquid in the distilling flask.

Draw in air through the combined liquid for a minute to remove the last traces of petroleum ether.

(d) *If the test liquid contains less than 30% of alcohol* the salting out should be done with 10 gm dry NaCl instead of its solution.

After completion of the above procedures, the aqueous alcohol liquids are subjected to the process of distillation.

Distillation Process

Before distillation, distilling liquid is made up to 75 ml tight-fitting rubber stoppers are used for the distillation flask and condenser. The receiver (a 50 ml of volumetric flask) should be immersed in a vessel with cold water. For proper uniform boiling, few small beads of porcelain or pumice-stone are added to the distilling flask.

48 ml of distillate is collected in receiver. The temperature brought to room temperature and made up with water to its mark (50 ml volumetric flask). The distillate should be clear or slightly turbid. The specific gravity of the distillate is determined by a specific gravity bottle (also called pyknometer) and the corresponding alcohol contents in percents by volume read off in the alcoholometric table.

The alcohol content of the preparation is calculated in percent by volume from the formula: $X = 50 \times a/b$, where,

X = alcohol per cent of the preparation

50 = volume of the distillates in ml

a = alcohol content of the distillate

b = volume of test liquid taken for distillation

Determination of Weight per Millilitre

The weight per ml of liquid is the weight in gm of 1 ml of a liquid when weighed in air at 20°C.

The weight per millilitre (of a liquid) is determined by dividing the weight in air, expressed in grams, of the quantity of the liquid which fills a pyknometer (also called specific gravity bottle) at 20°C or 25°C, by the capacity of the pyknometer at 20°C or 25°C, respectively, expressed in millilitres.

The capacity of pyknometer at these temperatures is ascertained from the weight in gram of quantity of water required to fill the pyknometer. The weight of 1 ml of water in air at specified temperature is prescribed in the table:

Temperature	Weight of 1 ml of water
20°C	0.99719 gm
25°C	0.99602 gm
30°C	0.99462 gm

Ordinary deviations in the density of air do not affect the result of a determination significantly for pharmacopoeial purposes.

Examples

1. Glycerine, at 25°C = 1.252 – 1.257 gm
2. Almond oil, at 20°C = 0.910 – 0.915 gm
3. Olive oil, at 20°C = 0.910 – 0.913 gm
4. Simple syrup, at 20°C = 1.315 – 1.333 gm
5. White soft paraffin, at 60°C = 0.815 – 0.880 gm

Determination of Specific Gravity

A. *Definition of specific gravity*—The specific gravity of a liquid is the weight of a given volume of the liquid at the specified temperature compared with the weight of an equal column of water at the same temperature in air.

B. *Determination*—The specific gravity of a liquid can be determined by (i) Specific gravity bottle (or Pyknometer) and (ii) Common hydrometer.

(a) Determination of specific gravity of a liquid by a specific gravity bottle

Theory: By definition, Sp. Gr. of a liquid =

$$\frac{\text{Wt. of a given vol. of the liquid } (W_L)}{\text{Wt. of an equal vol. of water } (W_W)} = S$$

If temperature correction is applicable 'S' should be multiplied by the Sp. Gr. St of the water used.

Apparatus: (i) Sp. Gr. bottle, (ii) Common balance, (iii) Weight box, (iv) Experimental liquid (say, Methylated spirit or a water solution), (v) Water, (vi) Blotting paper or old soft cloth.

Observations

Wt. of the dry, empty bottle (with stopper) = + + + = ... g wt (W_1)

Wt. of bottle, filled with liquid = + + + = ... g wt (W_2)

Wt. of bottle, filled with water = + + + = ... g wt (W_3).

Calculations

Wt. of the liquid ($= W_2 - W_1$) = ... – ...... = ... g wt (W_L)

Wt. of same vol. of water ($= W_3 - W_1$) = ... g wt (W_W)

∴ Specific gravity of the liquid = (W_L / W_W) = ▬ = ...

Method followed

1. The bottle was cleaned and dried.
2. The empty bottle (with the stopper) was weighed after checking the balance.
3. The bottle was filled with the experimental liquid, made free of bubbles, stoppered, wiped, dried and weighed.
4. The liquid was thrown out and the bottle washed several times with water. It was then filled with water, made free of bubbles, stoppered, wiped dry and weighed.

Precautions

1. No bubbles are allowed to stay in the bottle.
2. The bottle was always held by the neck.

(b) Determination of specific gravity of a Liquid by common hydrometer

Requirements: (1) A big glass cylinder, (2) Common hydrometer and (3) The liquid in question.

Procedure: The experimental liquid is taken in the glass cylinder and the hydrometer is slowly and carefully inserted into it. It is seen that upper level of the liquid corresponds with the mark expressing 0.816.

Conclusion: The specific gravity of the experimental liquid is 0.816 and it may be strong alcohol.

Determination of Boiling Range

Definition of boiling range: The boiling range of a substance is the range of temperature within

Table 6.3: Specific gravities of some common substances

Substance	Sp. Gr.	Substance	Sp. Gr.	Substance	Sp. Gr.
Absolute alcohol	0.792	Glycerine	1.255	Rosemary oil	0.894 – 0.912
Strong alcohol	0.816	Almond oil	0.910 – 0.915	Lavender oil	0.875 – 0.888
Dilute alcohol	0.89	Olive oil	0.910 – 0.913	Spermaceti	0.94
Dispensing alcohol	0.840	Sandalwood oil	0.970 – 0.978	Soft paraffin	0.815 – 0.880
Rectified spirit	0.812	Seasame oil	0.916 – 0.921		

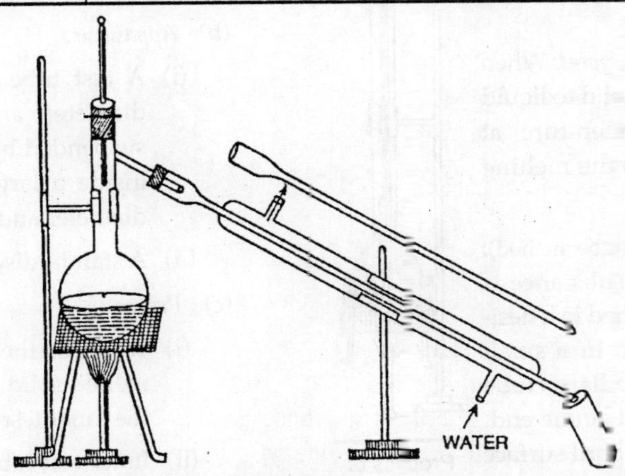

Process of boiling range

which the whole or a specified part of the substance distils.

Definition of boiling point: Boiling proceeds at a definite temperature for any single substance at a fixed pressure. This temperature is called boiling point. This is denoted usually at one atmospheric pressure.

Procedure: 100 ml of the test liquid is placed in a distillation flask and few glass beads or other suitable substance are added to it.

The bulb of the flask is placed centrally over a circular hole varying from 3-5 cm in diameter in a suitable asbestos board.

The thermometer is held concentrically in the neck of the flask by means of a well-fitted cork in such a manner that the bulb of the thermometer remains just below the level of the opening of the side tube. The flask is heated slowly in the beginning and, when distillation starts, adjusted heating in such a manner that the liquid distils at a constant rate of 4-5 ml per minute.

The temperature is read when the first drop runs from the condenser and again when the last quantity of liquid in the flask is evaporated.

Determination of Melting Range

Definition of melting range: The melting range of a substance is the range between the corrected temperature at which the substance begins to melt, as shown by formation of droplets and the corrected temperature at which it completely melts, as shown by formation of a meniscus.

Definition of melting point: When a change of state from solid to liquid takes place, the temperature at which it takes place is the melting point.

Procedure (Capillary tube method): The little of the drug substance is finely powdered and dried in a desiccator. A little is taken in a small thin-walled glass capillary tube about 5 cm long, sealed at one end. By gently tapping on a hard surface the powdered solid is forced down to the close end. The fine capillary tube is then attached by moistening it with the liquid of the bath to a calibrated thermometer so that the enclosed sample is as near as possible to the middle of the thermometer bulb. The thermometer held by a stand is introduced into a small Jena glass flask, containing a suitable liquid, e.g., conc. H_2SO_4, glycerol, high-boiling liquid paraffin, or castor oil. The bulb of the thermometer and about a half of the capillary tube are under the liquid surface. The flask is heated by a small non-luminous flame slowly (2°C – 3°C per minute). The temperature is noted when the substance begins to melt as shown by the formation of droplets, and again when the substance is completely melt as shown by formation of meniscus.

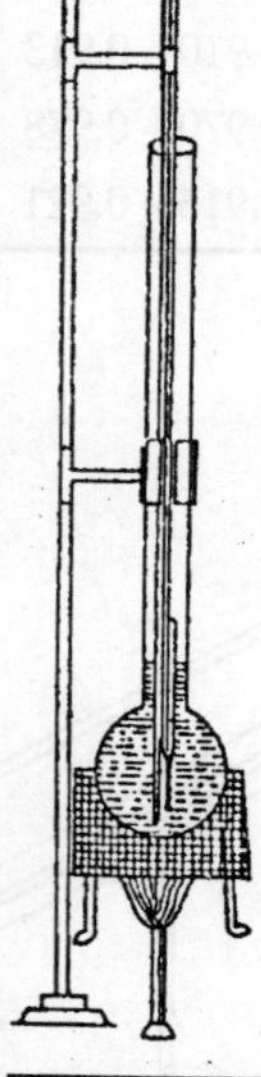

Process of melting range

Examples:

(i) Yellow or white soft paraffin: 38°C – 56°C
(ii) Bee's wax: 60°C – 65°C
(iii) Lanolin (anhydrous): 36°C – 42°C
(iv) Spermaceti: 42°C – 50°C.

Determination of Congealing Temperature

(a) *Definition:* The congealing temperature of a liquid or of a melted solid is the highest temperature at which it solidifies.

The congealing temperature of the liquid is same as the melting temperature of the solid, but since the liquid may be cooled to a temperature below its congealing temperature without assuming the solid form, the following method is employed to determine the congealing temperature of a liquid or a melted solid.

(b) *Apparatus:*

(i) A test tube of about 2 cm internal diameter and about 10 cm long, suspended by means of a bored cork, inside a larger tube, about 3 cm in diameter and 12 cm in length.

(ii) A standardised thermometer.

(c) *Process:*

(i) 10 ml of the liquid or 10 gm of the melted solid to be tested, is placed in the inner test tube previously dried.

(ii) Inner test tube is supended inside the outer tube and cooled together in water or in a suitable freezing mixture in a temperature about 5°C below the expected congealing temperature.

(iii) Temperature of water or freezing mixture is adjusted according to the congealing temperature with a standardised thermometer until it begins to solidify.

The highest temperature reached during solidification is regarded as the congealing temperature.

Determination of Refractive Index

(a) *Definition:* The refractive index (μ) of a transparent substance is the ratio of the velocity of light in vacuum to its velocity in the substance.

It is equal to sine of the angle of incidence made by a ray in air to the sine of the angle of refraction made by the ray in the material being tested.

(b) *Utility:* The refractive index (μ), is a physical property, which is characteristic of a particular substance.

So it is useful for identifying substances and establishing their purity such as liquids, especially those of more volatile ones—thus providing information for detecting adulterations.

Refractive index provides the basis for quantitative analysis of simple mixture as of alcohol and water. If the relationship of refractive index and concentration is known, it is easy to determine the refractive index of a liquid.

(c) *Method:* Both instruments are provided with polished prism with which the liquid to be examined is in contact and through which light that has been refracted through the liquid is also refracted through the prism. The last ray of light entering the prism provides a sharp demarcation between light and dark areas, is determined by refractive index of the liquid.

The index may be read directly, as in the Abbe instrument, or in terms of arbitrary scale, the reading on which may be converted to refractive index by referring to tables supplied with the instrument.

(d) *Examples:*

1. Glycerine, at 20°C = 1.471 to 1.473
2. Almond oil, at 20°C = 1.470 to 1.473
3. Olive oil, at 20°C = 1.468 to 1.471
4. Rosemary oil, at 20°C = 1.466 to 1.476
5. Lavender oil, at 20°C = 1.4590 to 1.4700
6. Sesame oil, at 20°C = 1.472 to 1.476.

Determination of Optical Rotation and Specific Rotation

Polarimeter or polariscope is an instrument for measuring the extent of rotation of polarised light passing through solution containing an optically active substance.

Ordinary visible light consists of rays of various wave lengths (4,000A° – 7,000A°); it vibrates in all directions in space at right angles to its path.

If a beam of monochromatic light (of a single wave length) is passed through transparent crystal of Iceland spar (calcite, $CaCO_3$), it splits up into two, each vibrating in one plane only. The light is said to be plane polarised; the two newly formed rays have different refractive indices. By combining two prisms of Iceland spar, suitably cut, it is possible to have total internal reflection for one of the rays and allow the other to pass on. Such a combination of prisms is called Nicol prism (after William Nicol, a British physicist).

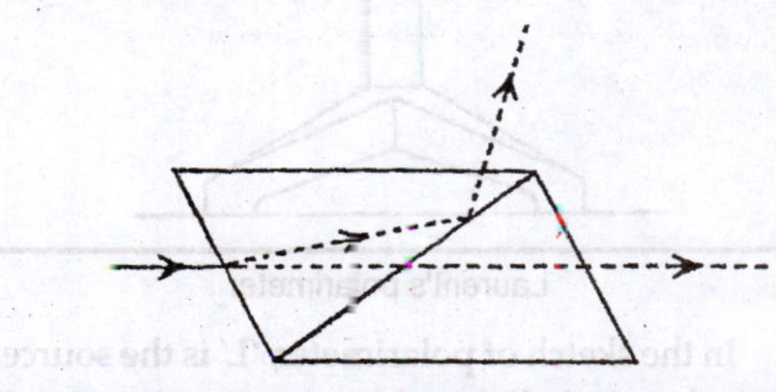

Nicol Prism

If another Nicol prism is placed in the path of the transmitted polarised ray, the effect becomes interesting. In case the axis of the 2nd prism is parallel to that of the first, the polarised beam passes through it with full intensity, but if the prism is rotated through 90°, the polarised ray is completely cut off due to total reflection. The 2nd prism analyser thus enables to find the plane of vibration of the polarised ray. In intermediate positions of the analyser, light of varying intensity will, of course, pass through.

The polariser (1st Nicol prism) and the analyser (2nd Nicol prism) are placed in the same axial line; the polarised ray passes through the analyser with undiminished intensity. Now, if between the two, a solution of certain drug substance is placed, the analyser has to be rotated through a certain angle in order to get the light of original intensity. It must have, therefore, rotated the polarised ray either to the left or to the right. The property by virtue of which many organic and some inorganic compounds turn the plane of plane polarised light to a clockwise or anticlockwise direction is known as optical activity or rotatory polarisation. Compounds which turn the plane towards the right are called dextrorotatory, while those which do so towards the left are Laevorotatory. The dextro- and Laevo-forms are denoted by the prefixes, d– and L– or by +ve and –ve sign, respectively. The construction of polarimeter (or polariscope) which measures such rotation is based on these facts.

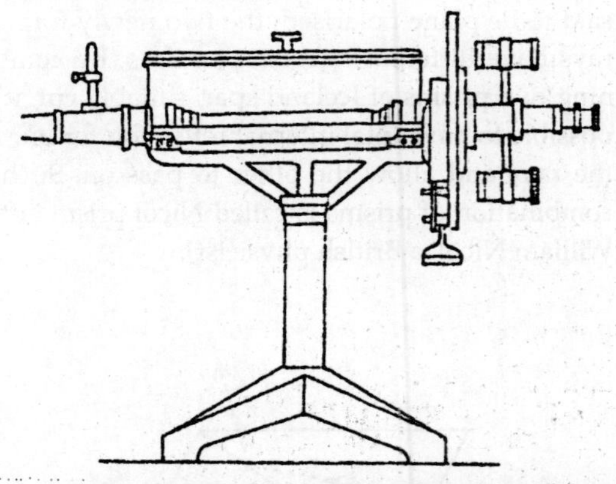

Laurent's polarimeter

In the sketch of polarimeter, 'L' is the source of monochromatic light which emerges out parallel after passing through the lens, A, and is incident upon the polariser, B. O, an observation glass tube with glass ends, contains the sample; D is the analyser. The field of view is observed through the telescope, EF, fixed to a graduated circular scale. C is a semicircular quartz plate of suitable thickness, which changes the phase of transmitted light by half a wavelength and facilitates the accurate determination of the extinction point. The analyser and the circular scale are rigidly connected and rotate simultaneously.

The zero reading of the circular scale is noted with water at the minimum (or maximum) illumination point. The tube is filled with the sample and the scale rotated until the minimum (or maximum) illumination point is again reached. The magnitude and the direction of rotation are known from the scale.

Definition of optical rotation: Optical rotation may also be defined as the angle through which the plane of polarisation is rotated when a layer of a liquid or solution of substance, 1 decimeter (dm) in thickness and at a temperature of 25°C, is examined by sodium light.

Optical rotation is expressed in degrees of either angular rotation (observed) or specific rotation (calculated with reference to the specific concentration of 1 gm of solute in 1 ml of solution measured under stated conditions).

Utility of optical rotation: This property may be utilised either for assaying or identifying a substance.

Procedure:

(i) For liquid drug substance: Minimum 5 readings of the rotation of the liquid and also for the empty tube at the specified temperature is taken.

(ii) For solid drug substance: Dissolve a suitable solvent and 5 readings of the rotation of the solution and the solvent used is taken.

Calculate the average set of 5 readings and find out the correct optical rotation from the observed rotation and the reading with the blank.

Specific Rotation (or Rotatory Power)

The specific rotation of a substance is defined as the rotation in degrees produced by a length of

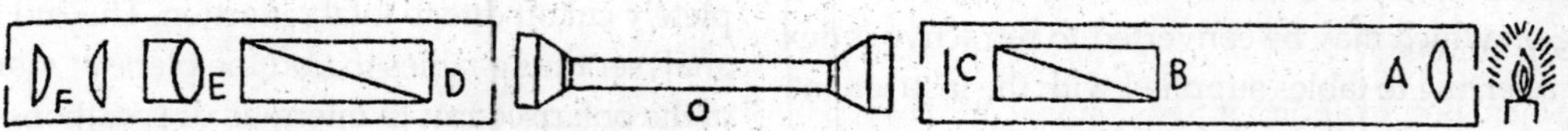

Optical parts of a Polarimeter

a decimeter of solution containing 1 gm of solute per ml.

The rotation varies for different substances. It is proportional to the concentration of the solution as well as the length of the tube. It also varies with temperature, nature of the solvent and wavelength of light used.

Calculations:

For solutions of solid: $[a]^{t}_{\pi} = \dfrac{\alpha^{obs} \times 100}{1 \times C}$

where, α^{obs} = The observed rotation in degrees

l = Length of the tube in decimeter

C = Concentration in gm per cent

$[a]^t/_\pi$ = Specific rotation (a) at temperature (t) and wave length π.

Examples of optical rotation:

1. Sugar of milk, at 20°C = +55.3°
2. Lavender oil, at 20°C = –3° to –10°
3. Rosemary oil, at 20°C = –5° to +10°
4. Simple syrup, at 20°C = +56° to +60°

Determination of Acid Value

Definition: It indicates the amount of free acid present in the fat or oil. It is defined as: 'The number of milligrams of KOH required to neutralise 1 gram of the fat or oil'.

Determination: A weighed quantity of oil or fat is dissolved in alcohol and titrated against standard KOH solution using phenolphthaline as an indicator.

Examples:

(i) Almond oil: Not more than 4.00

(ii) Olive oil: Not more than 2.00

(iii) Lanolin: Not more than 1.

(iv) Spermaceti: Not more than 10

(v) Sesame oil: Not more than 2.0

(vi) Yellow bee's wax: 17 to 23.

Determination of Saponification Value

(H.P.I. – Volume I)

The saponification value is the number of mg of KOH to neutralise the fatty acids, resulting from the complete required hydrolysis of 1 g of the oil or fat, when determined by the following method:

Dissolve 30 – 40 gm of KOH in 20 ml of water, and add sufficient alcohol to make 1,000 ml. Allow it to stand overnight and pour off the clear liquid. Weigh accurately about 2 g of the substance in a tared 250 ml flask, add 25 ml of the alcoholic solution of KOH, attach a reflux condenser and boil on a water-bath for one hour, frequently rotating the contents of the flask; cool and add 1 ml of solution of phenolphthalin and titrate the excess of alkalies with 0.5 (N) HCl. Note the number of ml required (a). Repeat the experiment with the same quantities of the same reagents in the same manner omitting the substance. Note the number of ml required (b). Calculate the saponification value from the following formula:

$$\text{Saponification value} = \frac{(b - a) \times 0.02805 \times 1{,}000}{W}$$

where 'W' is the weight of the substance taken.

Examples:

(i) Olive oil: 200

(ii) Almond oil: 188 – 196

(iii) Coconut oil: 250

(iv) Sesame oil: 188 – 195

(v) Lanolin: 96 – 106

(vi) Spermaceti: 120 – 135.

Determination of Esters

(From H.P.I. – Volume II)

Boil convenient quantity of alcohol (90%) thoroughly to expel CO_2 and neutralise it to solution of phenolphthalin.

Weigh accurately about 2 gm of the oil or ester and dissolve in 5 ml of the neutralised alcohol contained in a hard glass flask, and neutralise the free acid in the solution with 0.1 (N) alcoholic KOH using 0.2 ml of the solution of phenolphthalin as indicator. Add 20 ml of 0.5 (N) alcoholic KOH, attach the flask to a reflux condenser, boil on a water-bath for one hour add 20 ml of water and titrate the excess of alkali with 0.5 (N) H_2SO_4, using a further 0.2 ml of solution of phenolphthalin as indicator.

Repeat the experiment with the same quantities of the same reagents in the same manner, omitting the oil or ester. The difference between the titration figures is equivalent to the alkali required to saponify the esters.

Each ml. of 0.5 (N) alcoholic KOH is equivalent to:

0.1061 gm of benzyl benzoate.

0.09815 gm of bornyl acetate.

0.06959 gm of dibutyl phthalate.

0.1553 gm of ethyl oleate.

0.03637 gm of glyceryl triacetate.

0.09915 gm of methyl acetate.

0.07608 gm of methyl salicylate.

0.01312 gm of santalyl acetate.

Determination of Ester Value

(H. P. I. – Volume II)

The ester value of a substance is the number of mg of KOH required to neutralise the acids resulting from the complete hydrolysis of 1 gm of substance.

The ester value is determined by the method described for the determination of esters and is calculated from the following formula:

$$\text{Ester value} = \frac{m \times 28.05}{W}$$

where m = value in ml. of 0.5 (N) alcoholic KOH required to saponify the esters, and W = weight, in gm., of substance taken.

Determination of Iodine Value

It gives the degree of unsaturation of the acids present in oils and fats. It is defined as: 'The number of grams of iodine that combine with 100 gms of oil or fat'.

Determination: A known weight of fat or oil (0.1 gm) is taken in a flask and dissolved in CCl_4. A known volume of I_2 solution in C_2H_5OH with $HgCl_2$ is added to it and the contents kept for 24 hours (Hubl's method). The unused I_2 is titrated with standard $Na_2S_2O_3$ (Hypo) solution. From the amount of I_2 absorbed by 100 gms of fat or oil their iodine value can be calculated. Iodine monochloride solution in glacial acetic acid may also be used in the determination of Iodine value.

On the basis of Iodine value, fixed oils are classified into

Non-drying oil (Iodine value below 90) e.g.	Semi-drying oil (Iodine value between 90 & 120) e.g.	Drying oil (Iodine value above 120) e.g.
1. Olive oil (I.V.–168 to 204)	1. Cotton-seed oil (I.V.–90 to 119)	1. Linseed oil (I.V.–168 to 204)
2. Coconut oil (I.V.–10)	2. Sesame oil (I.V.–103 to 116)	2. China-wood oil. (I.V.–163 to 173)
3. Castor oil (I.V.–82 + 0.88)		

Determination of pH Values

The pH value of an aqueous solution may be defined as the negative logarithm of the hydrogen ion concentration, expressed in grams per litre. (Hydrogen ion concentration is a measure of the extent of acidity or alkalinity of a solution). Although this definition provides a useful practical means for the quantitative indication of the acidity or alkalinity of a solution, it is less satisfactory from a strictly theoretical point of view. No definition of pH as a measurable quantity can have a simple meaning which is also fundamental and exact. pH 7 is neutral, above it alkalinity increases, and, below it, acidity increases.

Different methods for determination: The hydrogen component or the pH of a solution can be determined experimentally by the following methods:

1. ***Potentiometric or Electromotive force (e.m.f.) method***

The pH value of a liquid is determined potentiometrically by means of the glass electrode and a suitable pH-meter.

The reagents used in the determination are:

Method—Operate the pH-meter and electrode system according to the manufacturer's instructions. Standardise the meter and electrodes with 0.05 (M) potassium hydrogen phthalate (pH – 4.00) when measuring an acid solution. At the end of a set of measurement take a reading of the solution used to standardise the meter and electrodes. This reading should not differ by more than 0.02 from the original value at which the apparatus was standardised. If the difference is greater than 0.05, the set of measurements must be repeated.

The pH/e.m.f. relationship of the particular glass electrode in use must be checked daily as follows: standardise with 0.05 (M) potassium hydrogen phthalate and measure the pH value of 0.05 (M) sodium borate. When the reading is higher by 0.02 or more, or lower by 0.05 or more than the appropriate value in the table, correct the pH value of all solutions measured on that day, assuming the e.m.f. of the glass electrode cell to be linearly related to the pH value of the solution, which it contains. Unless otherwise stated, all solutions must be brought to laboratory temperature prior to measurement.

Whilst the pH/temperature co-efficient of 0.05 (M) potassium hydrogen phthalate may be neglected, that of 0.05 (M) sodium borate must be taken into account in accordance with the value given in Table 6.4.

Table 6.4: pH values of 0.05 (M) sodium borate

Temp.	10°C	15°C	20°C	25°C	30°C
pH	9.29	9.26	9.22	9.18	9.14

When measuring pH values above 10.0, make sure that the glass electrode is suitable for use at the alkaline end of the pH scale and apply any correction that is necessary.

2. ***Colorimetric method***

Principle: When the colour of a known value of a fluid treated with a certain amount of a suitable indicator in a test tube matches that of the same volume of a standard buffer treated with the same amount of the indicator in a similar tube, the pH of the fluid is the same as that of the standard buffer solution.

Method: Several standard buffer solutions are prepared with different pH covering the effective range of the indicator selected. 5 ml of the buffer solution is taken in different test tubes of similar size, after labelling the tubes properly. 5 ml of the unknown solution is taken in another test tube. To each, 5 drops of the indicator is added and the colour of the unknown solution compared against those of the standards.

The pH of the unknown solution is the same as that of the buffer matching the unknown fluid.

Importance of pH value:

1. The acid-base balance of a fluid (mother tincture, mother solution or a mixture) carries much importance, if viewed from the standpoint of stability of the liquid, confirming its properties. Variations of temperatures and pressures and defects in mode of storage tend to alter the pH, thus causing the liquid to deviate from its indicated use.
2. It is also useful to detect any adulteration infused in a liquid.

CHROMATOGRAPHY

Introduction

The term chromatography (in Greek, *'kromatous'* meaning 'colour' and *'graphos'* meaning 'written') meaning colour writing. The credit for inventing chromatography goes to the Russian botanist, Mikhail Semyonovich Tsvet, who used it for the first time in 1901, while he was researching on plant pigments. Later on, many other scientists have developed several methods of chromatography following the basic principles.

Chromatography is one of the most important laboratory technique in which the components of a mixture are separated on an adsorbent in order to analyse, identify, purify, and or quantify the mixture or components. It is mostly implemented in science subjects such as chemistry and life-sciences, especially in biochemistry.

Basic Principles

The principle behind this technique is the differential adsorption of the various components of a mixture between two different phases i.e. mobile or moving phase and fixed or stationary phase. Stationary phase refers to the bed or support substance that are fixed, whereas mobile phase refers to the medium, through which the mixture to be separated moves in a particular direction. The mixture gets separated by distributing its component molecules between the two phases. Distribution may take place on the basis of their structure, size, shape, charge or molecular weight:

(i) Fixed or stationary phase: The adsorbent is termed the stationary phase. Suitable adsorbents that are commonly used are magnesium oxide, alumina, cellulose, paper, silica gel etc.

(ii) Mobile or moving phase: The liquid in which the substance is dissolved is termed the mobile phase or eluent. The eluents employed are petroleum ether, carbon tetrachloride, benzene, alcohol etc. Their selection depends upon the relative solubilities of the components of the mixture in them.

Uses of Chromatography in Homoeopathic Pharmaceutics

Chromatography is useful in qualitative and quantitative analysis of drugs especially mother tinctures and lower potencies. Thin Layer Chromatography (TLC) and Paper Chromatography (PC) are usually employed in the H.P.I. assays and tests.

Thin Layer Chromatography (TLC) is a simple, quick, and inexpensive procedure that gives a quick answer as to how many components are in a mixture. TLC is also used to support the identity of a compound in a mixture when the Rf of a compound is compared with the Rf of a known compound (preferably both run on the same TLC plate). Rf is the retention factor, or how far up a plate the compound travels.

HPTLC (High Performance Thin Layer Chromatography) is a sophisticated and automated form of TLC. The procedure simultaneously processes the sample and standard that results in better analytical precision and accuracy at a faster pace. It allows several analyses to be done at the same time.

Advantages of Chromatography

Chromatography technique has many advantages over other techniques in analytical studies. It is very sensitive and reliable (provided that the method is carried out carefully without any contamination). The main advantage is that a complex mixture can be separated accurately by using only a few micrograms of the sample. Also, separation takes less time as compared to other techniques. The other advantage is that equipment setups are simple and easy. Because of these advantages, chromatography has become an important technique for forensic science and other clinical studies. The disadvantage of chromatography is that since the method is very sensitive, improper setup or contamination, even in nanograms, will give different results.

Basic Types of Chromatography

A. **Liquid Chromatography (LC)**
(Mobile phase: Liquid)

Specific methods:

(a) **Adsorption chromatography** (Liquid-solid chromatography—LSC).
   (i) Column: HPLC.
   (ii) Plane: TLC & HPTLC.

(b) **Partition chromatography** (Liquid-liquid chromatography—LLC).
   (i) Column: HPLC.
   (ii) Plane: TLC & Paper chromatography.

(c) **Ion-exchange chromatography** (IEC).

(d) **Size-exclusion (Gel permeation) chromatography** (SEC).

B. **Gas Chromatography (GC)**
(Mobile phase: Gas)

(a) Gas—solid chromatography (GSC).

(b) Gas—liquid chromatography (GLC).

C. **Supercritical Fluid Chromatography (SFC)**
(Mobile phase: Supercritical fluid)

The Classification of Chromatography

1. **Classification Based on Mobile Phase:** The chromatographic methods are classified on the basis of physical nature of the mobile phase. The mobile phase can be a gas or a liquid which gives rise to the two basic types of chromatography, namely, gas chromatography (GC) and liquid chromatography (LC). Liquid

chromatography includes TLC and high performance liquid chromatography (HPLC).

2. **Classification Based on Stationary Phase:** The chromatographic methods are classified on the basis of shape of the stationary phase. There are basically two methods; first is **column chromatography**, where the stationary phase is in the form of a tube and second is **planar chromatography**, where the stationary phase is in the form of plane or present on a plane support.

The stationary phase can also take two forms, solid and liquid, which provides two subgroups of GC and LC, namely; gas-solid chromatography (GSC) and gas-liquid chromatography (GLC), together with liquid solid chromatography (LSC) and liquid—liquid chromatography (LLC).

Most thin layer chromatography (TLC) techniques are considered liquid-solid systems although the solute normally interacts with a liquid-like surface coating on the adsorbent or support or, in some cases an actual liquid coating.

3. **Classification Based on Mechanism of Separation:** In this category, the chromatographic methods are classified based on how the component molecules of the mixture are separated. The various chromatographic methods under this category include:
   (a) Adsorption chromatography.
   (b) Partition chromatography.
   (c) Ion-exchange chromatography.
   (d) Size-exclusion (Gel permeation) chromatography.

4. **Classification based on the main objective for which it has been followed:** The chromatography can be 'analytical' or 'preparative'—based on the main objective for which it has been followed.

Analytical Chromatography makes use of only a small amount of a mixture and determines the components of that particular mixture.

Preparative Chromatography, on the other hand, is followed as a purification process, where the components of a mixture are separated and used for further studies.

Liquid Chromatography

Liquid Chromatography (LC) is a chromatographic technique in which the mobile phase is a liquid. LC is a much older technique than GC, but was overshadowed by the rapid development of GC in the 1950s and 1960s. LC is currently the dominate type of chromatography and is even replacing GC in its more traditional applications.

Liquid chromatography can be carried out either in a column or on a plane [TLC or paper chromatography]. Modern liquid chromatography utilising smaller particles and higher inlet pressure was termed high-performance (or high-pressure) liquid chromatography [HPLC] in 1970. In 2004, ultra-performance liquid chromatography dramatically raised the performance of LC to a new plateau.

Advantages of LC compared to GC

LC can be applied to the separation of any compound that is soluble in a liquid phase.

LC more useful in the separation of biological compounds, synthetic or natural polymers and inorganic compounds. Liquid mobile phase allows LC to be used at lower temperatures than required by GC.

LC better suited than GC for separating compounds that may be thermally labile.

Retention of solutes in LC depend on their interaction with both the mobile phase and stationary phase.

GC retention based on volatility and interaction with stationary phase.

LC is more flexible in optimizing separations → change either stationary or mobile phase.

Most LC detectors are non-destructive and most GC detectors are destructive. LC is better suited for preparative or process-scale separations.

Disadvantage of LC compared to GC

LC is subject to greater peak or band-broadening. Much larger diffusion coefficients of solutes in gases vs liquids.

Adsorption Chromatography (Liquid-solid Chromatography—LSC)

Separation is based mainly on differences between the adsorption affinities of the sample components for the surface of an active solid.

Partition Chromatography (Liquid-liquid Chromatography—LLC)

Partition chromatography, or liquid-liquid chromatography, is a Chromatographic technique in which solute are separated based on their partition between a liquid mobile phase and a liquid stationary phase coated on a solid support.

Note: The partition chromatography involves separation between liquids while adsoption chromatography involves solid and liquid separations.

Ion-Exchange Chromatography (IEC)

Ion-exchange chromatography is a liquid chromatography technique in which solutes are separated by their adsorption onto a support containing fixed charges on its surface.

Size-Exclusion (Gel Permeation) Chromatography (SEC)

Separation is based mainly on exclusion effects, such as differences in molecular size and / or shape or in charge. The term Size-Exclusion Chromatography may also be used when separation is based on molecular size. The terms Gel Filtration and Gel-Permeation Chromatography (GPC) were used earlier to describe this process when the stationary phase is a swollen gel. The term Ion-Exclusion Chromatography is specifically used for the separation of ions in an aqueous phase.

Thin Layer Chromatography (TLC)

Introduction

TLC is a form of liquid chromatography consisting of a mobile phase (developing solvent) and a stationary phase (a plate or strip coated with a form of silica gel). Analysis is performed on a flat surface under atmospheric pressure and room temperature. This is one method that can be used in the quality testing of homoeopathic remedies.

Principles of TLC

TLC is one of the simplest, fastest, easiest and least expensive of several chromatographic techniques used in qualitative and quantitative analysis to separate organic compounds. The separations achieved may be based upon adsorption, partition or a combination of both effects, depending on its use with different solvents. Quantitative measurements are possible by removing the spots from the plate with a suitable solvent. For two-dimensional thin layer chromatography, the chromatographed plate is turned at a right angle and again chromatographed, usually in another chamber saturated with a different solvent system.

Common Classes of TLC

The two most common classes of TLC are:

1. **Normal phase:** Normal phase is the terminology used when the stationary phase is polar; for example silica gel, and the mobile phase is an organic solvent or a mixture of organic solvents which is less polar than the stationary phase.
2. **Reversed phase:** Reversed phase is the terminology used when the stationary phase is a silica bonded with an organic substrate such as a long chain aliphatic acid like C-18 and the mobile phase is a mixture of water and organic solvent which is more polar than the stationary phase.

Adsorbents for TLC

In thin layer chromatography, the adsorbent is a powdered material applied usually to a glass plate. Silica gel is slightly acidic and, therefore, is best applied to the separation of neutral and acidic substances. Alumina, on the other hand, is basic and should be used for the separation of basic compounds.

Operation Technique

Thin Layer Chromatography uses the different migration rates of individual constituents of mother tinctures or very low potencies on a thin film of inert material. This is applied to a glass plate which is then immersed in the mother tincture.

Various solvents have been used, such as butanol and acetic acid or methanol and chloroform, and migration distances of about 10 cm are used.

Characteristic bands are shown on a layer of silica gel of 25-250 microns thickness, and each band represents a specific chemical constituent of the mother tincture.

Because of the exquisite sensitivity of thin layer chromatography, mother tinctures from different countries can show considerable variation in composition, which is probably from the variation in the composition of soil in which the plant specimen is grown. Despite this, the therapeutic activity is usually the same:

(a) **Thin layer plate:** A neat and clean plate is arranged on the aligning tray, and secure them so that it will not slip during the application of the adsorbent.

(b) **Application of the adsorbant:** The proper quantity of adsorbent and liquid, usually water—are mixed, which when shaken for 30 seconds, give a smooth slurry that will spread evenly with the aid of spreader. Generally, an analytical plate has an adsorbent thickness of 250 micrometer to 500 micrometer, while a preparative plate has a thickness of 500 micrometer to 2,000 micrometer. Allow the plate to remain undisturbed for 15 minutes and then dry at 105°C for 30 minutes. The prepared plate is stored in a desiccator.

(c) **Application of the Sample:** The sample (e.g., mother tincture) to be separated is generally applied by means of suitable micro pipette as a small spot (1 to 2 mm diameter) of solution about 1 cm from the end of the plate. The adsorbent must not be disturbed while making the spot, since this will result in an uneven flow of the solvent. The starting position can be indicated by making a small mark near the edge of the plate and allowed to dry.

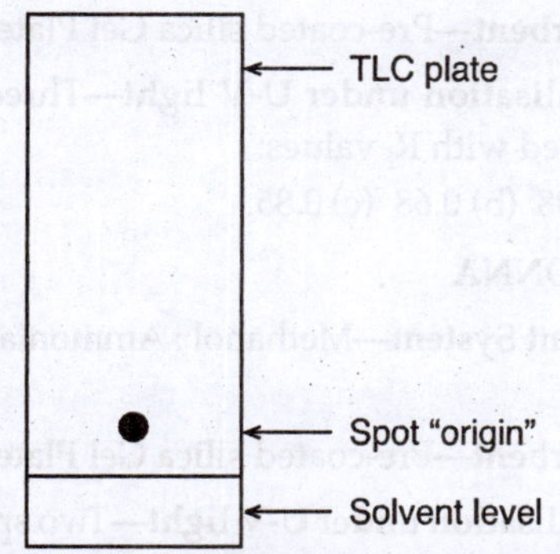

Position of the spot on a thin layer plate

(d) **Placing plate in developing chamber:** The plate is then placed in the developing chamber. The solvent in the chamber must be deep enough to reach the lower edge of the adsorbant, but must not touch the spot points. The solvent will then slowly rise in the adsorbent by capillary action. The developing chamber must be kept closed until the solvent front ascends; this commonly requires 15 minutes to 1 hour.

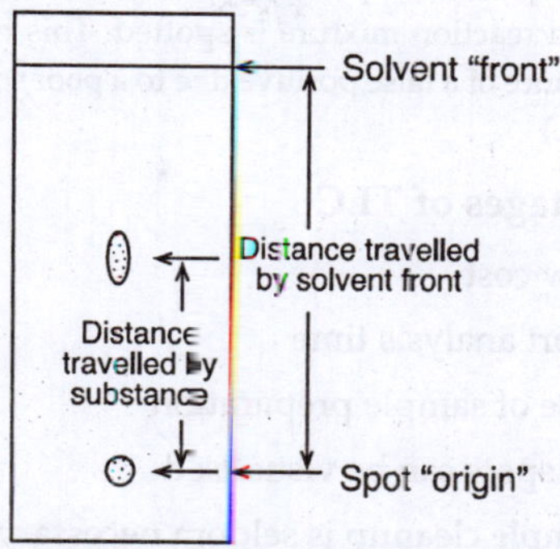

TLC plate showing distances travelled by the spot and the solvent after solvent front nearly reached the top of the adsorbent

(e) **Visualisation:** When the solvent front has moved to within about 1 cm of the top end of the adsorbent (after 15 to 1 hour), the plate should be removed from the developing chamber, the position of the solvent front marked, and the solvent allowed to evaporate. The spots are then observed first under ultraviolet light at 254 nm (shortwave UV).

(f) **Calculation of Rf Values:** Because the distance travelled by a substance relative to the distance travelled by the solvent front depends upon the molecular structure of the substance, TLC can be used to identify substances as well as to separate them. The relationship between the distance travelled by the solvent front and the substance is usually expressed as the R_f (= retention factor) value:

$$R_f \text{ value} = \frac{\text{distance travelled by the solute}}{\text{distance travelled by solvent front}}$$

The R_f values are strongly dependent upon the nature of the adsorbent and solvent. Therefore, experimental Rf values and literature values do not often agree very well. In order to determine whether an unknown substance is the same as a substance of known structure, it is necessary to run the two substances side by side in the same chromatogram, preferably at the same concentration.

Till such time the R_f of individual drug is prescribed, all mother tinctures should pass Co-TLC with the reported main constituents subject to the condition that they are not less than 1 per cent w/w in raw material. Co-TLC with tinctures made from authenticated raw material is also permitted.

Note: Co-spot (C—a spot on which both starting material and reaction mixture is spotted. This reduces the chance of a false positive due to a poor solvent front etc.)

Advantages of TLC

- Low cost
- Short analysis time
- Ease of sample preparation
- All spots can be visualised
- Sample cleanup is seldom necessary
- Adaptable to most pharmaceuticals
- Uses small quantities of solvents
- Requires minimal training
- Reliable and quick
- Minimal amount of equipment is needed
- Densitometers can be used to increase accuracy of spot concentration

Thin Layer Chromatography (TLC) of Some Mother Tinctures

ABROMA AUGUSTA

Solvent System—Chloroform : Methanol = 9 : 1(v/v)

Adsorbent—Pre-coated silica Gel Plate.

Visualisation under U-V light—Three spots are observed with R_f values:

(a) 0.08 (b) 0.68 (c) 0.85.

ABROTANUM

Solvent System—n-butanol : Acetic acid : Water = 4 : 1 : 1(v/v).

Adsorbent—Pre-coated silica Gel Plate.

Visualisation under U-V light—Three spots are observed with R_f values:

(a) 0.43 (b) 0.83 (c) 0.94.

ACALYPHA INDICA

Solvent System—Chloroform : Methanol = 9 : 1(v/v).

Adsorbent—Pre-coated silica Gel Plate.

Visualisation under U-V light—Six spots are observed with R_f values:

(a) 0.20 (b) 0.55 (c) 0.68 (d) 0.78 (e) 0.88 (f) 0.93.

AETHUSA CYNAPIUM

Solvent System—Chloroform : Methanol = 9 : 1(v/v).

Adsorbent—Pre-coated silica Gel Plate.

Visualisation under U-V light—Three spots are observed with R_f values:

(a) 0.13 (b) 0.27 (c) 0.84.

ANDROGRAPHIS PANICULATA

Solvent System—Chloroform : Methanol = 9 : 1(v/v).

Adsorbent—Pre-coated silica Gel Plate.

Visualisation under U-V light—Six spots are observed with R_f values:

(a) 0.05 (b) 0.30 (c) 0.53 (d) 0.67 (e) 0.75 (f) 0.83.

ARNICA MONTANA

Solvent System—Chloroform : Methanol = 9 : 1(v/v).

Adsorbent—Pre-coated silica Gel Plate.

Visualisation under U-V light—Three spots are observed with R_f values:

(a) 0.07 (b) 0.66 (c) 0.84.

AZADIRACHTA INDICA

Solvent System—Chloroform : Methanol = 9 : 1(v/v).

Adsorbent—Pre-coated silica Gel Plate.

Visualisation under U-V light—Three spots are observed with R_f values:

(a) 0.08 (b) 0.68 (c) 0.85.

BELLADONNA

Solvent System—Methanol : Ammonia = 100 : 1.5 (v/v).

Adsorbent—Pre-coated silica Gel Plate.

Visualisation under U-V light—Two spots are observed with R_f values:

(a) 0.64 (b) 0.73.

BELLIS PERENNIS

Solvent System—Ethyl acetate : Formic acid : Water = 8 : 1 : 1(v/v).

Adsorbent—Pre-coated silica Gel Plate.

Visualisation under U-V light—Two spots are observed with R_f values:

(a) 0.79 (b) 0.94.

BERBERIS VULGARIS

Solvent System—Methanol : Ammonia = 100 : 1.5 (v/v).

Adsorbent—Pre-coated silica Gel Plate.

Visualisation under U-V light—Spots corresponding to berberine appear.

BRYONIA ALBA

Solvent System—Chloroform : Methanol = 9 : 1(v/v).

Adsorbent—Pre-coated silica Gel Plate.

Visualisation under U-V light—Four spots are observed with R_f values:

(a) 0.28 (b) 0.48 (c) 0.82 (d) 0.93.

CACTUS GRANDIFLORUS

Solvent System—n-butanol : Acetic acid : Water = 4 : 1 : 1(v/v).

Adsorbent—Pre-coated silica Gel Plate.

Visualisation under U-V light—Three spots are observed with R_f values:

(a) 0.32 (b) 0.40 (c) 0.73.

CALENDULA OFFICINALIS

Solvent System—Ethyl acetate : Formic acid : Water = 8 : 1 : 1(v/v).

Adsorbent—Pre-coated silica Gel Plate.

Visualisation under U-V light—Three spots are observed with R_f values:

(a) 0.12 (b) 0.24 (c) 0.104.

RAUWOLFIA SERPENTINA

Solvent System—Chloroform : Methanol = 95 : 5 (v/v).

Adsorbent—Pre-coated silica Gel Plate.

Visualisation under U-V light—A spot corresponding to Reserpine appears.

RHUS TOXICODENDRON

Solvent System—Chloroform : Methanol = 9 : 1(v/v).

Adsorbent—Pre-coated silica Gel Plate.

Visualisation under U-V light—Six spots are observed with R_f values:

(a) 0.07 (b) 0.13 (c) 0.51 (d) 0.73 (e) 0.80 (f) 0.92.

RUTA GRAVEOLENS

Solvent System—n-butanol : Acetic acid : Water = 4 : 1 : 1(v/v).

Adsorbent—Pre-coated silica Gel Plate.

Visualisation under U-V light—Two spots are observed with R_f values:

(a) 0.50 (b) 0.93.

SABADILLA

Solvent System—Chloroform : Methanol = 9 : 1 (v/v).

Adsorbent—Pre-coated silica Gel Plate.

Visualisation under U-V light—A spot corresponding to Veratrine appears.

SABINA

Solvent System—Chloroform : Methanol = 9 : 1(v/v).

Adsorbent—Pre-coated silica Gel Plate.

Visualisation under U-V light—Five spots are observed with R_f values:

(a) 0.13 (b) 0.30 (c) 0.62 (d) 0.63 to 0.90.

SANGUINARIA CANADENSIS

Solvent System—Chloroform : Methanol = 9 : 1(v/v).

Adsorbent—Pre-coated silica Gel Plate.

Visualisation under U-V light—Eight spots are observed with R_f values:

(a) 0.16 (b) 0.22 (c) 0.31 (d) 0.34 (e) 0.59 (f) 0.88 (g) 0.91 (h) 0.96.

SECALE CORNUTUM

Solvent System—Chloroform : Methanol = 9 : 1(v/v).

Adsorbent—Pre-coated silica Gel Plate.

Visualisation under U-V light—Five spots are observed with R_f values:

(a) 0.6 (b) 0.20 (c) 0.53 (d) 0.71 (e) 0.97.

SENEGA

Solvent System—Chloroform : Methanol = 9 : 1(v/v).

Adsorbent—Pre-coated silica Gel Plate.

Visualisation under U-V light—Four spots are observed with R_f values:

(a) 0.11 (b) 0.19 (c) 0.25 (d) 0.44.

TERMINALIA ARJUNA

Solvent System—Chloroform : Methanol = 9 : 1(v/v).

Adsorbent—Pre-coated silica Gel Plate.

Visualisation under U-V light—Six spots are observed with R_f values:

(a) 0.05 (b) 0.12 (c) 0.37 (d) 0.45 (e) 0.72 (f) 0. 85.

THUJA OCCIDENTALIS

Solvent System—Chloroform : Methanol = 9 : 1(v/v).

Adsorbent—Pre-coated silica Gel Plate.

Visualisation under U-V light—Eight spots are observed with R_f values:

(a) 0.05 (b) 0.12 (c) 0.22 (d) 0.37 (e) 0.47 (f) 0. 68 (g) 0.84 (h) 0.93.

TRIBULUS TERESTRIS

Solvent System—Chloroform : Methanol = 9 : 1(v/v).

Adsorbent—Pre-coated silica Gel Plate.

Visualisation under U-V light—Six spots are observed with R_f values:

(a) 0.26 (b) 0.37 (c) 0.46 (d) 0.52 (e) 0.58 (f) 0. 66.

VERATRUM VIRIDE

Solvent System—Chloroform : Methanol = 9 : 1(v/v).

Adsorbent—Pre-coated silica Gel Plate.

Visualisation under U-V light—Three long spots are observed with R_f values:

(a) 0.05 to 0.21 (b) 0.25 to 0.35 (c) 0.41 to 47.

WITHANIA SOMNIFERA

Solvent System—Chloroform : Methanol = 95 : 5 (v/v).

Adsorbent—Pre-coated silica Gel Plate.

Visualisation under U-V light—Six spots are observed with R_f values:

(a) 0.03 (b) 0.15 (c) 0.42 (d) 0.82 (e) 0.89 (f) 0. 95.

High Performance Thin Layer Chromatography (HPTLC)

It is a sophisticated and automated form of TLC. The procedure simultaneously processes the sample and standard that results in better analytical precision and accuracy at a faster pace. It allows several analysis to be done at the same time.

HPTLC is a highly sophisticated equipment used for the qualitative (finger-printing) as well as quantitative analysis of drug ingredients i.e. glycosides, alkaloids etc. that are present in tinctures and extracts. It is also used for developing in-house standardisation of mother tinctures, and developing analytical methods for testing mother tinctures.

HPTLC method is very simple, powerful, rapid, reliable and cost-effective with respect to the accuracy of the result based on both qualitative and quantitative analysis.

For homoeopathic formulations, development of standard procedure through HPTLC is a new approach which may lead to proper standardisation of different homoeopathic tinctures based on

Table 6.5: Main differences of HPTLC and TLC-particle and Pore size of Sorbents

	HPTLC	TLC
Layer of Sorbent	100 μm	250 μm
Efficiency	High due to smaller particle size generated	Less
Separations	3–5 cm	10–15 cm
Analysis Time	Shorter migration distance and the analysis time is greatly reduced	Slower
Solid support	Wide choice of stationary phases like silica gel for normal phase and C8, C18 for reversed phase modes	Silica gel, Alumina and Kiesulguhr
Development chamber	New type that require less amount of mobile phase	More amount
Sample spotting	Auto sampler	Manual spotting
Scanning	Use of UV/Visible/Fluorescence scanner scans the entire chromatogram qualitatively and quantitatively and the scanner is an advanced type of densitometer	Not possible

fingerprinting characteristics. This investigation shows that these particular characteristics may be used as standardisation tool for homoeopathic tinctures more effectively and most accurately and is utmost essential which could enable the society in general to have quality homoeopathic formulations on one hand and to gain a momentum in homoeopathic medicine on the other.

However, these types of findings cannot rule out the need of further standardisation and evaluations of various homoeopathic formulations but definitely it may lead to a new way in the development of standard procedures for different homoeopathic mother tinctures as well as various other formulations.

The exclusive features of HPTLC include:

1. Simultaneous processing of sample and standard—better analytical precision and accuracy—less need for Internal Standard.
2. Several analysts work simultaneously.
3. Lower analysis time and less cost per analysis.
4. Low maintenance cost.
5. Simple sample preparation—handle samples of divergent nature.
6. No prior treatment for solvents like filtration and degassing.
7. Low mobile phase consumption per sample.
8. No interference from previous analysis—fresh stationary and mobile phases for each analysis—no contamination.
9. Visual detection possible—open system.
10. Non-UV absorbing compounds detected by post-chromatographic derivatisation.

The steps involved in HPTLC are:

(i) Selection of chromatographic layer.
(ii) Sample and standard preparation.
(iii) Layer pre-washing.
(iv) Layer pre-conditioning.
(v) Application of sample and standard.
(vi) Chromatographic development.
(vii) Detection of spots.
(viii) Scanning.
(ix) Documentation of chromatic plate.

High Performance Liquid Chromatography

HPLC is an acronym, which stands for High Performance Liquid Chromatography or high pressure liquid chromatography—a chromatographic technique to separate, identify, and quantify chemical compounds that are dissolved in solution. HPLC instruments consist of a **reservoir of mobile phase, a pump, an injector, a separation column, and a detector.**

Compounds are separated by injecting a sample mixture onto the column. The different components in the mixture pass through the column at differentiates due to differences in their partition behaviour between the mobile phase and the stationary phase. The mobile phase must be degassed to eliminate the formation of air bubbles.

Here a silica-based column (stationary phase) is used to separate the analytes by using a liquid (mobile phase), which is made to run through by means of a peristaltic pump. Finally, after entering and traversing the length of the column, the analytes are detected by means of a detector.

Components of HPLC

The components of a basic high-performance liquid chromatography [HPLC] system are shown in the following simple diagram:

A reservoir holds the solvent [called the mobile phase, because it moves]. A high-pressure pump [solvent delivery system or solvent manager] is used to generate and meter a specified flow rate of mobile phase, typically milliliters per minute. An injector [sample manager or autosampler] is able to introduce [inject] the sample into the continuously flowing mobile phase stream that carries the sample into the HPLC column. The column contains the chromatographic packing material needed to effect the separation. This packing material is called the stationary phase because it is held in place by the column hardware. A detector is needed to see the separated compound bands as they elute from the HPLC column. The mobile phase exits the detector and can be sent to waste, or collected, as desired. When the mobile phase contains a separated compound band, HPLC provides the ability to collect this fraction of the eluate

HPLC Column
Packing Material
Chromatogram
Peaks = Yellow, Red, Blue
Injector
Auto-sampler
Sample Manager
Computer Data Station
Solvent
(Mobile Phase)
Reservoir
Sample
Pupm
Solvent Manager
Solvent Delivery System
Detector
Waste

High-Performance Liquid Chromatography [HPLC] System

containing that purified compound for further study. This is called preparative chromatography.

Note that high-pressure tubing and fittings are used to interconnect the pump, injector, column, and detector components to form the conduit for the mobile phase, sample, and separated compound bands.

The detector is wired to the computer data station, the HPLC system component that records the electrical signals needed to generate the chromatogram on its display and to identify and quantitate the concentration of the sample constituents.

Uses of HPLC

This technique is used for research analysing complex mixtures, purifying chemical compounds, developing processes for synthesising chemical compounds, isolating natural products, or predicting physical properties. It is also used in quality control to ensure the purity of raw materials, to control and improve process yields, to quantify assays of final products, or to evaluate product stability and monitor degradation.

Ultraperformance Liquid Chromatography (UPLC)

In 2004, further advances in instrumentation and column technology were made to achieve very significant increases in resolution, speed, and sensitivity in liquid chromatography. Columns with smaller particles [1.7 micron] and instrumentation with specialised capabilities designed to deliver mobile phase at 15,000 psi [1,000 bar] were needed to achieve a new level of performance. A new system had to be holistically created to perform ultraperformance liquid chromatography, now known as UPLC technology.

Basic research is being conducted today by scientists working with columns containing even smaller 1-micron-diameter particles and instrumentation capable of performing at 100,000 psi [6,800 bar]. This provides a glimpse of what we may expect in the future.

Paper Chromatography

It is an analytical technique, where only a small amount of a sample is used for separating and identifying its components.

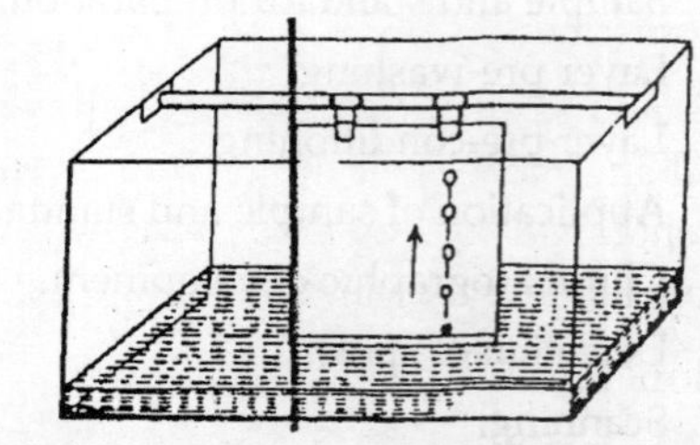

Paper Chromatography

Principle

The principle involved in separation is largely by partition (distribution) coefficient phenomenon and partly by adsorption mechanism. The constituents of the mixture are distributed between the water held on the filter paper (water acts as a stationary phase) and organic solvent (mobile phase).

Separation of components depends on both their solubility in the mobile phase and their differential affinity to the mobile phase and stationary phase.

Capillary Action—The movement of liquid within the spaces of a porous material due to the forces of adhesion, cohesion, and surface tension. The liquid is able to move up the filter paper because its attraction to itself is stronger than the force of gravity.

Solubility—The degree to which a material (solute) dissolves into a solvent. Solutes dissolve into solvents that have similar properties (like dissolves like). This allows different solutes to be separated by different combinations of solvents.

Separation of components depends on both their solubility in the mobile phase and their differential affinity to the mobile phase and the stationary phase.

Mobile and Stationary phase in Paper Chromatography

Like any other method of chromatography, paper chromatography has two phases: (1) the stationary phase, and (2) the mobile phase:

1. **The stationary phase:** In paper chromatography, porous paper serves as the stationary phase. Paper can be a filter paper or any special paper. However, it is better to use Whatman No.1 filter paper or chromatography paper, since they are pure and have uniform fibers.
2. **The mobile phase:** A solvent, either water or ethanol, serves as the mobile phase. The solvent travels through the fibres by capillary action, thereby carrying the sample with it.

Operation Technique

1. **Choice of filter paper:** Whatman filter papers are used as chromatography paper. In general, this paper contains 98-99% α-cellulose. There are various grade and types of paper available for separation of a sample.

   Factors that governs the choice of paper:

   Nature of sample and solvent used

   Based on quantitative or qualitative analysis

   Based on thickness of the paper.
2. **Preparation of paper:** Cut the paper into desired shape and size—depending upon the work to be carried out. The starting line is marked on the paper with an ordinary pencil 5 cm from the bottom edge. On the starting line, marks are made 2 cm apart from each other.
3. **Application of sample:** The sample mixture to be separated is applied as a small spot on the origin line. The spot is dried on the filter paper and is placed in developing chamber. Micropippete or glass capillary is used for sample application.
4. **Solvents:** A number of solvents can be used in the paper chromatography. The solvent selection depends upon nature of substance to be separated.

   Some example of solvents: Ethyl alcohol, N-Hexane, Benzene, Toluine, N-Butanol, Water, Methanol, Chloroform.

   These solvents are used in different ratio with different mixtures:
5. **Chromatographic chamber:** The chromatographic chambers are made up of many

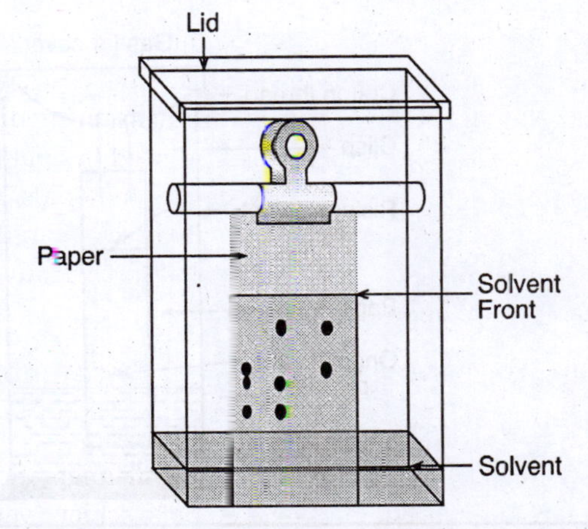

Chromatography jar

materials like glass, plastic or stainless steel. Glass tanks are preferred most. They are available in various dimensional size—depending upon paper length and development type. The chamber atmosphere should be saturated with solvent vapour.

6. **Development of chromatogram:** The paper is dipped in solvent in such a manner that the spots will not dip completely into the solvent. The solvent will rise up by capillary action. It is allowed to run 2/3rd of paper height for better and efficient result. After development is complete the paper is taken out of the chamber carefully.
7. **Drying of chromatogram:** The chromatogram is dried after its development. They are dried by cold or hot air, depending on volatility of solvents. A simple hair dryer is a convenient device to dry chromatograms.
8. **Location of spot:** If the substances are coloured they are visually detected easily. But for colourless substance, physical and chemical methods are used to detect the spot.

Physical method: In this method observations are done under U-V light, detection of fluorescence and radioisotope measurements

Chemical method: In this method the chemical reagent is used to develop the colour:

Amino acids—Ninhydrin reagent.

Alkaloids—Dragendroff's reagent.

9. **R_f Value:** In paper chromatography, the results are represented by R_f value which represents the movement or migration of solutes relative to the solvent front.

The R_f value is calculated as:

$$\frac{\text{Distance travelled by the solute}}{\text{Distance travelled by the solvent front}}$$

Development Technique

There are various methods of development of PC:

1. **Descending Chromatography:** In this method, solvent moves from top to bottom—so it is called descending chromatography.
2. **Ascending Chromatography:** In this method, the solvent migrates upward by capillary action.
3. **Ascending-Descending Chromatography:** A hybrid of above two technique is called Ascending-Descending Chromatography.
4. **Radial Chromatography:** In this method, a circular filter paper is taken and a cut is made in its centre to yield a wick or tongue. The spot of the material is placed at the centre of the circular filter paper. The paper is positioned horizontally on the petridish containing the solvent so that the tongue or the wick of the paper dips into the solvent.

The paper is covered by another petridish. The solvent rises through the tongue (or wick) and percolates evenly through the horizontally positioned filter paper and, as development proceeds, the components are separated in the form of concentric circular zones. Hence, this radial paper chromatography is also known as circular paper

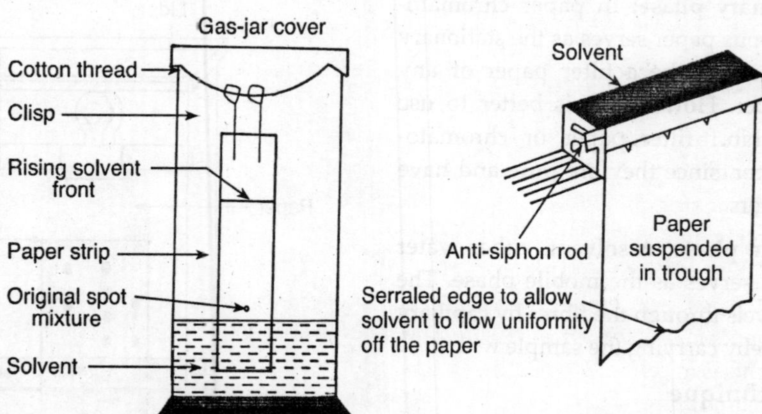

An experimental setup for paper chromatography

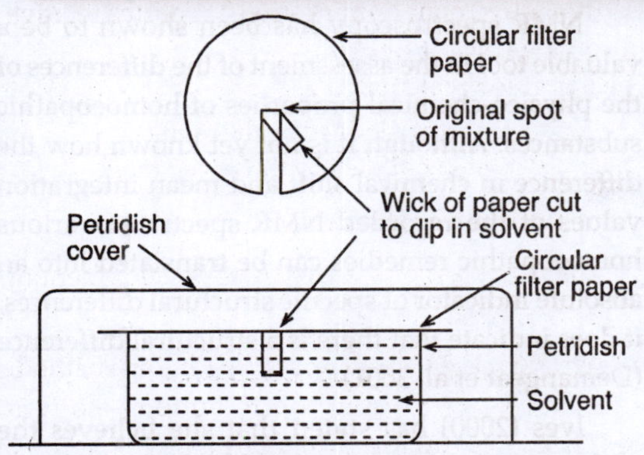

Radial or circular paper chromatography

chromatography. This technique is very useful for substances having low R_f values.

5. **Two-dimentional Chromatography:** In this method a square paper is taken and the sample is applied to one of the corners. Using solvent system the first development is carried as ascending method. The paper is taken out, dried, and second development is performed at right angles to the first dimensional development.

Advantages of Paper Chromatography

This analytical method is quick perform and easy to master. With a correctly chosen mobile phase (chromatographic solvent), an analyst can rapidly determine the number of constituents of a mixture sample. Sometimes, paper chromatography even allows one to positively identify these constituents. Another advantage of this method is that it requires a relatively small sample and is very inexpensive—a big plus in today's cost-conscious world.

Disadvantages of Paper Chromatography

Like all analytical methods, paper chromatography has its limitations. Some mixtures are very difficult to separate by paper chromatography; and any species that is not coloured is difficult to observe on the chromatogram. Also, paper chromatography is solely an analytical method, not a preparative one. Because the sample size is so small, it is difficult to perform further analysis after the sample's contents have been chromatographically separated. This is in contrast to methods such as column chromatography, which are frequently use to preparatively separate larger amounts of mixtures. Lastly, paper chromatography can only be used in qualitative analysis. It is not possible to extract meaningful information about the quantitative content of a mixture from a paper chromatogram.

Gas Chromatography

It is a highly efficient separation technique wherein the moving phase is gas such as hydrogen, helium, argon etc. and the stationary phase is a silica capillary column or very long length.

Gas chromatography methods have become important for moisture determination due to their specificity and efficiency. The water in the weighed, powdered sample can be extracted with dry methanol and subjected to chromatography on a column. The water separated by this means is readily determined from this chromatogram.

Gas chromatography are of two types: Gas-liquid chromatography (GLC), and Gas-solid chromatography (GSC).

Gas-Liquid Chromatography

This consists of a liquid stationary phase and a mobile gaseous phase. Some pharmacognostical examples of its application include examination of many volatile oils, camphor, etc.

Spectrometric/Spectroscopic Analysis

Introduction

Spectroscopy is a technique that uses the interaction of energy with a sample to perform an analysis. The data that is obtained from spectroscopy is called a spectrum. A spectrum is a plot of the intensity of energy detected versus the wavelength (or mass or momentum or frequency, etc.) of the energy. A spectrum can be used to obtain information about atomic and molecular energy levels, molecular geometries, chemical bonds, interactions of molecules, and related processes. Often, spectra are used to identify the components of a sample (qualitative analysis). Spectra may also be used to measure the amount of material in a sample (quantitative analysis). There are several instruments that are used to perform a spectroscopic analysis. In simplest terms, spectroscopy requires an energy source (commonly a laser but this could be an ion source or radiation source) and a device for measuring the change in the energy source after it has interacted with the sample (often a spectrophotometer or interferometer).

Common Types

1. **Ultraviolet-Visible Spectroscopy or Ultraviolet-Visible Spectrophotometry (UV-Vis):** It refers to absorption spectroscopy in the ultraviolet-visible spectral region. This means it uses light in the visible and adjacent [near-UV and near-infrared (NIR)] ranges. The absorption in the visible range directly affects the perceived colour of the chemicals involved. In this region of the electromagnetic spectrum, molecules undergo electronic transitions.

   It is used to perform quality control assays on drug substances obtained from different sources in order to compare their spectra with that of standard spectrum for the same drug substance.

2. **IR Spectroscopy:** It offers the possibility to measure diffe-rent types of inter-atomic bond vibrations at different frequencies. It is applicable in structure determination and identity of organic and inorganic compounds—quantitative analysis.
3. **Raman Spectroscopy:** Raman scattering of light by molecules may be used to provide information on a sample's chemical composition and molecular structure.
4. **Nuclear Magnetic Resonance (NMR) Spectroscopy:** Nuclear Magnetic Resonance is an analytical technique where a sample is immersed in a magnetic field and irradiated with radio waves. Using this technique to study a molecule enables the recording of differences in the magnetic properties of the various nuclei, protons, electrons and neutrons present, as well as what positions these hold within the molecule. This is directly influenced by the environment of, for example, a proton, and thus enables predictions concerning the structure of the liquid.

A variety of different tools have been used to investigate homoeopathic remedies, such as infrared spectra, electronic spectra and NMR spectroscopy (Sukul et al., 2001), diffraction, Raman spectroscopy (Berezin, 1994).

NMR spectroscopy has been shown to be a valuable tool in the assessment of the differences of the physico-chemical properties of homoeopathic substances. Although it is not yet known how the difference in chemical shift and mean integration values of the recorded NMR spectra of various homoeopathic remedies can be translated into an absolute indicator of specific structural differences, it does indicate that there is a structural difference (Demangeat et al, 2001).

Ives (2000) has stated that she believes the most promising line of research has come with the use of NMR spectroscopy. This is due to the fact that NMR spectroscopy can record energy transitions of protons, which are reliant on their precession rates and electronic environments.

NMR spectroscopy is a powerful tool used to determine the structure of molecules. The chemical environment of specific nuclei is deduced from information obtained about the nuclei. NMR takes advantage of the fact that the nuclei of these molecules have an intrinsic spin. The process of NMR entails placing the sample in a simple magnetic field and irradiating it with radio waves. NMR spectra then arise from the so-called spin property. The spin is a quantum effect where spin is quantised, i.e. having two directions, up or down.

Earlier research was conducted by **Smith and Boericke (1966)** on Sulphur potencies to evaluate homoeopathic drug structure. Distinct changes were noted in the hydroxyl part of the spectrum. They concluded that the solvent structure is changed in unsuccussed serial dilutions as compared to undiluted solvent. They established further differences in succussed serial dilutions, and the changes became more extreme as the potencies passed Avogadro's Limit. This led them to believe that there is a physical rearrangement in the solvent, most likely in the form of self-replicating polymers. A further study by **Smith and Boericke (1968)** with higher potency levels up to 60X level with bradykinin-triacetate, only compounded the evidence that the act of succussion increased the area of the hydroxyl spectrum as opposed to identical unsuccussed dilutions.

The employment of NMR spectroscopy as an experimental technique on homoeopathic potencies, has proven very useful (Schulte, 1999);

however problems have been reported by various investigators assessing this tool [Bol (1997), Demangeat and Poitevin (2001)].

Sukul et al (2001) conducted an experiment comparing the effects of Nux vomica 30c successed and unsuccussed on adult toads as well as the NMR spectra of the abovementioned compared to a range of variations. In the preparation of their samples they used 10 succussions except with the samples that were unsuccussed. They concluded that the ethanol-water mixture has the capability to imbibe some specific properties of drug molecules or particles during the dynamisation process, but that succussion is not an essential factor in producing an effective homoeopathic potency. The possibility remains that there is a threshold in the number of succussions that need to be used before its effect on the remedy will be evident.

The employment of NMR Spectroscopy as a method for the analysis of structure within homoeopathic potencies and as a method for the analysis of the differences between the respective homoeopathic potencies and a lactose-based control and differences between parallel potencies and a control has been well substantiated (Ross, 1997).

5. **Atomic Absorption Spectroscopy (AAS):** It is a spectro-analytical procedure for the qualitative and quantitative determination of chemical elements employing the absorption of optical radiation (light) by free atoms in the gaseous state. In analytical chemistry the technique is used for determining the concentration of a particular element (the analyte) in a sample to be analysed. AAS can be used to determine over 70 different elements in solution or directly in solid samples.
6. **X-ray Spectroscopy:** This technique involves excitation of inner electrons of atoms, which may be seen as X-ray absorption. An X-ray fluorescence emission spectrum may be produced when an electron falls from a higher energy state into the vacancy created by the absorbed energy.

Discussion

1. UV–VIS, IR, FTIR, and Raman Spectroscopy are used for the bulk "liquid" which, in most cases, is either water or a mixture of water and ethanol (95% ethanol). UV–VIS spectroscopy and Raman spectroscopy proved to be useful tools to investigate the subtle but significant changes in the structural parameters in both water and alcohol based remedies.
2. It should also be noted that different homoeopathic remedies and different dilutions of the same remedy have been distinguished from each other using Raman and infrared spectroscopy, even though all should theoretically contain nothing but water. Such findings may relate to complex processes such as the formation, during succussion, of colloidal nanobubbles that could contain the remedy source material.
3. In physical researches the most striking results indicating water memory were obtained from NMR UV and X-ray spectroscopy of ultrahighly diluted water (ultra-high dilution means a dilution of a substance in which there is high probability that not even one molecule of the substance is left; it is practically pure water).
4. Using Raman and Ultraviolet–visible (UV–VIS) spectroscopy Roy et al distinguished two different homeopathic medicines (Nux vom and Nat mur) and differentiated their 6c, 12c, and 30c potencies.
5. Potentisation may alter permanently the physical-chemical properties of the solvent water. It changes the structure of water molecule. Standard physico-chemical techniques, thermo-luminescence, Raman and UV–VIS spectroscopy and other methods have shown that water displays large changes in its physico-chemical properties.
6. **Heinz** studied the physical action of dilutions using the **infrared spectroscopy (IR)** and stressed on the specific value of succussion. He found the rhythmicity indicating some favourable points in the curve of dilution.

Conclusion

1. Homoeopathic remedies are spectroscopically distinct from the original solvent (water/ethanol).

2. Different potencies can be distinctly distinguished by the UV-VIS and Raman spectroscopy.
3. *Nat mur* and *Nux vomica* are distinctly different while the same potencies with different succussion also show a clear evidence of difference in the structure of the individual samples.
4. No studies/claims whatsoever on the clinical effects of the remedies are made.

Electro-chemical Techniques

1. **Potentiometry:** Potentiometry is the field of electroanalytical chemistry in which potential (or voltage) is measured under the conditions of no current flow. The measured potential may then be used to determine the analytical quantity of interest, generally the concentration of some component of the analyte solution. The potential that develops in the electrochemical cell is the result of the free energy change that would occur if the chemical phenomena were to proceed until the equilibrium condition has been satisfied.
2. **Conductometry:** Conductometry means measuring the conductivity—a conductometer measures the electrical conductivity of ionic solutions. This is done by applying an electric field between two electrodes. The ions wander in this field. The anions migrate to the anode and the cations to the cathode. In order to avoid substance conversions and the formation of diffusion layers at the electrodes (polarisation), work is carried out with alternating voltage. The rule of thumb is that the frequency of the alternating voltage must be increased as the ion concentration increases. Modern conductometers automatically adapt the measuring frequency to the particular measuring conditions.
3. **Polarography:** It is also called **polarographic analysis,** or **voltammetry** in analytic chemistry, an electrochemical method of analysing solutions of reducible or oxidisable substances. It was invented by a Czech chemist, **Jaroslav Heyrovský**, in 1922. In general, polarography is a technique in which the electric potential (or voltage) is varied in a regular manner between two sets of electrodes (indicator and reference) while the current is monitored. The shape of a polarogram depends on the method of analysis selected, the type of indicator electrode used, and the potential ramp that is applied.

   The majority of the chemical elements can be identified by polarographic analysis, and the method is applicable to the analysis of alloys and to various inorganic compounds. Polarography is also used to identify numerous types of organic compounds and to study chemical equilibria and rates of reactions in solutions.
4. **Titrimetry:** Chemical analysis by titration, the determination of a given component in solution by addition of a liquid reagent of known strength until a given end point (e.g., a change in colour) is reached.

   Moisture content in drug substance can be determined by this chemical method named Karl Fischer Titration.This is particularly applicable for drugs containing small quantities of moisture. The reagents and solutions used in this method are sensitive to water and precautions must be taken to prevent exposure to atmospheric moisture. The Karl Fischer reagent used for this purpose consists of a solution of iodine, sulphur dioxide and pyridine in dry methanol. This is titrated against a sample containing water, which causes a loss of the dark brown colour. At the end-point, when no water is available, the colour of the reagent persists.

Industrial Pharmacy

By definition, industrial pharmacy is a discipline which includes manufacturing, development, marketing and distribution of drug products including quality assurance of these activities. This broad research area relates to different functions in pharmaceutical industry and having contact areas with engineering and economics. Research in industrial pharmacy is done both locally at the Faculty of Pharmacy, Division of Pharmaceutical Technology, and in pharmaceutical industry as collaboration projects, licenciate thesis studies. All basic research is closely applicable to the benefit of industry. The research can either include laboratory work or be case-studies. The research topics are focused on solving current general problems in pharmaceutical industry, such as formulation and characterisation of sticky amorphous drugs, problem-solving for paediatric medicines and miniaturisation of manufacturing processes.

In pharmaceutical industry some examples of licenciate thesis topics are: implementation of the marketing authorisation procedures in the accession countries of the European Union, evaluation of implementation of GCP directives in countries within EU, outside EU and in accession countries.

SCHEDULE M-I [See Rule 85-E(2)]

Good Manufacturing Practices (GMP) and Requirement of Factory premises, Plant and Equipment for Homoeopathic Medicine

Central Government has notified the draft of rules for **Good Manufacturing Practices** and Requirement of Premises, Plant and Equipments for Homoeopathic medicines. Rule shall be replacing the Schedule M-1 of the Drugs and Cosmetics Rules, 1945. The draft is notified in consultation with the Drugs Technical Advisory Board [DTAB]. It is an exhaustive document touching all aspects of Homoeopathic manufacturing. Draft was notified on 2nd August 2005 and Government has invited response in the form of objections or suggestions from any person within 45 days of its publication.

Draft rules are divided in to eleven parts, these are being reproduced in part for the benefit of concern persons who can read and react so that any discrepancy can be corrected before these rules are taken as being final.

1. GENERAL REQUIREMENTS

Location and surroundings — The premises shall be situated in a place which shall not be adjacent to open drains, public lavatory or any factory producing pollution of any kind, garbage dump, slaughter house or any other source likely to cause contamination from the external environment. The premises shall be located away from railway lines so that the performance of sensitive electronic equipment is not affected by vibrations. There shall be no open drains inside or outside the manufacturing premises. It shall be so designed that the entry of rodents is checked. The drains shall facilitate easy flow of the effluent and shall be cleared periodically.

Building: *The premises shall not be used for any purpose other than manufacture of homoeopathic drugs and no part of the manufacturing premises shall be used for any other purpose.* Other facilities, if needed, could be provided in separate building(s) in the same campus. Crude raw materials, packing materials, etc. shall be stored and handled in places earmarked for them and shall not be taken inside areas where critical operations of manufacture are done excepting processed raw material. *Heating, washing, drying, packing and labelling, etc. shall be done in dedicated ancillary areas adjacent to the manufacturing sections concerned.* The walls and floorings of manufacturing areas shall be smooth and free from chinks, cracks and crevices and shall be washable. The design of the windows, window-panes and all fittings shall be such that they will not facilitate accumulation/lodging of dust and other contaminants:

(a) *Rooms:* The rooms should be airy and clean and the temperature of the rooms should be moderately comfortable. Sections which are required to be sterile, air-conditioned and provided with air handling systems should be designed accordingly. All sections should be free from insects, birds, rodents, worms etc. and suitable measures shall be taken to prevent the same from finding ways to the sections and equipment.

(b) *Water Supply:* The water used in the manufacture shall be pure and of drinkable quality, free from pathogenic micro-organisms.

(c) *Disposal of Waste:* There should be adequate arrangement for disposal of waste water and other residues from the laboratory.

(d) *Factories Act:* The building used for the factory shall be constructed so as to permit production under hygienic conditions laid down in the Factories Act, 1948 (63 of 1948).

(e) *Medical services:* The manufacturer shall provide adequate facilities for First Aid, medical inspection of workers pertaining to manufacture of drugs including handling of raw materials, packing materials, packing and labelling of drugs, etc. at the time of employment and periodically check up thereafter at least once a year.

(f) *Safety measures:* First-aid facilities shall be provided in such a manner that they are easily accessible and the staff shall be imparted knowledge and training in first-aid measures as may be needed. Fire control equipment in suitable numbers shall be provided at easily accessible places near all sections including stores and warehouses.

(g) *Working benches:* Working benches shall be provide for carrying out operations such as filling, labelling, packing, etc. Such benches shall be fitted with smooth, impervious tops capable of being washed.

(h) *Container management:* Proper arrangements shall be made for receiving containers, closures and packing materials in secluded areas and for de-dusting the same, removal of wastes, washing, cleaning and drying. Suitable equipment shall be provided as may be needed, considering the nature of work involved. Where soaps and detergents are used to wash containers and closures used for primary packing, suitable procedure shall be prescribed and adopted for total removal of such materials from the containers and closures. *Plastic containers which are likely to absorb active principles or which are likely to contaminate the contents may not be used. Glass containers used shall be made of neutral glass.* The closures and washers used shall be of inert materials which shall not absorb the active principles or contaminate the contents or which may otherwise be likely to cause deterioration of quality. The containers, closures and packing materials shall protect the properties of the medicines. Tablets, if blister-packed, shall have secondary protective packaging to protect the medicines from moisture, odour etc. Neutral glass phials and epoxy-coated closures shall be used for eye-drops. Transparent plastic containers may be used for eye-drops containing only aqueous preparations. Sterile plastic nozzles may be provided to eye-drops, separately along with the medicine, whatever needed.

2. PLANTS AND EQUIPMENTS

2.1 General: The design of the plant shall be suitable for the nature and quantum of the activities involved. Equipment shall be installed in such a manner as to facilitate easy flow of materials and to check crisscross movement of the personnel. The entry to all manufacturing sections shall be regulated and persons not associated with the activities in the sections shall not have access to them. There shall be arrangements for personal cleanliness of workers and toilets. These shall be separate for men and women workers. There shall be suitable arrangement, separate for men and women, to change from their outside dress and footwear into the factory dress and footwear. Uniforms of suitable colours and fabric which facilitate proper washing and which do not shed fibres other contaminants shall be provided. Suitable head-covers and gloves shall be provided to the workers. The manufacturing premises shall not be used for dining. There shall be separate area for the personnel to take food or rest. Toilets shall not be located in or adjacent to any of the areas concerned with any manufacturing activity. Spitting, smoking, chewing, littering, etc. in the manufacturing or ancillary areas shall not be permitted. *Standard operating practices (SOPs) for cleaning and sanitation, personal hygiene of the workers, general and specific upkeep of the plant, equipment and premises and every activity associated with manufacture of drugs including procurement, quarantine, testing and warehousing of materials shall be written and adopted.*

No person with any contagious disease shall be involved in any of the manufacturing activities. There shall be proper arrangements for maintenance of the equipment and systems. The performance of every equipment and system shall be properly validated and their use shall be monitored. Dos and donts in the matter of the use of the plant and equipment as may be applicable shall be written and displayed in all places. There shall be separate dedicated areas for each ancillary activity such as receipt, cleaning, warehousing and issue of raw materials, packaging materials, containers and closures, finished goods etc. Adequate measures shall be taken to prevent entry/presence etc of insects, rodents, birds, lizards and other animals into the raw material handling areas.

Every material shall have proper identification and control numbers and inventory tags and labels displaying status of the quality being used, etc. There shall be proper arrangements and SOPs for preventing mix-up of materials at every stage of handling. There shall be separate arrangements for handling and warehousing of materials of different origins. Materials with odour shall be kept in tightly closed containers and shall be well protected from other materials. Fresh materials and odorous materials shall, preferably be stored in separate dedicated areas. Where bonded manufacturing and or warehousing facilities are required as per Excise laws, the facilities required shall be provided without compromise on the requirements specified above. A well-equipped laboratory for quality control/quality assurance of raw materials and finished products and for carrying out in-process controls shall be provided.

2.2 Personnel: Manufacture of drugs shall be under the control of approved technical staff that shall possess the qualifications prescribed in Rule 85.

3. REQUIREMENTS OF EQUIPMENTS AND FACILITIES

3.1 Mother Tinctures and Mother Solutions: The following equipment and facilities shall be provided:

(i) Disintegrator;

(ii) Sieved separator;

(iii) Balances, weights and fluid measures, all in metric system;

(iv) Chopping board and knives;

(v) Macerators with lids;

(vi) Percolators;

(vii) Moisture determination apparatus;

(viii) Filter press/sparkler filter (all metal parts shall be of stainless steel);

(ix) Mixing and storage vessels (Stainless steel of grade 304);

(x) Portable stirrers (Rod, blades and screws shall be of stainless steel);

(xi) Water still/water purifier;

(xii) Macerators and percolators for preparing mother solutions of materials of chemical origin. These shall be of material which will not react with the chemicals used and which do not bleach;

(xiii) Filling and sealing machine.

Notes: 1. As far as possible metal contacts may be avoided once the drug is processed.

2. An area of 55 sq. meters is recommended for basic installations.

3. Adequate separate storage facility should be provided for raw material quarantine, storage and bonded room for alcohol where applicable.

4. Separate and suitable storage facility should be provided for fresh herbs and odorous raw materials.

5. Adequate laboratory facility shall be provided for testing of raw materials & finished products.

3.2 Potentisation Section: The following arrangements are recommended for potency preparation section, namely:

(i) Working tables with washable top.

(ii) Facilities for separate storage of different grades of back potencies.

(iii) Suitable measuring devices for discharge of drug and diluent in potentisation vial.

(iv) Potentiser with counter or suitable manual arrangement.

An area of 20 sq. meters is recommended for basic installation.

Notes: 1. Different droppers shall be used for different drug potencies.

2. All measuring devices shall be metric system and be made of glass and shall be free of metallic contents.

3. It is desired that glass droppers, etc. intended for re-use after cleaning should be sterilised by autoclave or by heating in a hot air oven.

4. Plastics, rubber tubes, bulks, etc. coming in contact with tinctures or back potencies should not be re-used for other tincture and potencies.

5. Method of potentisation will be adopted as specified in Homoeopathic Pharmacopoeia of India, Volume I.

3.3 Containers and Closures Section: Separate area for preparation of containers and closures shall be provided adjacent to the potentisation section. This area shall have the following facilities:

(i) Washing tanks with suitable mechanical or manual facilities for cleaning.

(ii) Rinsing tanks. Purified water shall be used for rinsing.

(iii) Closures washing or macerating tanks.

(iv) Drying chambers.

Notes: 1. Different droppers shall be used only for each different medicine and different potency.

2. All measures shall be in metric system. Measures used shall be of neutral glass. Metal droppers and plastic droppers shall not be used.

3. Glass droppers shall be reused only after proper cleaning and sterilisation.

4. Potentisation shall be done by the method(s) prescribed in the HPI.

3.4 Trituration, Tableting, Pills and Globules making Section: The following arrangement are recommended:

(i) Triturating machine of suitable device.

(ii) Disintegrator.

(iii) Mass mixer.

(iv) Granulator.

(v) Electrical oven.

(vi) Tablets punching machine.

(vii) Kettle (steam, gas, or electrically heated) for preparing solutions.

(viii) Dryers for drying granules and tablets.

(ix) Sieved separator (stainless steel).

(x) Tablet counters.

(xi) Balances.

(xii) Coating Pan with spray-gun.

(xiii) Multi-sifter.

(xiv) Mill with perforations.

Note: Tablet section shall be free from dust and floating particles. An area of 55 sq. meters is recommended for basic installations.

3.5 Syrups and other Oral Liquids Section: The following arrangements are recommended:

(i) Mixing and storage tanks.

(ii) Portable mixer.

(iii) Filter press/Sparkler filter (all metal parts shall be of stainless steel).

(iv) Filling and sealing machine; pH meter.

An area of 20 sq. meters is recommended for basic installations. The section shall be free from dust and other floating particles, cobwebs, flies, ants and other insects, birds, lizards and rodents.

1. Adequate number of work benches shall be provided.
2. Visual inspection table shall be provided. This shall comprise of a colour contrast background with lamp for providing diffused light, mounted on a suitable table.

3.6 Ointments and Lotions Section: The following arrangements are recommended:

(i) Mixing tanks (Stainless steel).

(ii) Kettle (steam, gas, or electrically heated) for preparing solutions.

(iii) Suitable powder mixer.

(iv) Ointment mill.

(v) Filling and sealing machine/Crimping machine.

(vi) Filtering equipment.

(vii) Balance and weights.

An area of 20 sq. meters is recommended for basic installation. An ancillary area for washing vessels and equipment shall be provided. An ancillary area for heating purposes shall also be provided.

3.7 Ophthalmic Preparations Section: The following equipment is recommended for manufacture under aseptic conditions of Eye Ointments, Eye Drops, Eye Lotions and other preparations for external use only, namely:

(i) Hot air oven, electrically heated, with thermostatic control.

(ii) Laminar Air Flow Bench.

(iii) Air Handling Unit with HEPA filters to provide filtered air and positive pressure to the section and air-locks.

(iv) Ointment mill, colloidal mill.

(v) Mixing and storage tanks of stainless steel or of other suitable material.

(vi) Pressure vessels, as may be needed.

(vii) Sintered glass funnels, Seitz filter or filter candle.

(viii) Vacuum pump.

(ix) Filling machines for liquids ointments etc.

(x) Autoclaves with pressure and temperature gauges.

(xi) Necessary workbenches, visual inspection bench, etc.

Area: An area of 20 sq. meters is recommended for basic installations.

Notes:
1. The section shall have a clean room facility of Class 100 specification.
2. The section shall be air-conditioned and humidity controlled.
3. Entry to the sections shall be regulated through air-locks with differential air pressures with the air-lock adjacent to the section having higher pressure and the first one through which entry is made with the least pressure.
4. Materials shall be passed to the sections through suitable hatches.
5. The personnel shall wear sterile clothing including head-gear, which shall not shed fibre.
6. Washing of phials shall be done in separate areas with proper equipment. Proper facilities shall be provided in the area for washing vessels.
7. Separate area shall be provided for packing and labeling.

4. QUALITY-CONTROL DIVISION

4.1 Functions. A separate quality-control division shall be provided in the premises. The section shall be under the control of an approved technical officer, independent of the manufacturing division and directly responsible to the management. The section shall be responsible for ensuring the quality of all raw materials, packing materials and finished goods. The section shall also carry out in-process quality-checks of the products. The section shall be responsible for the stability of the products and for prescribing their shelf life wherever applicable.

The function of this division is divided in to 8 parts which include:

(i) To test the identity, quality and purity of the raw materials and to recommend rejection of the materials of poor quality and approve materials of the prescribed quality only.

(ii) To test the identity, quality and purity of the finished products and to recommend rejection of the materials of poor quality and to approve materials of the prescribed quality only.

(iii) To prepare and validate the methods of analysis, validate the equipments, monitor their use, take steps for proper maintenance, etc.

(iv) To approve or reject containers, closures and packaging materials in accordance with the prescribed norms.

(v) To exercise/carry out in-process-control of products.

(vi) To prescribe SOPs on all matters concerning quality of materials and products.

(vii) To monitor the storage and handling of raw materials, finished products, containers, closures and packaging materials.

(viii) To investigate complaints on quality of products and take/recommend appropriate measures and to examine returned goods and recommend their proper disposal.

4.2 Personnel: The quality control staff shall be full-time personnel. Analysis and tests of drugs, raw materials, etc. shall be done by qualified and approved technical staff. The technical staff shall have the minimum qualification or degree in Homoeopathy, Pharmacy or Science with Chemistry or Botany as the principal subject and experience of not less than two years in the test and analysis of medicines including handling of instruments.

4.3 Equipment: The following equipments shall be provided:

(i) Microscope of suitable magnification and photographic device;

(ii) Dissecting microscope;

(iii) TLC apparatus;

(iv) UV lamp viewer;

(v) Monopan Digital Electronic Balance;

(vi) Hot air oven;

(vii) Distillation apparatus;

(viii) Water Bath;

(ix) Polarimeter;

(x) Refractometer;

(xi) Melting point apparatus;

(xii) pH meter;

(xiii) Magnetic stirrer;

(xiv) Table Centrifuge;

(xv) Muffle furnace/electric Bunsen;

(xvi) Moisture determination apparatus;

(xvii) UV Spectro-photometer;

(xviii) Rotary microtome/Section cutting facilities;

(xix) Tablet Disintegration Machine.

5. RAW MATERIALS

5.1 Raw materials of Plant Origin:

(a) The raw materials of plant origin used for manufacture of drugs shall be of the following specifications:

(i) the materials shall be those recently collected and dried and shall be free from moisture so as to eliminate the risk of deterioration and infestation with pests, moulds, etc. The materials shall be collected when the atmospheric temperature is suitable where its active constituents are not changed/damaged/destroyed;

(ii) when fresh materials are to be used, the time lapse from the time of collection to use shall be minimised to the extent possible;

(iii) the materials should be taken from healthy plants and shall be free from parasites, moulds, etc.;

(iv) the materials shall be free of inorganic or organic foreign matters;

(v) when dry materials are procured, they shall be from healthy plants and shall be in un-processed form, free from all extraneous matters such as fungus, insects, moulds, pathogenic organisms, etc. and should not be more than six months old. Plant materials of Agaricaceae, which are perishable, shall be used within one week of collection.

(b) To facilitate proper identification and purity of the material and to exercise proper quality control of the material, the following conditions must be satisfied:

(i) a small twig of the plant with leaves shall be available if the part used is bark of the plant;

(ii) an entire plant or part or aerial twig with leaves and some uncut roots/ rhizomes/bulbs shall be available if the part used is a root/rhizome/bulb;

(iii) if plants with flowers are to be used, a few dry flowers shall also be available with the aerial twig;

(iv) if the material used is a mould or of the plant families Agaricaceae, Polyporaceae/amanitacaea/Boletaceae/Russulaceae, a whole specimen plant/mould shall be available in properly dried form;

(v) the materials shall be free from insecticides, fungicides, etc.;

(vi) the materials shall be in open mesh bags or in suitable materials which permit the passage of air inside;

(vii) each consignment of the material shall be accompanied by a statement of the supplier's name; name of the plant with description of the part supplied; the pharmacopoeial reference, place of collection/harvest, date and time of collection, packaging and weight.

5.2 Raw materials of Chemical Origin: They shall be of respective pharmacopoeial standards and statements of their specification shall accompany the materials.

5.3 Raw materials of Animal Origin: The materials shall be those collected from healthy animals and shall be of pharmacopoeial specifications. The materials shall be those collected, packed and transported under proper hygienic conditions and well protected from all contamination. The materials shall be accompanied by statements as in para (a) above. In case of drugs derived from a whole insect, bulk of such drugs along with some uncut whole insect should be provided/maintained for records.

5.4 Sarcodes: The materials shall be those collected from healthy animals and shall be of pharmacopoeial specification. The materials shall be those collected, packed and transported under proper hygienic conditions and well protected from all contamination.

The materials shall be accompanied by statements as in the para (a) above. The materials shall be tested to see that they are free from pathogenic organisms such as E.coli, Salmonella, etc.

5.5 Nosodes: These shall be of pharmacopoeial specifications. As these are derived from diseased animals or human beings, they shall be autoclaved immediately after collection and preserved and transported under proper hygienic conditions and well protected from all contamination. Before use, these shall be sterilised by autoclaving and shall comply with the test for sterility as specified in the Homoeopathic Pharmacopoeia.

6. PROCEDURES

6.1 Manufacture of Mother Tinctures:

(a) Every material shall be identified and checked for its purity. They shall be cleaned and processed by cutting, chopping, etc. for use in macerators/percolators. A specimen of the material shall be preserved till approval of the product for release or for sale.

(b) The design and procedures adopted shall ensure reproduction of the product of the same quality every time.

(c) Mother tinctures shall be preserved in tight closed neutral containers at temperatures preferably below 25°C, protected from light.

6.2 Manufacture of Attenuations:

(a) Attenuations shall be prepared in a clean room environment with filtered air and positive pressure inside, suitable for the operations.

(b) The methods used shall be reproducible and shall be validated.

(c) The containers, tubings, etc. of the machines used for manufacture of attenuations shall be thoroughly washed, cleaned and dried after attenuation of a drug. Regular checks shall be carried out on the materials.

(d) The parts of the equipment that come into contact with the attenuation materials shall be of neutral quality and shall not cause any contamination to the material.

(e) Attenuations shall be preserved in properly labeled glass containers.

(f) Alcohol and other vehicles used shall be of Homoeopathic pharmacopoeia specification and shall be free from impurities.

6.3 Trituration: Trituration technique is used to manufacture drugs from insoluble strains. The procedure/method specified in the Homoeopathic pharmacopoeia shall be adopted.

6.4 Formulations: Compound formulations shall preferably be in liquid and solid forms and the potency of the ingredients shall be in detectable quantity preferably be in 3X except in case of highly poisonous materials and toxins which should not be below 6X.

The ingredients shall be compatible to each other Complete pharmacopoeial name of each ingredient shall be printed on the label along with composition.

6.5 Medicated Insert Pellets:

(a) Pellets shall be manufactured in clean rooms, free from particulate contaminants. The equipment used shall enable prevention of contamination and cross-contamination.

(b) The procedures shall be validated.

7. LABORATORY CONTROLS

Tests as per the pharmacopoeia and requirements shall be carried out on products and materials. The stability of the products shall be established by proper methods. Sterility tests, wherever applicable, shall be carried out. Control samples shall be preserved for not less than three years after the last sales.

8. PACKING AND LABELLING

A minimum area of 50 square meters shall be provided for packing and labelling section.

9. EXPIRY DATE

Not exceeding sixty (60) months from the date of manufacture.

10. STANDARD OPERATING PRACTICES

Standard Operating Practices (SOPs) shall be developed for various activities such as receipt, identification, cleaning, drying, warehousing, issue, handling, sampling, etc. of all materials. Labels and packing materials shall be examined for correctness and compliance with rules. Records shall be maintained for their printing, use, destruction, etc.

11. RECORDS AND REGISTERS

Records shall be maintained for all the activities. These shall include records of production, records of raw materials, records of testing, records of sales and other supplies, records of rejection, complaints and actions taken, SOPs and records in respect of compliance thereof, log books of equipment, master formula records, records of medical examination and fitness of personnel etc. All records shall be maintained for a period of one year after the expiry of a batch or for three years whichever is later.

Note: The principal rules were published in the Gazette of India vide notification number GSR F.28-10/45-H(1) dated 21.12.1945, and last amended vide notification number GSR 579(E), dated the 20 September 2006.

Homoeopathic Pharmacopoeia Laboratory (HPL)

Homoeopathic Pharmacopoeia Laboratory (HPL) was established in 1975 under the Ministry of Health & Family Welfare, Govt. of India, as a quality monitoring apex body. It is situated at Central Govt. Offices, Complex No. 1, Kamla Nehru Nagar, Ghaziabad. Its main functions are to set standards and testing of homoeopathic medicine at national level. It is an approved laboratory under Drugs & Cosmetics Act, 1940, with duties and functions of Central Drugs Laboratory for homoeopathic medicine under Section 6 of the Act and Rule 3A and Sub-Rule 7. The standard of homoeopathic medicines to be complied with for manufacture, sale or import are defined in Section 4A of Second Schedule of Drugs & Cosmetics Act. The laboratory is also recognised by the Department of Science & Technology, Govt. of India.

Worked out standards are released by the Ministry of Health & Family Welfare in the form of Homoeopathic Pharmacopoeia of India (HPI). Eight volumes covering standards for 916 drugs and 159 finished product have already been published. HPI is included in the Second Schedule of Drugs & Cosmetics Act, 1940. Recommendatory standards on two hundred fifty seven drugs have also been released. In the years to come, it has to cover additional 1,600 drugs.

Being an apex laboratory, HPL has also undertaking training of State Govt. officials engaged in quality control/quality assurance activities in the field of modern methods of drug testing. The laboratory also imparts training to the manufacturers and Principals of homoeopathic medical colleges. As a result, in the last decade, it has so far organised 36 training programmes covering approximately 300 trainees. In the last 15 years, remarkable improvements have taken place in the quality control of homoeopathic medicines.

Majority of HPL's functions have been switched over to computers and microprocessor based instruments, to achieve higher accuracy and outputs in the shortest possible time. It also undertakes research, evaluation and rationalisation of homoeopathic medicines and formulations. Plant introduction, maintenance of reference samples, survey and collection of data in respect of adulteration are its other functions. The laboratory must also have good collection of germ plasm/seeds of medicinal plants of both indigenous and exotic nature.

To achieve these, a multidisciplinary approach is adopted with high technology involvement. like Ultraviolet spectro-photometer (UV), Infrared spectro-photometer (IR), Gas Liquid chromatography (GLC), High Pressure Liquid Chromatography (HPLC), Atomic Absorption Spectrophotometer (AAS), Nuclear Magnetic Resonance and Scan Electron Microscope. It also had allied facilities like Microtomy, Thin Layer chromatography, Lyophilisation, Computer-data-processing, Museum, Library, Seminar room, Photography and Documentation unit, a Germ Plasm/Seed Bank and Tissue-culture facilities, an experimental herb garden and a nosode bank.

The laboratory receives samples from Drug Control Authorities, Central/State Govts. It is a notified laboratory for drug testing for states like Andhra Pradesh, Bihar, Union Territory of Delhi, Karnataka, Rajasthan, Uttar Pradesh, West Bengal and Tripura.

Dissemination of technical information and suggestions for remedial measures for quality improvement through survey sampling are being done at national level.

Standardisation of Homoeopathic Drugs

For laying down standards for identity, purity and testing of Homoeopathic Drugs, Govt. of India, Ministry of Health & Family Planning had constituted a Homoeopathic Pharmacopoeia Committee in 1962 with objectives:

1. To preserve a Pharmacopoeia of Homoeopathic Drugs whose therapeutic usefulness have been proved on lines of the American, German and British Homoeopathic Pharmacopoeia.
2. To lay down principles and standards for preparation of Homoeopathic Drugs.
3. To lay down tests of identity, quality and purity.
4. Such other matters as are identical and necessary for preparation of Homoeopathic Pharmacopoeia.

Functions of the Homoeopathic Pharmacopoeia Committee were further enlarged by The Ministry of Health & Family Planning also to prepare

1. A pharmaceutical codex in order to give such detailed information on drugs which are normally not given in pharmacopoeias e.g., constituents, uses etc. and
2. To prepare standards on nosodes.

For laying down standards for identity and purity and for testing of Homoeopathic Drugs, Govt. of India had set up a Homoeopathic Pharmacopoeia Laboratory at Ghaziabad in the year 1975.

Important functions which Homoeopathic Pharmacopoeia Laboratory is to discharge include:

1. Laying down of standards for identity and purity of Homoeopathic Drugs. Finding out indigenous substitutes for Foreign Drugs.

2. Verification of pharmacopoeial standards, done elsewhere, for adoption or improvement of standards or updation of standards.
3. Testing of samples of Homoeopathic Drugs for identity and quality under different provisions of Drugs and Cosmetics Act and Rules. Testing of samples referred by Drug Control Authorities, Port Authorities, State Government, etc.
4. Survey and collection of samples of Homoeopathic Drugs for verification of quality and adulteration trends of drugs marketed.
5. Maintenance of a Medicinal Plants Garden with preference to plants used in Homoeopathy. Cultivation and introduction of medicinal plants.
6. Survey and collection of Medicinal Plants.
7. Maintenance of a preference herbarium and a museum.
8. To import orientation to all India State/Central Government Drug Authorities, Drug Inspectors, Drug Analysts, Pharmacists etc. In methods of standardisation, identification and testing of Homoeopathic Drugs and application of various provision of Drugs Act.
9. To act as Central Drugs Laboratory for Homoeopathic Drugs for whole of India.
10. To perform functions of Government analyst for State Government and when desired by them.

For correct identity, enforcement and maintenance of quality of Homoeopathic Drugs, suitable provisions have been made in the Drugs and Cosmetics Act 1940 and Rules 1945.

Status of Homoeopathic Medicines in Drugs and Cosmetics Act, 1940 and Rules, 1945, and Status of Homoeopathic Pharmacopoeia Laboratory.

1. Homoeopathic Medicines are defined under Rule 2 (DD) of Crugs and Cosmetics Rule, 1945.
2. Standards of Homoeopathic Medicines to be complied for manufacture, for sale, distribution or import are covered under second schedule of the Drugs and Cosmetic act (item no. 4A).
3. New Homoeopathic Medicines are included under Rule 30AA and Rule 85C.
4. Minimum requirement for good manufacturing are included in schedule M-1.
5. Standards of ophthalmic preparations come under schedule FF (Rule 126A).
6. Homoeopathic Pharmacopoeia Laboratory, Ghaziabad is to function as Central Drugs Laboratory w.r.t. Homoeopathic Drugs under section 6 of the Act under Sub Rule 7 of rule 3A.
7. Anybody can get medicines tested under sections 26.
8. Under section 26A Central Govt. can cancel the license of manufacturing of drugs, if therapeutic claims are not genuine.
9. Procedures for labelling and packing of Homoeopathic Medicines are included in Rule 32A, Rule 106A and Rule 105B (Part ix-A).
10. Rule 85B covers manufacture of Mother Tinctures, potencies or potencies from back potencies. Application for which is made under form 24C.
11. Rule 85C and 30AA covers manufacture of new Homoeopathic Drugs.
12. Manufacture by pharmacists (shop keepers) of potencies is allowed only from back potencies under Rule 85D,
13. Retail is covered under Rule 67C. Application be made under form 20C. Single Drugs.
14. Though wholesale is covered under Rule 67C, but application is made under form 20D. Single Drugs.
15. Licensing Authority for issue of license for Homoeopathic Medicines lies with the State Government as per Rule 67A and 85B.
16. Schedule K, item 31 provides permission for sale of some selected Homoeopathic Drugs through any registered retail dealer of medicine licensed under Rule 61. Item 31 (schedule K) includes some 32 single Homoeopathic Medicines in pills in 30C potency in original sealed packs; 12 biochemics tissue remedies; 4 ointments and Arnica hair oil.

Chapter 08

Hospital Pharmacy (Institutional Pharmacy)

Introduction

Hospital Pharmacy may be defined as the practice of pharmacy in hospitals, health maintenance organisations and nursing homes.

Hospital Pharmacy is a discipline concerned with the objects of planning, organising, directing, motivating, communicating and controlling all aspects related to drugs with a view to contributing to the overall objectives of the homoeopathic hospital as an organisation of health care. Its scope ranges from drug procurement to drug administration.

A hospital pharmacy is a drug procurement, processing and dispensing, a storage, distribution and administration centre, depending upon the size and nature of the hospital in which it is set up.

The practice of pharmacy in a homoeopathic hospital set up is not as complicated due to the simplicity of the nature of medicines. Homoeopathic medicine chests also do not include narcotic substances as well as poisonous substances in their crude form for dispensing purposes. The different dosage forms in homoeopathy are quite simple to store, handle and dispense. Homoeopathic pharmacy also does not employ compounding of mixtures in prescriptions. It is desirable that all records right from the procurement of drugs up to the drug administration be stored in an electronic form. This improves the overall efficiency of the hospital and also helps in planning and research.

Unlike its counterpart in the West, the 'Hospital pharmacy' service has not established itself in India to its full/rather desired bloom form, as such, it is not popular enough among the hospital administrators and clinicians.

It is also not correct to compare with the Western pharmacies and pharmacists as they are not equals and at the same time there is no level playing.

However, to put it optimistically: "There is a great potential in the Indian hospitals to establish and develop 'Hospital Pharmacy' service".

Hospital pharmacy concerns itself with the drug logistics—supply chain management that includes policy, planning, warehouse management, procurement and dispensing/distribution.

Hospital pharmacies typically provide medications for the hospitalised patients only, and are not retail establishments. They typically do not provide prescription service to the public. Some hospitals do have retail pharmacies within them, which sell over-the-counter (OTC) as well as prescription medications to the public, but these are not the actual hospital pharmacy.

Functions

1. The primary function of the hospital pharmacy is to support the medicinal treatment for hospitalised patients.
2. To estimate needs for facilities, supplies, and equipment and to implement a system for evaluation, control and maintenance.
3. To supply medicines and necessary accessories to user departments in out-patient department (OPD) or the clinics and the in-patient department (IPD) or the hospital wards.
4. To fill up of those prescriptions where receipt demands dispensing.
5. To fill up prescriptions in OPD and IPD.
6. To receive, store and issue drugs.
7. To participate in the coordination of the functions of the department with the functions of all other departments and services of the hospital.
8. Statistical and research work.

Location

Hospital pharmacies can usually be found within the premises of the hospital at such a place that all the user departments and patients have an easy access to it. It should be prominently, conveniently and centrally located. The pharmacy with the dispensing and the billing section should ideally be located on the main floor. The pharmacy and the dispensing area should not be located close to the public lavatory or unsanitary filthy surroundings. The general environment should be non-polluting. Though the room should be well-ventilated with a constant circulation of fresh air, entry of direct sunlight should be avoided. There should be an arrangement for exhaust, and should be air-conditioned, if possible.

Drug Procurement

Homoeopathic pharmaceuticals and other accessories for the hospital may be purchased in one of the following ways:

1. By direct purchase from the manufacturer.
2. By direct purchase from a wholesaler.
3. By purchase from a local retail pharmacy.

It is always cost-effective to procure bulk orders of medicines or other dispensing accessories from the manufacturer. As a manufacturing unit may not handle smaller orders, purchase from a wholesaler is usually resorted to. The local retail homoeopathic pharmacy can always be a ready source for procurement of drugs on demand, as the fulfillment of the orders by the manufacturer and the wholesaler may consume time.

Storage, Distribution and Administration

After the receipt of the stock, the most important part is storage of the stock in such a way that it is easily procurable. Centralised storage facilities facilitate reduction in labour and record keeping, as well as tight control, and all the time are easily accessible.

Medical Stores

Medical stores maintain the medicines and other accessories in proper conditions. It issues the drugs and other accessories to the hospital wards and user departments. Proper care should be taken in the preservation of homoeopathic medicines. Separate arrangements should be kept for potentised medicines and other odorous substances. The stock should be properly labelled. If coded or computerised data is maintained, the corresponding reference number should be attached to the stock.

Medical stores have the following objectives:

1. Procurement of drugs.
2. To stock all the drugs and accessories.
3. Issue of drugs to user departments.
4. To carry out all operations economically and with proper statutory compliance.

Stock Arrangement

While arranging the stock, the following should be considered:

1. The movement rate of the various homoeopathic medicines.
2. The therapeutic category of the product.

3. The dosage form type of classification (solid or liquid).
4. The accessibility factor.
5. The visibility factor.

As a method of inventory control, the medicines should be classified as:

1. Fast moving.
2. Medium moving.
3. Slow moving.

The movement factor should be determined on the basis of

1. The total volume needed within specified time.
2. Frequency with which orders are placed.
3. Period for which the drugs remain in the stores.
4. Disease pattern.

Depending upon the rate of usage, the orders for these products should be carefully placed and sufficient quantities should be carefully ordered.

Shelf Stripping

Shelf stripping consists of attaching a strip of tape to the front run of the shelf and marking upon it pertinent information relating to the product being stored. The usual information placed on the tape consists of the name and strength of the product, unit size, and a reference number that is simultaneously maintained in records. Floor marking consists of preparing a stencil with the necessary information and painting it on the store room floor. By marking and identifying the storage areas it helps in providing a fixed place for the storage of a particular product.

Issue System

The medicines must be issued against an authorised prescription signed by a registered homoeopathic practitioner. This must then be accounted for in the issue register. In a homoeopathic hospital, usually, a proper set-up is required for dispensing as well as for administrative service.

Pharmaceutical Services in Out-patient Department (O.P.D.)

The clinics or the OPD must be very conveniently located, generally on the ground floor, in the main wing of the hospital. The issue of case papers must be the first point of location. In hospitals too, the principles underlying dispensing of prescriptions for out-patients are essentially the same as those in routine dispensing. The main difference in the form of hospital prescriptions is that, generally the length of time and duration of the treatment is specified rather than the actual quantity of the medicine that is to be supplied.

Pharmaceutical Services in In-patient Department (I.P.D.)

Normally, physicians prescribe, pharmacists dispense and the nurses administer. But the overall drug distribution and utilisation process involves many procedures. In addition to the traditional physician-pharmacist-patient relationship that exists in private clinical practice, there is a physician-pharmacist-nurse-patient relationship in a hospital.

The in-patient departments are generally divided into wards and each ward is in charge of a responsible medical and nursing officer on whose authorisation the stores issue them the necessary medicines—brought in trolleys to the concerned departments.

Hospital Prescriptions

For in-patients, supply of medicines in hospital has a different form of dispensing. Prescriptions for in-patients are written on the in-patient case-sheets under the follow-up record and on a sheet where the daily record of medicines administered to the patient is kept. This is called the 'physician's order sheet'. This, in turn, is sent to the hospital pharmacy for dispensing.

Ward Stock Medicines

The matron should maintain the bare minimum stock of essential medicines in the ward. As soon as the supplies are depleted, they should be replenished from the stores. The medicines consumed must be properly accounted for.

Chapter 09

Brief Study of Standardisation of Drugs

Introduction

The acceptability of any material is always established by prescribing a standard.

It is a numerical value which "quantifies" a parameter and thus denotes the "quality & purity" of material, thereby enhancing its "efficacy".

Any standard product definitely possesses certain amount of *stability or shelf life.*

Stability of a pharmaceutical product may be defined as the capability of a particular formulation, in a specific container/closure system, to remain within its physical, chemical, microbiological, therapeutic, and toxicological specifications for a prescribed period.

The concepts of standardisation in the current day practice is emphasised mainly due to the industrialisation of homoeopathic pharmaceutics so as to meet the global needs and standards for uniformity in procedures, quality, quantification.

Stability

It is defined as the extent to which a product retains—within specified limits and throughout its period of storage and use (i.e its shelf life)—the same properties and characteristics that it possessed at the time of its manufacture.

There are five types of stability that must be considered for each drug:

1. **Physical:** The original physical properties including appearance, palatability, uniformity, dissolution, suspendability are retained.
2. **Chemical:** Each active ingredient retains its chemical integrity and labelled potency, within the specified limits. Uninfluenced by storage conditions, temperature, light and humidity.
3. **Microbiological:** Stability or resistance to microbial growth is retained according to the specified requirements. Antimicrobial agents that are present retain effectiveness within the specified limits.
4. **Therapeutic:** The therapeutic effect remains unchanged.
5. **Toxicological:** No significant increase in toxicity occurs. The pioneers of R & D wings and Research Institutes are entrusted in standardisation works.

Aim

The ultimate aim of standardisation is to produce homoeopathic drugs that are highly efficacious in:

Quality

Safety.

DIFFERENT METHODS OF DRUG STANDARDISATION

A. Organoleptic evaluation

B. Microscopic evaluation

C. Physical evaluation

D. Chemical evaluation

E. Biological evaluation

A. Organoleptic Evaluation

It refers to evaluation by means of organs of senses, e.g. eyes (to see), nose (for odour), tongue (to taste), skin (by touch) and includes the macroscopic appearance, its odour and the taste and feel of drug to touch. Occasionally, the group of the fracture of the plant material is also considered:

1. **Shape and Size:** The underground plant part includes—rhizomes, roots, corms, bulbs, tubers etc. and they occur in entire longitudinal slices, oblique or transverse slices, cut in small cubical pieces or broken into pieces.

   Different shapes: (i) Conical: ACONITE; (ii) Cylindrical: SARSAPARILLA; SUMBUL; (iii) Sub-cylindrical: PODOPHYLLUM; RHEUM; (iv) Cylindrical or somewhat tapering: RATANHIA; RAPHANUS; (v) Cylindrical-ovoid: FILIX MAS; (vi) Cylindrical in older parts but flattened dorsiventrally: IRIS VERSICOLOR; (vii) Fusiform, ovoid and pyriform: *JALAPA*.

   Sizes are described in length and breadth or diameter, measuring in mm or cm.

2. **External colour:** They vary from white to yellow, yellowish, grey-yellowish, brown reddish-orange to brownish-black.
3. **External markings:** These may be furrows; parallel; wrinkles; ridges and valleys; transverse markings of various types; annulated etc.
4. **Fractures:** To study the way how the plant breaks, when subjected to a sufficient pressure.
5. **Flowers and leaves:** Usual botanical terms are used to identify and describe them.
6. **Odour:** Such as aromatic; balsamic spicy alliaceous; camphoraceous; teribinthinate; ethereal etc.
7. **Taste:** These are termed as—acids (sour); saline (salty); saccharine (sweet); alkaline; bitter; insipid (tasteless); astringent; pungent; starchy; gritty etc.
8. **Colour:** The terms are standardised according to recommendations of Inter-Society Colour Council (I.S.C.C.); National Bureau of Standards and Technology (N.I.S.T.).

B. Microscopic Evaluation

Microscopic examination of drugs has been used since 1847. Microscopic examination helps for searching adulterants in powdered plant and animal drugs and also in the identification of pure powdered drugs.

Details of histology with microscopic appearance of drug in sectional view and powdered form has been given in the monograph of the respective drug in pharmacopoeia.

1. **Plant parts:** These are made up of numerous tissues. Histology refers to the arrangement and individual characters of these tissues. These histological studies are done with very thin transverse or longitudinal sections properly mounted in suitable stains or reagents or mounting media.
2. **Powdered drugs:** Gives very few microscopic features for identification. Since the complete structure is not available, powdered drug should be reduced to not less than No. 40 powder. The cells are mostly broken except those with lignified walls. The cell contents—calcium oxalate crystals, starch, aleurone, oil, gum, resin etc. remain scattered in the powder. They are the evidence of the source. Proper mounting and reagents can demonstrate cell walls, blast-fibres, stone-cell, leaf-epidermal tissues. The study of stomatal index also helps to determine the identity of the plant.

Micro-chemistry

It comprises the study of the constituents of drugs by application of chemical (and physical) methods to small quantities, a few mg of the powdered drug or to histological section of drug.

By these methods various constituents of drugs can be isolated and identified.

Outline of the Principal Techniques

1. **Isolation of constituents of drugs by**
   (a) Micro-sublimation: A small quantity of the drug is heated to evaporation. The vapours of this are collected in crystallised form by using method of condensation. When these crystals are formed they represent the characteristic pattern of structure of the pure constituent. The crystallography will determine the identity, e.g., red droplets of cinchona bark.
   (b) Chemical solvents: (i) Micro-extraction—Separation of the constituents from a small quantity of drugs, (ii) Micro-filtration, (iii) Micro-crystallisation.
2. **Identification of constituents of drugs by**
   (a) Crystallography: It is the science of the forms, structures, properties and classification of the crystals which helps in identifying the constituents of drugs.
   (b) Melting point determination.
   (c) Confirmative tests: (i) Physical test, (ii) Chemical test—colour reaction test.

Colour reaction test: These are very valuable aids for the identification; though by themselves they may not be authoritative, some total tests will decide upon the purity, e.g.

Alkaloid	Reagent	Colour/ppt.
1. Anthraquinone alkaloid (present in Rheum, Senna)	Alkali	Red
2. Aqueous solution of alkaloid	Auric chloride	Yellow ppt.
3. Aqueous solution of alkaloid	Iodine in KI	Brown ppt.
4. Aqueous solution of alkaloid	Na_2CO_3 or Tannic acid	White or yellow ppt.

C. Physical Evaluation

1. Chromatographic study of drugs: Details of this test described in Chapter 6.
2. Fluorescence test: The reaction of certain drugs either in powdered form or on the smooth sectioned surfaces with filtered UV light help in determining adulterants. e.g.
   (i) *Rheum emodi* shows deep violet fluorescence.
   (ii) 1% tincture of *Rauwalfia* fluorescence blue in UV.

Many alkaloids show distinctive colours under this UV light. e.g.

(i) Aconitine: Light blue
(ii) Berberine: Yellow
(iii) Emetine: Orange.

The application of physical constants is largely employed to the active principles of drugs, e.g., alkaloids and fixed oils.

Generally applied physical constants for such drugs are: (i) Solubility, (ii) Sp. Gr. (iii) Melting point, (iv) Congealing point, (v) Refractive index, (vi) Optical rotation, (vii) Water content or loss on drying.

D. Chemical Evaluation

Chemical methods of evaluation cover the isolation, identification, purification and characteristic determination of non-cellular drugs of animal origin and drugs of plants having active principles.

Chemical assay is done to assess the potency of the vegetable and animal source materials in terms of their active principles.

The chemical assays include: (i) Colour reaction test, (ii) Molisch and Barfoed's test, (iii) Acid value, (iv) Iodine value, (v) Saponification value, (vi) Ash value, (vii) Sulphated ash value, (viii) Determination of acid insoluble ash, (ix) Determination of water soluble ash.

These tests help to determine the identity and adulterations.

E. Biological Evaluation(Bio-Assays)

Pharmacological activity of certain drugs has been applied to evaluate and standardise them. The assays on living animals and on their intact or cut-off organs can indicate the strength of the drug or their preparation.

As living organisms are used, these assays are known as Biological Assays or Bio-Assays.

Using these Bio-Assays we can evaluate or standardise the following drugs e.g., *Cascara sagrada; Verat viride; Cannabis indica; Cannabis sativa; Sec. cor; Nosodes; Sarcodes.*

ANALYSIS OF VEGETABLE AND ANIMAL DRUGS—ANALYTICAL PHARMACOLOGY

1. *Foreign organic matter:* Refers to any other part of the plant or animal tissues. The permissible p.c. of the foreign organic matter in drugs are usually specified in their respective official monographs.
2. *Foreign inorganic matter:* Refers to the adhering soil, clay, sand, dirt etc. for determining which ACID–INSOLUBLE ASH METHOD is applied. However, some drugs, naturally, contain acid-insoluble ash. Maximum 2% of acid insoluble ash is officially permitted, unless otherwise prescribed in the monograph.
3. *Moisture Content:* is usually from 5 to 10% in all dried drugs; an excess of moisture, if present, is an adulterant.

Systemic Analysis

1. At first analyst will perform the organoleptic examination with special traces to the morphological features—size, odour, taste etc.
2. Then, if necessary, he/she will proceed to the microscopic examination for histological study.
3. After that, he will determine the foreign organic matter, by official method.
4. Next, he will take the proper amount of official sample and following tests will be done systematically: (i) Determination of total ash, (ii) Determination of acid insoluble ash, (iii) Determination of moisture content.
5. Lastly, he will determine the constituents of the drug sample.

Determination of Constituents

The quality of standards which is dependent upon the amount constituent present in drugs, capable of being extracted, have been prescribed for certain drugs. They are extracted in a continuous apparatus and the extracts thus obtained are determined by weight, after removing the solvents (common solvents used—strong alcohol, dilute alcohol, ether, petroleum, benzene and water).

Alkaloids: are recovered from drug sample by extraction, next purified with immiscible solvents and can be determined gravimetrically or volumetrically by titration of the quantity of the acid required to convert them into salts.

Volatile Oils: Amount of volatile oil present in a volatile oil containing plant can be determined by distilling with water in the proper clevenger apparatus, which is a continuous distillation apparatus, wherein the separated volatile oil is obtained in a trap and is then determined by volume.

In some cases, special assays for drugs containing some definite chemical constituents have been deviced. In other cases where no extraction, chemical or physical assay has been devised, the quality is determined by proper Bio-Assays.

STANDARDS OF MOTHER TINCTURES, MOTHER SOLUTIONS AND ATTENUATIONS

Same tests may be applied as in case of mother tinctures. A few such standards have been worked out by the Homoeopathic Pharmacopoeia Laboratory (H.P.L.), Ghaziabad (It is a subordinate office of Ministry of Health and Family Welfare. It is situated at Central Govt. Office Complex, Kamla Nehru Nagar, Ghaziabad 201 002).

A. **Aethusa cynapium:** Mother tincture; IX

1. Sp. Gr.: 0.894 to 0.918
2. Alcohol content: 52 to 62%
3. Total solid: Not less than 0.3%
4. pH: 5.3 to 6.2
5. Identification: Preparation of solution 'S'. Shake 2 ml with 5 ml. of CCl_4. Allow the layers to separate. Evaporate the CCl_4 layer in a dish to dryness on a water-bath. Dissolve the residue in water by little warming:

   (a) The solution 'S' is discoloured when a few drops of $KMnO_4$ solution added.

   (b) To the solution 'S' add a drop of alcoholic $FeCl_3$ solution—yellowish-green colour is produced.

6. T.L.C.: Carry out the method for T.L.C. using Silica gel G as the coating substance and a mixture of $CHCl_3$ and CH_3OH (9 : 1 v/v) as the mobile phase. The R_f of the spots when detected under UV light are 0.13; 0.27; 0.84.

B. **Avena sativa:** Mother tincture; IX

1. Sp. Gr.: 0.906 to 0.916
2. Alcohol content: 56 to 62% (v/v).
3. Total solid: Not less than 0.3%
4. pH: 5.6 to 6.5
5. P.C. (Paper chromatography): Carry-out p.c. using n-butanol: Acetic acid: Water (4 : 1 : 1 v/v) and spraying reagent 0.1% ninhydrin in acetone. These spots corresponds to cystine (0.04); lysin (0.095), dihydroxy phenyl alanine (0.20) and tryptophan (0.37) and valine (0.54).

C. **Belladonna:** Mother tincture; IX

1. Sp. Gr.: 0.931 to 0.948
2. Alcohol content: 40 to 46% v/v
3. Total solid: Not less than 1%
4. Total alkaloid: Not less than 0.03% and not more than 0.04% of total alkaloids calculated as hyoscyamine.
5. pH: 6.8 to 7.0
6. Identification: Evaporate 35 ml to dryness. To the residue add 5 drops of HNO_3 (fuming) and evaporate on the water bath. The residue cooling and moistening with a freshly prepared 10% w/v solution of KOH in acetone produces a violet colour.
7. T.L.C.: Carry out the method for T.L.C., using silica gel G as the coating substance and $CH_3OH : NH_3$ (100 : 15 v/v) as the mobile phase. The R_f value of spots when detected under UV light are 0.73 and 0.64.

D. **Calendula officinalis:** Mother tincture; IX

1. Sp. Gr.: 0.933 to 0.970
2. Alcohol content: 37 to 43% v/v
3. Total solid: Not less than 1.8%
4. pH: 5.1 to 6.1
5. Identification: Shake 10 ml with 20 ml. of $CHCl_3$. To $CHCl_3$ layer add 1 ml of H_2SO_4. The $CHCl_3$ layer becomes red and acid layer gives green fluorescence.
6. T.L.C.: Carry out the method for T.L.C. using silica gel G as the coating substance and ethyl-acetate, formic acid and water (8 : 1 : 1 v/v) as the mobile phase.

The R_f value of the spots, when detected under UV light before and after spraying with Boric and Oxalic acid, are 0.104; 0.12 and 0.24.

E. **Kali bichromicum**

1. Mother solution, IX

   Sp. Gr.: 1.069

   Assay: 9.5 to 10.5% of $K_2Cr_2O_7$
2. Potency: 2X

   Sp. Gr.: 1.007

   Assay: 0.95 to 1.05% of $K_2Cr_2O_7$
3. Potency: 3X

   Sp. Gr.: 1.003

   Assay: 0.095 to 0.105% of $K_2Cr_2O_7$.

F. **Mercurius dulcis**

1. Potency—1X

   (a) Water insoluble residue—Shake 5 gm with 10 ml of water and filter. Then dry the insoluble residue to a constant weight. The residue is not less than 0.48 gm.

   (b) Identification:

   (i) It is blackened by dil. NH_3 solution.

   (ii) When heated with an equal weight of anhydrous Na_2CO_3, a sublimate of metallic mercury is obtained. The residue in the tube is treated with dil. HNO_3, filtered; filtrate gives the reaction characteristic of chloride.

   (c) Assay: 9.5 to 10.5%
2. Potency—2X

   Assay: 0.95 to 1.05%

STANDARDISATION OF VEHICLES

Sugar of Milk

1. Identification:
   (i) When heated, it melts, swells and burns, evolving an odour of burnt sugar and leaving a bulky carbonaceous residue.
   (ii) When heated with potassium cupri-tartarate solution, a copious precipitate of cuprous oxide is formed.
   (iii) Optical rotation: It is dextro-rotatory, $[\alpha]D = 55.3°$ (Final value).
2. Acidity or Alkalinity: 5 gm of sugar of milk is dissolved in 50 ml of freshly boiled water, requires for neutralisation not more than 0.5 ml of 0.1 (N) NaOH, phenolphthalin solution being used as indicator.
3. Clarity, colour and odour of solution: 3 gm of sugar of milk is dissolved in 10 ml of boiling water—the solution is clear, colourless and odourless.
4. Arsenic: Not more than 1 part per million.
5. Copper: 2 gm sugar of milk is dissolved in 20 ml of water. Then 1 ml of dil. HCl and 10 ml of a solution of H_2S is added. No colour is produced.
6. Sulphated ash: Not more than 0.1%.
7. More soluble sugars: 5 gm of sugar of milk is shaken with 20 ml of alcohol (90 p.c. v/v) for 10 minutes and filtered. Then evaporate 10 ml of the filtrate to dryness and dry at 105°C. The residue weights not more than 7 mg.

Alcohol

1. Identification:
   (i) Iodoform test: To about 10 ml of a 0.5% v/v solution, 2 ml of 4% v/v solution of NaOH is added. Then about 4 ml solution of Iodine is added slowly. The odour of iodoform develops, and a yellow precipitate is produced:
   $CH_3CH_2OH + 4I_2 + 6NaOH \rightarrow CHI_3 + 5NaI + HCOONa + 5H_2O$.
   (ii) Refractive index (n) D^{20}: 1.3637 to 1.3639.
   (iii) Sp. Gr. at 15.6°C or 60°F: 0.816.
2. Acidity or Alkalinity: 20 ml requires not more than 0.2 ml of N/10 NaOH to give a pink colour with phenolphthalin solution, or not more than 0.1 ml of HCl. to give a red colour with methyl red solution.
3. Aldehyde: To 10 ml., 5 ml of a solution of NaOH is added, shaken and allowed to stand for 5 minutes. No yellow colour is produced.
4. Ketones: To 1 ml., 3 ml of purified water and 10 ml of a solution of mercuric sulphate added and heated on a boiling water bath. No ppt. is produced in 3 minutes.
5. Fusel oil and allied impurities: Allow 25 ml to evaporate spontaneously to a porcelain dish, protected from dust until the surface of the dish is barely moist no foreign odour is perceptible and, on addition of 1 ml of H_2SO_4, no red or brown colour is produced.
6. Oily or resinous substances: Dilute 5 ml to 100 ml with water in a glass cylinder. The solution remains clear when examined against a black background.
7. Non-volatile matter: When evaporated and dried at 105°C, leaves not more than 0.005% of residue.

Glycerine

1. Identification:
   (i) When heated with potassium hydrogen sulphate ($KHSO_4$), gives off irritating vapours which blackens a filter paper moistened with a solution of ammonaical silver nitrate.
   (ii) When heated on a borax bead in a Bunsen flame it gives a green flame.
   (iii) When diluted with six times its volume of purified water it gives no precipitate with solution of barium chloride, $AgNO_3$ and of lime or with sulphureted HCl.
2. A 10.0% w/v solution is neutral to solution of litmus.
3. Weight per ml: At 25°C, 1.252 to 1.257 gm, corresponding to 98.0 to 100.0% of $C_3H_8O_3$.
4. Refractive index: At 20°C, 1.471 to 1.473.

It should comply with the standards, as specified in H.P.I., in respect of: (a) Certain reducing substances, (b) Fatty acids and Esters, (c) Sucrose, (d) Sulphated ash etc.

Olive Oil

1. Acid value: not more than 2.0
2. Iodine value: 79 to 88
3. Saponification value: 190 to 195
4. Refractive index: At 20°C, 1.468 to 1.471
5. Weight per ml: At 20°C, 0.910 to 0.913.
6. Arachis oil: 1 ml of oil is boiled in a flask with reflux condenser with 5 ml of 1.5 (N), alcoholic KOH for 10 minutes, 50 ml of alcohol (70%) and 0.8 ml of conc. HCl is added. The solution is gradually cooled and in pure olive oil no turbidity appears above 9°C. This is the test of finding that the olive oil is free from Arachis oil (peanut oil).
7. Sesame oil: To ascertain the purity of olive oil, little olive oil is shaken with an equal volume of a mixture of 9 parts of alcohol (90%) and 1 part of strong ammonia and heated on a water-bath until free from alcohol and ammonia. Now, 2 ml of the oil is shaken with 1 ml of HCl containing 1% w/v of sucrose and set aside for 5 minutes. The acid layer is not coloured pink or faintly pink.

Almond Oil

1. Identification:
   (i) It remains clear after exposure to a temperature of -10°C for 3 hours; does not congeal until the temperature has been reduced to about -18°C.
   (ii) Solubility: Almost insoluble in alcohol (95%), miscible with $CHCl_3$, solvent ether and light petroleum.
   (iii) Sp. Gr.: At 20°C, 0.910 to 0.915
   (iv) B. P.: 40°C to 60°C
   (v) Freezing point: 18°C
   (vi) Refractive index: At 20°C, 1.470 to 1.473
   (vii) Acid value: Not more than 4.00
   (viii) Iodine value: 95 to 102 (Iodine monochloride method)
   (ix) Saponification value: 188 to 196
   (x) Weight per ml: At 20°C, 0.910 to 0.915 gm.
2. Arachis oil: compiles with the test for the absence of cotton-seed oil in other oils.
3. Sesame oil: compiles with the test for the absence of sesame oil in other oils.

Sesame Oil

1. Solubility: slightly insoluble in alcohol (90%), miscible with solvent ether, chloroform and light petroleum.
2. Sp. Gr.: 0.916 to 0.921, at 20°C
3. Acid value: Not more than 2.0
4. Iodine value: 103 to 116.
5. Refractive index: At 20°C, 1.472 to 1.476
6. Saponification value: 188 to 195

Rosemary Oil

1. Solubility: soluble in one volume of alcohol (90% v/v) but, upon further dilution, may become turbid.
2. Sp. Gr: 0.894 to 0.912
3. Optical rotation: –5° to +10°, in 100 mm tube
4. Refractive index: At 20°C, 1.466 to 1.476.

Lavender Oil

1. Solubility: Soluble in alcohol (90%) and absolute alcohol; sparingly soluble in alcohol (60%) and 1 in 4 of alcohol (70%)
2. Sp. Gr.: At 25°C, 0.875 to 0.888
3. Refractive index: At 20°C, 1.4590 to 1.4700
4. Optical rotation: –3 to –10°, in a 100 mm tube.

Simple Syrup

1. Weight per ml: At 20°C, 1.315 to 1.333 gm
2. Optical rotation: +56° to +60°.

Bee's Wax

1. Solubility: Insoluble in water; sparingly soluble in cold alcohol; completely soluble in $CHCl_3$, ether, fixed and volatile oils.
2. Melting point: 60°C to 65°C

3. Acid value: 17 to 23
4. Iodine value: 8 to 11 (Iodine monochloride method)

Lanolin (Anhydrous)

1. Identification: Dissolved 0.5 gm in 5 ml of $CHCl_3$, and added 1 ml of Acetic anhydride and 2 drops of H_2SO_4; a deep green colour is produced.
2. Solubility: Insoluble in water; sparingly soluble in cold alcohol (90%); freely soluble in solvent ether and in $CHCl_3$.
3. Melting range: 36°C to 42°C
4. Acid value: Not more than 1
5. Iodine value: 18 to 32
6. Saponification value: 92 to 106

Spermaceti (U. S. P.)

1. Solubility: Insoluble in water, nearly insoluble in cold alcohol and slightly soluble in cold petroleum and benzene; but is soluble in boiling alcohol, in ether, in $CHCl_3$ and in fixed and volatile oils.
2. Sp. Gr.: About 0.94
3. Melting range: 42°C to 50°C
4. Acid value: Not more than 1.0
5. Iodine value: Not more than 5
6. Saponification value: 120 to 136.

Soft Paraffin (Vaseline)

1. Solubility: practically insoluble in $CHCl_3$ and solvent ether and in light petroleum.
2. Sp. Gr.: At 20°C, 0.815 to 0.880
3. Melting range: 38°C to 56°C
4. Wt. per ml.: At 60°C, 0.815 to 0.880 gm.
5. Reaction: Boil 5 gm with 10 ml of alcohol previously neutralised to solution of litmus. The alcohol is neutral to litmus.
6. Fixed oils, fats and resins: Digest 10 gm. with 50 ml solution of NaOH at 100°C for 30 minute and allow the aqueous layer to separate. On acidifying the aqueous layer with dilute H_2SO_4, no ppt. or oily matter is produced.
7. Foreign organic matter: volatilises when heated, without emitting an acrid odour.
8. Sulphated ash: Not more than 0.1%.

Starch

1. Identification: yields, when boiled with 15 times of its weight of water and cooled, a translucent viscous fluid or jelly, which is coloured deep blue by iodine solution; the colour disappears on warming and reappears on cooling.
2. Acidity: Add 10 gm to 100 ml of alcohol (70%) previously neutralised to phenolphthalin solution, shake well, drying one hour, filter and titrate 50 ml of the filtrate with 0.1 (N) NaOH, using phenolphthalin solution as indicator, not more than 2.0 ml of 0.1 (N) NaOH is required.
3. Iron: Mix 0.5 gm with 10 ml of water and add 0.5 ml of HCl and 0.3 ml of K–ferrocyanide solution; the mixture does not become blue within one minute.

   Ash: Not more than 0.3% (maize starch), 0.6% (rice-starch), 0.3% (potato starch) and 0.3% (wheat-starch).
4. Loss on drying: When dried to constant weight at 105°C, loses not more than 14.0% of its weight (maize-starch, rice-starch and wheat-starch) or not more than 20.0% of its weight (potato starch).

Centres undertaking Drug Standardisation Studies

At present, pharmacognostical and physicochemical studies are being undertaken at two centres:

1. Drug Standardisation Unit (H), C/o Central Research Institute, A1/1, Sector 24, Noida 201 301
2. Drug Standardisation Unit (H), O.U.B. 32, Room 4, Vikram Puri, Habsiguda, Hyderabad (A.P.) 500 007

The pharmacological studies under Drug Standardisation Programme have been suspended since July 1999 due to certain conditions imposed by the Ministry of Social Justice and Empowerment for conducting animal experimentations.

Publications of monographs: (i) Hydrocotyle asiatica, (ii) Abroma augusta, (iii) Aegle folia, (iv) Aegle marmelos, (v) Cynodon dactylon, (vi) Atista indica, (vii) Cassia sophera, (viii) Kali mur, (ix) Boerhaavia diffusa, (x) Carica papaya, (xi) Terminalia chebula.

CCRH

The Council has undertaken pharmacognostical studies on 297 drugs, physico-chemical studies on 304 and pharmacological studies on 149 drugs (as on 23.10.2017) and all the three aspects on 142 drugs have been studied.

The standards of the drugs worked out by the Council are definite gains and are important for preparation of quality Homoeopathic Medicines.

Books: Standardisation

1. **Standardisation of Homoeopathic Drugs Vol. I:** Contains pharmacognostical, physico-chemical and pharmacological profiles of 11 drugs, viz. Acorus calamus, Alfalfa, Capsicum annum, Cassia fistula, Ficus religiosa, Iberis amara, Juncus effusus, Mimosa pudica, Psoralea corylifolia, Thea sinensis, and Withania somnifera.
2. **Standardisation of Homoeopathic Drugs Vol. II:** Contains pharmacognostical, physico-chemical and pharmacological profiles of 12 drugs, viz. Bixa orellana, Cissampelos pareira, Citrus decumana, Coffea arabica, Foeniculum vulgare, Lawsonia inermis, Magnolia grandiflora, Ocimum canum, Persia americana, Siegesbeckia orientalis, Tamarindus indica, and Theobroma cacao.
3. **Standardisation of Homoeopathic Drugs Vol. III:** Contains pharmacognostical, physico-chemical and pharmacological profiles of 11 drugs, viz. Allium cepa, Anacardium orientale, Cocculus indicus, Cochlearia armoracia, Fagopyrum esculentum, Gymnema sylvestre, Holarrhena antidysenterica, Hypericum perforatum, Origanum majorana, Robinia pseudo-acacia, and Tylophora indica.

Legislations: Homoeopatic Medicines

1. Rule 2 (dd) of Drugs and Cosmetics Rules, 1945: Homoeopathic medicines are defined. Include any drug which is recorded in Homoeopathic provings or therapeutic efficacy of which has been established through long clinical experience as recorded in authoritative literature of India and abroad and which is prepared according to the techniques of homoeopathic pharmacy and covers combinations of ingredients of such Homoeopathic Medicines but does not include a medicine which is administered by parenteral route.
2. Standards of Homoeopathic Drugs are covered under Second Schedule of Drugs and Cosmetics Act, 1940.
3. Under item 4A of the Second Schedule, under Sections 8 and 16 of D&C Act, 1940.

   Standards included in HPI, which include information on characterisation/identification/testing of standards and preparation of Homoeopathic Medicines.

   Statutory requirements to be followed by all the manufacturers of drugs for maintenance of quality of Homoeopathic Drugs.

Status of Homoeopathic Medicines in Drugs and Cosmetics Act, 1940, and Rules, 1945, and Status of Homoeopathic Pharmacopoeia Laboratory

1. Homoeopathic Medicines are defined under Rule 2 (DD) of Drugs and Cosmetics Rule, 1945.
2. Standards of Homoeopathic Medicines to be complied for manufacture, for sale, for distribution or for import are covered under Second Schedule of the Drugs & Cosmetic Act (item no. 4A).
3. New Homoeopathic Medicines are included under rule 30AA and Rule 85-C.
4. Minimum requirement for good manufacturing are included in Schedule M1.
5. Standards of ophthalmic preparations come under Schedule FF (Rule 126A).
6. Homoeopathic Pharmacopoeia Laboratory, Ghaziabad, is to function as Central Drugs Laboratory w.r.t. Homoeopathic Drugs under Section 6 of the act under Sub Rule 7 of Rule 3A.
7. Anybody can get medicines tested under Section 26.

8. Under Section 26A Central Govt. can cancel license of manufacturing a drug, if therapeutic claims are not genuine.
9. Procedures for labeling and packing of Homoeopathic Medicines are included in Rule 32A, Rule 106A and Rule 105B (Part ix-A).
10. Rule 85B covers manufacture of mother tinctures, potencies or potencies from back potencies. Application for which is made under form 24C.
11. Rules 85C and 30AA cover manufacture of new Homoeopathic Drugs.
12. Manufacture by pharmacists (shopkeepers) of potencies is allowed only from back potencies under Rule 85D.
13. Retail is covered under Rule 67C. Application be made under form 20C. Single Drugs.
14. Though wholesale is covered under rule 67C, application is made under form 20D. Single Drugs.
15. Licensing Authority for issue of license for Homoeopathic Medicines lies with the State Government as per Rule 67A and 85B.
16. Schedule K, item 31, provides permission for sale of some selected Homoeopathic Drugs through any registered retail dealer of medicine licensed under Rule 61.
17. Item 31 (Schedule K) includes some 32 single Homoeopathic Medicines in pills in 30C potency in original sealed packs; 12 Biochemics Tissue Remedies; 4 ointments and Arnica hair oil.

Standardisation Types

There are two types of standardisation :

In the first category, "true" standardisation—a definite phyto-chemical or group of constituents is known to have activity. Ginkgo with its 26% ginkgo flavones and 6% terpenes is a classic example. These products are highly concentrated and no longer represent the whole herb, and are now considered as phyto-pharmaceuticals. In many cases they are vastly more effective than the whole herb.

The other type of standardisation is based on manufacturers guaranteeing the presence of a certain percentage of marker compounds; these are not indicators of therapeutic activity or quality of the herb. Strict guidelines have to be followed for the successful production of a quality drug.

Chapter 10

Quality Control in Homoeopathy

Introduction

Quality can be defined as the status of a drug that is determined by identity, purity, content, and other chemical, physical, or biological properties, or by the manufacturing processes. Quality control is a term that refers to the processes involved in maintaining the quality and validity of a manufactured product.

Quality control is not only the analytical testing of the finished product, but also the procedures beginning with receipt of raw materials and continuing throughout the production and packaging operations, finished product testing, documentation, surveillance and distribution. An Analytical Control Laboratory is responsible for testing and approving raw materials, the work-in-process and the finished product.

Quality control procedures are procedures for standardisation, by which the quality of a commodity may be assessed by ascribing numerical values. The quality should not only be tested at the end but must be carried out right from the moment of receipt of raw materials, right through processing, till the final packaging.

Long before, Hahnemann fully depended on the pure quality of Homoeopathic Medicines which he mentioned in his "Organon of Medicine" in the following words: "The true physician must be provided with genuine medicines of unimpaired strength, so that he may be able to rely upon their therapeutic powers; he must be able, himself, to judge of their genuineness." (Sec. 264, 6th edition, Organon of Medicine)

"It should be a matter of conscience with him to be thoroughly convinced in every case that the patient always takes the right medicine and therefore he must give the patient the correctly chosen medicine prepared, moreover, by himself." (Sec. 265, 6th edition, Organon of Medicine).

Aim

Quality control is the total procedure for providing the standard medicines to the patients.

Quality control for efficacy and safety of homeopathic products is of paramount importance.

Objective of Quality Control

The objectives of quality control are that, the finished product:

(a) Complies with quality specifications (experiment design).

(b) Contains the correct ingredients in the correct proportions.
(c) Maintains uptodate purity.
(d) Has been correctly processed as specified in different pharmacopoeias (HPI, HPUS, BHP, GHP/HAB).
(e) Is packaged in proper container.
(f) Bears the proper label.
(g) Is properly stored for maintaining proper quality.

Factors (Parameters) for Quality Control

Various factors are related to quality control process which has great role in obtaining standard quality, starting from raw materials to finished products.

Prime factors are:

1. **Materials:** Qualities of all materials, from the raw products, to finished products, including the packaging materials, must be carefully controlled and supervised. A proper system must be evolved for purchase and receipt of materials and raw products, their testing, storage and finally, their issue for manufacture of dosage forms. At the same time, proper records should be maintained for all such transactions. All drug substances as well as vehicles and other non-drug components must conform to the specified standards as in the pharmacopoeia of purity, quality, and freedom from toxicity.

Similar procedures are adopted with respect to containers, closures, cartons, labels, etc.

2. **Personnel:** The peoples involved in processing and packaging the products and other related jobs are the most significant factors in quality control.

Every manufacturer must have a proper system of selection of personnel and of their training. High quality standard products are only possible if one can rely on the integrity, the involvement, the training, experience and the commitment of all concerned.

Homoeopathic pharmaceutical preparations involve medicaments that are difficult to evaluate and standardise. The 'personnel', hence, become a vital aspect in the preparation of Homoeopathic Medicines—the reliability of the product depending upon the motivation of the staff.

With the instrumentation of manufacturing techniques, the human error is relatively reduced. But pharmaceutical units that strictly follow Hahnemannian techniques of hand succussion need to ay stress on this variant of quality control.

3. **Equipments:** The equipments used in the manufacturing process are important to maintain the quality of the products. Equipments must be accurate and capable of reproducing quality as per specifications.
4. **Environments:** The environments under which the raw materials are stored, processed, and packaged are also very important. The environments in which the processing is done is important because any contamination of pollutants may deteriorate the quality of products.
5. **Methods:** Methodology for the manufacture of Homoeopathic Medicines must be in conformation of homoeopathic principles. Modified techniques in homoeopathic pharmaceutics are introduced due to increased demands of the profession. Hahnemannian methods should be followed as far as possible. The pharmacopoeial guidelines for procedures of identification, collection, preservation, preparation, and its analysis must be clearly indicated. Preparation of potencies needs to be standardised. Methods employed for processing, packaging, etc. also have important contributions to make to the qualities of products.
6. **Infrastructure:** Quality of products also depend on suitable infrastructure. The infrastructure should be constructed as per GMP rules.

Quality Control Department

Quality control is a total procedure for providing the standard medicines to the patients.

Quality control is not only a laboratory procedure but also the procedures through which a raw material is transformed to a drug and the finished product—till it is used by the patient. One important function of quality control department is to establish specifications for raw materials, packing materials, intermediates, and finished products to assure the proper quality.

Quality Control Monitoring Apex Body

In India, the quality of Homoeopathic Medicines are controlled by the Drugs and Cosmetics Act, a Central legislation. The Homoeopathic Pharmacopoeia Laboratory (HPL), Ghaziabad, was set up in Sept 1975 under the Ministry of Health and Family Welfare, Government of India, as a quality monitoring apex body, as a Plan Scheme under 5th Plan (1975-80). It is a subordinate institute of Department of ISM & Homoeopathy.

It is recognised by Dept. of Science and Technology, Government of India, as Scientific, Technological and Research Institution. It is recognised as Central Drugs Laboratory for testing of Homoeopathic Drugs (under Rule 3A, under Section 6 of D & C Act). Its main functions are to set standards and drug testing laboratory at national level. Worked out standards are released by the Ministry of Health and Family Welfare in the form of Homoeopathic Pharmacopoeia of India (HPI). The laboratory releases, from time to time, recommendatory standards for raw materials and common finished products for comments of the manufacturers and allied scientists. Homoeopathic Pharmacopoeia Committee (Sept 1982) of Government of India then subsequently examines them before they take shape of mandatory standards.

Total number of monographs in HPI = 1,111.

Homoeopathic Pharmaceutical codex published in 2002 contains detail of 101 drugs.

Homoeopathic Pharmacopoeia of India (HPI)

Volumes	Year of Publication	No. of Drugs
1	1971	180
2	1974 (revised edn. 1982)	100
3	1978	105
4	1984	107
5	1986	114
6	1990	104
7	1999	105
8	2000	101
9	2007	100
10	2013	101

Monograph of each drug contains details for identification, collection, part used, method of preparation, assessment of purity, limits of impurity etc. It is essential that these instructions be strictly followed to obtain mother tinctures of desired standards.

Modern techniques and systems of quality control do not invalidate the original Hahnemannian concept, nor replace the classical procedures. Indeed, they are enhanced.

Sampling

Sampling of raw materials, in-process products or the finished products, in order to determine any of its attributes, is a very significant step in the overall quality control of the dosage forms.

Scientifically, a true sample should consist of appropriate number, quantity from a batch which determines the true nature of the entire product.

There may be a variety of sampling plans. The commonly used sampling plans are the single sampling and double sampling. In single sampling, only one sample is analysed to determine the whole batch. In double sampling plan, if the first sample gives a 'rejection' result, a second sample is tested to determine the acceptability of the batch. Multiple sampling plans may also be used.

Method of Official Sampling for Analysis

A. **Process:** The correct sampling is an essential part for proper maintaining of the quality standard.

Sampling of raw plant products are usually done in the following way:

(a) **Where the component parts of gross samples are less than 1 cm or less in any dimension and all powdered or ground drugs:**

Taken with the help of sampler which removes a core from the top to the bottom of the container, not more than two cores being taken in opposite directions.

When the total weight of the drug sample is:

1. Less than 100 kg (200 lb) → Official Sample = at least 250 g.

2. More than 100 kg → Official Sample = at least 250 g. It should be taken in repeated samples by the same way. Next, they are mixed and divided into four equal quarters. Reject 2 of the diagonal quarters, combine and carefully mix the remaining quarters and again subject the drug to a quartering process in the same manner until two of the quarters weigh at least 250 gms. These latter quarters constitute an Official sample.

(b) **Where the component parts of gross samples are more than 1 cm in any dimension:**

They are collected by hand:

When the total weight of the drug sample is

1. Less than 100 kg (200 lb) → Official Sample = at least 500 g.
2. More than 100 kg → Official Sample = at least 500 g. It should be taken in repeated samples by the same way. Next, they are mixed and divided into four equal quarters. Rejecct 2 of the diagonal quarters, combine and carefully mix the remaining quarters and again subject the drug to a quartering process in the same manner until two of the quarters weigh at least 500 gms. These latter quarters constitute an Official sample.

(c) **Where the total weight of the drug sample is less than 10 kg:**

Same process is to be followed but somewhat smaller quantities be collected.

The Official Sample weighs at least 125 g.

B. **Preparation of crude raw materials for analysis:** Following methods are followed where there is no specific directions given in the text:

The Official samples are collected by the quartering process as described, as much as may be necessary. In case of unground and unpowdered drugs the collected sample is grinded so that it will pass through No. 20 standard mesh sieve. If the sample cannot be ground, it should be reduced to as fine a state as possible. Then it is mixed by rolling on paper or sampling cloth and spread out in a thin layer and collected for analysis.

Parameters for Quality Control and Standardisation of Drugs

Of raw materials and vehicles.

Of manufacturing process (Processing methods or "In-process" quality control)

Of finished products, and

Of storage and packaging.

Quality Control of Raw Materials

Raw material standardisation is the only way for all the drug manufacturers to produce the drugs in same quality and to maintain the uniformity. It has to be developed as a routine procedure. In homoeopathy the raw materials are the crude drug substances. Following steps are properly followed for quality control:

(i) All in-coming raw materials are transferred to the store.

(ii) Each in-coming material is marked with a coding reference for proper identification.

(iii) Samples of raw materials are analysed.

(iv) Identification of adulterants in raw materials is done.

(v) The raw materials are compared with standards and analysed.

(vi) Purity testing is done.

(vii) Equipments are inspected for ensuring any microbial contamination before starting manufacturing process.

(viii) After completion of manufacturing process, representative sample of finished product is analysed.

Schematic representations

Incoming raw material transfer to store → Sampling of raw materials → Identification of adulterants → Comparison with standards and analysed → Testing of purity → Equipments inspected → Manufactury → Finished products → Analysis of finished products.

The raw materials may be:

1. **Medicinal**
   - Plants and animals
   - Minerals
   - Microbes, pathological products, healthy tissues, drugs.
2. **Non-medicinal (vehicles)**
   - Alcohol
   - Lactose
   - Sugar
   - White petroleum jelly (WPJ)
   - Maize starch
   - Coconut oil
   - Wax.

The quality of raw materials are ascertained and standardised as specified in HPI. In case of raw material resources it is mandatory to follow the guidelines of Good Agricultural Practices (GAP), Good Harvesting Practices (GHP), and Good Laboratory Practices (GLP).

Evaluation of Standard of Raw Materials

In general, three important factors are related for evaluation of crude raw materials:

(i) **Identity** (physical and chemical): Morphological, sensory and microscopical characters; microchemical tests.

(ii) **Purity** (microbial and chemical): Against any chemical and microbial contaminations.

(iii) **Quality**: Physical, chemical, and biological methods.

Evaluation of crude raw materials of plant source

1. Organoleptic evaluation.
2. Microscopic evaluation.
3. Physical evaluation.
4. Chemical evaluation.
5. Biological evaluation.

Evaluation of crude raw materials of chemical source

1. Viscosity
2. Surface tension
3. Ultraviolet light absorptions
4. Light diffraction
5. Chemical tests
6. Assay.

Quality Control of Vehicles and Bases

Vehicles are the important solvents or mediums in homoeopathic pharmacy. They are nessasary in every step starting from preparation (mother tincture to dilutions), preservation, purification, to dispensing of medicines. So purity test has to be assured.

In an industrial pharmacy following vehicles are used:

(i) Solid vehicles: Sugar of milk.

(ii) Semi-solid vehicles: Wax, starch, white petroleum jelly.

(iii) Liquid vehicles: Purified water, strong alcohol, glycerine, coconut oil, almond oil, olive oil.

Choice of vehicles depends upon the purpose of use and nature of application.

Monographs of raw materials (vehicles) in HPI

Monographs of HPI	Volume	Page
Purified water	HPI—Vol 1	178
Strong alcohol	HPI—Vol 1	37
Saccharum lactis	HPI—Vol 1	184
Glycerine	HPI—Vol 1	250
Starch	HPI—Vol 1	254
Bases	HPI—Vol 2	App xiv
Vehicles internal use	HPI—Vol 5	App xiv

"IN-PROCESS" Quality Control (IPQC)

The "in-process" quality control includes 'every step of the preparation' from raw materials to finished products. It is critical in ensuring the purity and safety of Homeopathic Medicines. The system of quality control is even more vital in the manufacturing process than with their allopathic counterparts. In case of highly diluted and potentised medicines, care should be taken in every step of manufacture to maintain the quality and reliability of the final product. It is mandatory for the manufacturers to have **GMP (Good Manufacturing Practices) Certificate** and to follow their guidelines in order to produce quality drugs. GMP guidelines as described in Schedules MI, rule 85 – E(2), are designed for the **Drug Manufacturing Units** to ensure quality, efficacy and safety of their products for the benefit of the consumers.

Finished Products Quality Control

Finished homoeopathic products must meet the quality standard. As such, finished products should also undergo all possible sorts of physical and chemical tests. Homoeopathic Pharmacopoeia Laboratory (HPL) suggested some preliminary standards for finished products.

The standardisation includes:

(a) Mother tinctures
(b) Potentised dilutions
(c) Triturations (powders)
(d) Biochemic tablets
(e) Globules
(f) Ointments
(g) Oils
(h) Eye drops
(i) Ear drops

Mother Tincture Analysis: The Homoeopathic Pharmacopoeia Laboratory (HPL) suggested preliminary standards for mother tinctures which were approved by the Homoeopathic Pharmacopoeia Committee (HPC) for inclusion in the Homoeopathic Pharmacopoeia of India (HPI), using following parameters:

1. Specific Gravity.
2. Alcohol content (expressed in p.c.)
3. Assay for constituents.
4. Weight per ml.
5. pH value.
6. pk value.
7. Total solids.
8. Viscosity in case of oils.
9. Ultraviolet absorbance.
10. Identification.
11. Refractive index.
12. Optical rotation.
13. Chromatography: Thin Layer Chromatography (TLC), Paper Chromatography (PC), and HPTLC.

Only mother tinctures apart from the raw products, are subjected to a more comprehensive analysis—both qualitative and quantitative. Additionally, there is the problem of chemical complexity of the natural extract contained in the original mother tincture. These may be inorganic or organic, with complex mixtures including minerals, amino acids, proteins, steroids, vitamins, organometallic compounds, alkaloids, etc.

Potency analysis: Quality control of homoeopathic potencies is a difficult task. For extremely high dilutions of homoeopathic potencies, which do not contain any molecules of the drug, it is almost impossible to apply analytical tests by conventional methods in the laboratory. All the existing tests are ineffective for testing high dilutions. The personnel involved in the analytical laboratory requires dedication and sincerity in every step of preparation of potencies. However, modern analytical techniques are adopted for standardisation of homoeopathic potencies (as per HPL).

(a) **Spectroscopic analysis**

(i) Infrared (IR) Spectroscopy
(ii) Ultraviolet & Visible Spectroscopy
(iii) Raman Spectrometry
(iv) Atomic Absorption Spectroscopy
(v) Nuclear Magnetic Resonance (NMR) Spectroscopy
(vi) Inductive Couple Plasma Atomic Emission Spectroscopy
(vii) Scanning Electron Microscopy (SEM)
(viii) X-ray Diffraction
(ix) Flourescence Analysis of Crude Drugs.

(b) **Chromatography**

(i) Thin Layer Chromatography (TLC)
(ii) High Performance Thin Layer Chromatography (HPTLC)
(iii) Paper Chromatography (PC)
(iv) Gas Liquid Chromatography (GLC)
(v) High Pressure/Performance Liquid Chromatography (HPLC)

Table 10.1: Widespread application of Spectrometry and Chromatography

Methods	Purpose
1. Infra-red Spectrometry	Quantitative analysis of organic and inorganic compounds
2. Ultraviolet and Visible Spectrometry	Quantitative analysis/end methods in chemical analysis schemes
3. Raman's Spectrometry	Identification of organic compounds and solid state symmetry of molecular groups
4. Atomic Absorption Spectrometer	Quantitative analysis of heavy metal contents.
5. X-ray Diffraction	Identification of inorganic crystalline substances, polymers
6. Column Chromatography	Identify pesticidal contamination
7. Gas Chromatography	Quantitative analysis of volatile organics
8. Thin Layer Chromatography	Finger-printing pattern of herbal drugs, identify aflotoxins, volatile oil identity
9. Culture Tests	Microorganisms
10. X-ray Crystallography	Quantitative analysis of trace elements.

Testing of Trituration and Biochemics

1.	Ash Value	Not more than 1.0%
2.	Starch	Present
3.	Presence of talc, chalk and kaolin	Absent
4.	Sugar of milk	Present 96%
5.	Binder	Not more than 3.0%
6.	Lubricants	Not more than 3.0%
7.	Insoluble matters	Not more than 5.0%
8.	Sucrose	Absent
9.	Disintegration/ Dissolution time	5 minutes

Testing of Globules

1. Pharmaceutical Grade Cane Sugar
2. Size of the Globules
3. Ash Value
4. Absence of Foreign Matters
5. Hardness
6. Porosity
7. Solubility

Schedule FF Ophthalmic Preparations

1. Name and quantity of preservatives.
2. Should be used within one month after opening.
3. Should be sterile.
4. Should be isotonic.
5. Neutral or acidity within limit.
6. Warnings as per Schedule FF.

Testing of Hair Oil

1. Test for vegetable oil-arachis oil.
2. Test for mineral oil.
3. Test for acid value.
4. Test for saponification value.
5. Test for iodine value.
6. Test for ingredients by TLC.
7. Test for stability.

Testing of Ointments

1. Test for homogenecity.
2. Test for consistency.
3. Test for ingradients by TLC.
4. Alcohol contents.
5. Ash value.

Packaging and Labelling Homoeopathic Medicine

RULE 106-A

No Homoeopathic Medicine shall be imported unless it is packed and labelled in conformity with Rules in Part IX-A (Rule 106A).

Manner of Labelling of Homoeopathic Medicine:

The following particulars shall be either printed or written in indelible ink and shall appear in a conspicuous manner on the label of the innermost container of any Homoeopathic Medicine and on every other covering in which the container is packed:

1. The words 'Homoeopathic Medicine'.
2. The name of the 'Medicine'–
   (a) Pharmacopoeial name as given in: HPI, HPUS, BHP, GHP/HAB.
   (b) For other drugs, descriptive name.
3. Potency in decimal, centesimal and 50-millesimal (in case of two or more medicines, potency and percentage of each ingredient in metric system).
4. Name and address of Manufacturer or seller.
5. Alcohol percentage in volume, for packings bigger than 30 ml.
6. Batch No. and Manufacturing License No.
7. Single ingredient shall not bear proprietary name on its label.

RULE 106-B

1. Homoeopathic medicine having more than 12% alcohol shall be packed in 30 ml only.
2. For hospitals/dispensaries 100 ml packing is allowed.

Chapter 11

Vehicles (Menstrua or Solvents)

Etymology

The term vehicle comes from Latin—*vehiculum* from *vehere* means 'to carry'.

It acts as solvent, diluent, preserving agent, medium for administration of medicine.

Definition

Vehicle means 'transmission' or 'conveyance'. Vehicles are those substances which are almost chemically neutral (neither acidic nor alkaline), therapeutically inert, having no medicinal property of their own (or if there is any that is negligible) but they are intended to carry the dynamic powers of a drug safely to the interior of the human organism to fight the disease force.

They are the medium for purification, preparation, preservation, internal administrations—either by oral or olfaction route, and external application as the case may be.

Properties of an Ideal Vehicle

1. Chemically neutral (neither acidic nor alkaline).
2. Therapeutically inert.
3. It has no medicinal property of its own.
4. It should be capable of carrying the dynamic powers of a drug safely to the interior of the human organism to fight the disease force.
5. Harmless as regards to its action on human organism. Pharmaceutical message of the original drug is in balanced condition.
6. It must have the power of preservation of drug substances and medicines. It must not undergo any change or decomposition.
7. Sterilising property.
8. Edible and palatable.

Uses or Utility of Vehicles

1. For the preparation of mother tincture, mother solution and mother substance from crude drug materials.
2. Used for further trituration and potentisation.
3. Used as the bases for preparing external applications of medicines.
4. Vehicles like olive oil, vaseline, glycerol etc. are themselves applied externally as a mechanical aid only.
5. Preservation of medicines (Section 268 F.N.). Vehicles like alcohol (spirit of wine) is mixed in certain proportion with the freshly expressed juices of the plants.
6. For dispensing of the medicines to the patients as per physician's prescription.
7. As diet—in sick baby, e.g. sugar of milk.
8. Used as 'placebo' or 'phytum' or 'rubrum'.

Classification of Vehicles

A. *Solid (or dry) vehicles*

1. Sugar of milk (lactose)
2. Cane sugar (sucrose)
3. Grape sugar (glucose, dextrose)
4. Globules
5. Cones
6. Tablets or tabloids
7. Pellets or pilules.

B. *Liquid vehicles*

1. Purified water
2. Alcohol
   - (i) Absolute alcohol
   - (ii) Dilute alcohol
   - (iii) Strong alcohol
   - (iv) Dispensing alcohol
   - (v) Rectified spirit.
3. Solvent ether
4. Glycerine
5. Simple syrup
6. Oils
   - (a) Fixed oil
     - (i) Olive oil
     - (ii) Almond oil
     - (iii) Sesame oil
     - (iv) Hydnocarpus oil
     - (v) Chaulmoogra oil.
   - (b) Volatile oil
     - (i) Sandalwood oil
     - (ii) Lavender oil
     - (iii) Rosemary oil.

C. *Semi-solid vehicles*

1. Vaseline (soft paraffin):
   - (i) Yellow soft paraffin
   - (ii) White soft paraffin.
2. Waxes:
   - (a) Beeswaxes
     - (i) Yellow beeswax
     - (ii) White beeswax
   - (b) Spermaceti
   - (c) Lanonin (anhydrous).
3. Soap:
   - (a) Vegetable origin:
     - (i) Hard soap
     - (ii) Soft soap.
   - (b) Animal origin: curd soap
4. Prepared lard
5. Isinglass
6. Starch.

Vehicles used for Potentisation only

A. *Liquid vehicles*

1. Alcohol:
   - (i) Strong alcohol
   - (ii) Dilute alcohol
   - (iii) Dispensing alcohol
   - (iv) Absolute alcohol
   - (v) Rectified spirit.
2. Purified water.

B. *Solid vehicles (dry vehicles)*

1. Sugar of milk
2. Cane sugar
3. Grape sugar.

Vehicles used for Mother Tinctures or The First Trituration

Mostly, the abovementioned vehicles are used for mother tinctures or the first trituration. But in some cases, in addition to the above glycerine and simple syrups are also used.

Vehicles used for External applications

A. *Liquid vehicles*

1. Purified water
2. Glycerine
3. Almond oil
4. Olive oil
5. Sesame oil
6. Rosemary oil.

B. *Semi-solid vehicles*

1. Vaseline (soft paraffin)
   - (i) Yellow soft paraffin
   - (ii) White soft paraffin.

2. Waxes
   (a) Beeswaxes
      (i) Yellow beeswax
      (ii) White beeswax
   (b) Spermaceti
   (c) Lanonin (anhydrous).
3. Prepared lard
4. Isinglass
5. Soap:
   (i) Soft soap
   (ii) Hard soap
   (iii) Curd soap.
6. Starch

Vehicles used for Dispensing Medicines

1. Purified water (Aqua dist.)
2. Sugar of milk (Sac. Lac.)
3. Globules
4. Tablets
5. Pilules.

SOLID (DRY) VEHICLES

SUGAR OF MILK

(*Saccharum lactis* or *lactose*)

Etymology

'*Saccharum*' means 'sugar' and '*lactes*' means 'milk'.

Source

It is prepared from goat's milk.

Chemical nature

It is disaccharide.

1 unit beta-galactose + 1 unit Levo-glucose = SAC. LAC.

Chemical formula

$C_{12}H_{22}O_{11}H_2O$

Preparation of Sugar of Milk

A convenient graphic representation of preparation of pharmaceutically pure sugar of milk—from raw materials to final stage.

Goat's milk: Composition—
(i) Protein (Lacto-albumin + Lacto-globulin + caseinogen)
(ii) Fats (iii) Lactose
← Skimming (iv) Minerals (v) Salts
(vi) Water.

↓

Proteins + H_2O + Minerals + Salts + Lactose → Fat (Removed)

↓

Lactose + H_2O (Fluid portion) + Proteins + Salts + Minerals (Solid portion)

+ HCl (dil.) to remove solid portion
+ Filtration.

↓

Lactose + H_2O (whey) (Filtrate)

+ purified water
+ Filtration through charcoal bed

↓

Clear solution of whey

+ Boiled on direct heat
+ Made semi-solid
+ Process repeated 3 – 4 times by adding purified water

↓

Semi-solid Lactose

+ Strong alcohol
+ Purified water
+ Boiled in direct heat and then indirect heat with water bath

↓

Crystal Lactose

+ Slight alcohol
+ Dried

↓

Pure crystal of Lactose

+ Grinding with mortar and pestle

↓

Pure powder of Sugar of milk.

Purification of Sugar of Milk

(Johann Ernst Stapf's process)

Method adopted in Laboratory: Crystallisation

Steps

1. 450 gm crystals of commercial lactose is dissolved in about 2 litres of boiling purified water in a clear flask.
2. Then the mixture in hot state is filtered by a filter paper.

3. The filtrate is then thoroughly mixed with 2 litres of absolute alcohol.
4. The whole flask is kept closed tightly for 3–4 days, in cold environment, so that sugar may crystallise.
5. After 3–4 days, a thin layer of crystals of lactose will be seen deposited at the bottom of the flask.
6. The crystallised mass is to be collected and washed in purified water to which some alcohol is already added.
7. These crystals are dried by pressing between filter paper and kept in well-closed container for use.

Characteristics of Sugar of Milk

A. **Physical properties**

(i) Hard, crystalline mass, milky white in colour.
(ii) It is odourless, faintly sweet in taste.
(iii) Sandy or gritty feeling on touching in-between fingers.
(iv) Solubility: one gram lactose is soluble in 5 ml of water, whereas it is soluble in 2.6 ml of boiling water. Insoluble in alcohol.
(v) Optical rotation: +55.3° at 20°C.

B. **Chemical properties**

(i) Molecular weight: 360.3
(ii) Its solution is neutral to litmus paper
(iii) It may produce 'water of crystallisation' at 150°C (302°F).

Impurities of Sugar of Milk

1. Starch (arrowroot, barley etc.)
2. Cane-sugar (Sucrose)
3. Acid+ (i.e. milk had become sour)
4. Alum
5. PO_4^+
6. Cl^-
7. Copper.

Purity test of Sugar of Milk

Theory: The sugar of milk to be used in homoeopathic laboratory and prescriptions must be in a pure and unadulterated form (except placebo).

Requirements

1. Sample of sugar of milk
2. Blue litmus paper
3. Iodine solution
4. Purified water
5. NaOH solution
6. Potassium ferrocyanide solution
7. Silver nitrate solution
8. Test-tubes with holder.

Procedure

Experiment	Observation	Inferences
A. *Physical Test*		
1. Sample of sugar of milk is taken in-between the fingers and smelled	Sandy or gritty feeling, odourless	May be pure
2. Taste	Faintly sweet in taste	May be pure
3. Colour and consistency	Milky white, hard crystalline mass	May be pure
B. *Chemical Test*		
1. Litmus test—In a test tube containing aqueous solution of sugar of milk—a blue litmus paper is added	Blue litmus paper remains unchanged	Absence of acid
2. Iodine test: In a test tube, solution of Iodine is prepared. Now, a few drops of Iodine solution is added to the sugar of milk	The colour not changed into blue	Absence of starch
3. A weak solution of sugar of milk is prepared in clean test tube with purified water	The colour remains unchanged	Absence of starch
4. Sugar of milk solution + NaOH soln.	No white ppt is formed	Absence of Alum
5. Sugar of milk solution + Potassium ferrocyanide solution	No reddish-brown ppt is formed	Absence of Copper
6. Sugar of milk solution + Silver nitrate solution	No light yellow ppt is formed	Absence of Cl^- & PO_4^+

N.B.: All physical tests and litmus test as well as Iodine test may be employed by a physician in his chamber by a simple technique.

Conclusion

The supplied sugar of milk is pure and unadulterated.

Preservation of Sugar of Milk

1. It should be preserved in air-tight plastic containers or bottles in dry state and in dry place.
2. It should not be preserved for a long time as it may go rancid.

Uses

1. Preparation of triturations from mother substances, which are not soluble in liquid vehicle (purified water and alcohol).
2. It is extensively used in biochemic preparations.
3. For preparations of potentised medicines in decimal potency.
4. It is used as a 'placebo' (placebo is the second-best remedy in the Materia Medica as per Dr. Stuart Close).
5. It is used for dispensing medicines to the patients.
6. For the preparation of mother powders.
7. It is devoid of fat and, as such, may be used as a temporary diet to the babies who cannot tolerate milk.

Is placebo and Sac. Lac. same?

Placebo: Stuart Close: Placebo is the second-best remedy in the Materia Medica, without which no good homoeopathist could long practice medicine.

Synonym: Nihilinum; Phytum; Rubrum; Lactopen.

Definition: The doctrine of placebo, from the Latin *placere,* to please or satisfy.

When the physician does not like to administer any homoeopathic medicine to his patient, or in other words, when there is no necessity for administering any medicine, he gives some UNMEDICATED SUBSTANCE (such as powders of sugar of milk, globules, tablets, purified water etc.) to satisfy the patient and to create confidence that he has been using the medicine regularly. These unmedicated substances are called placebo.

Different forms of placebo

(a) Solid: (i) Sugar of milk, (ii) Cane sugar globules, (iii) Tablets, (iv) Cones.

(b) Liquid: (i) Alcohol, (ii) Purified water, (iii) Purified water with alcohol.

Utility of placebo

1. Both in acute or chronic diseases, when a well-selected medicine continues its action (in centesimal and decimal scale of potency), we should not disturb the case. During this period, we have to give placebo to keep the action of the medicine undisturbed. At the same time the patient also knows that he is taking medicine (psychological effect).
2. Most of the medicines start their action with homoeopathic aggravation (Kents 3rd obs., when medicine administered in centesimal and decimal scale). During this aggravation, the patient rushes to his doctor, being a bit perturbed due to this aggravation. Sometimes the aggravation is so severe that even the doctor becomes perplexed. But any experienced homoeopathic physician can easily differentiate it from other types of aggravation (i.e. medicinal and disease aggravation). In these circumstances no medicine should be administered to the patient. But, for the satisfaction of the patient, we should give placebo because this type of aggravation subsides within few hours to few days.
3. When a patient comes to us after being overdrugged from allopathic or homoeopathic system, generally it is found that the case does not give any clear indication for the selection of the similimum. Here, we should prescribe placebo at least for ten to fifteen days. In this time, the vital force can annihilate the medicinal symptoms due to overdrugging and we will get the true picture of the disease.
4. We have some medicines which start their action even after two to three weeks. If it is found after reviewing the case that the selection of the remedy is correct, then we have nothing to do but to wait. During this waiting period, we should give placebo as we should not disturb the case hurriedly.

5. In Homoeopathy, we give minimum quantity of medicine to the patient. So if we give only 2-4 doses to any patient and ask him to come after a long time (esp. in chronic diseases), the patient will not be happy. So, a number of placebo doses is given along with the medicine so that the patient will think that he is taking medicine regularly.
6. Placebo may be given to a patient who has imaginary illness.
7. It gives more time to the physician to study the case and select a medicine, and thereby keep his honour.

Hahnemannian view regarding placebo

1. **Sec. 91 (5th edition of Organon)**

"When the disease is of chronic character and the patient has been taking medicine up to the time he is seen, the physician may with advantage leave him some days quite without medicine, or in the meantime administer something of an unmedicinal nature."

2. **Sec. 96 (5th edition of Organon)**

"A pure fabrication of symptoms and sufferings will never be met with in hypochondriacs, even in the most impatient of them; a comparison of the sufferings they complain of at various times when the physician gives them nothing at all, or something quite unmedicinal."

3. **Sec. 281 (6th edition of Organon)**

"In order to be convinced of this, the patient is left without any medicine for eight to fifteen days, meanwhile giving him only some powders of sugar of milk."

Sac. Lac:

Saccharum Lactis = Sugar of milk

Chemical formula—$C_{12}H_{22}O_{11}$

It is prepared from goat's milk by chemical process.

Why do we use Sugar of milk instead of other solid vehicles for the purpose of trituration?

For trituration, Sugar of milk is used instead of other solid vehicles—because sugar of milk is the best crystalline substance, scentless, gritty to touch, faintly sweet.

It has been found by experiment that it is quite competent to ground down to an inconceivably fine powder, the particles of such mineral substances which are insoluble either in purified water or in alcohol.

CANE SUGAR

(Sucrose; Sucrosum)

Synonym: Saccharum purificatum; Refined sugar; Misri; Chini

Chemical Formula: $C_{12}H_{22}O_{11}$

Sources: (i) Sugarcane (15 – 20%)
(ii) Beetroot (12 – 15%)
(iii) Others: pineapples, coffee, almonds, and honey.

The main sources are sugarcane and beetroot, while the cane grows in tropical countries and 'beet' grows only in cold climates. In India, cane sugar is mostly obtained from the sugarcane.

Preparation of Sucrose or Cane Sugar

The process consists of:

1. *Extraction of the juice:* Sugarcane is crushed in iron roller mills, which gives more than 75% of juice leaving behind the cellulose residue.
2. *Purification of the juice:* The juice is heated with lime (CaO) when most impurities will be collected as scum at the top, which is removed. Then CO_2 and SO_2 are passed one after another when the calcium will be precipitated as $CaCO_3$ and $CaSO_4$. The juice is then filtered to remove the precipitate.
3. *Concentration and crystallisation:* It is usually done by boiling under reduced pressure and allowing to crystallise after cooling.
4. *Separation of crystals:* The liquid is now whirled in a centrifuge machine, when the crystals will be separated from the mother liquor.
5. *Drying of crystals:* It is done by dropping through a chamber containing hot air.

Properties of Cane Sugar

1. Colourless or slightly white crystals: Odourless and sweet to taste than other sugars. Its solution is neutral to litmus.
2. Solubility: easily soluble in water but sparingly soluble in alcohol.
3. Optical rotation: not less than +65.9° at 20°C.

Uses

1. For the preparation of globules, pellets and tablets.
2. For the preparation of simple syrup.
3. Used as a vehicle for trituration by some.

GRAPE SUGAR

(Glucose or Dextrose)

Chemical Formula: $C_6H_{12}O_6$

Sources: (i) Starch, (ii) Cane sugar, (iii) Lactose.

Preparation: Globules formed by the hydrolysis of Polysaccharides, Cane sugar, Lactose etc.

Commercially it is prepared by boiling starch with dilute H_2SO_4. Also it can be produced by the hydrolysis of Cane sugar with HCl in alcoholic solution:

$$C_{12}H_{22}O_{11} + H_2O \rightarrow \underset{\text{(Glucose)}}{C_6H_{12}O_6} + \underset{\text{(Fructose)}}{C_6H_{12}O_6}$$

Glucose is separated out as it is less soluble in alcohol.

From Starch: $(C_6H_{10}O_5)n + nH_2O = n(C_6H_{12}O_6)$

Uses: Glucose is gradually coming into use for potentisation because some are of opinion that glucose is better than sugar of milk. They say that lactose has slight medicinal property while glucose has the least. Moreover, glucose will be most easily absorbed.

GLOBULES

Source: It is prepared from:

1. Pure Cane sugar (12 – 13%) or Sucrose ($C_{12}H_{22}O_{11}$). It is more commonly used.
2. Beetroot (15 – 25%) or Sugar beet.

Preparations (From Cane sugar)

1. Granulated cane sugar is placed in a rotating stainless steel globule-making pan or pill-tubes and rolled until the granules are formed to spherical shape.
2. The purified water is injected while the tube is rotating. The size of the globule shall be bigger if the water spray is more, i.e. water spray is directly proportional to the size of globules.
3. When the required size globules are formed they will be removed to a hot chamber, where they become dry.
4. When the drying is completed, the globules are made to pass through sieve screen which has various size meshes.

Characteristics

1. Shape: Round.
2. Size: The sizes of globules vary from 8 to 80. In homoeopathy, globules Nos. 10, 15, 20, 25, 30 and 40 are generally used. These numbers denote the numbers in millimeters required to accommodate ten equal sized globules placed diameter to diameter.
3. Colour and odour: white in colour; odourless.
4. Taste: sweeter than sugar of milk as it is prepared from cane sugar.
5. Consistency: neither too hard nor too soft.
6. Solubility: soluble in water but insoluble in alcohol.
7. Melting point: 160°C, decomposes on further heating.

Impurities in Globules

1. Starch
2. Flour
3. Glucose
4. Glycerine
5. White colouring materials.

They can be detected through proper chemical testing.

Testing of Globules

1. They are sweeter in taste—as made from cane-sugar.
2. Conc. H_2SO_4 decomposes gradually and chars them—the charred mass froths up.
3. Conc. HNO_3 converts then into oxalic acid.
4. They do not react with aldehyde or ketones.
5. They are not easily fermentable by yeast.

Uses of Globules

1. Frequently used for the dispensing of medicines.
2. Best media for preserving medicines. By this vehicle (i.e. globules) medicines can be preserved for a pretty long period—as they are capable of retaining medicinal property for a longer period.

Preservation of Globules

1. The globules should be dried before storing—otherwise globules will be dissolved.
2. Globules should be kept in airtight vessels or bottles as they readily absorb moisture from humid weather.
3. The globules retains their medicinal virtue for many years, if protected against sunlight and heat (Sec. 272, 6th edition).

Measurement of Globules

1. **Theory:** The space of a scale (mm) occupied by ten unknown size of globules is the number of these globules.
2. **Requirements**
   (i) A mm measuring scale.
   (ii) The globules of equal size which are to be measured.
   (iii) A clean sheet of paper.
   (iv) Paste or gums.
   (v) Stationeries—Pen, papers etc.
3. **Procedure**
   (i) The paper sheet is folded.
   (ii) The gum is attached along the folded line of paper.
   (iii) Then ten given globules of uniform size are attached in such a way—to avoid inter-globular spaces.
   (iv) Then with the help of a millimetre scale, space occupied by the globules are measured.
   (v) The process is repeated three times.
   (vi) The average of the reading is noted.
4. **Calculations**

No.	Space occupied by globules (in mm scale)	Mean
1.	22	
2.	23	22
3.	21	

Hence, the number (No.) of globules is 22.

Medication of Globules

A. **Process of medication of globules**

1. *In large scale:* A large porcelain bowl is taken. It is filled with globules keeping one-third vacant. Required potency of the medicine is poured over it, in order to moisten them thoroughly for a minute or two. The contents are then poured off on a dry clean filter paper so that the excess quantity of the medicine should be absorbed and the globules, when dry, may be kept into a phial duly marked with the name and potency of the medicine and corked tightly. They are then ready for use.
2. *For emergency or limited quantity:*
   (i) A perfectly dry, clean, round phial and a new non-porous velvet cork is taken after careful cleaning.
   (ii) Name of the medicine and its potency (e.g. Bell. 30) is written over the top of the cork.
   (iii) Then fresh non-medicated globules poured in the phial filling up to ¾th part of it.
   (iv) Then requisite quantity of the liquid medicine (here, Bell 30) poured upon the globules, to moisten them uniformly. Then the phial is closed by the

cork—and the phial kept standing on the cork for 8 hours.

(v) After this period the excess liquid medicine (if any) is drained out by loosening the cork a little.

(vi) Then the cork is again closed. A label is pasted over the body of the phial, writing the name of the medicine and the potency.

(vii) These medicated globules are kept for 48 hours (2 days) and then they become ready for use.

3. ***According to instruction of Hahnemann:* (In Chronic Diseases,** Vol. I, Page 187)

"The globules are poured into a clean porcelain bowl rather deep than broad, and enough of the required potency dropped upon them to moisten completely every globule in the space of one minute. The contents of the bowls are then emptied on a piece of clean, dry filtering paper, so that any excess of liquid may be absorbed and the globules spread out so that they may soon dry. The dry globules are then poured into a vial duly marked with the name and potency and securely corked."

B. **Reasons why the globules do not stand medication in certain cases:** Globules do not stand medications in certain cases due to the presence of considerable quantities of water in the medicines which are to be mixed with globules:

1. The vegetable ingredients from which mother tincture are prepared (from Class I to Class III) contains large quantities of water.
2. The potencies (say, 1X, 2X, 3X, 6X etc.) prepared with water or dilute alcohol under decimal scale, also contain large quantities of water.

In both the above cases, globules do not stand medication as these melt away by the solvent power of the water e.g.:

(i) We cannot prepare doses of Antim crude 3X, either in purified water or in globules, because it is in the triturated form and will not be dissolved in water.

(ii) We can prepare doses of Arg. nit. 3X in purified water but not in globules, because the mother solution of Arg. nit. is an aqueous solution which corresponds to 1X. The 2nd and subsequent potencies are prepared with dilute alcohol which contains three parts of water in every ten parts of the preparation (30%), therefore the globules will be dissolved.

PELLET

It is a small sphere and made of Cane-sugar, synonym for globule. Method of its medication is same as that of globule.

CONES

Preparation: These are prepared from Cane sugar added with egg-albumin, i.e. two kingdoms—vegetable and animal—both become its source.

Characteristics

(a) Shape—conical or semi-globular.

(b) Size—commonly size used in homoeopathy is No. 6. The size is determined by the diameter of the base in millimeters.

(c) Consistency—harder than globules.

(d) They absorb small quantity of liquid medicines.

Medication of Cones: The process of medication is same as that of globules. They are medicated by pouring sufficient quantity of medicine upon them and pouring off the excess. One No. 6 cone can absorb drops of dispensing alcohol.

Preservation: Should be kept in dry place to prevent fermentation due to dampness.

Uses: They are used for preserving very highly potentised medicine for a longtime.

Advantages

1. They are harder than globules and as a result, they absorb very small quantity of liquid medicine. So we may dispense very small quantity of medicine to our patients.
2. They are harder than globules, due to presence of egg-albumin. So they do not

absorb atmospheric moisture as readily as the globules do and hence they remain intact for a long time.

3. Administration of very small dose is possible in the case of medicated cones as they are very small in size.

TABLETS OR TABLOIDS

Tablets are unit forms of solid medicinal substances with or without suitable diluents prepared by compressing or moulding.

Source: These are prepared from pure refined sugar of milk.

Characteristics

1. *Shape:* Discoid in form; round but flat, white colour.
2. *Size:* They are found in size of 1 grain or 65 mg size.
3. *Consistency:* Softer than globules or pilules as they are made of sugar of milk; They are less sweeter.
4. *Solubility:* More easily soluble in water than globules or pilules. Insoluble in alcohol.

Medication: They are medicated by the same process as globules but small quantities of medicine are used to medicate the tablets, as there is every chance of these being dissolved.

1 grain tablet is medicated with a drop of medicine poured upon it and 2 grain tablets with two drops.

Preservation: Should be preserved in well-closed containers and not to be tightly packed.

LIQUID VEHICLES

PURIFIED WATER

Formula: H_2O Molecular weight = 18

Water was shown to be a compound by Cavendish (1781).

Synonyms: Distilled water; Aqua distillata; Aqua purificata.

Preparation

1. For Small scale:
   a) Distillation process
   b) Deionisation process
2. For Large scale: by electrically operated automatic water distillator.

I. Distillation process

In this process firstly volatile water is converted into its vapour by boiling and then the vapour is again converted back to the liquid state by cooling.

$$\text{Volatile water} \xrightarrow{\text{boiling}} \text{vapour} \xrightarrow[\text{by cold}]{\text{condensation}} \text{liquid state}$$

(a) *Apparatus*

(i) *Liebig's condenser:* This condenser is the two-chambered vessel having a central tube jacketed by a water-tube. This water-tube has two side-tubes near the ends. The lower side-tube is attached with a water-tap by means of a rubber tube. When the tap is opened, water enters into the jacket-tube, cools the central tube and comes out through the second side-tube at the upper side.

(ii) *Flask:* 2 in number—one distilling flask and one receiving flask (to collect the distillate).

(iii) Bunsen burner.

(iv) Tripod stand and wire-gauze.

(b) **Procedure**

(i) The ordinary water to be distilled is taken in a round-bottomed distilling flask. This distilling flask has a side-tube at the top. This side-tube is connected by means of a bored cork to one end of the Liebig's condenser, the other end of the condenser is inserted into a vessel, called the receiver, to collect the distillate.

(ii) The mouth of the distilling flask is closed with a rubber cork and a thermometer is inserted into the cork for noting the temperature of the issuing vapour.

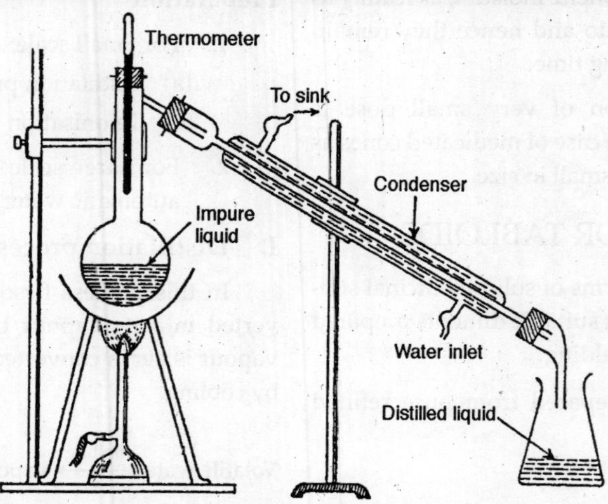

Distillation

(iii) The distilling flask is placed on a tripod stand over wire-gauze and kept in position with the help of a clamp and a stand. A few glass-beads or small pieces of porcelain ware were dropped in, to avoid unusual bumping of the liquid during boiling.

(iv) The water in the distilling flask is heated. When a boiling point of a particular liquid is reached, its vapours are produced which come out of the side-tube of the flask and pass through the condenser, where they cool down and condense to a liquid and collect in the receiver, which is called the purified water.

II. Deionisation process

There are some synthetic substances, called ion-exchange resins, which can exchange other cations and anions from a solution by hydrogen ions and hydroxyl ions, respectively. Those resins which replace other cations by hydrogen ions are called cation-exchangers or cation-exchange resins and the others which replace other anions by hydroxyl-groups, are called anion-exchangers or anion-exchange resins.

The cation-exchangers are generally sulphonated organic compounds of high molecular weights, like zeocarb H, and the anion exchangers are hydroxyl compounds derived from organic amines of high molecular weights, like Amberlite IRA 400.

When impure water, containing calcium or magnesium salts, is passed through columns containing a cation exchanger (H.R.), all the metallic ions (including even the alkali metal ions, if present in water) are replaced by hydrogen ions, with the formation of an equivalent amount of acids of the

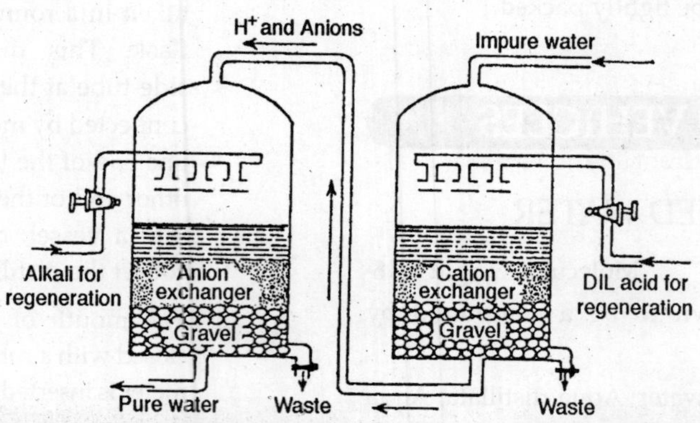

Ion-exchange process, using both cation and anion-exchanger in succession

corresponding anions of the metal salts. Chlorides and sulphates of metals react:

$$CaCl_2 + 2HR = R_2Ca + 2HCl$$

$$MgSO_4 + 2HR = R_2Mg + H_2SO_4$$

The water coming out of this column is, therefore, acidic (though completely free from metal ions) and, as such, is hardly suitable for most purposes. The resultant acids are, therefore, removed by passing this water again through a column containing an anion-exchanger (RN.OH) which removes the anions of the acids by hydroxyl groups, forming water:

$$HCl + RN.OH = RN.Cl + H_2O$$

$$H_2SO_4 + 2RN.OH = (RN)_2SO_4 + 2H_2O$$

RN.OH represents an anion exchanger

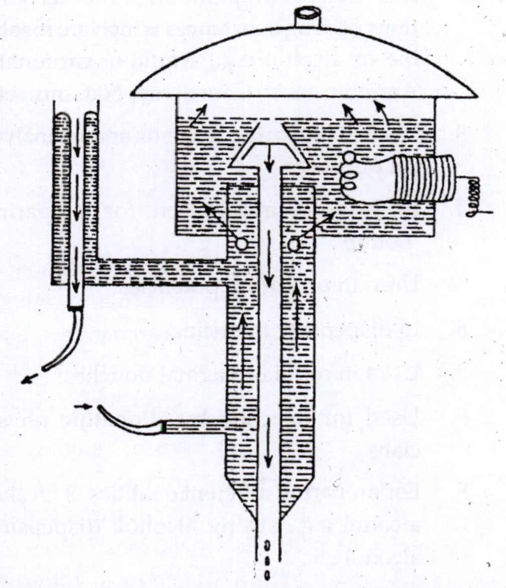

Automatic Water Distillator

The combined effect of the passage of impure water through the cation and anion exchangers in succession results in the production of very pure water, practically free from ions. Such water is called de-mineralised or deionised water and it is as good as purified water for all practical purposes.

Preparation of purified water by automatic water distillator

For commercial purpose in large scale manufacture, an automatic water distillator and stainless steel vessel known as 'still' is used.

In this process, the distillation and cooling is done by the same water. A portion of the cooling water will go through some holes into the heating chamber. The steam will be produced here which will pass into the inner chamber through the special passage at the top and come down for cooling purpose. The cooling water will exit through an overflow. The instrument needs little care.

Note: Electric stills are profitable as the process is quick and can be connected to the general water supply. The required quantity of purified water can be obtained as fresh and when needed.

Properties

(i) It is neutral and pH does not vary more than 6 to 7

(ii) Specific gravity at 25°C: 1.000

(iii) Freezing point: 0°C

(iv) Boiling point: 100°C

(v) Temperature of maximum density: 4°C

(vi) Ionic product at 25°C: 1×10^{-14}

(vii) Latent heat of fusion at m.p: 79.72 cal/g

(viii) Latent heat of vapourisation at b.p: 539.4 cal/g

(ix) Heat of formation at 25°C: 68.32 K. cal/mol

(x) Critical temperature: 374.2°C

(xi) Surface tension at 25°C: 71.97 dynes/cm

(xii) Viscosity at 25°C: 8.937 millipoises

(xiii) Refractive index nD^{20}: 1.33300

(xiv) It is a clear, colourless liquid, tasteless and odourless.

(xv) It is practically a non-conductor of electricity due to its negligible ionisation into hydrogen and hydroxyl ions:

$H_2O \rightleftharpoons H^+ + OH^-$. It is also a bad conductor of heat.

(xvi) Water readily forms crystalline hydrates with many compounds, e.g., $CuSO_4.5H_2O$ (Blue vitriol); $Na_2SO_4.10H_2O$ (Glauber's salt); $FeSO_4.7H_2O$ (Green vitriol); $C_2H_2O_4.2H_2O$ (Oxalic acid dihydrate).

(xvii) It is a good ionising solvent for acids, bases and salts. It is an amphiprotic solvent.

(xviii) Water is absorbed by many substances, of which the important ones are concentrated H_2SO_4; fused $CaCl_2$; P_2O_5; CaO (quicklime); Magnesium percolate; Silica gel and anhydrous NO_2SO_4. These substances are generally called dehydrating or desiccating agents or desiccants.

Impurities in Water

I. Various kinds of Impurities

(a) Insoluble substances: Clay, sand and vegetable matters.

(b) Soluble substances:

(i) Non-volatile substances: Chlorides, carbonates, bicarbonates, sulphates of Na, K, Ca, Mg, Fe.

(ii) Volatile substances: Air, CO_2, H_2S, NH_3, NO_2, SO_2 etc.

II. Detection of purity in water

1. Purified water may be detected by the physical properties such as:
   (i) It is a clear colourless, odourless and tasteless liquid
   (ii) pH shall not vary more than 6 to 7
   (iii) Boiling point: 100°C
   (iv) Freezing point: 0°C
   (v) Temp. of maximum density: 4°C
2. No changes when blue or red litmus paper is in contact with water.
3. Purified water leaves no residue on evaporation.
4. Anhydrous copper sulphate ($CuSO_4$) powder reacts with water to form blue colour.
5. Potassium reacts with water to form hydrogen which spontaneously undergoes combustion:

$$K + 2H_2O = H_2\uparrow + KOH$$

6. The purified water must be free from chloride, calcium, sulphate and ammonia etc. which can be tested by the following experiments:

Test for	Reagent added	Ordinary or Tap-water	Purified water
1. Chloride	Silver nitrate ($AgNO_3$) soln.+ Dilute Nitric acid (HNO_3)	White turbidity	Nil
2. Calcium	Ammonium oxalate soln. + Dilute Acetic acid	White turbidity	Nil
3. Sulphate	Barium chloride($BaCl_2$) soln. + dil. Hydrochloric acid(HCl)	White turbidity	Nil
4. Ammonia	Nessler's reagent (alkaline K_2HgI_4)	Brown colour or precipitate	Nil

Uses

1. It is used for final cleansing of utensils or equipments.
2. It is used for preparation of mother solutions of drug substances which are insoluble in alcohol e.g., Ammon. carbonate; Ammon. caust; Causticum; Nat. mur. etc.
3. Used in preparing reagents and in analytical purposes.
4. In external application for preparing 'Lotion'.
5. Used in preparing potencies.
6. In dispensing medicines.
7. Used in rectal or vaginal douches.
8. Used for injection by allopathic physicians.
9. For preparing different qualities of weaker alcohol e.g., strong alcohol; dispensing alcohol etc.

Storage: The purified water should always be stored in pyrex glass bottles which are previously thoroughly cleansed in hot water.

Demerits: The medicines dispensed with purified water cannot be preserved for a long period as aqueous solutions are unstable.

ALCOHOL (Alc)

The alcohols are the hydroxyl derivatives of hydrocarbons. They are theoretically obtained by replacing one or more hydrogen atoms from the hydrocarbons by hydroxyl groups (OH).

Classification:

(Depending on the number of OH groups present in its molecules).

1. *Monohydric alcohol:* The general formula of saturated monohydric alcohol is $CnH_{2n+1}OH$ or briefly R–OH. The –OH is obviously the functional group of alcohols. They are primary, secondary or tertiary according as the –OH group is attached to a primary, secondary or tertiary carbon atom:
   (i) Primary alcohol—contains CH_2OH group and they may be represented by the general formula $R.CH_2OH$, e.g., $H–CH_2OH$ (methyl alcohol); $CH_3–CH_2OH$ (ethyl alcohol).
   (ii) Secondary alcohol—contains > CHOH group and they may be represented by the general formula $R_1 R_2 > CHOH$
   e.g. $CH_3 CH_3 > CHOH$ (Isopropyl alcohol)
   $CH_3 \; CH_3{\cdot}CH_2 > CHOH$ (Secondary butyl alcohol)
   (iii) Tertiary alcohol—contains C–OH group and they may be represented by the general formula
   $R_1 R_2 R_3 > C–OH$
   e.g. $CH_3 CH_3 CH_3 > C–OH$ (T-butyl alcohol).
2. *Di-hydric alcohol:* Alkaneols or glycols contain two hydroxyl groups on different carbon atoms. The simplest, methylene glycol, $CH_2(OH)_2$, is unknown in the free state; an aqueous solution of formaldehyde, HCHO, is believed to exist as methylene glycol. 1, 2 – or vicinal glycols are the most important. Ethylene glycol or ethane –1, 2 – diol, $CH_2OH–CH_2OH$, is the first representative number of the series. Glycols have the general formula $C_nH_{2n}(OH)_2$. The common names of 1, 2 – glycols are obtained from the corresponding alkene by adding 'glycol' to it, e.g., propylene glycol, $CH_3–CHOH–CH_2OH$.
3. *Tri-hydric alcohol:*

   CH_2OH
   |
   $CHOH$ (glycerol)
   |
   CH_2OH

ETHYL ALCOHOL

Chemical formula: C_2H_5OH

Molecular weight: 46.07

Synonyms: Ethanol; Spirit of wine; Grain alcohol

Sources

1. Molasses, a waste byproduct from sugar factories. In India, it is the main source of ethyl alcohol.
2. Substances rich in starch $(C_6H_{10}O_5)n$, e.g. rice, wheat, maize, potato etc.
3. Substances rich in sugar. e.g. beet, carrot, grapes, sugarcanes etc.
4. From sugars, e.g. beet-sugar, cane-sugar etc.
5. Synthetically—from ethylene.

Preparations

A. **From Molasses**

Molasses is the mother liquor left after crystallisation of cane-sugar from cane juice. It contains about 50% fermentable sugar (sucrose, glucose, fructose). It is a thick dark-coloured liquid. It is the chief source for manufacturing of alcohol.

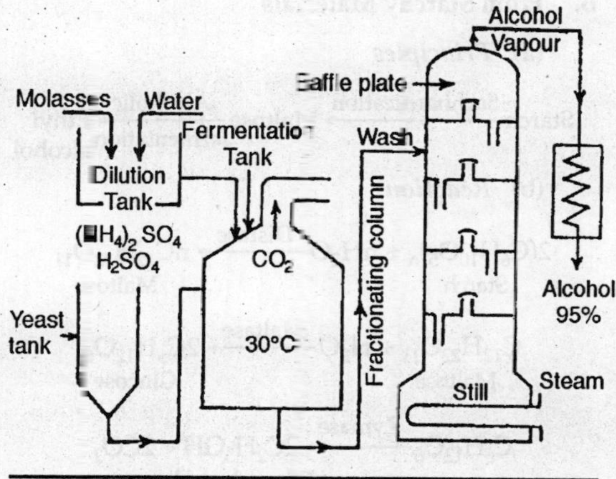

Dilution Tank, Fermentation Tank, Still and Condenser

The various steps involve are:

(a) *Preparations of Wash:*

(i) Molasses is diluted with water to prepare a 10% solution of sugar. A small amount of $(NH_4)_2SO_4$ is added to it as a food for the ferment.

It is acidified with small amount of H_2SO_4.

(ii) It is warmed at 25°C – 30°C and yeast ferment added to it.

(iii) Fermentation starts with the evolution of CO_2 and is completed in 2 – 3 days.

(iv) The enzymes invertase and zymase present in yeast bring about the decomposition of cane-sugar into ethyl alcohol as:

$$\underset{\text{Sucrose}}{C_{12}H_{22}O_{11}} + H_2O \xrightarrow{\text{Invertase}} \underset{\text{Glucose}}{C_6H_{12}O_6} + \underset{\text{Fructose}}{C_6H_{12}O_6}$$

$$C_6H_{12}O_6 \xrightarrow{\text{Zymase}} 2C_2H_5OH + 2CO_2$$

The fermented liquor is known as 'wash'.

(b) *Distillation of Wash:*

The wash contains 15% alcohol. It is subjected to fractional distillation in a special type of fractionating column known as **Coffey's still.**

The vapours of almost pure alcohol from the head of the fractionating column are lead to the condenser.

The distillate so obtained is known as crude rectified spirit and contains about 95% v/v or 92% w/w of ethyl alcohol.

B. From Starchy Materials

(a) ***Principles***

$$\text{Starch} \xrightarrow{\text{Sachharification}} \text{Maltose} \xrightarrow[\text{fermentation}]{\text{Alcoholic}} \text{Ethyl alcohol}$$

(b) ***Reaction***

$$\underset{\text{Starch}}{2(C_6H_{10}O_5)_n} + nH_2O \xrightarrow{\text{Distase}} \underset{\text{Maltose}}{nC_{12}H_{22}O_{11}}$$

$$\underset{\text{Maltose}}{C_{12}H_{22}O_{11}} + H_2O \xrightarrow{\text{Maltase}} \underset{\text{Glucose}}{2C_6H_{12}O_6}$$

$$C_6H_{12}O_6 \xrightarrow{\text{Zymase}} \underset{\text{Ethyl alcohol}}{2C_2H_5OH + 2CO_2}$$

(c) ***Process:*** It consists of the following steps:

1. Sachharification: The process of converting starch into maltose is known as Sachharification.

It consists of the following steps:

(i) Malting: Barley is allowed to germinate in the dark, at 15°C, when enzyme diastase is developed in it. After a few days, germination is stopped by the action of heat and the malt so obtained is extracted with water. The malt extract contains diastase in solution.

(ii) Mashing: Suitable starchy material is suspended in water and agitated with superheated steam under pressure to get a pasty mass. This suspension of starch is known as 'mash'.

(iii) Hydrolysis: Mash is mixed with malt extract and the temperature maintained between 50°C to 60°C. Fermentation starts and, under the influence of diastase, starch is hydrolysed into maltose.

2. Alcoholic fermentation: The solution of maltose so obtained is mixed with yeast at 30°C – 35°C and kept for 3 – 4 days. Maltose is converted into glucose by the enzyme maltose contained in the yeast. Glucose is converted to

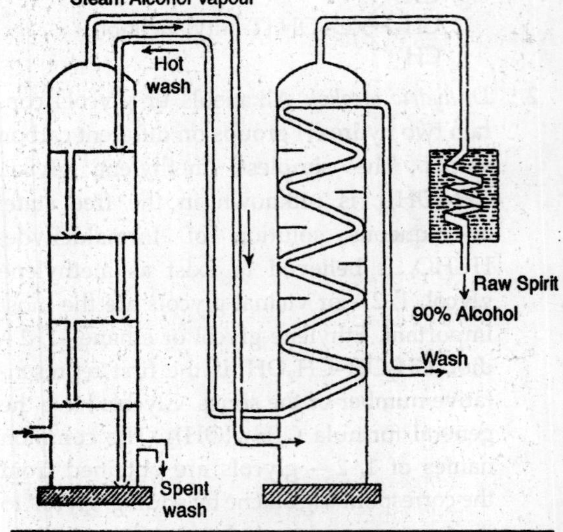

Alcoholic Fermentation

C_2H_5OH and CO_2, by the enzyme zymase contained in yeast. A 15% solution of C_2H_5OH is obtained by this process—technically known as 'wash'. It is subjected to fractional distillation in a special type of fractionating column known as "Coffey's still". The vapours of almost pure alcohol from the head of the fractionating column are led to the condenser. The distillate so obtained is known as crude rectified spirit and contains about 95% v/v or 92% w/v of C_2H_5OH.

Properties of alcohol

1. It is a colourless, neutral, transparent volatile liquid (boiling point 78.5°C) with a pleasant smell and burning taste.
2. It is lighter than water (Sp. Gr. 0.789) and miscible with it in all proportions with evolution of heat and contraction in volume.
3. It freezes at –114°C and so it is used in 'alcohol thermometer' for measuring low temperatures.
4. It is highly hygroscopic and inflammable; it burns with a pale blue smokeless flame.
5. In small doses, alcohol is a stimulant but, in excess, a poison.
6. Alcohol is a good solvent for organic compounds.

Advantages of alcohol

1. Non-expensive, as it is prepared from waste product—'molasses'.
2. It has no medicinal property of its own.
3. Neutral in reaction, i.e. neither acidic nor alkaline.
4. Not spoiled by long storage.
5. Soluble with almost all common fluids.
6. Edible in small doses, acts as a stimulant and is non-poisonous.
7. Preparation is not much difficult.
8. It possesses great extracting power for the medicinal properties from crude and mucilagenous substances.
9. A 70% strength, it acts as a great preserver of animal and plant tissues.
10. It is used in increasing strengths for dehydration of animal and plant tissues.

Disadvantages of alcohol

1. It evaporates easily. So it should be kept in air-tight bottles.
2. Highly inflammable, if kept near fire. So it should be kept in cool place away from fire, with fire-fighting arrangements.
3. Ordinary corks are easily discoloured if in contact with alcohol by over-filling the bottle.
4. It is a highly taxable item.
5. Not easily procurable, as it is strictly controlled by every Govt.'s Excise Departments.
6. It cannot dissolve many inorganic salts directly. Albuminous and starchy substances are not dissolved in alcohol.
7. In large doses it is poisonous.

Precautions in preserving or using alcohol

1. It must be stored in cool dark place and in air-tight closed container—as it evaporates easily and absorbs moisture from atmosphere or air.
2. Bottles made up of pyrex glass (81%, SiO_2; 5% Na_2O; 2% Al_2O_3; 12% B_2O_3) should be preferred. Bottles must be well-cleansed.
3. Alkaline bottles should be avoided.
4. It is highly inflammable. So it should be kept in cool place away from fire, with fire-fighting arrangements.

Uses of alcohol

1. It is added to the juice of plants in fresh state, to prevent their deterioration (Sec. 267, **Organon of Medicine**). It also prevents moulds, yeast and fermentation of materials inside.
2. For preparing mother tinctures (Class I to Class IV under old method) and mother solutions (Class VI) from crude drug materials.

By Schematic representation

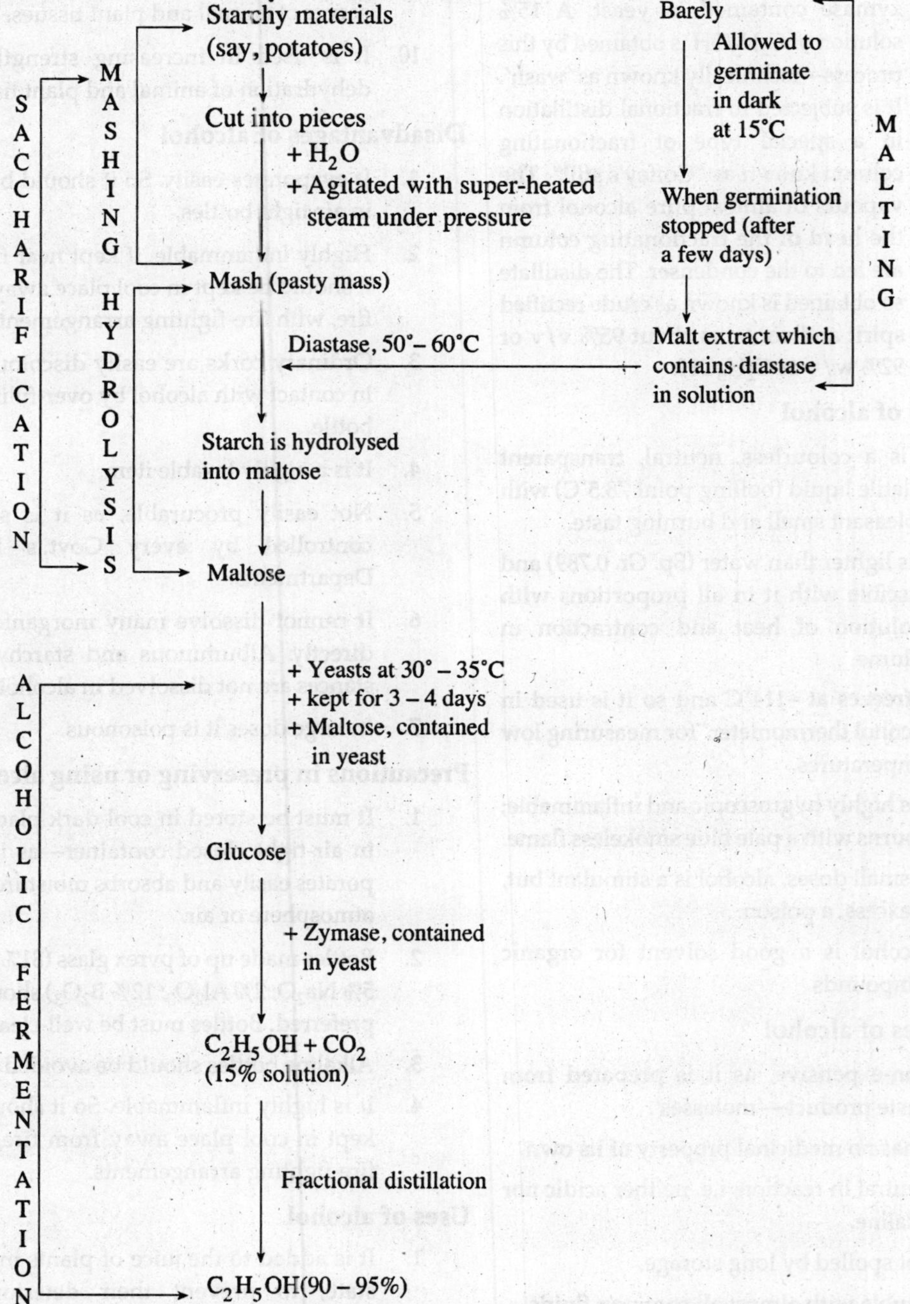

3. For preparing dilutions and higher potencies.
4. It is easy to prepare medicines and medicate globules with alcohol.
5. It is used for preparing medicines from gums, resins, oleo-resins, resinoids, alkaloids, and many volatile oils.
6. It is employed for making methylated spirit (for varnishes, lacquers etc.), ether, ethylene, chloroform, iodoform, acetic acid, etc. and also for transparent soaps, hair washes.
7. It is a solvent in the dye and rayon industries.

8. Ethyl esters make fruit essences and perfumes.
9. It works as an antiseptic, at a strength of above 10%.
10. It has a cooling effect and so applied on burns and over forehead to soothe burning sensation and headache, respectively.

The Food value of alcohol

The alcohol may be regarded as a food, within certain limit. The chief point is whether it can be regarded as a protein sparer.

The proteins help in formation and repair of tissues. Carbohydrates and fats are sources of heat and energy. Since alcohol does not contain nitrogen, it cannot replace protein and, therefore, has no power to build tissues. Whereas about 90% of alcohol taken disappears in the body and is converted into CO_2 and water; by virtue of the chemical energy thus liberated it can replace carbohydrate and fats in the diet—in this sense it is a non-nitrogenous food.

But, when taken with other foods, it economises the use of fat and carbohydrate, which, in their turn, are stored in the body, the carbohydrate as glycogen and fat in tissues. As alcohol does not require digestion, it is in a sense superior to other foods. Moreover, it does not require more energy for absorption than other foods.

Though it cannot replace protein, alcohol will, under certain conditions, spare the protein in the same way as fat and thus prevent tissue waste. Alcohol, therefore, is regarded as a food in the sense that it will, when given with other foods, replace carbohydrate and fat for a short time and would supply energy and spare protein and prevent tissue waste. But the value of alcohol as a food is limited because the supply of energy is fixed and cannot be adjusted according to the needs of the body, nor can it be increased to meet a sudden emergency, because it cannot be stored in the body like fat or carbohydrate as reserve.

The caloric value of alcohol in diet lies in between carbohydrate (4.3 cal/gm) and fat (9.3 cal/gm) whereas alcohol supplies 7 calories—as such, a pint of whisky will supply 1,400 calories (approx).

Impurities of Alcohol

1. **Various kinds of impurities**
   (a) Fusel oil: It is the commonest impurity in alcohol. It is a bright-yellow liquid (from the last runnings in the distillation of crude spirit), is chiefly iso-amyl alcohol or iso-butyl carbinol, $(CH_3)_2CH–CH_2–CH_2OH$, (boiling point –131°C) with traces of two propyl alcohols, butyl alcohols, some esters etc.

   Fusel oil comes from the amino-acids such as valine and leucin present in starch.

   (b) Acids e.g. succinic acid.
   (c) Water (H_2O).
   (d) Other inferior qualities of alcohol: Amyl alcohol, Propyl alcohol, Butyl alcohol; Glycerine.
   (e) Aldehydes and Ketone bodies: e.g. Acetaldehyde.
2. **Detection of impurities** (shown in Table 11.1)
3. **Method of removal of impurities (purification of alcohol)**

   After detection of impurities in alcohol (such as fusel oil, aldehyde, ketone, water, low quality alcohol etc.), the impure alcohol is purified by distillation with purified animal charcoal.

Chief varieties of Alcohol

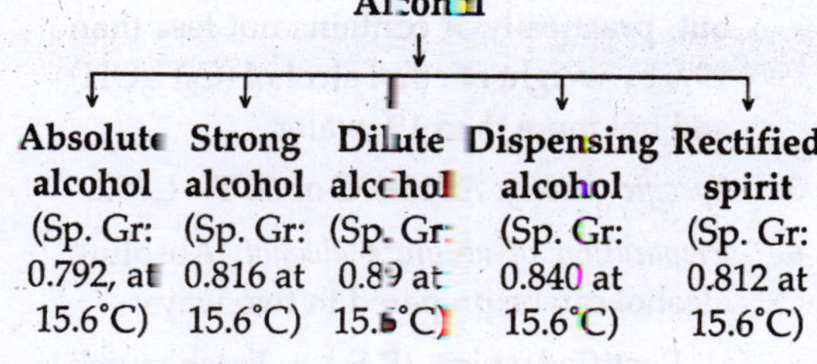

Absolute Alcohol

1. *Synonyms:* Anhydrous alcohol; Alcohol dehydrated.
2. *Definition:* By the term 'Absolute alcohol' is meant alcohol entirely free from water, i.e. 100% pure alcohol.

   Strictly, this is an incorrect name, for it may contain 1 per cent by weight of water.

Table 11.1: Detection of impurities in Alcohol

Experiment	Observation	Inference
(a) The given sample of alcohol is soaked with blue litmus paper	It turns red	Presence of acid
(b) Purified water is added to the sample of alcohol in equal volume	A foreign smell is found	Impure alcohol
(c) A few drops of Silver nitrate ($AgNO_3$) is added to the sample of alcohol in a clean test tube and exposed to bright light	A reddish colour is noticed	Presence of fusel oil
(d) Equal amounts of conc. H_2SO_4 and the sample of alcohol mixed	Appearance of red or brown colour $C_2H_5OH + H_2SO_4 = C_2H_5HSO_4 + H_2O$	Presence of fusel oil
(e) A small quantity of alcohol is made to evaporate from a porcelain dish. This is protected from dust	After evaporation of alcohol, there is foreign odour from the evaporaing dish	Presence of fusel oil
(f) (i) 10 cc of alcohol is shaken vigorously with 0.5 gm of anhydrous Copper sulphate	(i) The powder will assume blue colour	Presence of water
(ii) Calcium carbide is added to the sample of alcohol	(ii) Produces acetylene gas $CaC_2 + 2H_2O \rightarrow Ca(OH)_2 + C_2H_2$	
(g) Oil of Wintergreen test: 3-4 ml of alcohol is taken in a test tube and 1 gm of Sodium salicylate or Salicylic acid is added and then 1 ml of conc. H_2SO_4 is added and warmed.	A characteristic fragrant smell of Methyl salicylate (Oil of Wintergreen)	Presence of Methyl alcohol

Theoretically, it is 100% of ethyl alcohol (C_2H_5OH) by volume (v/v) or by (w/w) but, practically, it contains not less than 99% by weight of ethyl alcohol (C_2H_5OH) and not more than 1% water.

3. *Specific gravity:* At 15.6°C or 60°F—0.792.
4. *Preparation of absolute alcohol:* Absolute alcohol can be prepared in two ways:
   (a) Rectified spirit (R.S.) + Fresh quick lime (CaO)

↓

Heated, due to which most of water is removed

↓

Distillation

↓

Distillate now contains about 0.6 to 1% water—so to remove the traces of water

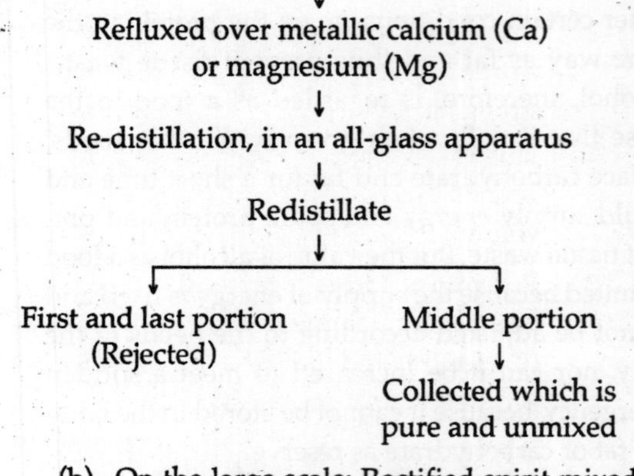

(b) On the large scale: Rectified spirit mixed with little Benzene (C_6H_6)

↓

Distillation

↓

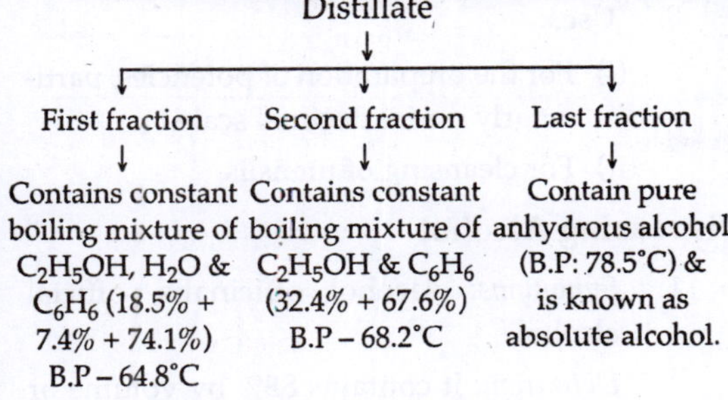

5. *Difference between absolute alcohol and homoeopathic alcohol:* The homoeopathic alcohol is of 87% strength and is used in making many homoeopathic attenuations. Absolute alcohol, theoretically, should be 100% proof. Practically 95% is about the highest it ever attains, as it constantly absorbs water from the atmosphere. 95% alcohol may be reduced to homoeopathic alcohol by adding to 7 parts of 95% alcohol 1 part of purified water.

6. *Purity test of absolute alcohol:* As regards the traces of water (0.3%), 10 ml of the sample of alcohol is taken in a test tube and vigorously shaken with 0.5 gm of anhydrous copper sulphate, which will turn blue, if water is present in the sample.

7. *Uses:* It is used in Stapf Process for the purification of Sugar of milk.

Strong Alcohol

1. *Synonyms:* Alcohol fortior; Alcohol fortis.

2. *Definition:* In homoeopathy, when the word 'alcohol' is only used it means strong alcohol.

   This is obtained after second distillation and its strength becomes appr. 95% by volume.

3. *Preparation:* It is prepared by mixing 94.9 p.c. by volume of pure ethyl alcohol (C_2H_5OH) and 5.1 p.c. by volume of purified water.

   It may be diluted to any extent with purified water.

4. *Properties:*

   (a) Specific gravity: At 15.6°C or 60°F—0.816.

   (b) Refractive index (n_D^{20}): 1.3637 – 1.3639.

   (c) It is colourless, transparent, mobile, volatile liquid, with pleasing aroma and burning taste

   (d) It is neutral to all indicators when pure.

   (e) It is miscible with purified water, acetone ($CH_3–CO–CH_3$), chloroform ($CHCl_3$), ether and many other organic solvents.

   (f) Iodoform test: Take 2-3 ml of the solution in a test tube, add equal volume of a strong solution of iodine in potassium iodide (KI), warm gently, take it out of the flame and add a solution of NaOH drop by drop until the colour is pale yellow. Cool the test tube, a yellow crystalline ppt. of Iodoform separates out:

   $$C_2H_5OH + 4I_2 - 6NaOH = CHI_3 + HCOONa + 5NaI + 5H_2O$$

5. *Uses:*

   (a) It is used for the preparation of mother tinctures from vegetable and animal substance under Hahnemannian old method as well as in new method.

   (b) For the preparation of mother solutions (i.e. alcoholic solutions) as in Class VI under old method, where the drug substance is soluble in alcohol.

   (c) For the preparation of absolute alcohol, dilute alcohol and dispensing alcohol.

6 *Storage:* It should be kept in well-stoppered glass bottle, in cool dark place, away from fire, as it is very inflammable.

Dilute Alcohol

Different authorities differ as regards the specification of dilute alcohol:

1. **As per H.P.I. (Vol I):** Dilute alcohol (66%) contains 62.5% v/v or 60.6% w/w of alcohol. Dilute 695 ml of strong alcohol to 1,000 ml with purified water. Specific gravity: At 20°C, 0.9139 to 0.9169.

2. **As per A.H.P.:** It consist of 7 parts of alcohol (Sp. Gr: 0.83) and 3 parts of purified water. Specific gravity: At 15°C, 0.89.
3. **As per B.H.P.:** It consist of equal quantity of rectified spirit, 60 o.p and purified water.
4. **As per M. Bhattacharya's Pharmacopoeia:** 7 parts in volume of rectified spirit 60 o.p is added to 3 parts in volume of purified water. Specific gravity: 0.89.
5. **As per Drs. Buchner, Gruner, Jahr, J. Hampel:** It is prepared by adding equal parts in volume of alcohol and purified water.
6. **As per Dr. K. P. Majumder:**
   (i) It is prepared by adding 7 parts of alcohol (Sp. Gr: 0.816) with 3 parts of purified water in volume. Specific gravity: 0.935 to 0.937.
   (ii) Equal volume of strong alcohol (Sp. Gr: 0.816) and purified water (for official dilute alcohol).
7. **As per Dr. Dewey:** It is prepared by adding 7 parts of 87% alcohol with 3 parts of purified water.

Note: When alcohol is mixed with purified water there is rise of temperature with shrinkage in volume to an extent of 3%. So little more purified water should be added to make the specific gravity stand at 0.89.

8. **Uses:**
   (i) For the preparation of potencies, particularly under decimal scale.
   (ii) For cleansing of utensils.

Dispensing Alcohol

1. *Synonyms:* Alcohol officinalis, official alcohol.
2. *Definition:* It contains 88% by volume or 83.1% by weight of ethyl alcohol (C_2H_5OH) and 12% by volume of purified water.
3. *Preparation:* It is prepared by mixing:
   (a) 10 parts by weight of strong alcohol (Sp. Gr: 0.816) and 1 part by weight of purified water, or
   (b) 12.25 parts by volume of strong alcohol (Sp. Gr: 0.816) and 1 part by volume of purified water.

   The specific gravity of the resulting dispensing alcohol, at 15.6°C or 60°F is 0.840.

Note: Actually 12.75 parts by volume of strong alcohol (Sp. Gr: 0.816) should be added, which, after mixing is reduced to 12.25 due to shrinkage. Normally, 55% shrinkage occurs when equal quantities of strong alcohol and purified water is mixed.

4. *Uses:* It is mostly used for potentising the drugs from their mother tincture state, as it is more readily absorbed by globules, sugar of milk or tablets.

Table 11.2: Conversion of Rectified Spirit into Absolute Alcohol

1.5 ounce (43 cc) of potassium carbonate (K_2CO_3) is poured in a glass stoppered bottle and 1 pint of rectified spirit 60° o.p. is added to it.

↓

The mixture is kept well-stoppered in that bottle for two days shaking briskly every now and then.

The spirit is very carefully decanted to the flask so that the ppt. may not come to the flask.

10 (284 cc) ounce slaked lime or Calcium hydroxide [$Ca(OH)_2$] is taken in a covered crucible

↓

Heated for at least 30 minutes. It is allowed to become cool.

↓

When perfectly cooled it is transferred to a big flask.

↓ A condenser is fixed to the flask. It is kept without giving heat for 24 hrs.

↓

Then it is heated gently.

↓

Allowed the spirit to distil.

↓

The distilled spirit, thus obtained, is absolute alcohol.

Note: In India, for dispensing purpose, alcohol of this strength is not used. Rectified spirit 60 o.p., which is 3.29% stronger than the dispensing alcohol, is used.

Rectified spirit (60°O.P.)

1. *Definition:* Rectified spirit 60° o.p. means that 100 volumes of the alcohol, diluted with purified water, will give 160 volumes of proof-spirit.

   In other words, it means pure rectified spirit contains 160 per cent of proof-spirit.

   It contains 91.29% by volume of C_2H_5OH having specific gravity at 15.6°C: 0.8294.

2. *Preparation:* It is prepared by mixing 375 ml of purified water with 1,000 ml of strong alcohol.

3. *Uses:*
   (i) It is used for potentisation of medicine under centesimal scale.
   (ii) For cleansing of utensils.

Note: Rectified spirit 60° o.p. was recommended by B.H.P. It is popularly used in India and Commonwealth countries for dilution purposes, in place of dispensing alcohol (H.P.I and H.P.U.S.). It is 3.29% stronger than dispensing alcohol and difference in Sp. Gr. is approximately 0.01.

Q. State the type, strength, source and common impurities of the alcohol generally Indian pharmacists are supplied.

Type: Rectified spirit.

Strength: 60°o.p.

Source: Molasses

Common impurity: Fusel oil.

Rectified spirit (40°O.P.)

It is prepared by mixing 7 parts of strong alcohol with one part of purified water, both by volume. It contains 73.37% by weight of strong alcohol, Sp. Gr. 0.8646 at 15.6°C.

Rectified spirit (20°O.P.)

It is prepared by mixing 6 parts of strong alcohol with 2 parts of purified water, both by volume.

It contains 60.85% by weight of strong alcohol. Sp. Gr: 0.8936.

Denatured spirit (Alcohol)—Methylated spirit

Alcohol is largely used as solvent and also as intoxicating drinks. To make it unfit for unlawful human consumption, poisonous or bad smelling substances are mixed in small quantities with the rectified spirit. The mixture is known as denatured spirit. The substances usually mixed for this purpose are methyl alcohol, benzene, bone oil, crude pyridine and caoutchoucine etc. The product is also slightly coloured by adding some dye to indicate its nature. This, however, does not prevent its use as a solvent in industries.

Rectified spirit, denatured by mixing methyl alcohol, is known as methylated spirit. Nowadays, however, 0.5% light caoutchoucine (obtained by distilling vulcanised rubber) and 0.5% pyridine bases are used as denaturants, although the old name (methylated spirit) is still used.

Proof-spirit (Alcoholometry)

Definition: Proof-spirit is defined by Act of Parliament as: "being such as shall, at a temperature of 51°F, weighs exactly $^{12}/_{13}$th part of an equal measure of purified water". In other words, proof-spirit is a mixture of alcohol and purified water, weighing $^{12}/_{13}$th of an equal volume of purified water at 51°F.

Standard strength: The proof-spirit is 57.1% of ethyl alcohol (C_2H_5OH) by volume or 49.28% of C_2H_5OH by weight and 42.9% of purified water by volume with specific gravity 0.91976 at 60°F.

It is fixed by the Excise Department and is measured by a special type of graduated hydrometer (i.e. alcohol hydrometer).

Designation: This spirit of standard strength (i.e. proof-spirit) is expressed in terms of degrees under- or over-proof.

The alcohol which is stronger in strength than this proof-spirit is called 'over-proof' (o.p.) and the weaker one 'under-proof' (u.p.)

Significance: Above percentage is considered as the proof-strength of alcohol and according to them it is decided whether any liquid is stronger or weaker.

Examples

1. *Over-proof (O.P.):*
   (i) 10° over-proof (o.p): means that 100 volumes of the liquid (Alcohol/Spirit), diluted with purified water, will give 110 volumes of proof-spirit.

(ii) 30° over-proof (o.p): means that 100 volumes of the liquid (Alcohol/Spirit), diluted with purified water, will give 130 volumes of proof-spirit.

(iii) 60° over-proof (o.p): means that 100 volumes of the liquid (Alcohol/Spirit), diluted with purified water, will give 160 volumes of proof spirit.

2. *Under-proof (U.P.):*

(i) 10° under-proof (u.p): means that 100 volumes of the liquid contains 90 (100 – 10) volumes of proof-spirit.

(ii) 30° under-proof (u.p): means that 100 volumes of the liquid contains 70 (100 – 30) volumes of proof-spirit.

(iii) 60° under-proof (u.p): means that 100 volumes of the liquid contains 40 (100 – 60) volumes of proof-spirit.

Determination of proof strength of alcohol

Proof strength of alcohol means the standard strength of alcohol.

Alcohol freely mixes with water. Almost all the Governments of the world have imposed some sort of duty on alcohol and alcohol preparations. As a result it is necessary to know the strength of alcohol. Formerly, the strength was roughly determined by pouring alcohol over gun powder and firing it. If the sample contained much water, it did not take fire and if the quantity of water was small it took fire easily.

For convenience, a special type of hydrometer has been invented by the Excise Authority to ascertain the strength of alcohol. For this purpose a mixture containing 57.1% by volume of ethyl alcohol and 42.9% by volume of purified water is called the standard proof-spirit. The strength is measured in terms of degrees.

The hydrometer is graduated specially, corresponding to the upper level of the standard proof spirit, above and below of the standard mark there are equal graduations.

When the strength of an unknown quality of alcohol is to be determined, the alcohol is taken in a big glass cylinder and the hydrometer is dipped into it carefully and the upper level of alcohol is read.

If it is seen that the upper level is 60 marks above the standard mark, expressing its lowered density and, hence, strong due to less amount of water, it is called 60°o.p.

On the other hand, if the upper level corresponds with a line 20 marks below the standard mark it is called 20°u.p.

Formula for conversion from percentage to proof-strength, or vice versa:

(i) $90\% = (90 \times 1.75) - 100 = 57.5$ or 57.5 o.p.

(ii) $50\% = (50 \times 1.75) - 100 = -12.15$ or 12.5 u.p.

(iii) $60°\text{o.p.} = \dfrac{60 + 100}{1.75} = 91.45\%$

(iv) $60°\text{o.p.} = \dfrac{-60 + 100}{1.75} = 22.86\%$

SOLVENT ETHER (Aether Solv.)

Synonyms: Ethyl oxide; Ethylic ether; Sulphuric ether.

Chemical formula: $C_2H_5–O–C_2H_5$ or (C_2H_5) or $(C_2H_5)_2O$.

Source: It is diethyl ether (96% to 98%), remainder consists of alcohol and water.

It is prepared by distilling a mixture of Ethyl alcohol (C_2H_5OH) and Sulphuric acid (H_2SO_4) and rectifying the distillate.

$$\underset{\text{Ethanol}}{2C_2H_5OH} \xrightarrow{H_2SO_4} \underset{\text{Ethyl ether}}{C_2H_5–O–C_2H_5 + H_2O}$$

Properties

1. A colourless, transparent, very mobile liquid.
2. Sweet smell and burning taste.
3. It is very inflammable, boils at 34.5°C and burns with a white flame. It is extremely volatile.
4. Specific gravity: 0.72.
5. Solubility: Soluble in 8.5 volumes of water; miscible in all proportions with alcohol (90 p.c.), Chloroform, fixed and volatile oils.

   Most of the alkaloids, resins, balsams, tannic acid etc. are easily dissolved by it. It dissolves bromine and iodine readily but sparingly dissolves phosphorus and sulphur. The corrosive sublimate ($HgCl_2$) is very quickly dissolved by it.

Precautions

1. As solvent ether is highly inflammable and volatile, it should be always kept away from fire and the bottle kept tightly corked.
2. It should never be used as an anesthetic.

Uses

1. It is used only when alcohol in its varying properties with water cannot extract the drug substance from plant.
2. It is a good solvent for many organic compounds, e.g. resins, gums, fats, oils, cellulose esters, etc.

GLYCERINE (Glycer)

Synonym: Glycerol

Chemical formula: $CH_2OH.CHOH.CH_2OH$ or $C_3H_5(OH)_3$

Molecular weight: 92.1

Boiling point: 290°C

Specific gravity: 1.26

Introduction: It is an important tri-hydric alcohol. It contains not less than 98% w/w of $C_3H_8O_3$ (H.P.I.):

It is the commonest constituent of all animal and vegetable oils and fats, e.g. olive oil, coconut oil, cod-liver oil etc.

Preparation

A. **From sugars by fermentation**

When sugars are fermented with yeast, about 3% glycerol is formed along with alcohol:

$$\underset{\text{Glucose}}{C_6H_{12}O_6} \longrightarrow \underset{\text{Glycerol}}{C_3H_5(OH)_3} + \underset{\text{Acetaldehyde}}{CH_3CHO} + CO_2$$

B. **Synthetic Process (From propylene)**

Large quantities of glycerol are now manufactured in USA and CIS from propylene obtained as a by-product during cracking of petroleum. This synthesis is carried out in the following steps:

It is prepared from propylene, a petroleum product. It is chlorinated to form Allyl chloride which is converted to Allyl alcohol. Then it is treated with Hydrochlorous acid (HOCl) when 'Chlorhydrin derivative' is produced. Extraction of HCl with soda lime, followed by hydrolysis, yields glycerine.

C. **From spent soap Lyes**

Fats and oils are hydrolysed with NaOH solution (lye) when glycerol and sodium salts of fatty acids (soaps) are formed:

The soap is salted out while glycerol remains in solution known as 'spent lye'. Spent lye contains 3 – 5%, glycerol, small amount of free alkali, NaCl, dissolved soap, proteinous matter, inorganic salts, and colouring matter.

Glycerol is recovered from it as:

(i) The spent lye is allowed to settle in iron tanks where heavy impurities settle down.

(ii) The clear liquid is pumped into 'treating tank' fitted with steam coils. It is treated with HCl to neutralise about three-fourth of the free alkali present in the lye. It is now treated with alum or basic ferric sulphate which neutralises the remaining alkali and also converts the traces of sodium soaps as well as the free acids still present into the insoluble iron soaps. A gelatinous precipitate of $Fe(OH)_3$ and insoluble iron soaps is formed:

$$6NaOH + Fe_2(SO_4)_3 \longrightarrow 2Fe(OH)_3 + 3Na_2SO_4$$
$$6C_{17}H_{35}COONa + Fe_2(SO_4)_3 \longrightarrow 2(C_{17}H_{35}COO)_3Fe + 3Na_2SO_4$$

(iii) The liquid along with the precipitate is filtered through filter-presses under pressure. The clear liquid so obtained is concentrated in vacuum pans to about

$$\underset{\text{Propylene}}{\begin{matrix}CH_2\\ \| \\ CH\\ | \\ CH_3\end{matrix}} \xrightarrow{Cl_2} \underset{\text{Allyl chloride}}{\begin{matrix}CH_2\\ \| \\ CH\\ | \\ CH_2Cl\end{matrix}} \xrightarrow[150^\circ,\ 12\ \text{Atom}]{Ag{\cdot}NO_2CO_3} \underset{\text{Allyl alcohol}}{\begin{matrix}CH_2\\ \| \\ CH\\ \| \\ CH_2OH\end{matrix}} \xrightarrow[Cl_2\text{—water}]{HOCl} \underset{\text{Glycerol β-chlorohydrin}}{\begin{matrix}CH_2Cl\\ \| \\ CHOH\\ \| \\ CH_2Cl\end{matrix}} \xrightarrow{NaOH} \underset{\text{Glycerol}}{\begin{matrix}CH_2OH\\ \| \\ CHOH\\ \| \\ CH_2OH\end{matrix}}$$

80% of glycerol. During evaporation, common salts separate out and are removed from time to time from the bottom:

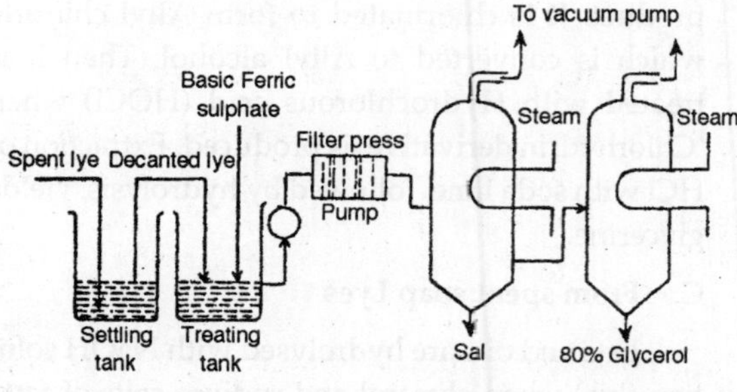

Preparation of crude glycerol from spent lye

(iv) The crude glycerol so obtained is decolourised with animal charcoal and purified by distillation with superheated steam under reduced pressure.

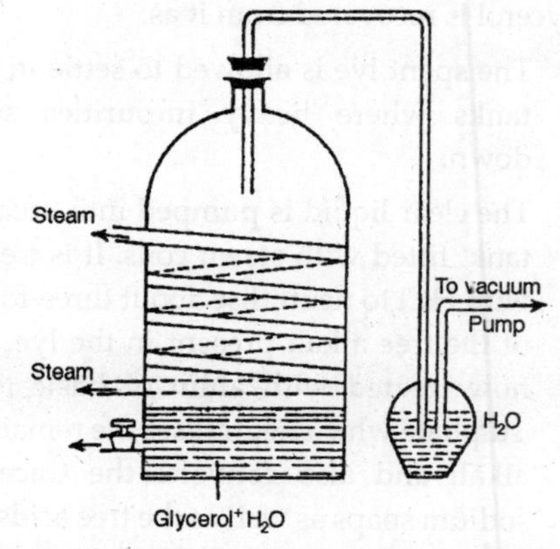

Purification of crude glycerol by distillation

(v) The distillate containing water is then concentrated in vacuum pans until the glycerol has specific gravity 1.26. It is 99.9% pure.

Properties

1. *Physical*

(i) A clear, colourless, syrupy liquid; odourless.

(ii) Tastes sweet, followed by sensation of warmth.

(iii) Hygroscopic i.e., absorbs moisture from atmosphere or air.

(iv) Solubility: Miscible with water and alcohol (90 p.c.), insoluble in chloroform ($CHCl_3$), in solvent ether and in fixed oils.

(v) Pure glycerol boils at 290°C but impure decomposes at its boiling point.

(vi) When kept for some time at a low temperature, it may solidify, forming a mass of colourless crystals which do not melt until the temperature reaches about 20°C.

(vii) Its specific gravity is 1.255 to 1.266 at 20°C. It is commonly obtained by the hydrolysis of fats and fixed oils or by synthesis.

2. *Chemical*

(i) When heated with dehydrating agents, like $KHSO_4$, forms acrolein, a pungent-smelling unsaturated aldehyde.

(ii) It crystallises on cooling, if kept at a low temperature for some time, it may solidify forming a mass of colourless crystals, which melts at about 17°C.

Purity test of Glycerine

1. *Acrolein test:* Two drops of glycerine is taken in a test tube and a little powdered potassium hydrogen sulphate ($KHSO_4$) is added to it. Then it is heated cautiously at first and then more strongly. A vapour with a very irritating and pungent smell of acrolein is produced, which blackens a filter paper moistened with a solution of ammoniacal silver nitrate ($AgNO_3$).

$$\begin{array}{c} CH_2OH \\ | \\ CHOH \\ | \\ CH_2OH \\ \text{(Glycerine)} \end{array} \xrightarrow[\text{Heat}]{KHSO_4} \begin{array}{c} CH_2 \\ || \\ CHCHO \\ \\ \text{(Acrolein)} \end{array}$$

2. **Dunstan's test (Borax-Phenolphthalein test)**

About 6 ml. of 0.5% solution of Borax

↓ ← Added drop by drop, enough of 1% alcoholic solution of phenolphthalein

Appearance of distinct red colour

↓ ← Added 20% Glycerol, drop by drop

Disappearance of red colour

↓ ← On boiling/heating.

Reappearance of red colour.

Sodium borate (borax) in aqueous solution is partially hydrolysed to the boric acid and sodium hydroxide. The solution is alkaline, as boric acid is a weak acid. Glycero-boric acid formed on addition of glycerol, being strong acid, turns the solutions acidic. On heating or boiling glyceroboric acid hydrolyses to glycerol and boric acid, turning the solution alkaline.

3. **Copper hydroxide test:** A suspension of cupric hydroxide [$Cu(OH)_2$] is made by mixing 2.5% $CuSO_4$ solution with 3 ml of 5% NaOH. A few drops of glycerine is added to this suspension. A blue colour is obtained. Glycerine prevents the precipitation of cupric hydroxide. No change occurs on boiling the solution.
4. **Borax-bead test:** When heated on a borax bead in a Bunsen burner flame it gives a green flame.

Storage: It should be kept in dry well-closed containers.

Uses

1. **Externally**
   (i) It is an antiseptic, emollient, and demulcent.
   (ii) As an emollient (substances which soften or relax the skin upon which they are applied) glycerine is the best application for chapped lips and hands, rough, dry, furfuraceous skin, and for every kind of skin disease, such as herpes, eczema etc.
   (iii) It is used as an application on superficial ulcers of tongue and the mouth.
   (iv) It is used in ear discharges, as it absorbs the pus easily.
   (v) As glycerine is an excellent solvent for numerous bodies, such as fixed alkalies, large number of salts, vegetables, acids, pepsin, tannin, some active principles of plants, gums, etc., it is a good vehicle for applying these substances to the skin and to sores.
2. **Internally:** Used as a suppository in constipation. For evacuation of the bowels in simple constipation, especially when the feces are in the sigmoid flexure and rectum, it may be introduced by a special metal syringe per rectum, being mixed with olive oil and tepid purified water.
3. **For preparation**
   (i) It is used for preparing mullein oil.
   (ii) It is used for preparing 'Glycerole'.
   (iii) It is used for preparation of mother tinctures and lower dilutions of certain poisonous products e.g. *Apis mellifica; Naja tripudians; Tarentula hispanica.*
4. **For preservation:** It is used for preserving poisonous animal products, e.g. *Lachesis; crotalus horridus; Elaps corallianus.*
5. **Others**
   (i) It is used in cosmetics for its softening action on the skin.
   (ii) In the manufacture of Nitroglycerine (the homoeopathic drug Glonoinum).
   (iii) For the treatment of chronic simple open-angle glaucoma.
   (iv) In the preparation of stamp inks, shoe polishes etc.
   (v) In leather, rubber, plastics, and textile industries.

SIMPLE SYRUP Or SYRUP SIMPLEX (Syr)

Source

It is a solution of sucrose (or Cane-sugar) and purified water.

Preparation

450 ml of purified water is taken in a flask and heated to boiling

↓

550 gm. of sucrose is added to it

↓

The mixture is heated cautiously with constant stirring until the whole of the sucrose is dissolved

↓

Resultant solution is filtered through purified cotton or a suitable filter

↓

Ringed the vessel with hot purified water till the final solution admeasures 1,000 ml. When cooled this mixed thoroughly.

Storage

It should be kept in well-closed clean neutral glass container. It should not be exposed to undue fluctuations in temperature.

Uses

It is used as a sweet vehicle. During prescription of homoeopathic mother tinctures, these syrups are the best vehicles to combine with, which is the odour or taste of these tinctures.

OLIVE OIL
(Oleum olivae; Ol. oliv.)

Source

It is a fixed oil, expressed from the ripe fruits of olea europoea (family—oleaceae) found in southern Europe and countries near about Mediterranean sea.

Composition

Olive oil is composed of:

(i) Olein, glyceride of oleic acid (93%);

(ii) Linolein, glyceride of linoleic acid (7%);

(iii) Palmitin, a solid oil composed of palmitic acid and glycerol;

(iv) Arachin.

Method of preparation

Ripe olive fruits are crushed in mill. The remaining portion is mixed with a solvent like carbon disulphide (CS_2) and boiled. Then the residual oil is extracted by expression.

Properties

(i) Pale, yellow but its colour may vary from colourless to green or greenish-yellow.

(ii) Odour: slight but not rancid.

(iii) Taste: bland in taste.

(iv) At low temperatures it may be solid or partly solid.

(v) Specific gravity: 0.910-0.913 at 20°C.

(vi) Boiling range: 40°C to 60°C.

(vii) Solubility: almost insoluble in alcohol (95 p.c.); miscible with solvent ether, with chloroform ($CHCl_3$) and light petroleum.

(viii) If exposed to air and heat, it gradually loses colour and becomes rancid.

Storage

It should be kept in well-closed container.

Uses

1. **Externally**

(i) Olive oil-being a bland unirritating

Table 11.3: Purity test of Olive oil

	Experiment	Observation	Inference
1.	1 ml. olive oil is taken in a flask with reflux condenser ↓← 5 ml of 1.5(N) alcoholic KOH. Boiled for 10 minutes. ← 50 ml of alcohol (70%) ↓← 0.8 ml of conc. HCl. The solution is gradually cooled	If above 9°C: (a) No turbidity (b) Turbidity present	 (a) Pure olive oil (b) Olive oil is mixed with the arachis oil or peanut oil (i.e. *cheena-badam tel*)
2.	Little olive oil is shaken with equal volume of a mixture of 9 parts by volume of alcohol (90 p.c.) and 1 part by volume of strong ammonia solution ↓ Heated on water-bath until free from ammonia and alcohol Now, 2 ml of the olive oil is shaken with 1 ml HCl, containing 1% w/v of sucrose ↓ Set aside for 5 minutes.	If the acid layer: (a) Does not colour pink or faintly pink (b) Coloured pink	 (a) Pure olive oil (b) Olive oil is mixed with the sesame oil (or teel oil)

fixed oil—usually applied as an emollient in dry skin diseases. It is a common soothing protective to burns and may be mixed with poultices to prevent their stickings to the skin.

(ii) Used to apply for getting smoothing effect on superficial ulcers.

(iii) It is rubbed, after mixing with cod-liver oil, over the skin of the patients suffering from Rickets and Marasmas. It renders the skin softer, smoother and more flexible.

2. **Internally**

(i) Because olive oil retards the flow of the gastric juice, it is an excellent food in cases of gastric ulcer, for the acid prevents the healing of the ulcers.

(ii) It is a good mild laxative and can be taken at bedtime.

(iii) In constipation, it is introduced per rectum through a specially made syringe.

3. For preparation: It is used for preparing 'liniment'.

ALMOND OIL
(Ol. amygdal)

Synonyms

Oleum amygdalae; oleum amydalae expressum, *Badam tel*.

Source

Almond oil is the fixed oil obtained from the seeds of Prunus amygdalus var. dulcis, or of Prunus amygdalus var. amara, by macerations with water and subsequent distillation with steam.

Composition

It contains not less than 80% benzaldehyde, composed mainly of olein with some linolein, but no stearin present.

Properties

(i) A pale-yellow, non-drying oil.

(ii) Nearly inodorous.

(iii) Bland, musty taste.

(iv) Solubility—Miscible with solvent ether, with chloroform, slightly soluble in alcohol (90 p.c.)

(v) Specific gravity — 0.910 to 0.915 at 20°C.

Adulterations

It is commonly adulterated with peach-kernel oil. It may be rarely adulterated with arachis oil, sesame oil and cottonseed oil.

Test for peach-kernel oil: 5 ml of oil is vigorously shaken with 1 ml of a fresh mixture of equal parts by weight of H_2SO_4, HNO_3 and water. The mixture is kept cool while cautiously mixed. After 15 minutes the whitish mixture is produced, showing no pink colour.

Test for arachis oil and sesame oil: Already described in 'Olive oil', as it is same as olive oil.

Storage

It should be kept in well-filled, well-closed container.

Uses

1. **Externally**

(i) Almond oil is a demulcent and emollient, and being a bland oil makes a good basis for the preparation of 'Liniment' in place of olive oil.

(ii) It is a soothing application for chapped hands, excoriations and irritable skin diseases.

2. **Internally:** The oil is a mild purgative in 120 to 240 ml doses.

SESAME OIL
(Ol. sesam.)

Synonyms

Oleum sesami; Teel oil; Gingelli oil; Benne oil.

Source

It the refined fixed oil, expressed from the seeds of one or more cultivated varieties of sesamum indicum, Linn. (family—pedalicacae), native in India, China and most other tropical countries.

Composition

(i) Sesamin, a crystalline substance and sesamolin

(ii) Liquid fats, 70 p.c. consisting of glycerides of oleic acid and linoleic acids.

(iii) Sesamol, a phenol.

(iv) Solid fats; (12 – 14%) stearin, palmitin etc.

Properties

(i) A limpid oil of a pale-yellow colour.

(ii) Faint odour; bland taste.

(iii) Solubility: Slightly soluble in alcohol (90 p.c.), miscible with solvent ether, with chloroform and with light petroleum.

(iv) Specific gravity 0.916 to 0.921 at 20°C.

Uses

(i) Used instead of Olive oil in the preparation of liniment.

(ii) Used in the preparation of hair oil.

(iii) An edible oil.

HYDNOCARPUS OIL
(Ol. hydnocarp)

Synonym

Oleum hydnocarpi.

Source

Hydnocarpus oil is a fatty oil obtained by cold expression from the fresh, ripe seeds of *Hydnocarpus wightianus*, Blume (family—Flacourtiaceae). The tree grows in Southern India, where it is called 'Marroti'.

Composition

(i) Glycerides of chaulmoogric acid, $C_{18}H_{32}O_2$.

(ii) Glycerides of palmitic acids and fatty acids.

(iii) Hydnocarpic acid.

Properties

(i) A yellowish or brownish yellow oil, or soft cream-coloured fat.

(ii) Characteristic odour and slightly acrid taste.

(iii) Solubility: partially insoluble in cold alcohol (90 p.c.), freely soluble in hot alcohol (90 p.c.); miscible with solvent ether, chloroform and carbon disulphide.

Uses

It is used as an external application in skin diseases, especially in 'Leprosy'.

CHAULMOOGRA OIL
(Ol. chaulmoog.)

Synonyms

Oleum chaulmoogra; Gynocardia oil; *Chaulmoogra tel.*

Source

Chaulmoogra oil is the fatty oil obtained by cold expression from the fresh, ripe seeds of *Hydnocarpus kurzii* or other species of Hydnocarpus, a native of Sikkim, Assam, Chittagong, Sylhet, Upper Mayanmar (Burma) and the Malaya peninsula.

Composition: Same as Hydnocarpus oil.

Properties

(i) Yellow or brownish-yellow oil. Below 25°C, a whitish soft solid.

(ii) Odour: characteristic, resembling that of rancid butter.

(iii) Taste: somewhat acrid.

(iv) Solubility: sparingly soluble in alcohol (90 p.c.), soluble in benzene, in chloroform and in solvent ether.

Uses

(i) The oil and its derivatives are to a certain extent effective in the treatment of leprosy, especially in early cases.

(ii) It is used as a rubefacient.

Storage

Should be kept in a tight well-closed container in a cool place protected from light.

SANDALWOOD OIL
(Ol. santal)

Synonyms

Oleum santali; oil of Sandalwood; Santal oil; *Chandaner tel.*

Sources

Oil of Sandalwood is the volatile oil distilled from the dried heartwood of *Santalum album*, Linn (family–Santalaceae). The tree grows in India (specially Mysore, some parts of Kerala district and southern parts of Tamil Nadu), as well as Germany and England.

Composition

The chief constituents are (i) Santalol, a mixture of two sesquiterpene alcohols, (ii) An aldehyde, Santalal, (iii) Esters, free acids, etc.

Properties

(i) Thick, pale-yellow or nearly colourless volatile oil
(ii) Odour: Strongly aromatic
(iii) Taste: Pungent, aromatic
(iv) Solubility: Readily soluble in alcohol, ether or chloroform
(v) Reaction: Slightly acidic
(vi) Specific gravity: 0.973 to 0.985 at 20°C.

Adulterations

It is commonly adulterated with Castor oil and other fixed oils.

Test for Castor oil: If 10 ml of a mixture of 3 volumes of alcohol and 1 volume of water be added to 1 ml of the oil, a perfectly clear solution should result.

Storage

It should be kept in well-stoppered bottles in a cool place, protected from light.

Uses

(i) It is mixed with other oils and applied externally.
(ii) Due to its sweet smell it is generally used in cosmetics and perfumes.

LAVENDER OIL
(Ol. lavand.)

Synonyms: Oleum lavendulae; Oil of Lavender.

Source

It is a volatile oil, obtained by distilling from the fresh flowering tops of *Lavendula officinalis* of L. vera (family—Labiatae), grows in Germany, France, Spain, Italy and also cultivated in the Union Territory of Jammu and Kashmir in India. It contains (English oil) 7.0–12.0 p.c. w/w, or (foreign oil) not less than 35.0 p.c. w/w. of esters, calculated as Linalyl acetate, $C_{12}H_{20}O_2$.

Composition

(i) Linalol, an alcohol and its acetic ester, Lynalyl acetate, are the principal constituents.
(ii) Pinene, $C_{10}H_{16}$, present in some samples but is not a constant constituent.
(iii) Limonene, geraniol and a sesquiterpene.

Properties

(i) A colourless, pale yellow or yellowish-green liquid.
(ii) Odour, that of the flowers.
(iii) Taste pungent and slightly bitter.
(iv) Solubility: Miscible with alcohol (90 p.c.) and absolute alcohol; sparingly soluble in alcohol (60 p.c.) and 1 in 4 of alcohol (70 p.c.).
(v) Specific gravity 0.875 to 0.888 at 25°C.
(vi) Refractive index: at 20°C, 1.4590 to 1.4700.
(vii) Optical rotation 3 to –10°, in a 100 mm tube.

Adulterations

It may be adulterated with (i) Glycerine monoacetate, (ii) Alcohol, (iii) Salicylic acid ester, (iv) Benzoic acid ester:

(i) Test for Glycerine monoacetate: It may be detected by shaking with 4 – 5 volumes of petroleum ether, in which the glycerine monoacetate is insoluble and glycerine may be further identified by its specific tests.
(ii) Test for alcohol: It may be detected by shaking the oil with purified water in equal volumes, the volume of oil should not be diminished.
(iii) Test for Salicylic acid ester: It may be detected by purple-red coloration produced on addition of a solution of Ferric chloride after saponification.
(iv) Test for Benzoic acid ester: It may be confirmed by a solution of Ferric chloride.

Storage

It should be kept in a cool place, protected from light, in well-closed container.

Uses

(i) It can be applied on superficial ulcers without alcohol.

(ii) It is used with alcohol for soothing effect in headache.

ROSEMARY OIL
(Ol. rosmarin.)

Synonyms: Oleum Rosemarini; Oil of Rosemary.

Source

It is a volatile oil, steam distilled from the fresh flowering tops of *Rosemarinus officinalis*, Linn. (family – Labiatae), native in England and Southern Europe.

It contains not less than 2% w/w of esters, calculated as bornyl acetate, and not less than 9% w/w free alcohols, calculated as borneol, $C_{10}H_8O$.

Composition

(i) Borneol, 8 – 16%

(ii) Bornyl acetate and other esters, about 2–5% camphor, cineole, pinene and camphene.

Properties

(i) A colourless or pale-yellow volatile oil

(ii) Odour: Characteristic odour of rosemary

(iii) Taste: Warm, aromatic

(iv) Solubility: 1 in 1 of alcohol (90 p.c.)

(v) Specific gravity: 0.894 to 0.912

(vi) Optical rotation: –5° to +10°C, in a 100 mm tube

(vii) Refractive index: At 20°C, 1.466 to 1.476.

Storage

The oil should be kept in well-closed container, in a cool place, protected from light.

Uses

(i) It is a component of Liniment, Saponin etc.

(ii) It is a stimulant and rubefacient to the skin and is commonly used in the form of hair oil.

SEMISOLID VEHICLES

VASELINE
(Soft-paraffin)

Synonyms

Petroleum jelly, Paraff. moll.; Paraffinum molle.

Definition

It is a semi-solid mixture of hydrocarbons obtained from crude petroleum, after kerosene oil, gas oil, fuel oil or diesel oil have been separated. It is then bleached and purified.

Varieties: It is available in two varieties — (i) White soft paraffin and (ii) Yellow soft paraffin. The white soft paraffin is better than yellow variety.

1. **White Soft Paraffin (White soft paraff.)**

Synonyms: White petroleum jelly; Paraff. moll. alb; Paraffinum mole album.

Source: It is a mixture of semi-solid hydrocarbons obtained from petroleum and bleached.

Properties

(i) A white translucent, soft mass; unctuous to touch.

(ii) Odourless, when rubbed on the skin; Tasteless.

(iii) Not more than slightly fluorescent by daylight, even when melted.

(iv) Solubility—Practically insoluble in $CHCl_3$ and solvent ether and in light-petroleum (b.p.: 40°C to 60°C).

(v) Specific gravity: 0.815 to 0.880 at 20°C.

Uses

(i) It is used for the preparation of emulsifying ointment, paraffin ointment and simple ointment.

(ii) It is used as lubricant and applied on ulcers or wounds in dressing.

2. **Yellow Soft Paraffin (Yellow soft paraff.)**

Synonyms: Yellow petroleum jelly; Paraff. molle flavum; Paraffinum molle flavum.

Source: It is a semi-solid mixture of hydrocarbons obtained from petroleum.

Properties

(i) A pale-yellow to yellow, translucent, soft mass; unctuous to touch.

(ii) Almost free from odour and taste.

(iii) Not more than slightly fluorescent by daylight even when melted.

(iv) Solubility: Practically insoluble in water and alcohol (90%); soluble in $CHCl_3$, in solvent ether and in light petroleum (b.p: 40°C to 60°C).

(v) Specific gravity: 0.815 to 0.880 at 20°C.

Uses: It is used for the preparation of paraffin ointment, simple ointment and wool-alcohol ointment.

WAXES
(Simple lipid)

Definition

Waxes are solid esters of higher monohydric alcohols and higher fatty acids other than glycerol.

Varieties

The three common waxes are:

1. Beeswax.
   (i) Yellow beeswax
   (ii) White beeswax.
2. Lanolin (anhydrous).
3. Spermaceti.

Beeswax: It is available in two varieties:

1. **Yellow Beeswax**

Synonym: Cera flava; Cera flav.; Beng–Mom.

Source: Yellow beeswax is a secretion formed by the hive-bee, Apis mellifica, L and possibly other species of Apis (Family: Apidae) and is used by the insect to form the cell of the honeycomb.

Preparation

Honeycomb
↓
Comb—after removal of honey
↓
Melted with hot water, which washes away any honey remaining
↓
Cooled
↓
Bees wax is separated at the surface as a solid cake
↓
Extracted.

Composition

(i) Myricin (Myricyl palmitate—$C_{15}H_{31}COO C_{30}H_{61}$)—80%.

(ii) Cerotic acid (15%)

Properties

(i) A yellow to greyish brown solid

(ii) Odour—honey-like

(iii) Taste—faint and characteristic

(iv) Brittle when cold but becoming plastic when warm

(v) Insoluble in water, sparingly soluble in cold alcohol; completely soluble in $CHCl_3$, ether, fixed and volatile oils

(vi) Melting point—60°C to 65°C

(vii) Contains 70% of ester's, the chief being myricyl palmitate.

Identification

(i) Acid value—17 to 23

(ii) Iodine value—8 to 11 (Iodine monochloride method)

Uses: Used as a stiffening agent and as an ingredient of yellow ointment.

2. **White beeswax (Cera. alba.):** It is the bleaching variety of yellow beeswax. Used as component of cerates and ointments.

LANOLIN
(anhydrous)

Synonyms: Wool fat; Adeps lanae; Adepes lan.

Preparation

It is a purified anhydrous fat-like substance, obtained from the wool of the sheep, ovis aries (family: Bovidre). The natural grease is extracted from the wool by treating with dilute alkali, with which it readily forms an emulsion; next the emulsion is acidified and the wool-fat separates as a distinct layer at the surface of the liquid.

Purification may be effected by repeated treatment with water in a centrifuge.

Properties

(i) A pale yellow, tenaceous, unctuous substance.

(ii) Odour, faint and characteristic.

(iii) Solubility: insoluble in water, sparingly soluble in cold alcohol (90%); freely soluble in solvent ether and in $CHCl_3$.

(iv) Melting range: 36°C to 42°C.

(v) Acid value: Not more than 1.

(vi) Iodine value: 18 to 32.

(vii) Saponification value: 92 to 106.

(viii) Contains not more than 200 parts per million of butylated hydroxyanilose or butylated hydroxytoluene.

Uses

Due to penetrating power within the skin, it is extensively used in ointments.

Storage

In well-closed container at a temperature not exceeding 30°C.

SPERMACETI (U.S.P.)

Synonyms: Cetaceum, sp. Esperma de ballena.

Source

It is a waxy substance obtained from the head of the sperm whale physeter macrocephalus Lirin. (family: Physeteridae).

Constituents

It is a mixture of several constituents of which cetin or acetyl palmitate ($C_{15}H_{31}COOC_{16}H_{33}$) predominates. When recrystallised from alcohol, cetin is obtained, while the mother liquor on evaporation deposits an oil, cetin plain, which, when saponified, yields cetin elaic acid, an acid resembling but distinct from oleic acid.

Preparation

It is obtained by the forcible expression of the oleaginous material found in the head of the sperm whale to separate the liquid portion which is known as sperm oil, which is a liquid wax. The solid fat is termed cetin (acetyl palmitate) and also belongs to the class of waxes.

Properties

(i) A white somewhat translucent, slightly unctuous mass with a crystalline fracture and pearly lustre.

(ii) Faint odour; a bland milk taste and free from rancidity.

(iii) Specific gravity: 0.94 (approx.).

(iv) Melting range: 42°C to 50°C.

(v) Acid value: Not more than 1.0.

(vi) Iodine value: Not more than 5.

(vii) Saponification value: 120 to 136.

(viii) Solubility: insoluble in water, nearly insoluble in cold water and slightly soluble in cold petroleum benzene but is soluble in boiling alcohol, in ether, $CHCl_3$ and in fixed and volatile oils.

Uses

It is one of the solid fatty substance employed to give consistency to cerates and ointments, as in the well-known water ointments.

Storage: It is preserved in well-closed container.

PREPARED LARD

Synonyms: Adeps lard; Adeps praeparatus; Sukar charbi.

Source: It is the purified internal fat of the abdomen of hog, sus scrofa, Linn, Var. domesticus Gray.

Preparation: It is prepared by careful removal of membranes and adhering flesh and then rendered.

Composition: (i) Olein (60%), (ii) Stearin, (iii) Palmitin.

Properties

(i) A soft, white, unctuous mass.

(ii) Faint odour and a bland taste, free from rancidity.

(iii) Solubility: insoluble in water, very slight soluble in alcohol (90%); soluble in solvent ether, in $CHCl_3$ and in light petroleum.

(iv) Melting point: 36° to 42°C, forming a clear liquid, from which no water layer separates.

Uses: It is used as an ingredient in ointments.

Precaution: Must be protected from conditions favouring rancidity.

ISIN GLASS

Source: It is a collagen derived from the thin, inner silver shiny layer of the air-bladder of some fishes, particularly sturgeons, carps and cat fishes.

Method of preparation: The air-bladder is collected, washed thoroughly and then the outer thick and fibrous layer of the wall is separated from the inner layer which is exclusively Isin glass raw material. Then they are cut into small pieces and after maceration, pressed into sheets by means of large roller.

Properties: It is light whitish or yellowish, semi-transparent, tough, fibrous, tasteless and odourless solid.

Uses: It is a component of Calendula and Arnica plasters.

SOAP

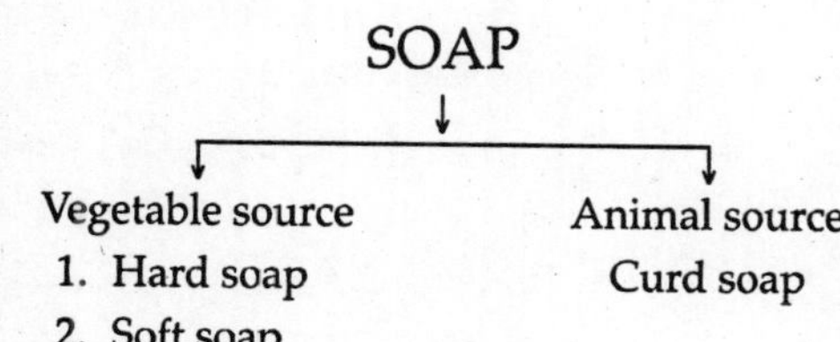

Hard Soap

Synonyms: Sapo durus; Sap. dur.; Castile soap; Olive oil soap; Sodium oleate.

Source: Hard soap is made by the interaction of sodium hydroxide (NaOH) with a suitable vegetable oil or oils or with fatty acids derived therefrom.

Properties

(i) A greyish white or yellowish white substance.

(ii) Nearly odourless, becomes horny and pulverisable when dried.

(iii) Solubility: soluble in water; almost completely soluble in alcohol (90%) and more readily soluble when warmed.

Storage: Preserved in well-closed containers.

Category: Detergent.

Soft Soap

Synonyms: Sapo. mollis; Sap. moll.; Green soap; Potassium oleate.

Source: Soft soap is made by the interaction of potassium hydroxide (KOH) or sodium hydroxide (NaOH) with a suitable vegetable oil or oils or with fatty acids therefrom. It yields not less than 44% of the fatty acids.

Properties

(i) A yellowish-white to green, or brown unctuous substance.

(ii) Solubility: Soluble in water and in alcohol (90%).

Storage: Preserved in well-closed container.

Category: detergent.

Preparation: soap liniment.

Curd Soap

Synonyms: Sapo. animalis; Sap. animal; Sodium stearate.

Sources: Curd soap is made from sodium hydroxide (NaOH) and purified solid animal fats.

Properties: A greyish-white or yellowish-white substance, nearly odourless. Becomes horny and pulverisable when dried. Soluble in water; almost completely soluble in alcohol (90%) and more readily soluble when warmed.

Uses: It is a component of opodeldocs.

STARCH

Synonyms: Amylum; snetsar.

Chemical formula: $(C_6H_{10}O_5)n$

Source

(i) Maize or Indian corn (Zea mays L.): 65 to 70%.

(ii) Wheat (Triticum sativum Lam): 60 to 65%

(iii) Potato (Solanum tuberosum. L): 15 to 20%.

(iv) Paddy (oryza sativa L): 75 to 85%.

Method of Preparation

1 From maize or Indian corn: The germs are separated mechanically. The cells are made soft so as to permit the escape of the

starch granules, which is done by allowing them to become sour and decomposed, stopping the fermentation before the starch is affected.

2. From potato: Firstly grating them and then washing the soft mass upon a sieve which separates the cellular substances and permits the starch granules to pass through by decantation.
3. From wheat: At first a stiff ball-like dough is made and kneading it while a small stream of water trickles upon it. The starch is carried-off with the water while the 'gluten' remains as a soft elastic mass, which, being purified, may be used for other purposes.

Properties

It is a white, tasteless, odourless, hygroscopic powder, insoluble in cold water and all organic solvents except formamide and dimethyl sulphoxide.

Uses: It is a component of 'Glycerole of Starch'.

Chapter 12

Different Scales of Preparations of Drugs

Scales of Potentisation

(a) *Scales for trituration:*

1. Decimal Scale.
2. Centesimal Scale.

(b) *Scales for Succussion:*

1. Decimal Scale.
2. Centesimal Scale.
3. 50-millesimal Scale.

Today, all three scales are used, though the 50-millesimal scale is used relatively seldom. In France, the centesimal scale is exclusively used. In English-speaking countries, predominantly the centesimal scale, is in use and in Germany on the whole the decimal scale is very popular.

DECIMAL SCALE

Inventor: This scale was introduced by Dr. Constantine Hering (1800-1880, German-born physician, emigrated to USA) to potentise snake-venoms. Dr. Vehsemeyer of Berlin gave a more detailed description of this scale in 1836.

Ratio: 1 : 9

Drug strength: $\frac{1}{10}$

Principle: This scale is based on the principle that first potency should contain $\frac{1}{10}$th part of the original drug and each succeeding potency should contain $\frac{1}{10}$th part of the previous potency.

Designation: The decimal potency is denoted by suffixing the letter 'X' to the number indicating the potency, i.e. the first potency is 1X, the second potency is 2X, and so on.

Application of this scale: Decimal scale is applicable in old method (established by Hahnemann) for the process of potentisation. This scale is usually used to make the lower potencies or strength, especially up to 6X. In modern method (new method) for preparation of mother tincture, it is the only scale that is used.

Preparation of potencies under this scale

1. **Liquid potencies:** A well-cleaned and round phial of 15 ml capacity is taken. It is fitted with a new velvet cork. The cork is marked with the name and the potency 1X. Then the cork is removed. Next, name of the mother tincture or solution to be potentised, is checked. 1 ml of the tincture or solution poured in the phial, and then 9 ml of rectified spirit (60 o.p.) i.e. dispensing alcohol is added to the phial. This $\frac{1}{3}$rd of the phial remains empty for succussion. Then it is corked and ten downward strokes of equal strength are given. The 1X is now ready. A level on the wall of

the phial is pasted, marking the name of the medicine with potency 2X.

All succeeding potencies are prepared under this scale by mixing one part of the preceding potency to nine parts of dispensing alcohol.

2. **Solid potencies:** For making 1X potency, one part by weight of the crude drug is triturated with nine parts by weight of sugar of milk, for the period of one hour, including three stages, each consuming 20 minutes, and dividing the nine parts sugar of milk in three equal parts.

All the following potencies are made by taking one part of the preceding potency with nine parts of sugar of milk. Trituration is done up to 6X potency, and then 8X liquid potency is prepared.

CENTESIMAL SCALE

Inventor: This scale was introduced by the founder of homoeopathy, Samuel Hahnemann, in 5th edition of Organon of Medicine (1833) in Sec. 270.

Principle: This scale is based on the principle that first potency should contain $\frac{1}{100}$th part of the original drug and each succeeding potency should contain $\frac{1}{100}$th part of the preceding potency.

One part by volume or weight of drug or previous potency + ninetynine parts by volume or weight of vehicle.

Designation: This scale is denoted by simply affixing the numericals after the name of the drug, e.g. Apis mel. 3, Apis mel. 6, denote 3rd and 6th centesimal potency of Apis mel. These may be denoted by 3C or 6C, but this kind of denotation may bring confusion with 'C' which means 100 as 2C = 200th potency. Some of these potency strengths are designated by Roman numericals, e.g. 200 as cc; 1,000 as M or 1M; 10,000 as 10M; 50,000 as 50M or L.M; 100,000 as C.M; 500,000 as D.M; 1,000,000 as MM and 500,000,000 as DMM.

Application of this scale: This scale is applicable in old method (established by Hahnemann) for the process of potentisation. This scale is used to make higher potencies or strength. Centesimal scale has been discarded by the new official pharmacopoeia due to the uniformity of drug-strength (10%). In the new method, only decimal scale is used.

Preparation of potencies under this scale

1. **Liquid potencies:** A well-cleaned round phial of 150 ml capacity is taken. It is fitted with new velvet cork. The cork is marked with the name and potency 1. Then the cork is removed. Next, name of the mother tincture or solution to be potentised is checked. 1 ml of the tincture or solution is poured in the phial, and then 99 ml of dispensing alcohol is added to the phial. Thus, $\frac{1}{3}$rd of the phial remains empty for succussion. Then it is corked and ten downward strokes of equal strength are given. This first potency of this scale is now ready. A label on the wall of the phial is pasted, marking the name of the medicine with potency 1.

All succeeding potencies are prepared under this scale by mixing one part of the preceding potency, and ninetynine parts of dispensing alcohol.

2. **Solid potencies:** For making first potency, one part by weight of the crude drug is triturated with ninetynine parts by weight of sugar of milk, for the period of one hour, including three stages, each consuming 20 minutes as in decimal scales and dividing the ninetynine parts of sugar of milk into three equal parts (33 + 33 + 33). For the second potency, one part of the first potency is triturated with ninetynine parts of sugar of milk in the usual way. Trituration is done up to 3rd potency and the fourth liquid potency is prepared.

Relation between Decimal and Centesimal scale of potency

In decimal scale, the first potency contains $\frac{1}{10}$th part of the original drug, whereas in centesimal scale the first potency contains $\frac{1}{100}$th part of the original drug. Therefore, in decimal scale second potency contains $\frac{1}{10} \times \frac{1}{10} = \frac{1}{100}$ equal to first potency of the centesimal scale. Similarly, second centesimal scale corresponds to fourth decimal scale and the third centesimal scale corresponds to the sixth decimal scale.

Note: Both the centesimal and the decimal scales have their protagonists. In my experience (unsupported by statistical analysis) the decimal scale is better for low potencies up to 6X, whilst the centesimal scale provides more rapidly acting medicines in the higher potencies (Gerhard Koehler).

50-MILLESIMAL SCALE OR L.M. SCALE

Introduction: This is the finer and latest scale of potency, introduced in the 6th edition of Organon of Medicine, prepared in the ratio 1 : 50,000 and was mentioned clearly about its preparation, preservation, and administration. In fact, this name was not given by Hahnemann but by Pierre Schmidt of Geneva. Hahnemann himself termed this new method as, "Renewed Dynamisation" (Sec. 161).

In footnote 1, Sec. 132 he writes: "new altered but perfected method"—*"New dynamisation method"* etc. The details of this method was incorporated in his 6th edition of Organon. Potencies prepared under this method are named by Schmidt as "fifty-millesimal potencies" because of the fact that the material part of the medicine was said to be decreased by 50,000 times for each degree of dynamisation. The physicians are not in the habit of using this scale but recently some physicians are using it.

History of preparation of 50-Millesimal scale of potency

1838: On 19th Feb. 1838, Hahnemann, in Paris, wrote the introduction of Chronic Disease. In 5th part of **Chronic Disease** he wrote about the new dynamisation methods.

1842: Hahnemann completed the manuscript of 6th edition of Organon of Medicine including the preface in Feb. 1842, after 18 months' work. The two versions of 6th edition of Organon—one in German and another in French, was ready for publication. Hahnemann wanted to publish the French version at first, and followed by German version. But he could not publish it because of the bungling of his German publisher, Mr. Schaub, in Dusseldorf.

1843: Next year, on 2nd July 1843, the world lost Hahnemann and the 6th edition of Organon remained unpublished. The manuscript remained in possession of his 2nd wife Malanie. The 2nd wife of Hahnemann did not allow the publication of 6th edition because of her unexpected greed for money. Several attempts were made by different homoeopaths all over the world, to publish the 6th edition from the custody of Malanie. Some of these attempts are:

(i) *Von Boenninghausen:* In 1856, he tried to obtain her permission to publish the 6th edition of Organon. Though she allowed Boenninghausen to publish the manuscript of 6th edition, but omitted to state, the German or the French text, which will be given to him. However, later she rejected her consent.

(ii) *Suss Hahnemann*, the grandson of Hahnemann, made an attempt to publish the 6th edition but in vain.

(iii) *Constantine Hering* tried to publish English edition from the text, but terms and conditions compelled him to wait for future.

(iv) *Dunham* of New York took an attempt to publish the 6th edition of Organon but it was not possible due to his death.

(v) *Dayes* of London took an attempt to publish the 6th edition but Malanie did not accept his request on the ground, that an English homoeopath would be unable to translate the German text in exactitude.

1878: *Malanie* died on 27th May 1878.

1920: Long after the death of Malanie, *R. Haehl* managed to procure the German manuscript from the heirs of Hahnemann in the Boenninghausen's estate, and published it in original only in 1920.

1921: *William Boericke* of San Francisco, paid $ 10,000 and published a more precise and perfect retranslation of the 6th edition of Organon from the original German text. During this period, centesimal scale of potencies from 6 to CM, was fully established in the homoeopathic world. Therefore, even after the publication of the English version of 6th edition of Organon nobody gives any importance to this "New Dynamisation Method". But very unfortunately this highly beneficial work was in cold storage until *Charles Pahud* of France and *Pierre Schmidt* of Geneva brought out this lost contribution of Hahnemann to limelight in the first half of 1950s.

1950: *Charles Pahud* of France drew the attention of the world homoeopathic physicians to the 6th edition of Organon in his article "My experience about Hahnemann's 50-millesimal scale potency" issued in "The British Homoeopathic Journal".

1954: *Pierre Schmidt*, M.D., of Geneva, published an article entitled "The Hidden Treasure of the Last Organon", in "The British Homoeopathic Journal" July-October 1954. Another article was published by him in "The Journal of The Institute of Homoeopathy", December-January 1955-56.

In this way, these two learned and world-famous homoeopaths first opened the door of the hidden treasure of the 6th edition of Organon.

Introduction of 50-Millesimal scale in India

In India, many homoeopaths use 50-Millesimal scale of potency successfully, but few of them only narrates their experience, idea, and views in different books and journals.

1957: In March 1957 *S. M. Bhattacharyya* of Behrampur, West Bengal, wrote an article "Hahnemann's 50-Millesimal scale of potency" in "Hahnemannian Gleanings". Here, he has compared 50-Millesimal scale with centesimal scale, giving conversion table. In 1957, Hahnemann Publishing Company of Kolkata started to manufacture medicines in 50-Millesimal scale, and became pioneer in the world.

1960: In 1960, *R. P. Patel* of Kerala wrote a book entitled "My experience with 50-Millesimal scale of potencies".

1964: *Chandipada Chakravorty*, in collaboration with *Harimohan Chowdhury*, first published a book on this subject, under the title, "Sahasratamiker Prayog Vigyan" in 1964. They also started manufacturing drugs in this scale.

1968: In 1968, B. K. Basu wrote a Bengali book entitled, "Panchas Sahasratamik Shakti O Tahar Prayog Vigyan".

1971: First volume of H.P.I., published in 1971, mentions about "Fifty-millesimal potency" for its preparation (in page 12).

1972: *Harimohan Chowdhury* published a book in Bengali, "Panchas Sahasratamik paddhtir Oushadher Prayog Vigyan", in 1973, for wide circulation about the hidden treasures of the Organon 6th edition.

The same author wrote the English version of this Bengali book entitled "50-Millesimal potency in Theory and Practice".

1981: *S. P. Dey* of Kolkata, famous Hahnemannian homoeopath, wrote about 50-Millesimal potencies in his book "Essential of Principles and Practice of Homoeopathy".

How Hahnemann arrived at the Concept of 50-Millesimal potency?

Hahnemann's view of the highest ideal of cure was rapid, gentle and permanent. But during his practice life, he faced various problems with medicines prepared under centesimal scale of potency, as per 5th edition of Organon.

The main causes of dissatisfaction with centesimal scale are:

1. Rapid gentle cure is not possible at all, it takes a long time.
2. Undesirable homoeopathic aggravation comes even after the well-selected medicine is administered.
3. After administration of single dose, one has to wait for long, and watch helplessly the action of the medicine.
4. Too frequent repetition is not possible.

For this purpose Hahnemann concluded experimental research through clinical trial and came to minimise the quantity of the dose with maximum results. The laborious research for last 4-5 years of his life shows the light for the introduction of "new dynamisation method". Different advantages were observed by Hahnemann than centesimal scale which compelled him to introduce the 50-Millesimal scale, which he called, "new altered but perfected method" instead of, "so near to perfection".

With the new scale of potencies Hahnemann observed the following advantages:

1. The action of the selected medicine is rapid.
2. Homoeopathic aggravation can easily be avoided by minimising the quantity of the medicine.
3. Medicine can be repeated frequently both in acute and chronic diseases.
4. Medicine may be continued even after improvement starts.

5. A chronic disease can be cured within shortest period of time.

6. Within 4 to 5 days after administration of medicine, the physician can ascertain the action of the medicine.

So we see the different disadvantages after using centesimal scale, which dissatisfied Hahnemann "for rapid, gentle and permanent cure", and after his rectification by laborious work, how Hahnemann reached the goal of "the perfected method".

Designation

In India, it is designated as 0/1, 0/2, 0/3, 0/4, etc.

In Bangladesh, it is designated as M/1, M/2, M/3, M/4 etc.

In Western world, it is designated as 1/0, 2/0, 3/0, 4/0 etc.

Hahnemann used to write 0/1, 0/2, 0/3, 0/4, etc.

It would be better if we write LM/1, LM/2, LM/3 etc. Here, "L" stands for 50 and "M" for Millesimal. The potency of this scale my be denoted by using the simple Roman numbers as, I, II, III, IV etc.

The numerator "0" represents symbolically the poppy-sized globule employed in each dynamisation, as distinct from the drop of medicine utilised in the centesimal scale.

Materials and appliances (for preparation and dispensing)

A. *Ingredients*

(a) Crude drug substance. (b) Vehicles: (i) Sugar of milk, purest quality for potentisation. (ii) Purified water, purest quality, for potentisation and dispensing. (iii) Strong alcohol. (iv) Sugar globules, of purest quality, which are free from dust particles by passing them through a sieve. Then they are passed through another sieve which will allow only globules of such size—a hundred of which weigh one grain.

B. *Appliances*

(a) Porcelain mortar and pestle. (b) Horn-made spatula. (c) Balance with weight box. (d) Different containers for mother solution potentised medicines etc. (e) Dispensing phials of different quantity with washer and caps. (f) Pen, paper, gums, scissors etc. (g) Labelling marking dose.

Preparation of 50-Millesimal potencies

The mode of preparation according to new method (6th edition, Organon of Medicine) has not yet found any place in any Homoeopathic Pharmacopoeia. Hahnemann himself clearly explained about the mode of preparation in Sec. 270-271 and their footnotes of the Organon.

Preparation of 50-Millesimal potency is easier, in the sense that the range of potencies is less and the arrangements are not complicated. Moreover, these medicines can be prepared without any machine. The quality and quantity of the dose are properly measured as per Hahnemannian Doctrine (**Medicaments au globule**).

A detailed description of the method of preparation will be found in Pierre Schmidt's translation of the Organon (Sec. 270).

1. *Preparation of mother tincture*

(a) First, the drug-substances, soluble or insoluble, solid or liquid, juicy or dry (plants and animals as a whole) is triturated with sugar of milk up to 3rd centesimal potency, i.e. 1 grain of drug-substances with 300 grains of sugar of milk for three hours, in the usual manner of trituration.

The final drug strength is: $\frac{1}{10,00,000}$ or $\frac{1}{10^6}$

(b) Conversion of 3rd centesimal trituration into liquid form—to an approximately 60 ml bottle, one grain (0.063 gm) of that powder is dissolved (by necessary shaking) in 500 drops of a mixture of one part dispensing alcohol, and four parts purified water (500 drops = 100 drops of 20% alcohol + 400 drops purified water). Thus, the dry trituration is converted into liquid form. We call it "The mother potency of the new method" or mother tincture of the 50-Millesimal scale.

The drug-strength is $\frac{1}{500} \times \frac{1}{10^6} = \frac{1}{5 \times 10^8}$

2. *Potentisation*

(a) *Preparation of 1st potency* ($^0/_1$): Into a separate bottle (approximately 10 ml) containing 100 drops of 95% alcohol, one drop of the above-mentioned mother tincture from the 60 ml bottle is placed. The bottle must be large enough so that the solution does not fill more than ⅔rd of it.

The bottle is closed with a cork carefully, and 100 succussions are given by holding it in the hand, and pounding the hand rapidly on a leather-bound book— a surface which is resilient and elastic. This is the first degree of dynamisation or first potency (0/1, or LM/1 or M/1). The drug strength will be—

$$\frac{1}{5 \times 10^8} \times \frac{1}{100} = \frac{1}{5} \times \frac{1}{10^{10}} = \frac{1}{5} \times 10x$$

$$= \frac{1}{5} 5C \left[\frac{1}{10^{10}} = 10x;\ 10x = 5C\right]$$

Conversions in the form of globules: The small poppy sized globules (100 weighing 1 grain) are moistened with it, and spread quickly on a piece of blotting paper to dry. Then they are kept in a well-corked glass phial protected from heat and sunlight with mark $^0/_1$ on it. It is found that 500 standard globules of poppy seed size can hardly absorb one drop of alcohol for their saturation.

(b) *Preparation of 2nd potency* ($^0/_2$): Only one globule of the first potency is taken in a "second new phial," and one drop of purified water is added to dissolve it. To it, 100 drops of pure alcohol (95%) is added and dynamised with 100 powerful succussions as before.

Conversion in the form of globules: With this alcoholic medicinal fluid, globules are again moistened and spread upon blotting paper, and dried quickly. These are put into well-stoppered phials protected from heat and sunlight. This is the 2nd degree of dynamisation, or 2nd potency (0/2 or LM/2 or M/2 potency).

(c) *Preparation of next higher potencies:* The above-mentioned process is repeated with one globule to the previous potency, to increase it to next potency. The process is continued up to 0/30 or onwards up to 0/50 or 0/60 as per necessity.

Schematic representation of preparation of 50-Millesimal potencies (step by step)

I. Original substance 1 drop (1 grain) + 100 grains of sugar of milk + 1 hour trituration by grinding, pounding, scraping etc.

This is the first trituration $= \frac{1}{100}$

II. 1st trituration 1 grain + 100 grains of sugar of milk + 1 hour trit. = 2nd trituration.

$$= \frac{1}{100} \times \frac{1}{100} = \frac{1}{10{,}000}$$

III. 2nd trituration 1 grain + 100 grains of sugar of milk + 1 hour trit. = 3rd trituration

$$= \frac{1}{10{,}000} \times \frac{1}{100} = \frac{1}{10{,}00{,}000}$$

IV. 3rd trituration 1 grain + 500 drops of a mixture containing 1 part of 20% alcohol and 4 parts of purified water (100 drops of dispensing alcohol + 400 drops of purified water) = Mother tincture.

$$\text{Drug power} = \frac{1}{10{,}00{,}000} \times \frac{1}{500} = \frac{1}{50{,}00{,}00{,}000}$$

V. 1 drop of mother tincture + 100 drops of absolute alcohol + 100 succussions = LM/1, the 1st potency.

$$= \frac{1}{50{,}00{,}00{,}000} \times \frac{1}{100} = \frac{1}{50{,}00{,}00{,}00{,}000} = \frac{1}{5 \times 10^{10}}$$

VI. Conversion in form of globule: 1 drop of the first potency moistened with 500 globules and dried quickly.

VII. 1 globule of 1st potency + 1 drop purified water + 100 drops of pure alcohol + 100 succussions = LM/2, the 2nd potency.

VIII. In this way, LM/3 or 0/3 onwards will have to be prepared and potentised.

Comparison between 50-Millesimal Scale, Decimal Scale, and Centesimal Scale in Dilution

Comparison is valuable only in dilution. In succussions this is entirely wrong—as each potency needs 100 succussions in this new scale, while Centesimal potency needs only 10.

Mother tincture (Q)

$$= \frac{1}{5 \times 10{,}00{,}00{,}000} = \frac{1}{5 \times 10^8} = \frac{1}{5} \times 4C$$

1. **50 milles: 1 (50 M.L.-1)**

$$= \frac{1}{5 \times 10^8 \times 100} = \frac{1}{5 \times 10^{10}} = \frac{1}{5} \times 10x$$

Table 12.1: Conversion between 50-Millesimal Scale and Centesimal Scale in Succussion

50-Millesimal			*Centesimal*			
Potency	***Succussions***		***Potency***		***Succussions***	
1	100	Above	5	But	50	only
6	600	Approx.	17	...	170	...
12	1,200	"	31	...	310	...
30	3,000	"	73	...	730	...
100	10,000	"	238	...	2,380	...
200	20,000	...	473	...	4,730	...
500	50,000	...	1,178	...	11,780	...
1,000	1,00,000	...	2,352	...	23,520	...
10,000	10,00,000	Accurate	23,498	...	2,34,980	...
50,000	50,00,000	...	1,17,478	...	11,74,780	...
1,00,000	10,00,00,000	...	2,34,953	...	23,49,530	...

$= \frac{1}{5} \times 5C \; [\frac{1}{10^{10}} = 10x; 10x = 5C]$

From 2 upwards all potencies are on the 50-Millesimal scale, and are expressible in terms of the previous potency.

$$\frac{1}{50,000} = \frac{1}{5 \times 10,000}$$

$$= \frac{1}{5 \times 10^4} \text{ of the previous potency.}$$

2. **50 milles: 6 (50 M.L.-VI):**

$$\frac{1}{5 \times 10^{10}} \times \left[\frac{1}{5 \times 10^4}\right]^5 \text{ (there being 5 degrees)}$$

$$= \frac{1}{5 \times 10^{10}} \times \frac{1}{5^5 \times 10^{20}} = \frac{1}{5^6 \times 10^{30}}$$

Now, 5^6 expressed in powers of 10 = 10^4 approx. ($10^{4.1940}$ accurately).

$$\therefore \text{The sum} = \frac{1}{10^4 \times 10^{30}} = \frac{1}{10^{34}}$$

= 34x = 17C approx.

3. **50 milles: 12 (50 M.L.-XII):**

$$\frac{1}{5 \times 10^{10}} \times \left[\frac{1}{5 \times 10^4}\right]^{11} \text{ (there being 11 degrees)}$$

$$= \frac{1}{5 \times 10^{10}} \times \left[\frac{1}{5^{11} \times 10^{44}}\right] = \frac{1}{5^{12} \times 10^{54}}$$

Now, 5^{12} expressed in powers of 10 = 10^8 approx. ($10^{8.3880}$ accurately).

$$\therefore \text{The sum} = \frac{1}{10^8 \times 10^{54}} = \frac{1}{10^{62}}$$

= 62x = 31C approx.

4. **50 milles: 30 (50 M.L.-XXX):**

$$\frac{1}{5 \times 10^{10}} \times \left[\frac{1}{5 \times 10^4}\right]^{29} \text{(there being 29 degrees)}$$

$$= \frac{1}{5 \times 10^{10}} \times \frac{1}{5^{29} \times 10^{116}} = \frac{1}{5^{30} \times 10^{126}}$$

Now, 5^{30} expressed in powers of 10 = 10^{21} approx. ($10^{20.9700}$ accurately).

$$\therefore \text{The sum} = \frac{1}{10^{21} \times 10^{126}} = \frac{1}{10^{147}}$$

= 147x = 73C approx.

5. **50 milles: 100 (50 M.L.-C):**

$$\frac{1}{5 \times 10^{10}} \times \left[\frac{1}{5 \times 10^4}\right]^{99} \text{(there being 99 degrees)}$$

$$= \frac{1}{5 \times 10^{10}} \times \frac{1}{5^{99} \times 10^{396}} = \frac{1}{5^{100} \times 10^{406}}$$

Now, 5^{100} expressed in powers of 10 = 10^{70} approx. ($10^{69.9}$ accurately).

$$\therefore \text{The sum} = \frac{1}{10^{70} \times 10^{406}} = \frac{1}{10^{476}}$$

= 476x = 238C approx.

From the calculations it is evident that the differences between centesimal and millesimal scales are neither very wide nor spectacular. It is only about the ratio of 1 : 2.

Dudley W. Everitt has calculated that 50-Millesimal potencies can be compared, or equated theoretically on paper, to the traditional potencies (decimal and centesimal) as follows:

50-Millesimal		*Decimal*	*Centesimal*
I		16x	8C approx.
II	Between	20x and 21x	10C ...
III	...	24x and 26x	13C ...
VIII	...	44x and 51x	25C ...
X	...	52x and 61x	30C ...
XII	...	60x and 71x	35C ...
XVIII	...	84x and 101x	50C ...
XXIV	...	108x and 131x	65C ...
XXX	...	132x and 161x	80C ...

Administration of medicine in 50-Millesimal Scale of potency

A. **Medicinal solution**

(a) *Mode of preparation of medicinal solution for dispensing:*

(i) Firstly one brand new (unused) phial of 120/60/30 ml with new washer and cap are taken.

(ii) Then, ¾th part of the phial is filled up with purified or distilled water.

(iii) Only one medicated globule of no. 10 of selected medicine in desired potency is added.

(iv) To this solution 5/8/10 drops of rectified spirit are added as preservative agent.

(v) The phial is closed with cork tightly.

(vi) The phial is marked with 16/8/7/4 or less equal doses.

(vii) Now, this medicinal solution is ready for use.

(b) *Direction to the patient for taking of medicinal solution:*

(i) Before taking the medicine each time 8/10/12 downward succussions are given, according to the susceptibility of the patient—10 for a less sensitive patient, and 12 times for the least excited and sensitive patients.

(ii) After succussion, one dose (marked over the phial) is taken in ¾th glass of pure water.

(iii) Then stir it well, with a tea-spoon.

(iv) One or two tea-spoonful (as directed by the physician) from it should be taken by the patient, and the rest portion of the solution is to be thrown away.

(v) Each dose from the medicinal solution of each potency is to be applied in the same manner.

If there is any aggravation by taking the medicine in abovementioned process, then repetition of taking the medicine is to be stopped. The aggravation will be diminished gradually in a shortperiod and then the same remedy is diluted further in 2nd or 3rd or, if required, in the 4th glass of water (as the patient can stand) and only one tea-spoonful of it will be taken and rest portion will be thrown away.

B. **Dose**

(a) *The single medicine (or the simplex):* one single, simple medicinal substance to be administered at one time (Sec. 273, 6th edition).

(b) *Minimum dose (or infinitesimal dose):* Every dose should be as small as possible (Sec. 273, 6th edition).

(c) *Exceptions to the minimum dose (F.N., Sec. 282):* However, there is a very important exception in regard to minimum doses in the treatment of primary (cutaneous manifestations) psora, syphilis, and sycosis, namely:

For psora: recently developed itch.

" *syphilis:* untreated primary chancre (on the sexual organs, mouth or lips, and so forth).

" *sycosis:* condylomata.

In these three cases, large doses of their specific remedies of over higher and higher degrees of dynamisation daily (possibly also several times daily) must be administered.

(d) *Form:* Medicine of this new method must be administered in liquid form, only to establish the highest ideal of cure.

(e) *Application of medicine in many doses instead of single dose:* One small (no. 10) globule soaked with medicine, if placed on the tongue, touches only a few nerves. But a similar globule, crushed with some sugar of milk and dissolved in a good deal of water, stirred well before every administration will produce a more powerful medicine for the use of several days. Every dose, no matter how minute, touches, on the contrary, and many nerves. Therefore, it is most reasonable and scientific to administer medicine in liquid form, than giving in the form of pills, for achieving the quickest accomplishment of cure.

(f) *Potency problem:*

(i) Limitation of potency: Hahnemann has recommended potencies from 0/1 to 0/30 only (Sec. 270. 6th edition). Though limitation of potency has been extended up to 0/30, if majority of patients proceeds towards ideal of cure within 0/10, there is no reason to apply higher potency unnecessarily. On the other hand, in long-lasting and so-called incurable diseases, potencies beyond 0/30 may be necessary. R. P. Patel of Kerala has mentioned high experience of using this scale up to 0/50th potency. A complicated case of varicose ulcer of both lower limbs was completely cured by the author, Biman Mandal, using Graphites up to 0/43. Therefore, medicine is needed up to 0/60 or onwards for complete cure in this modern era—as per susceptibility of the patient.

(ii) From what potency to start treatment: The treatment must be started from the *lowest degrees of dynamisation*, i.e. with any potencies from 0/1 to 0/6, and advance to gradually higher as necessary, in any patient, either acute or chronic (F.N. 270). But to begin the treatment from a particular potency we should follow the susceptibility of the patient.

Note: 1. Practical experience shows that better results are obtained if we start treatment of acute disease (where susceptibility is high without h/o loss of vital fluids and not allergic or idiosyncratic) from 0/6 or 0/10 or 0/20. But in acute diarrhoea vomiting, severe bleeding treatment should begin from 0/1.

2. In many cases, to fulfil the susceptibility of the patient, and by applying the jumping potency such as 0/3, then 0/5, then after 0/7 it minimises the unnecessary killing of time than going through serial potencies.

(iii) How long the first prescription will continue: First prescription should be continued so long as the patient experiences continued improvement without encountering one or another complaint that he/she never had before in his/her life. In these cases, only the potency of medicine is to be changed from low to high, i.e. from 0/1 to 0/2; 0/2 to 0/3 and so on (Sec. 280).

(iv) Proper time of 2nd prescription: If new symptoms appear then another, one more homoeopathically related medicine must be chosen in place of the last and administered in the same repeated doses, modifying the solution of every dose with thorough vigorous succussions, thus changing its degree of potency and increasing it somewhat (Sec. 248).

(v) Potency of 2nd prescription: The potency of the newly selected medicine is to be started from the lowest degrees of dynamisation, i.e. with any potency from 0/1 to 0/6.

C. **Repetition of doses (Pharmacopollaxy)**

Repetition of doses, in 50-Millesimal potency, mainly depends upon the nature of disease which are:

(a) *In chronic diseases:* Once a day or once every alternate day (e.g. Bronchial asthma, Rheumatic diseases, Skin diseases, Cancer, Essential hypertension etc.)

Thus, in chronic diseases, every correctly selected homoeopathic medicine, even those whose action is of long duration, may be repeated daily for months with ever-increasing success.

(b) *In acute diseases:* Once every 2, 3, 4 or 6 hours (e.g. Diarrhoea, Dysentery, Malaria, Typhoid etc.)

(c) *In very urgent cases:* Every hour or oftener (e.g. Chicken pox, Tetanus, Cholera etc.).

In chronic diseases, if the medicinal solution is used up (in 7-15 days) then higher potency of the same medicine to be prepared, and administered in the same way so long as the patient experiences continued improvement.

D. Aggravation after administration of medicine

(a) *Disease aggravation:* If the new group of symptoms belonging to the disease (i.e. disease symptoms) appear during the course of treatment, then the medicine is to be changed according to the changed totality and to be administered in the same ways.

(b) *Medicinal aggravation:* If the new symptoms of the medicine appear which are not there in the patient earlier, the medicine should be discontinued. In such a case:

(i) If aggravation is very violent: It must be first partially neutralised as soon as possible by an antidote before giving the next remedy chosen more accurately according to similarity of action.

(ii) If aggravation is not very violent: The next remedy must be given immediately, in order to take the place of the improperly selected one.

(c) *Homoeopathic aggravation:* If towards the end of the treatment of chronic diseases "homoeopathic aggravation" of the existing symptoms only takes place, the doses must be reduced still further and repeated in longer intervals, then possibly stopped for several days, in order to observe the convalescence, need no further medication. The transient aggravation caused by the excess of the homoeopathic medicine will soon disappear, and the patient will be cured.

E. Proper time for administration of medicine

(a) The most appropriate and efficacious time for administration of the medicine in intermittent fever is immediately or very soon after the termination of the paroxysm (Sec. 236).

(b) There is a definite period of aggravation of the disease in acute or chronic cases and that is not the suitable time for the administration of medicines, e.g. the troubles of syphilitic patient aggravate at night. So night should be avoided for dministration of medicine in a syphilitic patient.

(c) There is also a period for medicinal aggravation, and that is not the proper time for administration of medicine, e.g. Ars alb< from 12.00 p.m. to 2.00 a.m. and 12.00 a.m. to 2.00 p.m.; Nat mur < 10.00 a.m. to 11.00 a.m.; Kali group < from 3.00 a.m. to 5.00 a.m.; Lyco < 4.00 p.m. to 8.00 p.m. and Sulphur < from 10.00 a.m. to 11.00 a.m.; (d) In menstrual disturbances—the best time is the post-menstrual period.

F. Routes of administration of medicine (Pharmaconomy)

There are four methods of administration of medicine to the patients:

(a) *By oral route* (ingestion through mouth).

(b) *By olfaction* (inhalation through nose and mouth): Adapted to patients who are unusually excited and sensitive.

(c) *By rubbing:* To massage on the body along with oral route with a view to expecting rapid and lasting cure. External application has been recommended only in case of figwort.

(d) *By mother's milk or milk of wet nurse:* For newborn and children.

G. Conditions for administration of medicine (Sec. 246, 6th edition)

(a) The selected medicine should be perfectly homoeopathic.

(b) It should be highly potentised.

(c) It should be dissolved in water.

(d) Medicine must be given in proper small dose.

(e) Every subsequent dose must be higher than the previous one.

(f) Repetition should be made at definite intervals for the quickest accomplishment of the cure.

Advantages and special characteristics of 50-Millesimal potencies over Centesimal and Decimals

1. *Minimum homoeopathic aggravation:* Homoeopathic aggravation may be avoided, minimised, and even controlled, due to less amount of material quantity. It can be safely used even in the most deplorable case without fear of dangerous and violent aggravation.
2. *Quick cure of chronic disease:* Long-lasting complicated and intractable chronic diseases may be cured within the shortest period of time. As said in Sec. 246, the period taken for cure can be diminished to one-half, one-quarter or even still less. Only this new system can face boldly any challenge with the so-called modern medicines in regard to quickest recovery.
3. *Frequent repetition permissible:* Medicine can be frequently repeated—both in acute as well as chronic disease—and also in emergency conditions. Even the long-acting anti-miasmatic constitutional medicines and nosodes can be repeated too frequently as per need without fear of aggravation. It can be repeated:
   (a) Daily or every 2nd day, in chronic disease.
   (b) Once every 2, 3, 4 or 6 hours, in acute disease.
   (c) Every hour or oftener, in very urgent cases. Deep acting constitutional medicines like *Lyco., Calc carb, Kali ars., Psor., Sulph., Thuja* may be administered and repeated several times for months together according to the need of the patient.
4. *Judge of appropriate medicine:* The correctness of the selected medicine can be judged within 2-4 days in chronic diseases, and within 2-4 hours or even earlier in acute cases by the use of this potency. So, we need not unnecessarily wait (long) for this purpose. After administering a dose of Thuja or Sulphur in 200th potency, we may have to wait for a fairly long period to watch for the action of the medicine. But in this potency, the action can be noticed after administration of only a few doses consecutively.
5. *Palliative and curative purposes simultaneous use:* The same constitutional medicine may be used both for palliative and curative purpose simultaneously. No separate medicine is essential for palliation when needed.
6. *Mental diseases:* Very useful in mental diseases where least aggravation may be very much harmful to the patient and confusing to the physician. This potency can effect the cure smoothly without the least aggravation.
7. *Change from incurable to curable stage:* The so-called incurable diseases may turn to be curable after few months of treatment by using this potency.
8. *Effective, for palliation, in incurable diseases:* In incurable diseases, where palliation is the only method of choice, this potency is infalliable for ideal palliation. Because, the least aggravation, even when palliation is essential, is certainly most unfortunate. Palliation without the least chance of aggravation, is quite possible in this potency.
9. *Effective, to bring back the suppressed state:* In cases of suppression which occurred long ago, this potency works marvellously, to bring back the suppressed state on the surface. Because, where one or two doses of centesimal potency fail to revive the suppressed symptoms, the repeated administration of 50-Millesimal potency can easily bring back the suppressed state within a short period of time.
10. *Primary manifestation of miasm:* In primary stage of psora, syphilis, and sycosis—where Hahnemann advises administration of large doses and repeated doses—this potency proves to be very helpful and efficacious.
11. *Highest development of latent power:* 100 succussions are given to develop the powers of medicine to the desired extent, for a more and long-lasting penetration. So, all the three ideals of potency activity: (a) rapid penetration, (b) gentle impression (minus medicinal aggravation), and (c) permanent restoration of health—can be maintained by the administration of medicine in 50-Millesimal potency.
12. This new system gives full freedom to both physicians and patients from the tyranny of

Centesimal scale. Thus, medicines can be used off and on, and when necessary. In case of wrong selection of medicine, new well-selected medicine can be used without antidoting previous one.

Disadvantages of 50-Millesimal scale of potency

1. Medicines must be administered in liquid form (i.e. in distilled water). So, to prevent the decomposition of water, rectified spirit (60 O.P.) is required.
2. Standard quality of phial and cork (machine-made) are essential to preserve the medicinal solution for long time (for fortnight or a month).
3. It is very difficult to regulate the effect of the medicine administered if the patient lives far away from the physician's residence/chamber. In such cases, the patient may continue the intake of the same medicine in spite of the disease aggravation, homoeopathic aggravation, because they fail to discriminate the changes even though proper direction were given to the patient earlier. As a result, the case may be complicated and become very difficult in making the second prescription. Close observation by the physician may easily solve the problem.
4. If the medicine administered is not "similimum" and covers only the local symptoms, it may act as a palliative and the symptoms take the wrong direction for cure. So, here a medicine is to be selected on the basis of totality of symptoms and immediately administered to the patient.
5. Repeated administration of partially selected homoeopathic medicine may give relief to the chief complaints of the patient, but the patient, as a whole, does not improve as the medicine does not cover the whole constitutional state of the patient. Prolonged administration of this partially selected medicine repeatedly may develop drug diseases or iatrogenic diseases, which are difficult to cure, sometimes incurable.
6. In simple and uncomplicated chronic diseases of dynamic pathology, it is easier to observe the effect of the medicine by administering a single dose of centesimal potency. It also helps to understand easily as to when the action of the dose comes to an end, and needs change of remedy or repetition. But this is not possible with the medicine of 50-millesimal scale of potency.
7. The intricacy of the mode of use of the medicine and regulation of the so-called aggravation, though very mild, lead to lack of enthusiasm amongst many of us.

Table 12.2: Differences between Centesimal and 50-Millesimal scale of potency

Features	*Centesimal scale*	*50-Millesimal scale*
Inventor	This scale was introduced by Hahnemann and followed up to 5th edition of Organon.	This scale was introduced by Hahnemann in 6th edition of Organon.
Synonyms	This scale is also known as drop method (Medicaments a la goutte) of preparing medicines.	This scale is also known as globule method (Medicaments au globule) of preparing medicines.
Abbreviations	The abbreviation for this scale is common, e.g., 3, 6, 12, 30, 200, 500, IM, <10M, 50M, CM., DM., MM etc. throughout the world.	The abbreviation for this scale varies in different countries, e.g. India 0/1, 0/2, 0/3. Bangladesh M/1, M/2, M/3. Western countries 1/0, 2/0, 3/0. Germany LM/1, LM/2, LM/3.
Ratio	Ratio between previous and next potency is 1 : 100.	Ratio between previous and next potency is 1 : 50,000.
Succussion	In this case only 10 succussions are given.	In this case only 100 succussions are given.

Contd.

Contd. table 12.2

Features	*Centesimal scale*	*50-Millesimal scale*
Gap between potencies	There is a long gap between the potencies like 30, 200, IM, etc. which creates galloping potency problem.	No such galloping method, rather we get always a series of potencies, e.g. 0/1, 0/2, 0/3, 0/4 etc.
Mother Tincture	Mother tincture is prepared as per the pharmacopoeia of different countries. In old method up to Class VI succussion process, and for Class VII, Class VIII and Class IX trituration process are adopted. The ratio varies as per the juicy contents of the material substances or by maceration and percolation.	In early phase of mother tincture, all the medicinal substances, whether dry or oily, are triturated up to 3rd centesimal potency. Then 1 grain of 3rd trituration dissolving in 500 drops of a mixture containing 1 part dispensing alcohol and 4 parts of purified water forms the mother potency —Drug power is 1/50,00,00,000.
Subsequent potencies	All subsequent potencies are prepared with 1 drop of the preceding potency to ninety-nine drops of dispensing alcohol.	All subsequent potencies are prepared by dissolving only one globule of the previous potency, in one drop of purified water followed by adding 100 drops of alcohol. To this, 100 downward succussions are given to produce next potency.
Medicinal quantity	The medicinal quantity is minimised but not as much as in 50-millesimal.	The medicinal quantity is minimised so that it produces highest development of power and mild action.
Homoeopathic aggravation	Medicine of this scale will cause aggravation at first part of treatment, and then it will be followed by amelioration.	Medicine of this scale will cause amelioration first and then it will be followed by aggravation only towards the end of the treatment (Sec. 248, 6th edition).
Control of homoeopathic aggravation	As soon as there is the slightest < after application of one dose of medicine or doses with succussion of the medicinal solution, any repetition of medicine shall have to be stopped immediately. So long as there is observed the slightest indication of action of the medicine applied, application of medicines is to be totally stopped.	Medicines are to be gradually continued with due succussion at necessary intervals so long as there is aggravation towards the end of the treatment. Medicine is to be administered at longer intervals or stopped totally, till the aggravation is over.
Medicinal aggravation	Medicinal aggravation for long time is the common feature, unless the potency is appropriate and exact quantity of medicine which is similimum is administered.	Medicinal aggravation is nominal and that too is controllable due to less amount of medicinal quantity.

Contd.

Contd. table 12.2

Features	*Centesimal scale*	*50-Millesimal scale*
Judge of appropriate medicine	After the administration of medicine, we may have to wait for a fairly long period to watch for the action of the medicine.	The correctness of the selected medicine can be judged within 2-4 days. In acute cases, with 2-4 hours or even earlier by the use of this potency. So, we need not unnecessarily wait for long interval for this purpose.
Time taken for cure	To cure a patient with the medicine of centesimal scale would take longer time.	This scale diminishes this period to "one-half", "one-quarter" and even still less, so that a much more rapid cure might be obtained (Sec. 248, 6th edition).
Scope for repetition	Too frequent repetition cannot be done in chronic diseases.	The medicine can be repeated daily and for months as and when necessary.
When to repeat	When the improvement comes to a standstill condition, the medicines are repeated.	Medicine can be repeated alongwith improvement of the patient.
Arrest versus freedom	After application of medicine, both the physician and the patient cannot remain apart from the influence of the medicine, both of them are arrested in the hands of medicinal force.	After the application of the medicine, both the physician and the patient are free as the medicine can be used as and when necessary. In this scale, antidoting of any remedy is seldom required.

Chapter 13

Methods of Preparing Homoeopathic Drugs (Old Method)

Hahnemann has given instructions for preparation of homoeopathic medicines from vegetable, animal and mineral drug-substances, in old method, under § 264 to § 271 of Organon of Medicine.

Drugs are prepared in old method by three ways:

1. By preparing mother tinctures e.g., Class I to Class IV.

Three ways according to the sources, solubility and moisture content of drug-substances

- By immersion of drug-substances of vegetable and animal kingdom in strong alcohol → **Mother tincture**
  - Most juicy plants (mostly European) → Class I
  - Medium juicy plants (also mostly European) → Class II
  - Least juicy plants (all American and some European) → Class III
  - Dried vegetable and animal substances and also from animals → Class IV
- By dissolving drug-substances of mineral and chemical in purified water or alcohol → **Mother solution**
  - Aqueous solution (Soluble in water) → Class V
    - Easily soluble in water → Class V(A)
    - Easily soluble in water, but soluble in larger quantity of water → Class V(B)
  - Alcohol solution (Soluble in alcohol) → Class VI
    - Easily soluble in alcohol → Class VI(A)
    - Easily soluble in alcohol but in larger quantity of alcohol → Class VI(B)
- By grinding, from all sources → **Trituration**
  - Dry, insoluble medicinal substances → Class VII
  - Liquid insoluble medicinal substances → Class VIII
  - Fresh vegetable and animal substances → Class IX (This method is now discarded)

2. By preparing mother solutions e.g., Class V and VI.
3. By preparing mother substances e.g., Class VII to Class IX.

Process involved in formation of drugs in all three methods are:

1. For mother tincture preparation: Extraction.
2. For mother solution preparation: Solution or dissolving.
3. For mother substance preparation: Trituration.

PREPARATION OF MOTHER TINCTURE (CLASS I TO CLASS IV)

Definition of Mother Tincture

It is a drug, pharmaceutically prepared from drug-substances of vegetable and animal kingdom, using strong alcohol as a vehicle (solvent) by the process of immersion, maceration, and percolation.

Designation of Mother Tincture

It is denoted as θ. It is the precursor of corresponding potency of the drug.

Drug Power of a Mother Tincture

By drug power of a tincture is meant the strength of the drug. It means amount of the drug in proportion to its solvent. It indicates the proportion of the drug contained in the medicinal preparation, e.g. D.P—$\frac{1}{6}$, it means in total 6 parts—1 part is medicinal substance and 5 parts are solvents (vehicles).

Estimation of the strength of homoeopathic tincture: By the proportion of the medicinal substance which it represents, just as the strength of a solution or trituration is estimated by the proportion of medicinal substance it contains.

Utility of a Drug Power of a Mother Tincture

Drug power is essential for potentisation from mother tincture to prepare 1st potency. Because, according to drug power, amount of vehicle and tincture is determined. Suppose, drug power of a mother tincture is $\frac{1}{2}$. Then potentisation is carried under centesimal scale by taking 2 minims of mother tincture and 98 minims of dispensing alcohol. Similarly, under decimal scale, it is done by taking 2 minims of mother tincture and 8 minims of alcohol.

Are Mother Tinctures Homoeopathic Medicines?

Mostly, the homoeopaths of today claim to have cured the patients suffering from various acute and chronic diseases with mother tinctures, that too, 'rapidly, gently and permanently'. They claim it only because they are followers (so-called) of Hahnemann who taught us: 'our vital-force, as a spirit-like dynamis, cannot be attacked and affected by injurious influences on the healthy organism caused by the external inimical forces that disturb the harmonious play of life, otherwise than in a spirit-like (dynamic) way ......' Hahnemann has claimed that diseases can not be removed by any other means, than by a spirit-like dynamic which is nothing else than a potentised Homoeopathic Medicine only. Further, Hahnemann tried to explain how the dynamic potentised medicines act through nerves of the organism. So, if Hahnemann's explanation is right, and his discovery is infallible then the claims made by the so-called homoeopaths are false. There is no other way to cure both acute and chronic diseases except through dynamic potentised medicines or any other form of dynamic energy.

Solvents (vehicles) generally used in the preparation of Mother Tincture or Solution

1. *Strong alcohol:* Almost all mother tinctures are prepared with strong alcohol because alcohol is a great solvent. No other solvent has so unique a power as alcohol in respect of extraction of medicinal properties from the crude drug ingredients. Moreover, it prevents decomposition, and the preparation will remain intact for good, if stronger qualities of alcohol is used.
Example: Aconite θ; Belladonna θ.
2. *Purified water:* Some acids (as in Class V) are not dissolved in alcohol, they are prepared with purified water; of course the higher potencies are prepared with dispensing alcohol (Rectified spirit 60 o.p.) e.g., Nitric acid mother solution.
3. *Glycerine:* Certain animal poisons (venoms) are prepared and preserved with the help of glycerine, e.g. Lachesis 0; Elaps 0; Crotalus 0 etc.

Table 13.1: Differences between Allopathic and Homoeopathic mother tinctures

Allopathic mother tincture	Homoeopathic mother tincture
1. These are made from dried plants, often with the introduction of foreign substances, e.g., tincture of Sanguinaria contains acetic acid; tincture of opium contains phosphate of lime; tincture of Rheum contains cardamom.	1. These are made from fresh plants, because their medicinal properties remain quite intact, they are far superior to dry ones. When the fresh plants are not available, dry ones should be used, e.g., tincture of Sanguinaria made from rhizome; Tincture of opium and Rheum are pure.
2. Allopathic tincture are standardised on the basis of the alkaloid, glucosides etc. content in the medicinal substances.	2. Homoeopathic tincture prepared with the whole plants, leaves, fruits etc., as the case may be, without considering alkaloid content in the medicinal substances.
3. Allopathic tinctures are generally reddish or brown in colour.	3. Homoeopathic tinctures are generally green when prepared from fresh plants etc. and sometimes reddish or brown when prepared from dry vegetables.

Different classes under Mother Tincture

Hahnemann classified the drugs obtained from vegetable kingdom (some from animal sources) for the preparation of mother tincture into four classes, depending upon their juicy contents:

(i) Class I (most juicy plants)

(ii) Class II (medium juicy plants)

(iii) Class III (least juicy plants)

(iv) Class IV (dried vegetable and animal substances and also from fresh animals).

CLASS I

Introduction: Most of the European plants are included in this class. The plants in this class contain large quantity of juice.

Tinctures prepared with equal parts by weight of drug juice and alcohol (i.e., 1 : 1).

Fundamental rule for this class has been described in Hahnemann's **Materia Medica Pura—** under **'Belladonna'**.

This is applicable to juicy but not viscid materials and not containing resins, terpins and volatile oils.

Preparation of Mother Tincture

A. Requirements

1. *Ingredients*

(i) Selected drug-substances (Fresh plants) whose mother tincture will be prepared

(ii) Strong alcohol.

2. *Utensils and apparatus*

(i) Wooden chopping board and knife.

(ii) Porcelain mortar and pestle.

(iii) Horn-made spatula.

(iv) Linen cloth—new and sterilised.

(v) A clean small beaker.

(vi) Glass-stoppered phial.

(vii) Glass funnel with stand.

(viii) Filter paper.

(ix) Another clean phial with a new, non-porous velvet cork.

(x) Balance with weight box.

(xi) Pen, paper, gums, scissors etc.

B. Procedures

1. The fresh plant (or part of a plant—root, bark, leaves etc.) are cut into small pieces with a well-polished steel knife, free from rust, on a clean chopping board and pounded to a pulp with mortar and pestle.

2. The pulp is now enclosed in a new linen cloth and the juice is expressed by means of a press, or by wringing the cloth.

3. Expressed juice is weighed and kept in a glass jar.

4. Equal quantity by weight of strong alcohol is added to it.

5. The mixture is shaken vigorously for some time, and then put into a well-stoppered bottle, and allowed to stand for eight days, in a cool, dark place and is then filtered.
6. Then it is poured in a clean phial provided with the best quality of new, non-porous, velvet cork.

C. Drug power (Calculation)

Drug substance	*Solvent/Vehicle (Strong alcohol)*	*Mother Tincture*
1 ml	1 ml	2 ml

In 2 ml mother tincture, the drug substance is 1 ml. In 1 ml mother tincture, the drug substance is ½ ml.

∴ Drug power (D.P.) = ½.

Potentisation (Succussion)

1. Centesimal Scale

2 minims of the mother tincture of the drug and 98 minims of dilute alcohol are mixed, and then 10 downward strokes of equal strength (succussion) are given. It gives the 1st potency.

1 minim of the 1st potency and 99 minims of dispensing alcohol and 10 downward stroke of equal strength will give the second potency.

All succeeding potencies are prepared by taking 1 minim of the preceding potency and 99 minims of dispensing alcohol.

2. Decimal Scale

2 minims of the mother tincture of the drug and 8 minims of dilute alcohol are mixed, and then 10 downward strokes of equal strength (succussion) are given. It gives the IX potency.

1 minim of 1X potency and 9 minims of dilute alcohol and 10 downward strokes of equal strength will give the 2X potency.

All succeeding potencies are prepared by taking 1 minim of the preceding potency, and 9 minims of dilute alcohol.

Drugs under this Class (Class I)

Vegetable Source

1. **Whole plant**

Aconitum napellus	Hyoscyamus niger
Anagallis arvensis	Lilium tigrinum
Asarum europeum	Menyanthes trifoliata
Belladonna	Millefolium
Bellis perennis	Petroselium sativum
Chamomilla	Plantago major
Chelidoneum majus	Rannunculus bulbosus
Convallaria majalis	Solanum nigrum
Cynodon dactylon	Taraxacum officinalis
Drosera	Thlaspi bursa pastoris
Dulcamara	Urtica urens
Gratiola officinalis	Verbascum thapsus

2. **Roots**

Arum dracontium	Cicuta virosa
Arum trifolium	Cyclamen europeum
Arum maculatum	Tannus communis
Bryonia alba	Rumex crispus

3. **Stem with leaves**

Clematis erecta

4. **Modified stem (bulb)**

Colchicum autumnale

5. **Leaves**

Bryophyllum calycinum	Lactuca virosa.
	Lamium album
Calendula officinalis	Sambucus nigra
Cephalandra indica	Sempervivum tectorum
Digitalis purpurea	Solanum arrebenta

6. **Flowers**

Cannabis sativa

7. **Fruits**

Rhamnus catherticus, Solanum mammosum

8. **Seeds**

Avena sativa

9. **Bark**

Granatum

Mineral and Chemical Source

e.g., Causticum

Instruction of Hahnemann

(According to Sec. 267 of 5th edition of Organon) Fresh juice of the freshly gathered indigenous plants is first extracted. In order to obtain the medicinal qualities in the most complete and certain manner as in fresh state, it is immediately mixed with equal parts of alcohol (of a strength sufficient to burn in a lamp). Now, it is kept in a well-stoppered bottle for a day and a night. This results in deposition of fibrinous and albuminous matters at the bottom of the bottle. Then the clear supercumbent fluid is to be decanted off for medicinal use.

Alcohol is added to prevent any fermentation of vegetable juice which is thus retained (perfect and uninjured) for ever by keeping preparations in well-corked bottles and protected from the sunlight, heat and strong smelling substance.

CLASS II

Introduction: This class includes those plants (European) which contain only a small quantity of juice.

Fundamental rule for this class has been described in Hahnemann's **Materia Medica Pura** under 'Thuja'.

This is applicable to non-mucilagenous materials containing resins, terpins, or volatile oils.

Preparation of Mother Tincture

1. **Principle:** The tincture is prepared by adding two parts of strong alcohol by weight to three parts of the juice of plant by weight (i.e. 2: 3).
2. **Requirements**
   (a) *Ingredients*
   (i) Selected drug-substance (the plant or its parts) whose mother tincture will be prepared.
   (ii) Strong alcohol
   (b) *Utensils and apparatus*
   (i) Wooden chopping board and knife.
   (ii) Porcelain mortar and pestle.
   (iii) Horn-made spatula.
   (iv) Linen cloth—new and sterilised.
   (v) A clean small beaker.
   (vi) A glass-stoppered phial.
   (vii) Glass funnel with stand.
   (viii) Another clean phial provided with best quality of new, non-porous velvet cork.
   (ix) Filter paper.
   (x) Balance and weight box.
   (xi) Pen, paper, gum, scissors etc.
3. **Procedure**
   (i) The fresh plant or parts thereof are cut into small pieces with well-polished steel knife on a clean chopping board, and pounded to a pulp with mortar and pestle.
   (ii) The chopped drug is weighed. For every three parts of the drug, two parts by weight of alcohol is taken.
   (iii) The whole quantity of the chopped drug is at first moistened with just the quantity of alcohol necessary to bring the whole mass into a thick pulp. Remaining portion of alcohol is now added to the drug and kept for two or three days.
   (iv) The whole quantity is now strained through a piece of new linen cloth.
   (v) The tincture thus obtained is allowed to stand eight days in a well-stoppered bottle, in cool-dark place and then filtered.
   (vi) Then it is poured in a clean phial provided with the best quality of new, non-porous velvet cork.
4. **Drug power**

   Ratio of medicinal substances: Strong alcohol = 3 : 2 But medicinal substance in 1 cc loss = $\frac{1}{3}$ cc.

   Medicinal substance in 3 cc loss $= \frac{1}{3} \times 3$ cc = 1 cc.

   So net medicinal substance = (3 – 1) cc. = 2 cc.

   There is no loss of vehicle (strong alcohol).

Net medicinal substance	*Solvent/Vehicle*	*Mother Tincture (Strong alcohol)*
2 cc	2 cc	4 cc

∴ In 4 cc mother tincture net medicinal substance = 2 cc.

In 1 cc mother tincture net medicinal substance = 2/4 cc.

∴ Drug power (D.P.) = 1/2

Potentisation (Succussion)

1. Centesimal Scale

2 minims of the mother tincture and 98 minims of dilute alcohol are mixed and then 10 downward strokes of equal strength are given. It gives the 1st potency.

1 minim of the 1st potency and 99 minims of dispensing alcohol and 10 downward strokes of equal strength will give the 2nd potency.

All succeeding potencies are prepared by taking 1 minim of the preceding potency and 99 minims of dispensing alcohol.

2. Decimal Scale

2 minims of the mother tincture and 8 minims of dilute alcohol are mixed, and then 10 downward strokes of equal strength are given. It gives the 1X potency.

1 minim of 1X potency and 9 minims of dilute alcohol and 10 downward strokes of equal strength will give the 2X potency.

All succeeding potencies are prepared by taking 1 minim of the preceding potency and 9 minims of dilute alcohol.

Drugs under this Class (Class II)

1. Whole fresh plant

Euphrasia (excluding root)	Thymus serpyllum
	Viola tricolor
Mercurialis perenis	Vinca minor
Thlaspi bursa pastoris	Veronica beccahunga

2. Leaves

Oleander	Rhus toxicodendron
Thuja occidentalis	Uva ursi
Laurocerasus	Viscum album

3. Fresh roots

Symphytum (G.H.P.)

4. Bark

Mezereum

5. Buds

Prunus spinosa

6. Twigs

Taxus baccata

7. Strobila (Cat kin)

Lupulus.

CLASS III

Introduction: This class includes those plants which are least juicy. Mostly American plants and some of the European plants are included in this class.

Preparation of Mother Tincture

1. **Principle:** The tincture is prepared by adding two parts by weight of alcohol, and one part of the plant, or part thereof, by weight.
2. **Requirements**

(a) *Ingredients*

(i) Selected drug-substance (plants or their part) whose mother tincture will be prepared.

(ii) Strong alcohol.

(b) *Utensils and apparatus*

(i) Wooden chopping board and knife.

(ii) Porcelain mortar and pestle.

(iii) Horn-made spatula.

(iv) Linen cloth—new and sterilised.

(v) A clean small beaker.

(vi) A glass-stoppered phial.

(vii) Another clean phial with new non-porous velvet cork.

(viii) Glass funnel with stand.

(ix) Filter paper.

(x) Balance with weight box.

(xi) Pen, paper, gums, scissors etc.

3. **Procedure**

(i) The fresh plant or parts thereof are cut into small pieces with a well-polished steel knife on a clean chopping board and pounded to a pulp with mortar and pestle.

(ii) Pulp is weighed and taken in a glass jar. Double quantity by weight of strong alcohol is added.

(iii) At first powder is moistened with 1/6th part of alcohol. Moistened drug is put into a stoppered bottle and rest of the alcohol added to it.

(iv) The whole mixture is allowed to stand for 8 days, in a cool dark place.

(v) After this period the tincture is decanted, strained through the new linen cloth and filtered.

(vi) Then it is poured in a clean phial provided with the best quality of new, non-porous velvet cork.

4. **Drug power (Calculation)**

Ratio of medicinal substance:

Strong alcohol = 1 : 2

But medicinal substance in 1c.c. loss = $2/3$ c.c.

∴ Net medicinal substance
= $(1 - 2/3)$ c.c. = $1/3$ c.c.

Vehicle in 1 c.c. loss = $1/6$ c.c.

∴ Vehicle in 2 c.c. loss = $2 \times 1/6$ c.c. = $1/3$ c.c.

∴ Net vehicle = $(2 - 1/3)$ c.c. = $5/3$ c.c.

Net medicinal substance	*Solvent/Vehicle (Strong alcohol)*	*Mother Tincture*
$1/3$ c.c.	$5/3$ c.c.	$(1/3 + 5/3)$ c.c. = 2 c.c.

∴ In 2 c.c. mother tincture, net medicinal subst. = $1/3$ c.c.

In 1 c.c. mother tincture, net medicinal subst. = $1/3 \times 1/2$ c.c. = $1/6$ c.c.

∴ Drug power (D.P.) = $1/6$

Potentisation (Succussion)

1. **Centesimal Scale**

6 minims of mother tincture and 94 minims of dilute alcohol and ten downward strokes of equal strength give 1st centesimal potency.

1 minim of the 1st potency and 99 minims of alcohol and ten downward strokes of equal strength will give 2nd centesimal potency.

All succeeding potencies are prepared with one minim of the preceding potency to ninetynine minims of dispensing alcohol.

2. **Decimal Scale**

6 minims of mother tincture and 4 minims of dilute alcohol and ten downward stroke of equal strength give 1X potency.

1 minim of the 1X potency and 9 minims of dilute alcohol, and ten downward strokes of equal strength give 2X potency.

All succeeding potencies are prepared with 1 minim of the preceding potency to 9 minims of dilute alcohol.

Drugs under this Class (Class III)

Vegetable Source

1. **Whole plant:** Absinthium; Acalypha indica; Achyranthes aspera; Adonis vernalis; Aethusa cynapium; anthoxanthum odoratum; Anthemis nobilis; Arnica montana; Chenopodium; Chimaphila umbellata; Cistus canadensis; Convallaria majalis; Echinacea angustifolia; Equisetum hyemale; Erigeron canadense; Hepatica triloba; Hypericum perforatum; Lil. tig, Lobelia inflata; Lycopus virginicus; Mentha pipertæ Mitchella repens; Nabalus serpentaria; Penthorum sedoides; Plantago major; Pulsatilla; Ranunculus bulbosus; Ruta graveolens; Thymus serpyllum; Urtica urens; Verbascum thapsus; Viola tricolor.

2. **Roots:** Actaea spicata; Aletris farinosa; apocynum cannabinum; Aralia racemosa; Artemisia vulgaris; Arum triphyllum; Asarum cannadense; Asclepias incarnata; Caladium seguinum; Caulophyllum thalictroides; Cimicifuga racemosa; Collinsonia canadensis; Ficus indica; Gelsemium sempervirens; Hydrastis canadensis; Iris versicolor; Inula helenium; Juncus effusus; Lappa major; Leptandra virginica; Menispermum canadense; Nuphar luteum; Nymphae odorata; Paullinia pinnata; Phytolacca decandra; Pimpinella saxifraga; Podophyllum peltatum; Pothos foetidus;

Raphanus sativus; Rumex crispus; Sabal serrulata; Sanguinaria canadensis; Symphytum officinale; Thaspium aureum; Trillium pendulum; Triosteum perfoliatum; Veratrum viride; Wyethia helenioides.

3. **Leaves:** Abroma augusta; Aegle folia; Agave americana; Cotyledon umbilicus; Ilex opaca; Eupatorium perfoliatum; Justicia adhatoda; Kalmia latifolia; Lachnanthes tinctoria; Mimosa humilis; Ocimum sanctum; Oxydendron arboreum; Plumbago littorale; Rhus toxicodendron; Rumex acetosa; Salvia officinalis; Sempervium tectorum; Thuja occidentalis; Tradescantia diuretica; Viscum album.
4. **Stems (only):** Cactus grandiflorus.
5. **Stem with leaves:** Rhus venenata; Sabina.
6. **Rhizome:** Piper methysticum.
7. **Bulb:** Allium cepa; Allium sativum; Scilla maritima.
8. **Herbs:** Buxus sempervirens; Gaultheria procumbens; Ledum palustre; Silphium laciniatum.
9. **Young shoots:** Artemisia abrotanum; Myrtus communis; Pinus sylvestris.
10. **Twigs:** Ficus religiosa; Juniperus virginiana; Taxus baccata.
11. **Flowers:** Cannabis sativa; Grindelia robusta; Melilotus alba; Melilotus oficinalis; Solidago virgaurea; Trifolium repens; Trifolium pratense.
12. **Fruits:** Aesculus hippocastanum; Aesculus glabra; Carica papaya; Crataegus oxyacantha; Gymnocladus canadensis; Ilex opaca; Prinos verticillatus; Xanthoxylum fraxineum.
13. **Seeds:** Avena sativa; Eugenia jambos.
14. **Bark:** Abies canadensis; Alnus serrulata; Baptisia tinctoria; Berberis aquifolium; Berberis vulgaris; Daphne indica; Gossypium herbaceum; Myrica cerifera; Populus tremuloides; Prunus padus; Ptelea trifoliata; Rhus aromatica; Rhus glabra; Salix nigra; Viburnum opulus; Xanthoxylum fraxineum.
15. **Algae:** Fucus vesiculosus.
16. **Fungi:** Agaricus muscarius; Sec.cor; Polyporus pinicola.
17. **Lichen:** Sticta pulmonaria.

Instruction of Hahnemann
(F.N. of Sec. 267, 5th edition, Organon)

In case of the plants that contain much thick mucus (e.g. Symphytum officinale; Viola tricolor etc.) or an excess of albumin (e.g. Aethusa cynapium; Solanum nigrum etc.) a double quantity of alcohol is to be mixed with freshly expressed juice.

Plants that are very deficient in juice (as Buxus sempervirens; Taxus baccata; Ledum palustre; Sabina etc.) must first be pounded up singly into a moist fine mass and then stirred up with a double quantity of alcohol so that the juice may combine with it, and—being thus extracted by the alcohol—may be pressed out.

CLASS IV

Introduction: This class includes dry plants, herbs, animal substances—dried or fresh.

Fundamental rule for this class has been described in Hahnemann's **Materia Medica Pura** under '**Staphysagria**' and '**Spigelia**'.

Preparation of Mother Tincture

1. **Principle:** The tincture is prepared by adding five parts by weight of strong alcohol to one part by weight of pulp or powder (medicinal-substance).
2. **Requirements**

   (a) *Ingredients*

   (i) Selected drug-substances whose mother tincture will be prepared.

   (ii) Strong alcohol.

   (b) *Appliances*

   (i) Wooden chopping board and knife.

   (ii) Porcelain or iron mortar and pestle.

   (iii) Horn-made spatula.

   (iv) A linen cloth—new and sterilised.

   (v) A clean small beaker.

   (vi) A glass-stoppered phial.

   (vii) Another clean phial with new non-porous velvet cork.

   (viii) Glass funnel with stand.

   (ix) Filter paper.

(x) A glass rod.

(xi) Balance with weight box.

(xii) Pen, paper, gums etc.

(c) *Procedure*

(i) The dried vegetable and animal substances are pulverised into fine powder, and fresh animal substances into fine pulp.

(ii) The powder or pounded drug-substances are weighed, and taken in a glass jar.

(iii) Five times its weight of strong alcohol is added to it, and the same mixed with the pulp or powder.

(iv) After thoroughly mixing, the whole mass is kept in a glass-stoppered bottle in cool-dark place for 15 days.

(v) The mixture is shaken well, two times a day.

(vi) After this period, the clear tincture is decanted, the residual substances are strained by a new linen cloth, and is added to the previously decanted tincture. It is again filtered by a filter paper and stored in a glass-stoppered phial.

(d) *Drug-power (Calculation)*

Drug-substance	*Vehicle (Strong alcohol)*
1 grain	5 grains

But, drug substance loss in 1 grain = $\frac{1}{2}$ grain

∴ Net drug substance = $(1 - \frac{1}{2})$ grain = $\frac{1}{2}$ grain

The vehicle loss in 1 grain = $\frac{1}{10}$ grain

" " " " 5 grains = $5 \times \frac{1}{10}$ grain = $\frac{1}{2}$ grain

∴ Net vehicle = $(5 - \frac{1}{2})$ grain = $\frac{9}{2}$ grains.

Net drug substance	*Net vehicle*	*Mother tincture*
$\frac{1}{2}$ grain	$\frac{9}{2}$ grain	$(\frac{1}{2} + \frac{9}{2})$ grain = 5 grains

In 5 grains mother tincture, drug substance = $\frac{1}{2}$ grain

In 1 grain mother tincture, drug substance = $\frac{1}{2} \times \frac{1}{5} = \frac{1}{10}$ grain

∴ Drug power (D.P.) = $\frac{1}{10}$.

On the other hand, for preparing 5 grains of mother tincture, 1 grain drug-substance, and 5 grains of vehicle required.

Potentisation (Succussion)

1. **Centesimal Scale**

10 minims of mother tincture and 90 minims of alcohol and 10 downward strokes of equal strength give first centesimal potency.

1 minim of the first centesimal potency and 99 minims of alcohol and 10 downward strokes of equal strength give 2nd centesimal potency.

All succeeding potencies are prepared by taking 1 minim of the preceding potency and 99 minims of alcohol.

2. **Decimal Scale**

As the drug power is $\frac{1}{10}$, it corresponds to 1X potency. Here 1X potency is same as the mother tincture of the drug.

1 minim of the mother tincture and 9 minims of alcohol and 10 downward strokes of equal strength give 2X potency.

All succeeding potencies are prepared by taking 1 minim of the preceding potency and 9 minims of alcohol.

Drugs under this Class (Class IV)

Vegetable Source

1. ***Whole plant:*** Arnica montana; Hydrocotyle asiatica.
2. ***Roots***
   (i) *Fresh:* Abroma angusta radix; Geum urbanum; Helleborus niger; Helonias dioica; Jalapa; Veratrum viride, Zingiber officinale.
   (ii) *Dried:* Calotropis gigantea; Ipecacuanha; Ratanhia; Rheum; Sarsaparilla; Senega; Sumbul; Valeriana officinalis; Veratrum album.
3. ***Leaves (dried):*** Eucalyptus globulus; Pilocarpus; Rhododendron chrysanthum; Senna; Tabacum.
4. ***Herbs:*** Gaultheria procumbens; Ledum palustre; Spigelia.

5. ***Flowers:*** Cannabis indica; Cina; Crocus sativus; Grindelia robusta; Helianthus annus; Melilotus officinalis.
6. ***Fruits:*** Aegle marmelos; Amloki; Capsicum annum; Carya alba; Colocynthis; Cubeba officinalis; Dolichos pruriens; Piper nigrum; Xanthoxyllum fraxineum.
7. ***Seeds:*** Cedron; Cocculus indica; Coffea cruda; Ignatia amara; Illicium anisatum; Jatropha curcas; Lathyrus sativus; Nux. moschata; Nux. vomica; Physostigma; Ricinus communis; Sabadilla; Sinapis nigra; Sinapis alba; Staphysagria; Syzygium jambolanum.
8. ***Bark (dried):*** Alstonia scholaris; Azadhirachta indica; Cerasus virginiana; Cinchona officinalis; Cinnamonum; Condurango; Jonosia asoka; Piscidia erythrina; Sassafras; Terminalia arjuna.
9. ***Juices:*** Aloe socotrina; Anacardium orientale; Opium.
10. ***Gums:*** Kino australiensis.
11. ***Gum-resin:*** Asafoetida; Euphorbium officinarum; Gombogia.
12. ***Algae:*** Fucus vesiculosus.
13. ***Fungi:*** Bovista; Ustilago maydis.
14. ***Lichen:*** Usnea barbata; Sticta pulmonaria.
15. ***Spores:*** Lycopodium clavatum.

Animal Source

Apis mellifica; Aranea diadema; Asterias rubens; Badiaga; Cantharis; Coccus cacti; Mygale lasiodora; Spongia tosta; Tarentula cubensis; Theridion.

PREPARATION OF MOTHER SOLUTION (CLASS V & CLASS VI)

Definition of Mother Solution (θ soln.)

It is the drug pharmaceutically prepared from drug-substances of mineral and chemical sources as the strongest alcoholic or aqueous solvent, by the process dissolving in alcohol or purified water or exposing—as the case may be.

Different Classes under Mother Solution

Two classes: Class V and Class VI

Class V (Aqueous Solution): It includes those chemical drugs which are soluble in purified water. Hahnemann classified them as Class V(A) and Class V(B) depending upon the solubility in the strength of 10% or 1%, respectively.

Class VI (Alcoholic Solution): It includes those chemical drugs which are soluble in alcohol. Hahnemann classified them as VI(A) and VI(B) depending upon their solubility in the strength of 10% or 1%, respectively.

CLASS V(A)

Introduction: It deals with the method of preparing aqueous solutions (with purified water). The substances included under this class are easily soluble in purified water.

Preparation of Mother Solution

1. **Principle:** 1 part by weight of medicinal substance is dissolved in 9 parts by weight of purified water.
2. **Requirements**
   (a) ***Ingredients***
   (i) Required medicinal substance
   (ii) Purified water
   (b) ***Appliances***
   (i) Porcelain mortar and pestle
   (ii) Horn-made spatula
   (iii) Clean glass phial with new cork
   (iv) Minim glass
   (v) Balance with weight box
   (vi) Conical flask
   (vii) Pen, gums, paper, scissors etc.
3. **Procedure**
   (i) Firstly the purity of the medicinal substances is tested. Then 1 part by weight of medicinal substances is taken in a well-cleansed round glass-phial, and 9 parts by weight of purified water is added to it—taking care that at least ¼th part of the phial remains vacant.
   (ii) The phial is closed by the cork, and a homogeneous solution is prepared by gentle shaking.

4. **Drug power (Calculation)**

Medicinal Subs.	*Vehicle* (Purified water)	*Mother Solution*
1 grain	9 grains	10 grains

In 10 grains of mother sol., the medicinal subs. = 1 grain

In 1 grain of mother sol., the medicinal subs. = $\frac{1}{10}$

∴ Drug power = $\frac{1}{10}$.

Potentisation (Succussion)

1. **Centesimal Scale**

10 minims of mother solution and 90 minims of purified water and 10 downward strokes of equal strength give the 1st centesimal potency.

∵ 1 minim of the 1st potency and 99 minims of alcohol and 10 downward strokes of equal strength give 2nd potency.

All succeeding potencies are prepared by taking 1 minim of the preceding potency and 99 minims of alcohol.

2. **Decimal Scale**

As the drug power is $\frac{1}{10}$, it corresponds to 1X potency.

1 minim of the 1X potency (i.e. mother sol.) and 9 minims of purified water and 10 downward strokes of equal strength will give the 2X potency.

All succeeding potencies are prepared by taking 1 minim of the preceding potency, and 9 minims of alcohol.

Drugs under this Class [Class V(A)]

Mineral and Chemical Source

1. *Acids:* Acetic acid; Chromic acid; Muriatic acid; Nitric acid; Phosphoric acid; Sulphuric acid.
2. *Inorganic compounds:* Ammon. carb; Ammon. caust; Ammon. mur; Ammon. nit; Baryta acetica; Baryta mur; Arg. nit; Aurum. mur; Cal. acetica; Cal. mur; Causticum; Ferrum. mur; Kali. carb; Kali. chlor; Kali. caust; Nat. mur; Nat. selenicum.

Vegetable Source

Balsam; Balsamum peruvianum.

CLASS V(B)

Introduction: This class includes those substances which are easily soluble in water. But they are soluble in greater quantity of water.

Preparation of Mother Solution

1. **Principle:** 1 part by weight of medicinal substance is dissolved in 99 parts by weight of purified water.
2. **Requirements**

   (a) *Ingredients*

   (i) Required medicinal substance
   (ii) Purified water

   (b) *Appliances*

   (i) Porcelain mortar and pestle
   (ii) Horn-made spatula
   (iii) Clean glass phial with cork
   (iv) Minim glass
   (v) Balance with weight box
   (vi) Conical flask
   (vii) Pen, pencil, gums, scissors, etc.

3. **Procedure**

   (a) Firstly, purity of the medicinal substance is tested. Then 1 part by weight of medicinal substances is taken in a well-cleansed round glass-phial, and 99 parts by weight of purified water is added to it—taking care that at least $\frac{1}{4}$th part of the phial remains vacant.

   (b) The phial is closed by the cork, and a homogeneous solution is prepared by gentle shaking.

4. **Drug power (Calculation)**

Medicinal Subs.	*Vehicle* (Purified water)	*Mother Solution*
1 grain	99 grains	100 grains

In 100 grains of mother sol., the medicinal subs. = 1 grain

In 1 grain of mother sol., the medicinal subs. $= \frac{1}{100}$

∴ Drug power $= \frac{1}{100}$

Potentisation (Succussion)

1. Centesimal Scale

As the drug power $= \frac{1}{100}$, it corresponds to 1st centesimal potency.

1 minim of 1st potency (i.e. mother solution) and 99 minims of dilute alcohol and 10 downward strokes of equal strength give 2nd potency.

All succeeding potencies are prepared by taking 1 minim of preceding potency and 99 minims of alcohol.

2. Decimal Scale

As the mother solution contains $\frac{1}{100}$ drug power, it will correspond to $\left(\frac{1}{100} = \frac{1}{10} \times \frac{1}{10}\right)$ 2X potency.

1 minim of the 2X potency (i.e. mother solution), and 9 minims of dilute alcohol and 10 downward strokes of equal strength give 3X potency.

All succeeding potencies are prepared by taking 1 minim of preceding potency and 9 minims of alcohol.

Drugs under this Class [Class V(B)]

Mineral and Chemical Source: Oxalic acid; Picric acid; Phosphoric acid; Fluoric acid; Bromium; Kali. bichromicum; Kali. bromatum; Merc. cyanatus; Hydrocyanic acid; Antim. tart; Kali. permanganicum; Platinum muriaticum; Cuprum aceticum; Kali. hydrobromicum; Plumbum aceticum; Kali. chloricum; Borax; Causticum.

CLASS VI(A)

Introduction: This class includes those substances which are soluble only in alcohol.

The fundamental rule for this class has been discussed in Hahnemann's **'Materia Medica Pura'** under **'Guaiacum'**.

Preparation of Mother Solution

1. Principle

(a) 1 part by weight of medicinal substance is dissolved in 9 parts by weight of strong alcohol (as per A.H.P.).

(b) 2 parts by weight of medicinal substance are dissolved in 9 parts by weight of alcohol (as per B.H.P.).

2. Requirements

(a) *Ingredients*

(i) Required medicinal substances

(ii) Strong alcohol

(b) *Appliances*

(i) Porcelain mortar and pestle

(ii) Horn-made spatula

(iii) Clean glass phial with new cork

(iv) Minim glass

(v) Balance with weight box

(vi) Conical flask

(vii) Pen, gums, paper, scissors etc.

3. Procedure

(a) Firstly the purity of the medicinal substances is tested. Then 1 part by weight of medicinal substances is taken in a well-cleaned round glass-phial, and 9 parts by weight of strong alcohol is added to it—taking care that at least $\frac{1}{4}$th part of the phial remains vacant.

(b) The phial is closed by the cork, and a homogeneous solution is prepared by gentle shaking.

4. Drug power (Calculation)

Medicinal Subs.	*Vehicle* (Purified water)	*Mother Solution*
1 grain	9 grains	10 grains

In 10 grains of mother sol., the medicinal subs. = 1 grain

In 1 grain of mother sol., the medicinal subs. $= \frac{1}{10}$

∴ Drug power $= \frac{1}{10}$

Potentisation (Succussion)

1. Centesimal Scale

10 minims of mother solution and 90 minims of strong alcohol and 10 downward strokes of equal strength give the 1st centesimal potency.

1 minim of the 1st potency and 99 minims alcohol and 10 downward strokes of equal strength give 2C potency.

All succeeding potencies are prepared by taking 1 minim of the preceding potency and 99 minim alcohol.

2. Decimal Scale

As the drug power $\frac{1}{10}$; so it corresponds to 1X potency. 1 minim of the 1X potency (i.e. mother solution) and 9 minims of strong alcohol, and 10 downward strokes of equal strength will give the 2C potency.

All succeeding potencies are prepared by taking 1 minim of the preceding potency, and 9 minims of alcohol.

Drugs under this Class [Class VI(A)]

1. **Mineral and Chemical Source:** Benzoic acid; Carbolic acid; Cal. caust; Camphora; Amyl. nitrosum; Glonoine; Carboneum hydrogenistum; Amyris gileadensis; Chloralum (chloral hydrate); Chinoidine; Chloroformum; Methyl alcohol; Myroxylon perniferum; Nicotinum; Nitri spiritus dulcis.
2. **Vegetable Source:** Abies nigra; Guaiacum officinale; Opopanax chironium.

CLASS VI(B)

Introduction: It includes those substances which are soluble in larger quantity of alcohol.

Preparation of Mother Solution

1. Principle

(a) 1 part by weight of the medicinal substance is dissolved in 99 parts by weight of alcohol.

(b) 1 part by weight of the medicinal substance is dissolved in 50 parts by weight of alcohol (As per G.H.P.).

2. Requirements

(a) *Ingredients*

(i) Required medicinal substances

(ii) Strong alcohol

(b) *Appliances*

(i) Porcelain mortar and pestle

(ii) Horn-made spatula

(iii) Clean glass phial with cork

(iv) Minim glass

(v) Balance with weight box

(vi) Conical flask

(vii) Pen, pencil, gums, scissors etc.

3. Procedure

(a) Firstly purity of the medicinal substances is tested. Then 1 part by weight of medicinal substances is taken in a well-cleansed round glass-phial, and 99 parts by weight of strong alcohol is added to it—taking care that at least $\frac{1}{4}$th part of the phial remains vacant.

(b) The phial is closed by the cork and a homogeneous solution is prepared by gentle shaking.

4. Drug power (Calculation)

Medicinal Subs.	*Vehicle* (Purified water)	*Mother Solution*
1 grain	99 grains	100 grains

In 100 grains of mother sol., the medicinal subs. = 1 grain

In 1 grain of mother sol., the medicinal subs. = $\frac{1}{100}$

∴ Drug power = $\frac{1}{100}$

Potentisation

1. Centesimal Scale

As the drug-power = $\frac{1}{100}$, it corresponds to 1st centesimal potency.

1 minim of the 1st potency (i.e. mother solution) and 99 minims of dilute alcohol, and 10 downward strokes of equal strength give 2nd potency.

All succeeding potencies are prepared by taking 1 minim of preceding potency and 99 minims of alcohol.

2. Decimal Scale

As the mother solution contains $\frac{1}{100}$ drug power, it will correspond to $\left(\frac{1}{100} = \frac{1}{10} \times \frac{1}{10}\right)$ 2X potency.

1 minim of the 2X potency.

1 minim of the 2X potency (i.e. mother solution), and 9 minims of dilute alcohol and 10 downward strokes of equal strength give 3X potency.

All succeeding potencies are prepared by taking 1 minim of preceding potency and 9 minims of alcohol.

Drugs under this Class [Class VI(B)]

1. **Mineral and Chemical Source:** Ars. alb; Benzoic acid; Carboneum chloratum; Carboneum sulphuratum; Eupion; Glonoine; Hydrocyanic acid; Iodum; Kali. iod; Kreosotum; Lactic acid; Merc. cor; Natrum hydroiodicum; Petroleum; Sulphur.
2. **Animal Source:** Mephitis; Tarentula cubensis; Trombidium; Muscae domestica; Upas antiaris.
3. **Nosodes:** Psorinum.
4. **Vegetable Source:** Croton tig; Oleum cajuputi; Oleum ricini; Terebinthinae oleum; Oleum santali; Opium; Oleum succini; Santoninum.

PREPARATION OF MOTHER SUBSTANCE (CLASS VII TO CLASS IX)

Definition of Mother Substance (O)

It is the drug pharmaceutically prepared from the drug-substance of any source insoluble in liquid vehicle as the strongest solid solvent by the process of trituration with sugar of milk.

Different classes under Mother Substance (O)

3 Classes: Class VII; Class VIII; and Class IX.

Class VII: Includes dry insoluble substances.

Class VIII: Includes liquid insoluble substances.

Class IX: Includes fresh vegetable and animal substances.

CLASS VII

Introduction: This includes those dry medicinal substances which, in their crude state, are neither soluble in purified water nor in alcohol.

The fundamental rule for this class has been described in Hahnemann's **'Materia Medica Pura'** under **'Arsenicum'**.

Trituration

1. **Principle:** 1 part by weight of the medicinal substance to 99 parts (in centesimal scale) or 9 parts (in decimal scale) by weight of sugar of milk gives 1st trituration.
2. **Requirements**
   (a) *Ingredients*
   (i) Required amount of crude drug-substance.
   (ii) Required amount of sugar of milk.
   (b) *Appliances*
   (i) One clean unglazed porcelain mortar and pestle
   (ii) One clean horn spatula
   (iii) An empty clean phial of required size
   (iv) A stop-clock or a watch
   (v) A freshly marked new velvet cork
   (vi) Label paper, paste, scissors, pen etc.
   (vii) Balance and weight box.
3. **Procedure**
   (a) *Centesimal Scale:* One part by weight of the medicinal substance to 99 parts by weight of sugar of milk gives the 1st trituration.
   All following triturations are prepared with one grain of the preceding trituration to 99 grains of sugar of milk.
   [For details see 'Trituration' under **'Potentisation'** chapter.]
   (b) *Decimal Scale:* One part by weight of medicinal substance to 9 parts by weight of sugar of milk, gives 1st trituration.
   All following triturations are prepared with one grain of the preceding trituration to 9 grains of sugar of milk.

Conversion of Trituration into Liquid Potency

1. **Centesimal Scale**

1 grain of the 3rd trituration dissolved in 50 minims of purified water, and mixed with 50 minims of alcohol gives the 4th potency.

1 minim of the 4th potency to 99 minims of alcohol gives the 5th potency.

All following potencies are prepared with 1 minim of the preceding potency to 99 minims of alcohol.

2. **Decimal Scale**

1 grain of the 6X trituration dissolved in 50 minims of purified water, and mixed with 50 minims of alcohol gives the 8X potency.

1 minim of the 8X potency to 9 minims of alcohol gives the 9X potency.

All following potencies are prepared with 1 minim of the preceding potency to 9 minims of alcohol.

[For details see 'Trituration' under **'Potentisation'** chapter.]

Drugs under this Class (Class VII)

1. **Vegetable Source**

Aloe socotrina; Aesculus glabra; Ammoniacum gummi; Benzinum; China; Coffea cruda; Condurango; Crocus sativus (G.H.P.); Ignatia amara; Nux vomica; Opium; Polyporus officinalis; Rheum (A.H.P); Sarsaparilla (G.H.P.); Ustilago.

2. **Animal Source**

Badiaga; Cantharis; Carbo. an; Corallium rubrum; Sepia; Spongia; Tarentula hispanica.

3. **Mineral and Chemical Source**

(a) ***Acids:*** Benzoic acid; Boric acid; Citric acid; Gallic acid; Oxalic acid; Picric acid; Salicylic acid; Tartaric acid.

(b) ***Elements:*** Alumina; Arg. met; Aurum met; Cup. met; Ferr. met; Iodum; Iridum met; Niccolum met; Palladium; Plumbum; Selenium; Stannum met; Sulphur; Tellurium; Zincum met.

(c) ***Compounds:*** Ammon. brom; Ammon. carb; Ammon iod; Ammon. phos; Ammon. picricum; Ammon. valerianicum; Ant. ars; Ant. iod; Ant. crud; Ant. oxydatum; Ant. sulphuratum aureum; Arg. mur; Arg. iodatum; Arg. nit; Ars. alb; Ars. iod; Ars sulphuratum flavum; Ars. sulphuratum rubrum; Aurum muriaticum; Aurum muriaticum natronatum; Aurum sulphuratum; Baryta carb; Baryta mur; Cal. ars; Cal. brom; Cal. sulphurica; Cup. ars; Cup. carb; Cup. sulph; Ferr. ars; Ferr. bromatum; Ferr. iod; Ferr. sulph; Ferr. carb; Ferr. magneticum; Ferr. phos; Carbo. veg; Kali. ars; Kali. bi; Kali. brom; Kali. carb; Kali. chloricum; Kali iod; Kali. nitricum; Kali. sulph; Kali. mur; Kali. phos; Mag. carb; Mag. mur; Mag. oxydata; Mag. phos; Mag. sulph; Merc. cyanatus; Merc. dulcis; Merc. solubilis Hahnemanni; Merc. sulph; Nat. ars; Nat. carb; Nat. phos; Nat. sulph; Nat. sulphurosum Paraffin; Naphthalinum; Aniline sulph.

(d) ***Minerals:*** Graphites; Hecla lava; Benzoaris lapis; Molybdenum sulphuratum; Adamas; Tetradymitum; Silicea.

CLASS VIII

Introduction: This class includes those medicinal substances which are neither soluble in purified water, nor in alcohol. They are subjected to trituration, with sugar of milk.

The fundamental rule for this class has been described in **Chronic Diseases** under 'Petroleum'.

Trituration

1. **Principle:** Same as Class VII.
2. **Requirements:** Same as Class VII.
3. **Procedure:** The process is same as Class VII, but some points must be known regarding this class, which differs from Class VII:

(a) In decimal scale, 9 parts of sugar of milk is taken to prepare medicine, but it should not be divided into 3 equal parts. Because sugar of milk in this case is very small in quantity, and hence, if it is again divided into 3 parts, the mixture of oily medicinal substances and vehicles will become paste-like preventing trituration.

So, the whole quantity of sugar of milk should be taken at a time in the mortar, but the trituration should be done thrice in twenty minutes.

(b) The adequate amount of sugar of milk should be taken at first in the mortar, and the medicinal substance should be poured over it for preventing sticking of the oily medicinal substance to the surface of the mortar.

Conversion of Trituration into Liquid Potency

(a) Centesimal Scale]
(b) Decimal Scale] Same as Class VII.

Drugs under this Class (Class VIII)

1. **Animal Sources**

   (a) Venoms: Crotalus; Elaps; Lachesis; Naja; Vipera; Apium virus; Bufo rana; Bungarus krait; Trigonocephalus atrox; Trigonocephalus jararaca.

   (b) Other animals: Araneninum.

2. **Vegetable Sources:** Myristica sebifera; Croton tig; Janipha manihot.
3. **Nosodes:** Lyssin; Malandrinum; Vaccininum; Variolinum.
4. **Minerals:** Petroleum.

Note: Nosodes (diseased products) and venoms (animals) etc. are included in Class VIII. Triturate those with sugar of milk and then convert those into liquid potencies (Hahnemann's direction). But A.H.P. includes some nosodes along with some fresh vegetable drug-substances in Class IX.

CLASS IX

Introduction: This class deals with preparation of medicines from vegetables and animal substances by trituration, in solid form.

The fundamental rule for this class has been discussed in the **Chronic diseases**, under 'Agaricus'.

Trituration

1. **Principle:** 2 parts by weight of medicinal substance to 99 parts (centesimal scale) or 9 parts (Decimal scale) by weight of sugar of milk gives 1st trituration.
2. **Requirements:** Same as Class VII.
3. **Procedure:** Same as Class VII but the ratio of medicinal substance and sugar of milk is 2 : 99 (centesimal scale) or 2 : 9 (decimal scale).

Note: Here, 2 parts of medicinal substance are taken because there is always some loss by evaporation during trituration.

Conversion of Trituration into Liquid Potency

(a) Centesimal Scale]
(b) Decimal Scale] Same as Class VII.

Drugs under this Class (Class IX)

1. **Vegetable Sources:** Anacardium orientale; Boletus satanus; Boletus suaveolens; Agaricus muscarius; Elaeis guineensis; Solanum oleraceum.
2. **Animal Sources:** Amphisboena vermicularis; Blatta americana; Blatta orientalis; Cervus brasiliensis; Cyprinus barbus; Delphunus amazonicus; Fel piscium; Fel tauri; Ovi gallinae pellicula; Spinguras martini; Vulpis fel; Vulpis hepar; Vulpis pulmo.
3. **Nosodes:** Anthracinum; Carcinosin; Leucorrhinum; Malandrinum; Medorrhinum; Psorinum; Syphilinum.

Note: Though the trituration is done, more or less in the same manner, in Class VII, VIII and IX, Hahnemann classified those into three different classes, instead of one, beause in all the three classes, different types of drug-substances are used.

For Class VII:	Insoluble solid drug-substances.
For Class VIII:	Insoluble liquid drug-substances.
For Class IX:	Fresh vegetable and animal drug-substances.

Alcohols used in Different Classes

For the preparation of mother tincture (Class I to Class IV), and mother solutions (except in Class V) strong alcohol is always used.

But for the preparation of potency, dilute or dispensing alcohols are used. But, in some cases, purified water is used.

Table 13.2: Hahnemannian Method of Preparation of Drugs

Class	Source	Nature of drug	Fundamental rule (M. M. pura)	Ratio (Drug: Menstrum)	Drug power	Medicinal loss	Duration	Process of potentisation
Class I	Vegetable kingdom	Most juicy plants. Non-mucilagenous, no resins, terpins or volatile oils.	Belladonna	1 : 1 (by weight)	½	–	8 days	Succussion
Class II	Vegetable kingdom	Moderately juicy plants. Non-mucilagenous but with resins, terpins or volatile oils.	Thuja	3 : 2 (by weight)	½	⅓ per cc	8 days	Succussion
Class III	Vegetable kingdom	Less juicy plants. Mucilagenous drug substances.	Scilla	1 : 2 (by weight)	⅙	⅔ per cc	8 days	Succussion
Class IV	Vegetable and animal kingdom	Dried vegetables, dried and fresh animal substances.	Staphysagria, Spigelia	1 : 5 (by weight)	$1/10$	½ per grain	15 days	Succussion
Class VA	Mineral	Substances soluble in less quantity of water.	Natrum mur	1 : 9 (by weight)	$1/10$			Succussion
Class VB	Mineral	Substances soluble in large quantity of water.	Acid phos	1 : 99 (by weight)	$1/100$			Succussion
Class VIA	Mineral	Substances soluble in less quantity of alcohol.	Guaiacum	1 : 9 (by weight)	$1/10$			Succussion
Class VIB	Mainly mineral rarely plant and animal	Substances soluble in greater quantity of alcohol.	Merc. cor.	1 : 99 (by weight)	$1/100$			Succussion
Class VII	Mineral, nosode and sarcode	Trituration of dried medicinal substances.	Arsenicum met.	1 : 99 (by weight centisimal) 1 : 9 (by weight decimal)	$1/100$ $1/10$			Trituration
Class VIII	Mineral, nosode and sarcode	Trituration of liquid-insoluble medicinal substances.	Petroleum (in Chronic diseases)	1 : 99 (by weight centisimal) 1 : 9 (by weight decimal)	$1/100$ $1/10$			Trituration
Class IX	Fresh vegetables and animals (A.H.P.—some nosodes)	Trituration of fresh vegetables and animals.	Agaricus (in Chronic diseases)	2 : 99 (by weight centisimal) 2 : 9 (by weight decimal)	$1/100$ $1/10$			Trituration

Decimal Scale

Class I	: Up to 3X, dilute alcohol	4X onwards dispensing alcohol
Class II	: Up to 2X, dilute alcohol	3X onwards dispensing alcohol
Class III	: Up to 2X, dilute alcohol	3X onwards dispensing alcohol
Class IV	: Mother tincture is same as 1X	2X onwards dispensing alcohol
Class V(A)	: Mother solution is same as 1X	2X potency prepared with purified water 3X potency prepared with dilute alcohol 4X onwards dispensing alcohol
Class V(B)	: Mother solution is same as 2X	3X potency prepared with dilute alcohol 4X onwards dispensing alcohol
Class VI	: All potencies are prepared with dispensing alcohol	
Class VII, VIII and IX	: Fluxion potency	6X to 8X, with dispensing alcohol 8X to 9X, with dilute alcohol 9X onwards dispensing alcohol
Centisimal Scale		
Class I to Class III	: 1C with dilute alcohol	2C onwards dispensing alcohol

Exceptions in Ratio's in Homoeopathic Pharmacy

Ratio's	Applications
1:4	The Ratio (Mother tincture: Olive oil) to prepare Liniments as per HPI
2:9	The Ratio (Drug substance: Sugar of milk) to prepare Mother triturations under Class IX
2:99	The Ratio (Drug substance: Sugar of milk) to prepare Mother triturations under Class IX
2:9	The Ratio ((Drug substance: Strong alcohol) to prepare Mother solutions as per Class VIA according to BHP
1:50	The Ratio (Drug substance: Sugar of milk) to prepare Mother solutions as per Class VIB according to GHP
1:3:5	The Ratio to triturate as per HPI (in Decimal scale)
11:33:55	The Ratio to triturate as per HPI (in Centesimal scale)
1:99	The Ratio (Mother tincture: Alcohol) to prepare Evaporating Lotion

Chapter 14

Methods of Preparing Homoeopathic Drugs (New Method)

Introduction

All pharmacopoeia should follow a standardised process for preparation of medicines whether in solution or in trituration, i.e. all triturations and all alcoholic medicinal solutions (e.g. tinctures, extracts etc.) and their dilutions might be made of uniform drug-strength to be represented by the dry crude drug as the unit of strength in case of mother tincture made from dried substances and the plant juice as the unit when made from fresh green drugs. For this purpose, Hahnemann introduced centesimal scale based on the principle that the 1st potency should contain $\frac{1}{100}$th part of the original drug and each succeeding potency should contain $\frac{1}{100}$th part of the one preceding it. This principle worked well so for as mother trituration, and potency triturations of dry drug substances were concerned.

But difficulty arises in standardising the drug strength in alcoholic solution (which was overlooked by Hahnemann), or dry substances and plant juice when collected from fresh green drugs, were noticed by the compilers of B.H.P. in 1876.

The lack of uniformity in drug-strength was due to different degrees of solvency of different kinds of drug substances in alcohol or water, and varying quantities of plant moistures, in different varieties of plants used in homoeopathy.

It is observed that water in the form of moisture present in plant is but a solvent, and a part of the vehicle or menstrum forms no part of the total medicinal substance. Hahnemann's view was that the plant moisture is a part of the drug substance but A.H.P. claims that it is only a solvent.

Previous editions of A.H.P. divided all vegetable and animal substances into four classes, for preparation of mother tincture, of which the first three classes treat of fresh plants and the fourth of animals and dried plants. The amount of drug substances was $\frac{1}{2}$, $\frac{1}{3}$, $\frac{1}{6}$ and $\frac{1}{10}$ in each of the respective classes according as the plants contain a large quantity of juice, or a small quantity of juice, or the plants are dry and animal products, fresh or dried.

Accordingly, nine different classes of formulae were adopted in the preparation of mother tincture, dilutions, and triturations of medicines, used in homoeopathic practice. To obviate these diversities and to bring out an uniformity in strength (drug strength) of all homoeopathic medicinal preparations, whether in tinctures or in triturations, the American Institute of Homoeopathy set up a special committee in 1888 on whose recommendations the Pharmacopoeia Committee has followed the directions of the B.H.P. to take in every instance of the dry crude substance, as the starting point from which to calculate its strength, and the tincture containing all the soluble matter of one gram of the dry plant and 10 cubic centimetre of the tincture. The tincture (θ), therefore, containing $^1/_{10}$th part medi-cinal substance, should represent the 1X($^1/_{10}$), thereby corresponding its strength with the 1X trituration.

In short, the dry crude drug has been made the unit, from which we estimate the drug-strength in all tinctures and triturations.

With the exception of a few drugs, H.P.U.S. (official) in 1941, prescribed the uniform standard of 10% drug strength in all cases of medicinal preparations. This standard eliminates the double standard of Hahnemann (in cases of alcoholic solutions or dry drugs, and fresh plant juices) the centesimal scale of potency, the previously adopted classifications of medicinal materials and different formulae in connection with the preparation of homoeopathic medicine and a uniform standard is thus secured.

Note: H.P.I. also accepts new method for the preparation of mother tincture, while the G.H.P. still holds to Hahnemannian methods, the drug strength differs from class to class.

Plant Moisture

1. **Definition:** Plant moisture is the juice contained in a plant.
2. **Utility to know the moisture content (or water percentage) of the vegetable drug substances:** It is to be noted that tinctures must be of uniform strength. The respective strengths vary greatly due to the 'variability' of moisture contained in the same plant at different seasons, and conditions of growth, procurement, time and storage. The variability of moisture contained in the plants causes great uncertainty in the strengths of tinctures and their dilutions. As such, moisture content or water content of each crude sample is ascertained beforehand.
3. **How the plant moisture is calculated?**
   (i) The drug substances are at first kept on the chopping board, and cut into different sizes with the chopping knife.
   (ii) The chopped drug-substance weighed and the weight is recorded. The weights of the empty porcelain crucible is taken.
   (iii) Then these pieces of drug-substances are placed on a crucible, which is then placed on a water-bath, so that by the gentle heat of the water-bath, the juice of the plant is evaporated.
   (iv) The chopped substances should be kept on the water-bath until the weight scale shows no further reduction of weight.
   (v) The substance is weighed after every 15 minutes after cooling for a minute until a constant weight is obtained.
   (vi) On obtaining a constant weight, which means there is no more water vapour left.
   (vii) Now, comparing the final weight, with that which is taken before, will give the amount of moisture content of the drug-substance.

After determining how much quantity of dry substance is present in the given quantity of the fresh moist materials, this is to be compared with the respective tincture formula for this drug, as specified in the pharmacopoeia.

If its weight falls below from that prescribed as the standard weight of the particular formula, sufficient quantities of purified water should be added to equalise with the standard weight.

But if its weight is above from that prescribed as the standard weight of the particular formula, then deduct sufficient quantity of purified water, required to be mixed with the strong alcohol to make it equal with the standard formula.

Preparation of Mother Tincture (Modern method)

1. **Peculiarity**
   (i) Uniform drug strength (1/10)
   (ii) Consideration of the moisture content of the drug-substances.
2. **Process**
   (i) Maceration
   (ii) Percolation.

MACERATION

1. **Definition:** It is a long process of preparation of mother tincture from vegetable and animal substances under N.T.P. according to new method.

2. **Substances taken for maceration**

Hard, gummy, mucilaginous substance of animal kingdom, those having much viscid juice, which do not allow alcohol (menstrum) to penetrate or permeate repidly, as in the process of percolation, are immersed in strong alcohol for a definite period of time, as per pharmacopoeia.

Hard, gummy and mucilaginous drug-substances do not allow the menstrum (alcohol) to penetrate rapidly due to the smallness of intermolecular space. Therefore, it takes long time to penetrate. The reason for cutting or pounding of the material is to increase the surface for penetration of alcohol.

3. **Conditions**

(a) Menstrum: Alcohol as well as purified water.

(b) Normal temp (15° – 20°C) and pressure (i.e. N.T.P.).

(c) Drug is in contact with vehicle for a long time.

(d) The merc is pressed after removing the liquid portion.

Menstrum: It is a liquid which is capable of penetrating the tissues of plant or animal substances and capable to dissolve the active principles.

Merc: It is the inert, fibrous and insoluble material remaining after expression of the juice from drug material or after maceration or percolation.

Magma: The thick residue of the soft doughy mass (molten mass) resulting from the expression of the fluid part of certain substances (pounded fresh plant).

Digestion: When the maceration is done in hot liquid it is known as digestion.

Procedure

(a) *Pre-process*

Moisture content of the drug-substances (i.e. excess or deficiency of water) is calculated with the help of water-bath.

(b) *Process proper*

(i) The drug substances are made into a pulp (magma), (or in its natural state if not reducible)

(ii) The pulp (magma) is placed in a macerating jar, preferably made of glass or stainless steel.

(iii) Prescribed quantity of alcohol (pre-calculated) is added to cover the whole mass of drug-substances.

(iv) The macerating jar is now carefully corked or sealed in order to prevent the evaporation of the menstrum (alcohol).

(v) The jar is kept in a cool dark place, free from dust, odour, heat or direct sunlight. The temperature be better within the range of 15°C to 20°C. The jar is kept for 2–4 weeks.

Note: The time required for proper extraction of medicinal substances varies considerably, it is, therefore, safe to allow the process of maceration to continue from 2–4 weeks according to the nature of the drug material.

(vi) The jar is powerfully shaken once daily.

(vii) After the lapse of this period, the supernatant fluid is decanted off in another clean glass-stoppered bottle.

(viii) The residue is pressed out through a piece of new clean linen cloth, and the same added to the former tincture. The total juice thus obtained is the mother tincture of the drug substance.

If the volume of the obtained mother tincture is less than the formula prescribed in the pharmacopoeia which is due to—(a) evaporation of alcohol, (b) contraction due to mixture of alcohol and water—required quantity of menstrum (alcohol) is added for standardisation.

If the volume of the obtained mother tincture is more than the formula prescribed in the pharmacopoeia, then volume is reduced by—(a) gentle heat (b) deducting the portion of water with the addition of calculated amount of strong alcohol.

In case of more viscid and mucilaginous substances, where alcohol does not act fully on the substance, the process is modified as:

(i) The drug-substance is made into a pulp.

(ii) The pulp is placed in a macerating jar.

(iii) Half-quantity of pre-calculated menstrum (alcohol) is added to the drug-substances.

(iv) Macerating jar is corked or sealed to prevent evaporation of alcohol.

(v) The jar is kept in a cool dark place for 2 to 4 weeks.

(vi) The jar is powerfully shaken once daily.

(vii) The supernatant fluid is decanted off.

(viii) The residue is pressed out thereafter.

(ix) The residual mass which remains behind, is taken in a clean porcelain mortar or pestle and double the quantity of green glass powder is added to it.

It is then thoroughly pulverised by a pestle. The pulp is now placed over the filter bed of a percolator, and percolated by that quantity of strong alcohol which was not used before. The resulting tincture, thus obtained, is mixed with the previously prepared tincture. It is filtered by a filter paper and stored in a glass-stoppered bottle, in a cool, dark place.

Note: In maceration process of preparing mother tincture, decantation prior to filtration is necessary. If filtration is carried out without decantation, the filter paper through which the filtration is performed will be choked up with the solid or semi-solid materials and the fluid substance will not be able to pass through the filter paper and there will be considerable loss by evaporation on account of delay.

PERCOLATION

Definition: It is a short process of preparation of mother tincture in a new method, where the vehicle is passed though the soft, non-gumming and non-mucilaginous drug-substance of vegetable and animal kingdom by an apparatus, percolator for a definite period of time as per the nature of drug-substance according to pharmacopoeia.

Preparation of Mother Tincture

1. **Principle**

When a liquid capable of dissolving only a portion of a powdered material is spread on porous material, and it passes through succeeding layers of powder, it gets saturated. This solution is subjected to two forces—one is the force of capillary attraction by which powder tries to retain it. The second is the force of gravity acting on it, and the column of liquid above it, resulting in downward displacement of this standard solution. The second force being stronger than the first, the liquid containing soluble parts of the powder gradually passes down through the porous material.

Physical forces acting in the process of percolation: (i) Gravitation, (ii) Viscosity, (iii) Adhesion, (iv) Friction; (v) Osmosis, (vi) Capillary attraction, (vii) Surface tension.

2. **Requirements**

(a) ***Ingredients***

(i) Drug-substances

(ii) Strong alcohol (menstrum)

(b) ***Appliances***

(i) Percolator with sieves and regulation cork-stopper

(ii) A glass rod with cork.

Diagrammatic Description of a Percolator

1. **Definition:** It is an apparatus, used for percolation, during the preparation of mother tincture in new method. There are different types of percolators in respect of their shape and material. They are made up of copper, stainless steel, some alloy, or of porcelain or glass.

2. **Parts:** It consists of two parts: (i) Percolator proper; (ii) Receiver.

These two parts are connected with rubber tubing and glass rod.

(a) ***Percolator proper:*** It is the 1st or upper part. It consists of two parts:

(i) *Head:* The upper end (conical or pear-shaped) is known as its 'head', fitted with a stop-cock on the top.

(ii) *Neck:* The lower end (narrowed) is known as 'neck', which is connected through rubber tubing and glass rod to the receiver vessel.

The cork within the orifice of the 'head' as well as that of the 'neck' below are very roughly rubbed, so that the cork and the upper body can very conveniently be fitted with one another. There are arrangements for the entry of air after complete closure.

(b) *Receiver:* It is the second or lower part. It is kept below the bottom of the percolator proper. It is a wide-mouth glass jar. The receiver is provided with a stop-cock. The apparatus is provided with arrangements for placing the powdered drugs, moistened with the solvent and a layer of coarse sand, and above all there is an arrangement for placing a white filter paper. A plug of an 'absorbent cotton' is inserted into the neck above the stop-cock. After arranging in this manner, the apparatus will be left alone for a full day or two, and then the requisite menstrum is poured on the drug powders. The tincture slowly falls through the neck drop by drop, and is collected in the receiver. When the collection is completed, the stop-cock of the receiver is loosened and the contents are taken out and filtered.

This is the desired mother tincture from the dry drug-substances.

3. **Procedure**

(a) ***Preparation of percolator***

A piece of fine well-washed muslin is tied to the neck in case of small percolators without stop-cock. A clean cork of best quality can be inserted in the neck in case of large percolators without stop-cock. If the percolator is not provided with stop-cock, insert a cork in the lower orifice, having first made a longitudinal small groove, so that by pressing the cork into the neck of the percolator with required force, the flow of the mother tincture may be regulated or stopped as desired.

A tow is placed on the muslin.

Tow: It is an obstruction made up of porous material, placed in or above the neck and below the powdered drug substance. It consists of the layers from below upwards:

(i) A plug of an absorbent cotton: inserted in the neck.

(ii) A layer of about ¼″ thick minimum coarse sand.

(iii) A layer of about ½″ thick medium coarse sand.

(iv) A layer of maximum coarse sand.

Powdered green glass may be used instead of sand. It controls the flow of liquid.

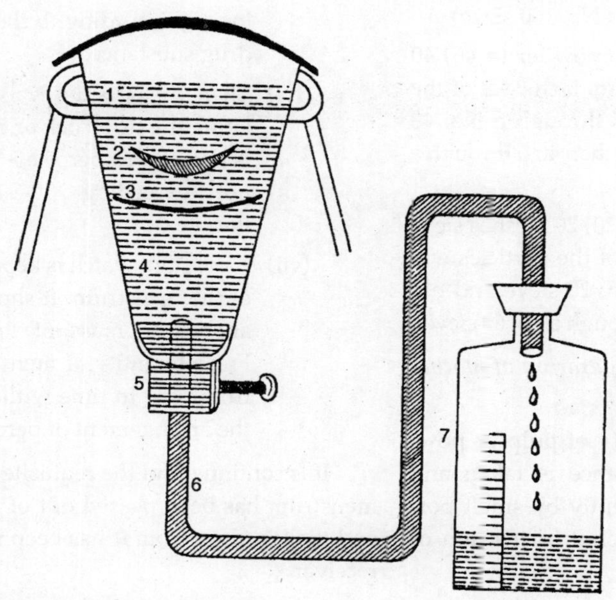

Percolator

(b) ***Preparation of drug-substances for percolation***

(i) If dry and hard, is finely powdered to give uniform consistency.

(ii) If fresh, is reduced to fine and uniform pulp.

(iii) Drug-substance is moistened by mixing it with sufficient menstrum with the help of a pestle or spatula in a mortar. This is done to make powder more absorbable by menstrum.

(iv) Preparation from fresh vegetables, in large scale.

The juice is pressed out from the pulp and the residue is uniformly mixed with equal quantity of powdered green glass. The expressed juice is put in the receiver of the percolator and is allowed to mix with the percolated fluid.

The fineness of powdered vegetable and animal drug-substances is expressed in the pharmacopoeia by the following terms:

(i) Very fine powder (≠ 80) 80 meshes sieve in a sq. inch. (All of the particles will pass through a No. 80 sieve)

(ii) Fine powder (≠ 60) 60 meshes sieve in a sq. inch. (All of the particles will pass through a No. 60 sieve and not more than 40% through a No. 100 sieve)

(iii) Moderately coarse powder (≠ 40) 40 meshes sieve in a sq. inch. (All of the particles will pass through a No. 40 sieve and not more than 40% through a No. 80 sieve)

(iv) Coarse powder (≠ 20) 20 meshes sieve in a sq. inch. (All of the particles will pass through a No. 20 sieve and not more than 40% through a no. 60 sieve).

(c) ***Actual process of preparation of mother tincture***

(i) Prescribed quantity of pulp or powdered drug-substance is taken and moistened sufficiently by small portion of strong alcohol (menstrum or solvent).

Moist pulp or powder is spread uniformly over the two (layers of sand), gradually passing it down gently by a broad flat cork fixed on the end of a glass rod, to get a uniform and compact mass, free from fissures or empty spaces. The pressing should be firm if the mass is coarse, and if strong alcohol is used, it should be light with fine powder.

(ii) Lastly, the upper surface of the mass is covered with the disc of a filter paper or a thin layer of finely powdered glass or sand.

(iii) Now, enough quantity of the prescribed menstrum is taken just to cover the mass, holding it by means of the flat cork attached to the glass rod, poured on the contents of the percolator, allowing the fluid to run gently and gradually down the glass rod, so that the fluid may fall on the cork and spread gradually over the surface, without disturbing or displacing the pounded glass or sand.

(iv) Then the rod and cork is removed and lid of the percolator is closed to prevent dust from contaminating, and evaporation, as soon as the fluid begins to drop. Now, the mouth is closed by pressing in the cork at the neck.

(v) It is allowed to stand for 24 hours or longer, according to the nature of the drug substance.

(vi) Then by opening valves and regulating the stop-cock or cork, the liquid is allowed to percolate drop by drop, not exceeding 10-30 drops per minute.

(vii) A constant watch is kept over the level of the menstrum. It should always be above the mass of drug-substance. Fresh quantity of menstrum is added from time to time without disturbing the arrangement of percolator.

It is continued till the requisite amount of the menstrum has been passed out of the percolator, and the last drop from it has been received in the receiver.

Once the last drop is received, sufficient amount of menstrum is added to cover the mass of the drug-substance in the percolator. The lid is closed to prevent percolation.

This arrangement is allowed to stand for 6 hours.

Then the cork is opened to allow the whole fluid to drop into the receiver as before. The tincture obtained is to be tested in laboratory to ascertain the drug-strength. The resulting tincture thus obtained in the receiver should then be drained out, and filtered through white filter paper or absorbent cotton directly into the glass bottles, which are to be tightly corked.

Potentisation

According to the new method, the drug power (d.p.) is one-tenth, therefore, it is equal to 1X potency of decimal scale.

The 2X potency will be prepared with 1 part of 1X potency (i.e. mother tincture), 9 parts of vehicle (purified water or alcohol) and 10 downward strokes of equal strength.

All succeeding potencies are prepared by taking 1 part of the preceding potency and 9 parts of dispensing alcohol.

Table 14.1: Differences between Maceration and Percolation

Maceration	Percolation
1. Long process; Time required: 2-4 weeks.	1. Short process; Time required: 24 hours.
2. Hard, gummy and mucilaginous drug substances are subjected.	2. Soft, non-gummy, non-mucilaginous drug-substances are subjected.
3. Fresh vegetable and animal drug-substances.	3. Dry or fresh drug-substances.
4. Mother tincture (θ) never obtained directly. Decantation prior to filtration is necessary.	4. Mother tincture (θ) is directly obtained. Decantation is not necessary.
5. Menstrum (strong alcohol) is added to standard drug-substances.	5. Menstrum is allowed to pass through drug-substances.

Table 14.2: Dissimilarities and similarities between Old and New methods

A. Dissimilarities

Old method	*New method*
1. This method was introduced by Hahnemann.	1. This method was introduced by American and British homoeopathic pharmacopoeia (A.H.P. & B.H.P.).
2. Always fresh drug-substances of vegetable and animal kingdom are required.	2. Air-dried drug-substances are required in place of fresh vegetable and animal drug-substances.
3. This method recommends nine classes in preparation of mother tincture, mother solution and mother substance, from drug-substances belonging to vegetable, animal and mineral kingdoms.	3. No such classification.
4. This method classified the vegetable and animal substances in 4 classes depending upon their juice content, e.g. most juicy, moderate juicy, less juicy and dry plant and animal drugs.	4. No such classification.
5. Prescribed different methods for mother tincture preparation from plant and animal substances: Class I: Plant juices to be used	5. Only two methods (i) Maceration (ii) Percolation

Contd.

Old method	*New method*
Class II: Plant substances are mixed with alcohol and then strained. Class III & IV: Drug-substances (dry vegetable and animal) are mixed with alcohol and the resulting mixture is allowed to stand for 8 days.	
6. Unit of drug strength or drug power variable: Class I and II: $\frac{1}{2}$ Class III: $\frac{1}{6}$ Class IV; V(A); VI(A): $\frac{1}{10}$ Class V(B) and VI(B): $\frac{1}{100}$	6. Uniform drug-strength of drug power excepting a few ones, depending on their solubilities e.g., (a) Hydrocyanic acid; Picric acid; Ambra grisea; Ammon aceticum; Arsenicum album; Bromium; Crotalus horridus; Crot. tig; Cup. aceticum; Elaps; Glonoinum; Kali ars; Kali chlor; Kali permanganicum; Mephitis; Mercurius cyanatus: D.P. = $\frac{1}{100}$. (b) Cactus; Moschus: D.P. = $\frac{1}{20}$ (c) Phosphorus: D.P. = $\frac{1}{667}$ (d) Sulphur: D.P. = $\frac{1}{5,000}$
7. Way of calculation of drug-strength: Hahnemann introduced double ways of calculation of drug strengths of mother tinctures, one for the cases of alcoholic tinctures of dry drugs, and other for the fresh plant juices, wherefrom to calculate the respective drug-strength e.g., from fresh plant juice and dry drugs.	7. The present day Pharmacopoeia Committee of United States of America has discarded the double way of calculation of drug-strengths of mother tincture of Hahnemann, and instead they have fixed one standard of calculation of respective drug power or drug-strength, taking the dry substance as the unit.
8. Consideration of moisture content: Moisture content of drug substances (i.e. water or juice) can not be considered. Hahnemann's view was that the plant moisture is part of the drug-substances.	8. Moisture content of drug substance is considered. A.H.P. claims that water in the form of moisture present in plant is a solvent, and a part of the vehicle or menstrum forms no part of the total medicinal substance.
9. Maintains two scales for the preparation: (i) Decimal scale (ii) Centesimal scale	9. Maintains only decimal scale.
10. Time required: Class I to III: 8 days Class IV: 15 days	10. Time required: (i) Maceration: 2 to 4 weeks (ii) Percolation: 24 hours.
B. **Similarities**	
1. Process adopted—Immersion	1. Process adopted—immersion.
2. In preparation of some drugs, Hahnemann was unique, which shows his originality and speciality, e.g., Causticum; Hepar sulph; Acid. phos; Calcarea carb; Merc. sol.	2. This method also includes those drugs of the Hahnemannian method, in full conformity with Hahnemann's particular direction as regards their mode of preparations.

Contd.

Old method	New method
3. In Class VA, VB, VIA, VIB of the old method, the respective amount of drug-power i.e. 1/10, 1/100 etc. of the requisite drugs have been calculated on the basis of the respective solubilities of them in purified water and alcohol. The Class VII includes all amorphous, crude or insoluble (or very sparingly soluble) drugs, which are insoluble in purified water or alcohol, or in a mixture of the both in any proportion. Here, the dry crude drug has been taken as an unit of medicinal strength from where the respective drug-power is ascertained.	3. The new method has followed the same.

Few Examples of Preparations

A. VEGETABLE KINGDOM

Aconitum napellus

(a) *Mother tincture θ,* Drug strength 1/10

Aconite napellus in Coarse powder	100 gm
Purified water	350 ml
Strong alcohol	368 ml

To make one thousand millilitres of the tincture.

(b) *Potencies*

2X to contain one part tincture, two parts purified water and seven parts strong alcohol; 3X and higher with *rectified spirit 60 o.p.*

Old method (for dilutions): Class I and II

Arnica montana

(a) *Mother tincture θ* Drug strength 1/10

Arnica montana in Coarse powder	100 gm
Purified water	400 ml
Strong alcohol	635 ml

To make one thousand millilitres of the tincture.

(b) *Potencies*

2X to contain one part of tincture, three parts purified water and six parts strong alcohol. 3X and higher with *rectified spirit 60 o.p.*

Old Method: Class III.

Belladonna

(a) *Mother tincture θ* Drug strength 1/10

Belladonna in coarse powder	100 gm
Purified water	567 ml
Strong alcohol	470 ml

To make one thousand millilitres of the tincture.

(b) *Potencies*

2X to contain one part of tincture, four parts purified water and five parts strong alcohol. 3X and higher with *rectified spirit 60 o.p.*

Old Method: Class I

B. MINERAL KINGDOM

Nitric acid

(a) *Solution* Drug strength 1/10

Acidum nitricum	141 gm

Purified water in sufficient quantity

To make one thousand millilitres of solution.

(b) *Potencies*

2X and 3X with purified water, to be freshly made for immediate use only.

4X and 5X with dilute alcohol.

6X and above with *rectified spirit 60 o.p.*

Old Method: Class Va.

Natrum muriaticum

(a) *Trituration IX* Drug strength $1/10$

Natrum muriaticum in crystals	100 gm
Saccharum lactis	900 gm

To make one thousand grams of the trituration.

(b) *Potencies*

2X and higher to be triturated.

6X may be converted to liquid 8X.

9X and higher with *rectified spirit 60 o.p.*

Silicea

(a) *Trituration IX* Drug strength $1/10$

Silicea in coarse powder	100 gm
Saccharum lactis	900 gm

To make one thousand grams of trituration.

(b) *Potencies*

2X and higher to be triturated.

6X may be converted to liquid 8X.

9X and higher with *rectified spirit 60 o.p.*

Zincum metallicum

(a) *Trituration IX* Drug strength $1/10$

Zincum metallicum in fine powder	100 gm
Saccharum lactis	900 gm

To make one thousand gram of the trituration.

(b) *Potencies*

2X and higher to be triturated.

6X may be converted to liquid 8X.

9X and higher with *rectified spirit 60 o.p.*

C. ANIMAL KINGDOM

Apis mellifica

(a) *Mother tincture θ* Drug strength $1/10$

Apis mellifica, moist magma containing 100 moisture 150 ml	250 gm
Glycerine	225 ml
Purified water	225 ml
Strong alcohol	425 ml

To make on thousand millilitres of the tincture.

(b) *Potencies*

2X to contain one part tincture, four parts purified water, five parts strong alcohol; 3X with dilute alcohol.

4X and higher with *rectified spirit 60 o.p.*

Old method: Class IV.

Cantharis

(a) *Mother tincture θ* Drug strength $1/10$

Cantharis in fine powder	100 gm
Strong alcohol in sufficient quantity	

To make one thousand millilitres of the tincture.

(b) *Potencies*

2X and higher with *rectified spirit 60 o.p.*

Old method: Class IV.

Sepia

(a) *Trituration IX* Drug strength $1/10$

Sepia in fine powder	100 gm
Saccharum lactis	900 gm

To make one thousand grams of the trituration.

(b) *Potencies:*

2X and higher to be triturated.

6X may be converted to liquid 8X.

9X and higher with *rectified spirit 60 o.p.*

D. NOSODES

Diphtherinum

The membrane, from a case of malignant diphtheria, is triturated with sugar of milk for an hour according to the old method laid down in Class VIII, and then to convert them into liquid potencies.

Hydrophobinum or Lyssin

The nosode of the virus of a rabid dog.

This drug was introduced and proved by Hering in 1833, fifty years before the crude experiments of Pasteur with the serum.

An empty flour-barrel was put from behind over a rabid dog, and to secure her saliva, the barrel was lifted on one side until the dog is trying to escape, put out her head, between the edge of the barrel and the ground. A quill was used to get saliva as much as possible from her mouth.

The collected saliva was divided into two parts:

(i) One part is triturated on the same day with sugar of milk according to Class VIII up to 3rd centesimal potency, later on up to 30th potency with alcohol.

(ii) From the tincture of the other part of the saliva put in alcohol, some weeks after, one drop was also potentised in the usual way for the purpose of comparative experiment (Ref: Allen, Mat. Med. Nosodes, 136-137; Allen's Encyclop. Mat. Med. X. 658).

Psorinum

The pus is collected from the itch pustule of an infected person, and kept in a phial adding some alcohol. After shaking it well, it is allowed to stand.

Now it is triturated with sugar of milk according to Class IX.

E. IMPONDERABILIA

Electricitas (Electricity)

The energy imparted by electricity (atmospheric or static). The potencies are prepared from sugar of milk which has been saturated with the current.

Magnetis Poli Ambo

It is prepared by exposing sugar of milk or purified water to the influence of an entire magnet stirring and thereby saturating the vehicle.

Potencies are prepared from the trituration. For preparing liquid potency, purified water is used instead of sugar of milk.

X-ray

It is prepared by exposing a phial containing alcohol to X-ray for half an hour. Dilutions are prepared according to centesimal scale of potency.

Chapter 15

Hahnemannian Method of Preparation of Drugs

Mercurius vivus

Chemical symbol: Hg.

Atomic weight: 200.

Synonyms: Hydrargyrum; Argentum vivum; Mercury.

Common name: Quicksilver.

Occurrence: Mercury sometimes occurs native, but its chief source is the ore Cinnabar, Mercuric sulphide, HgS, found at Almaden (Spain), Idria (Yugoslavia), Tuscany, in smaller amounts in California, Texas, Mexico, Peru, China, Japan, and India. The Almaden mine, worked since 415 B.C., is still the chief producer.

Preparation

(i) By roasting the ore (Mercuric sulphide, HgS), the sulphide sublimes, and the vapour being ignited by flame let into the chamber, the mercury is set free and is volatilised; by special arrangements, the vapourised mercury is condensed and collected in the liquid state.

(ii) The ore is also distilled with lime or blacksmith's scale, in closed vessels.

(iii) Metallic mercury comes in commerce in iron bottles or flasks, each holding about seventyfive pounds (30 kg), and is contaminated with small amount of other metals; it has to be purified by redistillation or by prolonged digestion with a mixture of equal parts of Nitric acid (HNO_3) and distilled water. The contaminating metals are thus oxidised, dissolved, and the mercury is separated from the acid solution, well washed with water and dried by means of bibulous paper.

Mercurius solubilis Hahnemanni

Chemical symbol: $Hg_4ONH_2NO_3 + NH_4NO_3$

Synonyms: Mercury oxide black Hahnemann; Ammoniated nitrate of mercury; Hahnemann's soluble mercury; Hahnemann's Quicksilver.

Preparation

(i) Purified mercury is dissolved in required quantities of common cold nitric acid, which requires several days to dissolve the mercury.

(ii) The resulting solution is concentrated and the salt is allowed to crystallise.

(iii) The resulting salt is dried on blotting paper and triturated for thirty minutes in glass mortar, adding one-fourth of its weight of the best alcohol. Next, the alcohol is thrown away, which has been converted into 'ether'. The trituration of mercurial is continued with fresh portions of alcohol for thirty minutes each time, until these fluids emit no longer the smell of ether. That being done, the alcohol is decanted, and the salt is dried on blotting paper, which is renewed from time to time.

(iv) The salt is then triturated in a glass mortar for fifteen minutes with twice its weight of purified water; the clear fluid decanted and the same process is repeated with fresh quantity of water, the clear fluid is added to the preceding, and thus we get an aqueous solution.

(v) Finally, dilute solution of ammonia is added to this aqueous solution, when the black precipitate of the 'Mercury oxide black Hahnemann' will be formed.

(vi) The black precipitate is collected by filtration, and dried in cool dark place.

Preparation for homoeopathic use

Mercurius solubilis Hahnemanni, prepared according to above formula, is triturated as directed under Class VII (old method).

Hepar sulphuris calcareum

Chemical symbol: CaS

Common name: Hepar sulphur; Impure calcium sulphide.

Synonyms: Liver of sulphur; Calcarea sulphuratum.

Description: It is a white, porous, friable mass or a white amorphous powder with the odour and taste of sulphuretted hydrogen. It is insoluble in cold water or strong alcohol but soluble in hot hydrochloric acid, with the evolution of sulphuretted hydrogen.

Preparation

(a) *Crude drug*

Hepar sulphur is an impure sulphide of calcium, obtained from calcined oyster shells and flowers of sulphur.

Hahnemann prepared it by mixing equal weights of clean and finely powdered oyster-shells and well-washed pure flowers of sulphur and placing them in a hermetically sealed crucible, and keeping the crucible at a white heat for at least ten minutes. The product is to be cooled and pulverised. It should be stored in glass-stoppered bottles, protected from light.

(b) *Trituration IX* Drug strength $1/_{10}$

Hepar sulphur (in coarse powder)	100 gm
Dry vehicle (Sac. lac)	900 gm

To make one thousand grams of powder.

Causticum (Hahnemann's Causticum)

Synonyms: Tinctura Acris Sine Kali.

Introduction: This preparation is peculiar to homoeopathy and has been introduced by Hahnemann, hence it should be prepared exactly according to Hahnemann's direction. It is of uncertain nature and strength. Probably, it is a weak solution of potassium hydrate.

Hahnemannian Technique of Preparation

(i) A piece of freshly burnt lime weighing about two pounds (1 kg) is immersed in purified water for one minute. It is then taken out of water and put in a dry cup. It pulverises itself into fine powder, giving out much heat.

(ii) 2 ounces (56 gm) of this powder is taken in a warm porcelain mortar and then 2 ounces of bi-sulphate of potash and 2 ounces of boiling purified water is mixed with it. The bi-sulphate of potash, before being dissolved is heated to a red heat, cooled and then pulverised.

(iii) This thick preparation is then taken in a glass retort, connected with a receiver dipped in water. The retort is heated gradually. The liquid that distills over is clear like water and measures about $1\frac{1}{2}$ ounce. This is Causticum in the concentrated form. It smells like potash lye and it has an astringent and burning taste. Causticum should not show any sign of the presence of sulphate when tested with solutions of the salts of Baryta and it should be free from any trace of lime-earth when tested with oxalate of ammonia.

Preparation

(a) *Tincture-θ* Drug strength

Causticum, in concentrated form	500 cc
Strong alcohol	500 cc

To make one thousand cubic centimetres of tincture.

(b) *Dilutions:* 2X and higher with dispensing alcohol.

(c) *Medications:* 2X and higher

Kali carbonicum

Chemical symbol: K_2CO_3

Synonyms: Potassium carbonate; Carbonate of Potassium; Kali carbonate; Pearl ash.

Description

(i) It is a dry, white, granular powder, or coarsely mass, or a white crystalline powder.

(ii) Odourless but having very strong alkaline taste.

(iii) It dissolves in dilute acids evolving CO_2 gas.

(iv) It is insoluble in alcohol but soluble in equal parts of water.

(v) It may be obtained from ashes of plants or by igniting nitrate of potash with powdered charcoal.

It can be obtained in pure state by heating the bicarbonate of potash.

Hahnemannian Technique of Preparation

(i) ½ ounce cream of tartar (potassium hydrogen tartarate) is moistened with little purified water and formed into a small ball, wrapped in filter paper and dried.

(ii) Then it is gradually heated to bright red by placing between the glowing coals or a good fire.

(iii) Next, the product is placed in a porcelain capsule, covered with linen and placed in a damp cellar for 2-3 weeks within which the last trace of calcareous earth would be precipitated.

Preparation

(a) *Triturations*

(i) A clear drop of the above preparation is used for making the 1st trituration according to Class VIII.

(ii) Decant the dissolved salt of the above preparation, add purified water, and filter; next evaporate to dryness, briskly stirring towards the closing of the process.

1 part by weight of the above is triturated with 99 parts of sugar of milk as per Class VII.

(b) *Liquid potencies:* According to Class VIII or Class VII as the case may be.

Calcarea carbonica

Chemical symbol: $CaCO_3$

Common name: Carbonate of lime; Impure carbonate of lime.

Synonyms: Calcarea carbonate of Hahnemann; Calcium carbonate of Hahnemann; Oyster shells.

Description: It is a fine white micro-crystalline powder, tasteless and odourless, almost insoluble in water, becomes slightly soluble in water containing carbon dioxide.

Hahnemannian Technique of Preparation

The drug substance which was used by Hahnemann was an impure carbonate of lime, as it exists in the oyster shell.

Clean, well-selected thick oyster shell is taken, and broken into small pieces in a wedgewood or porcelain mortar. The inner snow-white portions are carefully selected, next washed cautiously with purified water, dried over a water bath and powdered to a fine state.

Preparation

(a) *Triturations:* IX and upwards.

(b) *Dilutions:* Decimal and centesimal scale.

All the above preparations are made as directed under Class VII.

Carbo animalis

Common name: Animal charcoal.

Synonym: Leather charcoal; Carbon animal.

Preparation

(a) *Crude drug (Hahnemannian technique):* It may be prepared from thick cattle-leather (any animal or ox-hide). The hide is put on red-hot coals and allowed to burn with flame. As soon as the flame ceases, the red-hot mass is taken out and powdered by pressing between flat stones.

(b) *Powder θ*	Drug strength $^{1}/_{10}$
Animal charcoal	100 gm
Dry vehicle (sac lac)	900 gm

To make one thousand grams of powder.

(c) *Potencies:*

(i) *Trituraiton:* 2X and upwards

(ii) *Dilutions:* Decimal and centesimal scale.

Elaps corallinus

Zoo. name: Elaps corallinus.

Family: Elapidae

Common name: Coral snake, Coral viper.

Description

(i) The head of this snake is small, round and depressed with a short, broad muzzle but it has no neck.

(ii) It has sharp teeth, and the fangs stand alone in the upper jaw.

(iii) The body is covered with smooth scales, coloured to form bands of dark and deep red.

(iv) The rings of coloured bands are equi-distant.

(v) The length of the snake is about $2\frac{1}{2}$ feet (1 metre); it is very poisonous.

Distribution: Brazil

Parts used: The Venom.

Preparation

(a) *Mother solution*	Drug strength $^{1}/_{100}$
Coral snake venom	10 gm
Glycerine	990 ml

To make one thousand millilitres of the mother solution.

(b) *Dilution:* 3X and higher to contain one part solution, three parts purified water, and six parts glycerine.

In practice, all potencies above 6X are made with dispensing alcohol.

Mygale

Zoo. name: Mygale lasiodora.

Family: Mygalidae

Common name: Bird-spider.

Description: This is a kind of black spider. Its body is covered with brown hair. Generally, it feeds on ants and tiny birds.

Distribution: The spider is a native of Cuba, but it is also found in Texas and South America.

Parts used: The entire spider.

Preparation:

(a) *Tincture θ:*	Drug strength $^{1}/_{10}$ with dilute alcohol
Tin Mygale	100 gm
Purified water	525 cc
Strong alcohol	252 cc

To make one thousand cubic centimetres of tincture.

(b) *Dilutions:* 2X and higher with dispensing alcohol.

(c) *Medications:* 3X and higher.

Tarentula hispanica (Tarent. h)

Zoo name: Tarentula hispanica

Family: Lycosidae

Common name: Lycosa tarentula; Aranea tarentula.

Description

(i) Body stout, 3.8 - 5.1 cm long, colour greyish brown on upper surface, and deep saffron yellow on the under surface with a transverse black band.

(ii) A hairy-spider with six eyes and several pairs of legs, the third pair particularly being the shortest.

(iii) The margin of the thorax grey with a radiated dorsal line of the interior part of the dorsum, marked with triangular spots.

(iv) The poisons of the male and female are identical. The spider is most poisonous in July.

Distribution: South America and South Europe, especially Spain.

Parts used: The entire spider.

Caution: Poisonous, not to be prescribed below 3X.

Preparation

(a) *Tincture θ* Drug strength 1/10

Tarentula hispana	1 part
Purified water	3 parts
Glycerine	2 parts
Strong alcohol	5 parts

To make ten parts of Tincture.

(b) *Dilution:* 2X to contain one part tincture, four parts purified water, five parts alcohol; 3X and higher with dispensing alcohol.

(c) *Medication:* 3X and higher.

Tarentula cubensis

Zoo name: Tarentula cubensis

Family: Lycosidae

Common name: Cuban spider; C. tarentula.

Description: A large dark-brown hairy spider, found in Cuba and Mexico and belonging to the same family as T. hispana.

Parts used: The entire spider.

Preparation

(a) *Tincture θ* Drug strength 1/10

Tarentula cubensis	1 part
Purified water	3 parts
Glycerine	2 parts
Strong alcohol	5 parts

(b) *Dilutions:* 2X to contain one part tincture, four parts purified water and five parts alcohol; 3X and higher with dispensing alcohol.

(c) *Medications:* 3X and higher.

Chapter 16

Preparation of Medicines from Nosodes and Sarcodes

PREPARATION OF NOSODES

Introduction

Nosodes or biotherapeutic preparations are prepared from pure microbial culture obtained from diseased tissue, and clinical materials such as secretions, discharges etc. These are processed from original stock built from isolated microbes, diseased and clinical materials from whch the primary stocks are prepared.

Classification of Nosodes

Nosodes are divided into the four catagories, depending upon the nature of material used.

N-I: Preparations made from lysates of micro-organisms capable of producing bacterial endotoxins, e.g., Typhoidinum, paratyphoidinum, E. coli-bacillinum, Staphylococcinum.

N-II: Preparations made from micro-organisms capable of producing exotoxins, e.g., Diphterinum.

N-III: Preparations made from purified toxins.

N-IV: Preparations made from microorganisms/viruses/clinical materials from human convalescence or diseased subjects, e.g., Influenzinum, Morbillinum, Psorinum, Syphillinum and Variolinum.

General methods for Collection and Preparation of a Strain

1. Microbes available as pure organism, obtained from suitable clinical materials, from subjects suffering from the disease (comparatively virulent) are isolated, cultured, and identified.
2. Their properties are studied for complete identification and they are lyophilised (i.e., freeze-dry) to ensure preservation and stability of characteristics.
3. The culture media is prepared, most suitable for growth of the organism from which the homoeopathic nosode is to be prepared. Nutrient agar is usually recommended. In other instances, special solid culture media (enriched media) such as blood agar, serum agar are recommended. Freshly isolated organisms are recommended for use from which stock nosodes are made from recently isolated organisms only. If this is impractical, the culture should be kept below 50°C so that they retain their full antigenic value. Stock cultures are most often maintained in lyophilised state.

Repeated sub-cultures of the strain degenerates its antigenic value, and hence culture should be done from freshly isolated organisms.

4. Unless otherwise specified, the culture is allowed to incubate for 24 hours at 37°C. At the end of incubation, the microorganisms are harvested under aseptic conditions by pouring a sterile isotonic salt solution on the solid culture media, and then shaking or scraping until all the microorganisms have been suspended. If scraping is necessary, removal of culture media should be avoided.
5. The suspension is then centrifuged at 10,000 r.p.m. for 30 minutes. The supernatant fluid is discarded and bacterial pellets are resuspended in 0.9 per cent aqueous NaCl solution, shaken well and centrifuged again.
6. The suspension of bacteria is examined again for purity. It is essential that the purity of the strain is maintained during incubation, and handling. Purity is checked at different stages. In case of contamination, the lot is rejected and a fresh strain is used. After 24 hours of growth in incubation, colony is reexamined for checking the characteristics and purity of strain. The culture is then taken up in the 0.9 per cent aqueous NaCl solution.

Strength

The growth is suspended again in isotonic solution, shaken to break up the clumps and to make a uniform suspension. Number of bacteria in each ml of suspension is estimated, and is adjusted to 20 billion viable cells per millilitre. This forms the original stock in case of drugs of groups N-I and N-II. For group N-III and N-IV, the strength of IX should be 1 part of the pure material in 10 parts of the suspending/diluting material which may be sugar of milk or glycerine as suggested in individual monographs.

Preparation

Group N-I

Bacteriolysis of the suspension containing 20 billion viable cells per ml in distilled water is carried out by sonicator till most of the bacterial cells are ruptured. The material is centrifuged at 10,000 r.p.m. for 30 minutes. The supernatant fluid is filtered through a seitz filter (a bacterial filter made of asbestos), and the cell-free extract containing the endotoxin is treated with an equal volume of strong alcohol. This strength is sealed in a separate ampoule and is labelled as primary stock nosode. This serves as IX for preparation of homoeopathic dilutions. This is preserved at 4°C-6°C.

Group N-II

The toxigenicity of the strain is established before use. The suspension having 20 billion viable cells/ml is mixed with equal volume of strong alcohol and sealed under aseptic conditions. It is labelled as primary stock nosodes. This serves as 1X. This is preserved at 4°C-10°C. Further dilutions are made in dispensing alcohol in the ratio 1 : 9. This must comply with the test for sterility before being issued.

Group N-III

Preparations are made by trituration in sugar of milk with drug strength $\frac{1}{10}$. Attenuation up to 6X is kept in sealed ampoules, and stored in conditions prescribed under the individual monograph.

Group N-IV

Nosodes of this group are prepared as per Hahnemannian method of trituration, under Class IX, H.P.I., Vol. 1, P. 262.

Attenuation up to 6X should be stored between 4-6°C.

Notes:
1. In the above process, the centrifuge speed should not be below 10,000 r.p.m/minute, for 30 minutes.
2. The supernatant fluid should be filtered with a seitz filter.
3. No chemicals, antiseptic or bacteriostatic should be mixed with the material during preparation process. In cases where normal saline solution is used, full care should be taken to completely remove the same before attenuations.
4. All the products and potencies below 6X should be preserved in a refrigerator at 4°C-6°C.
5. The organisms should be handled with care, following aseptic conditions.
6. Bacterial count means total number of organisms/ml (live or dead).
7. The substance used in the original proving should be taken as the starting raw material, as far as possible.

8. To check the hygienic condition of the laboratory, plate count should be done from time to time.
9. Test for sterility, of both aerobic and anaerobic organisms should be made, before issue of any nosode, as per I. P. 1964.
10. All potencies below 3X of group N-I, N-II and N-III, should bear the date of manufacture and a life period of six months from the date of manufacture.

PREPARATION OF SARCODES

Sarcodes are obtained from healthy endocrine and exocrine glands, tissues, normal secretions and extracts especially of animals such as pigs, sheep or cattle. They are prepared as per homoeopathic specifications, provided that the basic substance is not altered and the final product is not adulterated by any pathogen or other deleterious substance. For collection and preparation, refer to the individual monograph.

Potentisation (Succussion)

(a) **Decimal Scale**

The fresh source material is coarsely ground. 1 part of it is combined with 9 parts of glycerine (85%) and homogeneously dispersed and succussed with ten equal and uniform downward strokes to produce 1X potency. It may be filtered if necessary.

1 part of the 1X potency and 9 parts of glycerine (85%) give 2X potency.

All succeeding potencies are prepared by taking 1 part of the preceding potency and 9 parts of diluent.

(b) **Centesimal Scale**

The fresh source material is coarsely ground. 1 part of it is combined with 99 parts of glycerine (85%) and homogeneously dispersed and succussed with ten equal and uniform downward strokes to produce 1C potency. It may be filtered if necessary.

1 part of the 1C potency and 99 parts of diluent give 2C potency.

All succeeding potencies are prepared by taking 1 part of the preceding potency and 99 parts of diluent.

Chapter 17

Methods of Preparation as per Homoeopathic Pharmacopoeia of United States (H.P.U.S.)

H.P.U.S. is the official and recognised pharmacopoeia in America. Homoeopathic preparation of mother tinctures and dilutions are done in the following headings:

1. **Liquid preparations of Drugs**
2. **Tinctures or Alcoholic solutions**
   A. Tinctures of Botanical substances
      (a) Maceration
      (b) Percolation
      (c) Incubation
      (d) Infusion
      (e) Decoction
      (f) Succus or Non-alcoholic solutions
      (g) Fermentation.
   B. Tinctures of Zoological substances
3. **Attenuations**
   (a) Decimal scale of attenuation
   (b) Centesimal scale of attenuation
4. **Liquid attenuations**
5. **Solid attenuations:** Triturations
6. **Attenuations from Microscopic fungal strains.**

1. Liquid preparations of Drugs

All substances soluble in vehicles are to be made into solutions or tinctures and their attenuations. But such moist and/or soluble substances may also be made into triturations with sugar of milk. All insoluble substances or partially soluble substances, below 8X, should be made into triturations only.

The first solution or tincture is made in the proportion of $\frac{1}{10}$ in water or alcohol of suitable strength, unless otherwise specified in the monograph.

Aqueous solutions are made of substances which are soluble in water, but insoluble in alcohol, or of those which, when soluble in alcohol, are subject to chemical change or decomposition. Aqueous solutions are unstable, and will keep but a short time.

Solutions of chemical substances are to be made on the decimal scale, where ratio is 1 : 9 i.e., 1 part by weight of soluble medicinal substance (solid or liquid) is mixed with 9 part solvent, and hence equal to 1X.

If not soluble in the proportion of 1 to 10, they should be made by adding 1 part by weight of medicinal substance to 99 parts by volume of solvent to make one hundred (100), and the solution marked 2X (or 1C).

If liquid substances contain water, this also should be deducted from that contained in the solvent, and the anhydrous substance taken as the unit of strength.

2. Tinctures or Alcoholic solutions

Most of the Homoeopathic Medicines can be prepared in the form of mother tinctures from botanical or zoological substances, which are wholly or partially soluble in alcohol.

A. Tinctures of Botanical Substances

Botanical substances comprise of plants or their parts. The mother tincture should be of uniform strength, though water content varies greatly, even in the same species of plants.

Fresh succulent plants and other substances containing water should be treated as follows: The dry crude material is taken as the starting point from which the strength of tincture is calculated.

Plant moisture is to be determined and proper allowance made in preparation of the solvent (or menstrua).

The dry crude material remaining after evaporation is taken as the unit of strength, the tincture being made to represent:

1 part by weight of dry crude matrial, in 10 parts by value of completed solution. In some cases, the tincture represents—1 part by weight of dry crude material, in 20 parts by volume of completed solution, or as otherwise specified in the monograph.

After determination of amount of moisture content in fresh moist material, the amount of strong alcohol and purified water to be added is calculated, according to the following general rules:

1. Tinctures with an alcohol content of 90% v/v: when the plant-substance is a gum or resin, or when it contains volatile oils, provided the moisture content is less than 42% (e.g.. *Asafoetida*).
2. Tinctures with an alcohol content of 65% v/v: when the plant-substance contains volatile oils, tanins or alkaloids, provided the moisture content is less than 79% (e.g., *Millefolium*, *Cinchona officinalis*).
3. Tinctures with an alcohol content of 55% v/v: when the plant substance contains volatile oils, tanins or alkaloids, provided the moisture content is not less than 83% (e.g., *Berb. vulgaris*, *Cynara scolymus*).
4. Tinctures with an alcohol content of 45% v/v: when the plant substance contains mucilage, sugars etc., provided the moisture content is less than 85% (e.g. *Allium cepa*).
5. Tinctures with an alcohol content of 35% v/v: when specified in the individual monograph (e.g. *Avena sativa*).

Plant substances with a moisture content more than 85%, such as mushrooms, succulent plants or fruits (e.g. *Citus limonum*) or fleshy roots (e.g., *Raphanus sativus*), cannot be used for preparing $\frac{1}{10}$ tinctures, as the alcohol content of such tinctures would not be high enough to enable them to be stored. Tinctures of such substances are therefore prepared with a drug content of $\frac{1}{20}$, and will be so noted in the appropriate monograph.

A tolerance of +/_ 5% of the stated alcohol strength is permissible.

Calculations of quantities of strong alcohol and purified water to be added to obtain a tincture at the desired alcohol strength.

—Tinctures at $\frac{1}{10}$: $A = DD - a$

$W = (DD - 10) - A - M$

—Tinctures at $\frac{1}{20}$: $A = DD - a - 2$

$W = (DD - 20) - A - M$

DD = weight of dry drug in the fresh moist material = weight of the moisture.

A = weight of strong alcohol to be added.

W = volume or weight of water to be added.

a = coefficient included in the following table:

Alcohol content of the tincture	Coefficient (W/W)
90% v/v	a = 9.27
65% v/v	a = 6.19
55% v/v	a = 5.11
45% v/v	a = 4.10
35% v/v	a = 3.13

The preparation of tinctures then is continued according to one of the following processes of maceration or percolation:

(a) Maceration

This process is effective for the treatment of large quantities of drug materials which require long time for the extraction of medicinal properties.

Hard, gummy, and mucilaginous substances, or those having much viscid juice, which do not allow the alcohol to penetrate or permeate rapidly due to the smallness of intermolecular space, as in the process of percolation, are immersed in strong alcohol for a definite period of time, as per H.P.U.S.

Moisture content of the drug substances is calculated with the help of water bath.

The drug substances are made into a pulp (magma, or in its natural state if not reducible). The pulp (magma) is placed in a macerating jar. The required quantity of alcohol is added to cover the whole mass of drug substance. The macerating jar is carefully corked or sealed in order to prevent evaporation. The jar is kept in a cool dark place, at temperature 15°C–20°C, for 2–4 weeks.

Note: The time required for proper extraction of medicinal substance varies considerably, it is, therefore, safe to allow the process of maceration to continue 2–4 weeks according to the nature of drug material.

The jar is powerfully shaken once daily. After the lapse of this period, the supernatant fluid is decanted off in another glass-stoppered bottle. The residue is pressed out and triturated in clean porcelain mortar, and double the quantity of green glass powder is added to it. It is then thoroughly pulverised by a pestle. The pulp is now placed over the filter bed of a percolator, and percolated by that quantity of strong alcohol which was not used before. The resulting tincture, is mixed with the previously prepared tincture. It is filtered by a filtered paper, and stored in a glass-stoppered bottle, in cool dark place.

(b) **Percolation**

This method is preferred for the extraction of dried substances that have been reduced to the proper degree of fineness.

The dried materials is carefully weighed and the menstrum is prepared as prescribed in the monograph under 'preparation and classification'.

The ground substance is carefully mixed with sufficient quantity of this menstrum and transferred to a suitable percolator. Then it is allowed to stand for 1 hour and packed firmly in the percolator. The percolator should be provided with a stop-cock to control the flow through the unit. A plug of absorbent cotton is inserted into the neck above the stop-cock, and covered with a suitable filter medium.

The powdered substances are firstly moistened with a portion of the menstrum, gradually, evenly upon the filter, and the mass pressed down with a broad, inert tamper. The surface of the mass is covered with a disc of filter paper. While holding down the mass by suitable means, the solvent is poured upon the contents of the percolator until the mass is covered, allowing the fluid to run gently down the rod so that the filter medium may not be displaced. The percolator is covered to prevent evaporation. The stop-cock is closed as soon as the fluid begins to drop, and allowed to stand 24 hours or longer, according to the nature of contents.

The fluid is allowed to pass through the percolator into the reciever, drop by drop, regulating it by means of the stop-cock so as to limit the flow to 10 to 30 drops per minute.

The menstrum should be cautiously and frequently added, so as to maintain a surface above the powder, thereby preventing access of air. The process is continued until the requisite quantity has passed into the receiver.

(c) **Incubation**

This process is applicable where drug materials required prolonged time for extraction, and where due to gradual rise of temperature complex carbohydrates break up into simple sugars.

Amount of moisture is calculated according to the rules in the H.P.U.S. The drug materials (reduced to magma or in its natural state if not reducible) are placed into a macerating jar or wide-mouthed bottle, required quantity of solvent is added to it and then the whole mass is covered, if possible.

The jar or bottle should be well corked or sealed to prevent evaporation, and heated at 37°C, kept for one hour. After cooling, the jar or bottle should be placed in a dark room at normal temperature and shaken at appropriate intervals. The time required for extraction and solution of the medicinal substance is variable, and it is safe to allow the further process of maceration to continue from 2–4 weeks. Thereafter decant the clear fluid and press out the residue.

All tinctures made by this process and all attenuations prepared from these tinctures must have the term 'incubation' on all labelling as a part of the name of the drug, just before the designation of the homoeopathic strength.

(d) Infusion

This process can be preferable in the treatment of dried plant materials containing large amount of aromatic principles.

The dried materials are carefully weighed and the amount of alcohol and water are calculated. The drug materials and alcohol are placed in a suitable container and allowed to stand for 15 minutes. After this time the water, previously heated to boiling, is poured over the preparation, and, under a reflux condenser, the entire mass is maintained at the boiling point for 5 minutes. After cooling, the container should be placed in a dark room at normal temperature and shaken at appropriate intervals. The time required for extraction and solution of the medicinal substances is variable, and it is safe to allow the further process of maceration to continue 2–4 weeks. Thereupon, decant the clear fluid and press out the residue.

All tinctures made by this process, and all attenuations prepared from these tinctures, must have the term 'infusion' on all labelling as a part of the name of the drug, just before the designation of the homoeopathic strength.

(e) Decoction

This process can be preferable in the treatment of fibrous drug materials, such as roots, barks, and woody substances.

The dried materials are carefully weighed and the amount of menstrum are calculated. The drug material and the menstrum are placed in a suitable well-stoppered container, and allowed to stand overnight. After this time, the entire mass is heated, under a reflux condenser and maintained at the boling point for 30 minutes. After cooling, the container should be well-stoppered and placed in a dark room at normal temperature, and shaken at appropriate intervals. The time required for extraction and solution of the medicinal substance is variable, and it is safe to allow the further process of maceration to continue 2–4 weeks. Thereupon, decant the clear fluid and press out the residue.

All tinctures made by this process, and all attenuations prepared from these tinctures must have the term 'decoction' on all labelling as a part of the name of the drug, just before the designation of the homoeopathic strength.

(f) Succus or Non-alcoholic solutions

Some drugs are prepared by the process of succus, as specified in the monograph. The succus may be used for oral, ophthalmic, or topical route, administration. Their preparation should strictly follow the guidelines of H.P.U.S. Two methods are adopted for preparation of tinctures:

(i) Succus-expressed: The fresh plant or parts thereof are chopped and pounded to a pulp. The pulp is then subjected to a pressure and the expressed juice collected in a clean container. The juice is then mixed with equal parts by weight of diluent (water, alcohol; etc.). The mixture is allowed to stand for 8 days or more. Then the liquid is decanted and filtered.

(ii) Succus-tapped: The exudations of living plants are collected by puncturing the bark or incising the plant part to be drained. The exudations are allowed to thicken. The inspisated juice is then processed as specified in the particular monograph.

All tinctures prepared by this process and all attenuations prepared from the tinctures must bear the term 'succus' on all labelling as part of the name of the drug just before the designation of the homoeopathic strength

(g) Fermentation

This process is preferable in the treatment of plant materials when the desired end product tincture should contain a minimal amount of ethanol or be alcohol-free. Thus, the normal dissolving action of ethanol, in the extraction of plant tincture must be replaced by the breaking down activity of the fermentation process. Either a lactic acid fermentation or an ethanolic fermentation can be used with suitable fermentation starters and aids.

B. Tinctures of Zoological Substances

Zoological substances comprise of living or dried insects or other animals, or parts of animals.

Tinctures of zoological substances are prepared by maceration in alcohol at 65% v/v, except in some cases specified in the monographs. These tinctures are made to represent 1 part by weight of the crude material in 20 parts by weight of completed solution.

The preparation of these tinctures is made according to the following process of maceration: The crude material is suitably divided and placed into the quantities of alchol, and water calculated to obtain a $\frac{1}{20}$ tincture with an alcohol strength of 65% v/v. The maceration process allowed to continue for not less than three weeks and shaken sufficiently. After decantation, the fluids are allowed to stand for 48 hours, and then filtered.

The tinctures obtained from maceration or percolation process from plant or animal substnaces are filtered and kept in a glass stoppered bottle, marked with the sign Q. Except in special cases specified in the monographs. The shelf life of the tincture is five years from the manufacturing date. The shelf life shall apply only to the tincture as a finished dosage form, and not to any subsequent dilution or product prepared from it.

Mother tincture should undergo analytical assay for proper standardisation and quality control before use.

3. Attenuations

The Pharmacopoeia Convention Committee of United States adopts three scales of attenuations—decimal, centesimal and 50 millesimal—under which each successive attenuation or trituration contains just $\frac{1}{10}$, $\frac{1}{100}$, and $\frac{1}{50,000}$ as much the drug substance as the preceding attenuation or trituration.

(a) Decimal Scale

1 ml of tincture, 1 ml of 1X aqueous solution, or 1 gm of 1X trituration represents 0.1 gm of dry crude medicinal substance.

1 ml of 2X attenuation, or 1 gm of 2nd trituration contains 0.01 gm of the dry crude medicinal substance.

Subsequent liquid or solid attenuations are prepared by serial progression, successing or triturating 1 part of preceding attenuation to 9 parts of the vehicle, and represents the following proportions of active principle (i.e., dried medicinal substance):

$2X = 10^{-2}$
$3X = 10^{-3}$
$4X = 10^{-4}$
$5X = 10^{-5}$
$6X = 10^{-6}$
$7X = 10^{-7}$
$8X = 10^{-8}$

(b) Centesimal Scale

1 ml of 1st centesimal liquid attenuation (1C) or 1 gm of 1st centesimal trituration (1C) represents 0.01 gm of dry crude medicinal substance.

1 ml of 2nd centesimal liquid attenuation (2C) or 1 gm of 2nd centesimal trituratiion (2C) represents 0.1 mg of dry crude medicinal substance.

Subsequent liquid or solid attenuations are prepared by serial progression, successing or triturating, 1 part of the preceding attenuation to 99 part of the vehicle, and represent the following proportions of active principle (i.e., dried medicinal substances):

$2C = 10^{-4}$
$3C = 10^{-6}$
$4C = 10^{-8}$

(c) 50-Millesimal Scale

1 ml of 1st 50-Millesimal attenuation (1 LM) represents 4.0×10^{-9} gm of dry crude medicinal substance.

1 ml of 2nd 50-Millesimal attenuation (2 LM) represents 8.0×10^{-4} gm of dry crude medicinal substance.

Method of Preparation

1. For solid substances, 3C trituration are prepared under centesimal scale. Initially, for liquid substances, sugar of milk is impregnated with liquid substance (mother tincture) in a proportion of 1 : 100. The 2nd and 3rd triturations are carried out in the same way as when starting with solid products.
2. 0.062 gm of 3C trituration is added to 500 drops of a mixture, composed of 1 part 95% v/v alcohol, and 4 parts purified water.
3. 1 drop from the result of step 2, mixed to 2 ml of 95% v/v alcohol and successed. The result is 1 LM.
4. 1 drop of the 1 LM poured on 0.575 gm # 10 pellets (500 # 10 pellets). 1 pellet from it is taken and dissolved in 2 ml of 95% v/v alcohol and successed. The result is 2 LM.

5. 1 drop of the 2 LM poured on 0.575 gm > # 10 pellets (500 # 10 pellets). 1 pellet from it is taken and dissolved in 2 ml of 95% v/v alcohol and succussed. The result is 3 LM.

4. Liquid Attenuations

- **Decimal scale:** In this scale, the original quantity of medicine is divided progressively by ten, so that first decimal (1X) contains $1/10$, the second decimal 2X) $1/100$, and the third decimal (3X) $1/1000$ of the oroginal substance suspended in, and attenuated or expanded by, the diluent (alcohol, water etc.) Each tincture (with some exceptions to be stated) is equal or equivalent in medicinal strength to the first decimal attenuation ($1/10$), designated as 1X.

Substances which are insoluble in the proportion of 1 to 10 and require more solvent (e.g., Ars. alb, Phos., Sulph.) their original solution shall be prepared in accordance with the respective monographs.

- **Centesimal Scale:** In this scale, the 1X solution or tincture is divided by 10 to produce the first centesimal (1C), then by 100 to produce each succeeding attenuation, 2C, 3C, 4C, etc.

Designations: Homoeopathic liquid attenuations are designated according to the method of attenuation. The designations, which must appear on the labels, are shown in the following table:

Designation	Scale	Method of attenuation
X or D	Decimal ($1/10$)	Hahnemannian
CH or C	Centesimal ($1/100$)	Hahnemannian
CK or K	Centesimal ($1/100$)	Korsakovian
LM	50-Millesimal ($1/50,000$)	Hahnemannian

- **Designation for decimal attenuation:** The preferred designation is X, which clearly indicate the scale used. All decimal attenuations are prepared according to Hahnemannian method.
- **Designation for Hahnemannian centesimal attenuation:** The preferred designation is CH, which clearly indicates both the scale used and the method of attenaution. As C is a synonym of CH, it can be only used to designate an attenuation that is prepared according to the Hahnemannian method.
- **Designation for Korsakovian centesimal attenuation:** The preferred designation is CK which clearly indicates both the scale used and the method of attenuation.
- The designatiion M refers to neither scale nor method of attenuation. M is equivalent to 1,000 and is used in place of the numeral 1,000 in Korsakovian centesimal attenuations. For example, 1M indicates a 1,000 CK attenuation, 10M indicates a 10,000 CK attenuation.

(a) **Hahnemannian attenuations:** Multiple flask method. A new well-cleaned glass-stoppered bottle of appropriate capacity is employed.

1 part (e.g. 10 ml mother tincture or 1X solution) is poured into this bottle. 9 parts (e.g. 90 ml) of diluent is added. This mixture is succussed thoroughly and labelled 2X.

10 ml of 2X attenuation is taken in a new, well-cleaned glass-stoppered bottle and 90 ml of diluent is added. This mixture is succussed thoroughly and labelled 3X.

(b) **Korsakovian attenuation:** Single flask method. A new well-cleaned glass-stoppered bottle of appropriate capacity is employed.

A measured volume of the tincture is added to the bottle. After thorough succussion of the bottle, it is emptied by turning it upside down or by suction. The emptying process employed must remove 99% of the original volume of the tincture, leaving 1% of the original volume in the bottle.

99 parts of diluent added to the 1 part tincture remaining in the bottle and thoroughly succussed. The resulting solution is the first Korsakovian attenuation (1 CK).

The bottle emptied once more. 99 parts of diluent added to the 1 part of the 1 CK remedy and thoroughly succussed. The resulting solution is the second Korsakovian attenuation (2 CK).

5. Solid Attenuations: Triturations

Attenuations of solid substances are prepared by trituration of the crude substance with sugar of milk, in a mortar and pestle for small amounts or in a mechanical triturator for large amounts, in the proportion of 1 part by weight of the crude substance, and 9 parts by weight of sugar of milk to produce the 1X trituration.

As with liquid attenuations, in the decimal scale, each step is accomplished by triturating 1 part of the original attenuation with 9 parts of sugar of milk. In the centesimal scale, 1 part by weight of the 1X trituration is triturated with 9 parts by weight of sugar of milk to produce the 1C trituration, then is divided by 100 to produce each succeeding trituration 2C, 3C, 4C etc.

Triturations may be dispensed in the form of powders or tablet triturates, either of which may be dissolved or mixed aqueous solutions.

6. Attenuations from Microscopic Fungal Strains

Given the risk of contamination during handling of fungal strains, these attenuations are prepared under a laminar flow hood.

- **Equipment for Each Strain** (to be sterilised the day before in a drying oven, for 1 hour at 150°C):

15 ml bottle	1
250 ml bottle	2
500 ml bottle	2
1 litre bottle	1
No. 3 sintered glass-funnel	1

- **Additional Equipment**

1.	A big jar filled with bleach in which the 15 ml bottle, 500 ml bottle, and sintered glass-funnel can be placed	1
2.	60 ml bottle of 30% v/v alcohol	1
3.	1 litre bottle of 70% v/v alcohol	1
4.	Platinum handle	1

Preparation of the 1C attenuation

5 ml alcohol (30% v/v) is placed in a 15 ml bottle. Then the carded cotton is placed near the burner. The culture tube is taken and, using pliers, the stopper is removed, close to the flame of a Bunsen burner.

Firstly, the platinum handle along its entire length are flamed and allowed to cool. Then it is used to scrape as much culture as possible and then put into the 15 ml bottle, while trying to crush the strain against the sides of the bottle in order to obtain a homogeneous suspension. Then the stopper is placed on the 15 ml bottle.

The platinum is flamed again. It should be passed through the flame in a horrizontal position, from left to right. This should be done slowly to avoid spluttering the strain.

By using the metal tongs, the carded cotton is flamed. The 15 ml bottle is potentised. The 1C attenuation is obtained.

Preparation of the 2C attenuation

400 ml (70% v/v) are placed in a 500 ml bottle. Then the 5 ml of the 1C fungal strain suspension is added. The 15 ml bottle is placed in the jar of bleach. It is not necessary to rinse the 15 ml bottle, containing the suspension.

The stopper and the rim of the 500 ml bottle are wiped with an alcohol-soaked piece of cotton to remove any possible fungal suspension.

Chapter 18

Methods of Preparation as per German Homoeopathic Pharmacopoeia (G.H.P.)

Different pharmaceutical methods are adopted as per German Homoeopathic Pharmacopoeia (GHP/HAB) for the manufacture of basic homoeopathic potencies and their dilutions.

Method 1: Mother tinctures and liquid dilutions

Principle: The tincture is prepared by adding equal part of ethyl alcohol (86%) and expressed juice of plant.

Procedure: The fresh plant is cut into pieces with a well-polished steel knife. The expressed juice is mixed with equal quantity by weight of ethyl alcohol (86%). The mixture is shaken, and put into a well-stoppered bottle and allowed to stand for not less than 5 days at a temperature not exceedig 20°C and is then filtered.

Dry residue or solid content of the above filtrate is determined. The amount of ethyl alcohol (43%) required is calculated by using the formula

$$E_1 \text{ (Ethyl alcohol \%)} = \frac{W(N_x - N_0)}{100} \text{ (kg)}$$

W = Weight of filtrate in kg.

N_0 = Dry residue or solid conent in per cent as required by monograph.

N_x = Dry residue or solid content of filtrate in per cent.

The filtrate is mixed with the required amount of ethyl alcohol (43%), and allowed to stand in a closed container for not less than 5 days at a temperature not exceeding 20°C and is then filtered.

Potentisation (Succussion)

(a) Decimal scale: 2 parts of the mother tincture and 8 parts of ethanol (43%) are mixed and 10 downward strokes of equal strength are given. It gives the 1X potency.

1 part of 1X potency and 9 parts of ethyl alcohol (43%) will give the 2X potency.

All succeeding potencies are prepared in the same way.

(b) Centesimal scale: 2 parts of the mother tincture and 98 parts of ethanol (43%) are mixed and 10 downward strokes of equal strength are given. It gives 1C potency.

1 part of 1C potency and 99 parts of ethyl alcohol (43%) will give 2C potency.

All succeeding potencies are prepared in the same way.

Method 2(a): Mother tinctures and liquid dilutions

Mother tinctures are prepared by the process of maceration.

The plants or parts of plants are finely minced. A sample is used to determine loss on drying.

The minced plant-material is mixed with not less than half the amount by weight of ethanol (86%), and stored in well sealed bottles at a temperature not exceeding 20°C.

The amount of ethanol (86%) required for the plant-material is calculated by formula and deducting the amount of ethanol, that has already been used, and adding the final amount to the mixture:

$$E_2 \text{ (Ethyl alcohol \%)} = \frac{MD}{100} \text{ (kg)}$$

M = Weight of plant-material in kg.

D = Loss on drying in sample, in per cent.

The mixture is then allowed to stand for not less than 10 days at a temperature not exceeding 20°C, and is then filtered.

Potentisation (Succussion)

Same as Method 1.

Method 2(b): Mother tinctures and liquid dilutions

Mother tinctures are prepared as per Method 2(a), using ethanol 62% (Ethanol content is approximately 30%). Ethanol (30%) is used to adjust to any concentration required as per monograph.

Potentisation

Decimal scale: 2 parts of the mother tincture and 8 parts of ethanol (30%) are mixed, and then it produces 1X potency.

1 part of 1X potency and 9 parts of ethanol (15%) will give the 2X potency.

All succeeding potencies are prepared in the same way.

Method 3(a): Mother tinctures and liquid dilutions

Mother tinctures are prepared as per Method 2(a) (ethanol content approximately 60%), with the following difference: The amount of ethanol (86%) required for the plant-material is calculated, by using the formula

$$E_3 \text{ (Ethyl alcohol \%)} = \frac{2MD}{100} \text{ (kg)}$$

M = Weight of plant-material in kg.

D = Loss on drying in sample, in per cent.

Ethanol (62%) is used to adjust to any concentration required as per monograph.

Potentisation

(a) Decimal scale: 3 parts of the mother tincture and 7 parts of ethanol (62%) are mixed and produce 1X potency.

1 part of 1X potency and 9 parts of ethanol (62%) will give the 2X potency.

All succeeding potencies are prepared in the same way. For potencies from 4X onwards, ethanol (43%) are used.

(b) Contesimal scale: 3 parts of the mother tincture and 97 parts of ethanol (62%) are mixed and produce 1C potency.

1 part of 1C potency and 99 parts of ethanol (43%) will give the 2C potency.

All succeeding potencies are prepared in the same way.

Method 3(b): Mother tinctures and liquid dilutions

Mother tinctures are prepared as per Method 2(a), using ethanol (73%). (Ethanol content is approximately 43%).

Ethanol (43%) is used to adjust to any concentration required as per monograph.

Potentisation

Decimal scale: 3 parts of the mother tincture and 7 parts of ethanol (43%) are mixed and produces 1X potency.

1 part of 1X potency and 9 parts of ethanol (15%) will give the 2X potency.

All succeeding potencies are prepared in the same way.

Method 3(c): Mother tinctures and liquid dilutions

Mother tinctures are prepared as per Method 2(a), using ethanol (43%). (Ethanol content is approximately 30%).

Ethanol (30%) is used to adjust to any concentration required as per monograph.

Potentisation

Decimal scale: 3 parts of the mother tincture and 7 parts of ethanol (30%) are mixed and produce 1X potency.

1 part of 1X potency and 9 parts of ethanol (15%) will give the 2X potency.

All succeeding potencies are prepared in the same way.

Method 4(a): Mother tinctures and liquid dilutions

Mother tinctures are prepared by the method of maceration, or percolation as described in the monograph of G.H.P.

1 part of the drug mixed with 10 parts of ethanol (unless otherwise stated in the monograph). If adjustment to a given value is necessary, the required amount of ethanol in the concentration used for manufacture is calculated according to the formula in Method 1. The calculated amount of ethanol is combined with the filtrate.

The mixture is then allowed to stand for not less than 5 days at a temperature not exceeding 20°C, and is then filtered.

Potentisation

(a) Decimal scale: The mother tincture is equivalent to 1X potency.

1 part of 1X potency and 9 parts of ethanol of the same concentration will give the 2X potency.

1 part of 2X potency and 9 parts of ethanol of the same concentration will give the 3X potency.

All succeeding potencies are prepared by mixing 1 part of the previous potency with 9 parts of ethanol (43%).

(b) Centesimal scale: 10 parts of the mother tincture and 90 parts of ethanol in the same concentration are mixed and produce 1C potency.

1 part of 1C potency and 99 parts of ethanol (43%) will give the 2C potency.

All succeeding potencies are prepared in the same way.

Method 4(b): Mother tinctures and liquid dilutions

Mother tinctures are prepared by the process of maceration or percolation as described in the monograph of G.H.P.

1 part of animal, part of animal or animal secretion is mixed with 10 parts of ethanol in suitable concentration. If adjustment to a given value is necessary, the required amount of ethanol in the concentration used for manufacture is calculated according to the formula in Method 1. The calculated amount of ethanol is combined with the filtrate.

The mixture is then allowed to stand for not less than 5 days at a temperature not exceeding 20°C, and is then filtered.

Potentisation

(a) Decimal scale: The mother tincture is equivalent to 1X.

1 part of 1X potency and 9 parts of ethanol of the same concentration will give the 2X potency.

1 part of 1X potency and 9 parts of ethanol of the same concentration will give the 2X potency.

1 part of 2X potency and 9 parts of ethanol of the same concentration will give the 3X potency.

All succeeding potencies are prepared by mixing 1 part of the previous potency with 9 parts of ethanol (43%).

(b) Centesimal scale: 10 parts of the mother tincture and 90 parts of ethanol in the same concentration are mixed and produce 1C potency.

1 part of 1C potency and 99 parts of ethanol (43%) will give the 2C potency.

All succeeding potencies are prepared in the same way.

Method 5(a): Solutions

Solutions are prepared from basic drug materials and a liquid vehicle.

Unless otherwise mentioned in the monograph, 1 part of basic drug materials is dissolved in 9 parts (= 1X) or 99 parts (= 1C or 2X) of the liquid vehicle and succussed. Absolute alcohol, purified water, glycerine (85%) and ethanol-water mixtures listed in the G.H.P. are used as vehicles.

If ethanol (15%) is the prescribed vehicle for the liquid preparations, the solution may also be produced by the following method:

1 part of the basic drug material is dissolved in 7.58 parts of purified water, to produce the 1X; 1.42 parts of ethanol is added to the solution.

1 part of the basic drug material is dissolved in 83.4 parts of purified water; 15.6 parts of ethanol is added to the solution.

Potentisation

(a) Decimal scale: 1 part of the mother tincture and 9 parts of ethanol (43%) are mixed and produce 2X potency (unless another vehicle is prescribed).

All succeeding potencies are prepared in the same way.

(b) Centesimal scale: 1 part of the 1C potency and 99 parts of ethanol (43%) are mixed and produce 2C potency (unless another vehicle is prescribed).

All succeeding potencies are prepared in the same way.

Method 5(b): Aqueous solutions

Solutions are made from basic drug materials and water for injections.

Unless otherwise mentioned in the monograph, 1 part of basic drug materials is mixed with 9 parts (= 1X) or 99 parts (= 1C or 2X) of water for injections and succussed.

Potentisation

Decimal scale: 1 part of the solution (1X) and 9 parts of water for injections are mixed and produce 2X potency.

Method 6: Triturations

By this method, trituration of basic drug materials are done, using sugar of milk as vehicle.

Trituration up to 4th dilution, by hand or machine are done in 1 : 10 or 1 : 100 ratio. Unless otherwise stated, the basic drug materials are reduced to the particle size given in the monograph. Quantities of more than 1 kg are triturated by mechanical means.

The duration and intensity of trituration should be such, that the resulting particle size of the basic drug materials in the 1X or 1C potency is below 10 μm at 80% level; no drug particle should be more than 50 μm.

Trituration up to and including the 4X or 4C are produced at the same duration and intensity of trituration.

Trituration by Hand

The sugar of milk is divided into three parts, and first part triturated in porcelain mortar. The basic drug material is added to it, and triturated for 6 minutes, followed by scraping for 4 minutes with porcelain spatula. Further trituration done for 6 minutes and scraping for 4 minutes.

The second part of sugar of milk is added to it, and triturated for 20 minutes as above.

The third part of sugar of milk added at the end of 40 minutes, and triturated in the same way. Total duration of trituration more or less 60 minutes (or one hour).

All succeeding potencies are prepared in the same way.

For trituration above 4X or 4C, 1 part of the previous potency mixed with 9 parts (in Decimal scale) or 99 parts (in Centesimal scale) of sugar of milk.

Trituration by Machine

Trituration up to 4th dilution made in a machine fitted with a scraping device.

By this method, ⅓rd part of sugar of milk is added to the basic drug material and triturated. Finally, the remaining sugar of milk is added in two equal portions and triturated.

Total duration for whole trituration process is 60 minutes (or one hour).

Trituration above 4X or 4C, 1 part of the previous potency mixed with 9 parts (in decimal scale) or 99 parts (in centesimal scale) of sugar of milk.

Method 7: Triturations

By this method, trituration of mother tinctures and solutions are done, using sugar of milk as vehicle.

The total amount of sugar of milk required is transferred to a suitable apparatus, and the prescribed amount of liquid preparation in the previous dilution stage is gradually mixed in. The moist homogeneous mixture is dried with care, grounded if necessary, and sieved before mixing again thoroughly.

The amount of sugar of milk used should be such that the preparation will have the prescribed total weight when the manufacturing process is complete.

For the preparation more than 1 kg, done by mechanical trituration: the type of mixer, mixing period, drying time, and length of the final mixing stage are determined in a single trial run, recorded and written down in the operating instructions for the production process.

Potentisation

Mother tinctures, solutions, and liquid dilutions are potentised in the relative quantities laid down for their production. Sugar of milk serves as the vehicle.

The amount of sugar of milk added must be such that the total weight is 10 parts for decimal and 100 parts for centesimal potencies.

Method 8(a): Liquid preparations made from triturations

Liquid dilutions from trituration done by Method 6.

(a) Decimal scale: To produce 6X liquid dilution, 1 part of the 4X trituration is dissolved in 9 parts of purified water and successed.

1 part of this dilution is mixed with 9 parts of ethanol (30%) to produce the 6X liquid dilution by succussion. The 7X liquid dilution is made from 5X trituration.

In the same way, 8X liquid dilutions are made from 6X trituration. For 9X liquid dilutions or above, 1 part of the previous potency mixed with 10 parts ethanol (43%).

(b) Centesimal scale: To produce 6C liquid dilution, 1 part of the 4C trituration is dissolved in 99 parts of purified water and successed.

1 part of this dilution is mixed with 99 parts of ethanol (30%) to produce the 6C liquid dilution by succussion.

The 7C liquid dilution is made from the 5C trituration. In the same way, 8C liquid dilution is made from 6C trituration.

For 9C liquid dilutions or above, 1 part of the previous potency mixed with 100 parts of ethanol (43%). The 6X, 7X, 6C and 7C liquid dilutions prepared by the above method must not be used to produce further liquid dilutions.

Method 8(b): Aqueous preparations made from triturations

Aqueous preparations made from trituration by the Method 6.

To produce a 6X liquid dilution, 1 part of the 4X trituration is dissolved in 9 parts of water for injections and successed.

1 part of this dilution is mixed with 9 parts of water for injections to produce the 6X liquid dilution by succussion.

The 7X liquid dilution is made from the 5X trituration. 8X liquid dilution is made from the 6X trituration. For 9X liquid dilutions or above, 1 part of the previous potency mixed with 10 parts of water for injections.

6X and 7X liquid dilutions prepared by the above method must not be used to produce further liquid dilutions.

Aqueous preparations prepared by this Method 8(b) are normally processed immediately; their use is limited to the manufacture of presentations by Methods 11, 13, 14, 15, 39(a) and 39(c), mixtures by Method 16, and potentised mixtures by Method 40(b).

Aqueous preparations must comply with the 'sterility test' of the G.H.P., if stored.

Method 9: Tablets

Tablets prepared solely from preparations produced by Method 6 or 7.

Except for 'uniformity of content', they must comply with the tablets monograph for uncoated tablets in the G.H.P.

Permitted excipients:

Starch up to 10%; Calcium bicarbonate or magnesium stearate up to 2%.

A saturated lactose solution or starch paste or ethanol in suitable concentration is used if granulation is required.

The tablets are usually 100 or 200 mg size. The weight of the excipients is additional to this.

Method 10: Globules (Granules)

They are prepared by transferring a dilution to sucrose granules (size 3: 110–130 granules weighed 1 gm) by moistening 100 parts of sucrose granules evenly with 1 part of dilution. Ethanol content of the dilution should not be less than 60 per cent. If this is not the case, it will be necessary to go against Methods 1 to 4b and produce the final potentisation of the decimal or centesimal dilution, which is to be used with ethanol 62 per cent.

Following impregnation in a sealed container, the globules are air-dried. They are labelled with the dilution stage of the dilution used to impregnate them.

Method 11: Parenteral preparations

This method adopted for the preparation of liquid dilutions for injections. They must comply with the parenteralia monograph in the G.H.P.

The only permitted additive, sodium chloride is used to make the preparations isotonic.

Parenteral preparations for human use are supplied in single dose glass ampoules.

'Uniformity of Content' tests are not required, with parenteral reparations produced from preparations containing ethanol, care is taken to keep the final ethanol content as low as possible.

This may be achieved by mixing and/or potentising with water for injections or the solutions of isotonising agent. For potentisation, an ethanol-free vehicle is used for the last two decimal dilution stages and the last centesimal dilution stage, respectively.

Method 12(a): Liquid external applications

Homoeopathic mother tinctures for external use are prepared in following process, based on different methods.

Mother tinctures for external use may contain up to 10% of Glycerine as an additive, and should not be used as internal remedies.

Method 12(b): Liquid external applications

Mother tinctures for external use are prepared, as per Method 2(a), with ethanol (73%).

The method differs from Method 2(a) in that, the amount of ethanol (73%) required (E) is calculated by using the following formula:

$$W = \frac{4MD}{100} \text{ (kg)}$$

M = Weight of plant-materials in kg.

D = Loss on drying in sample, in per cent.

Method 12(c): Liquid external applications

Mother tinctures for external use are prepared by maceration by following process:

The plants or parts of plants are finely minced. 1 part of plant-material mixed with 2.88 parts of purified water and 1.12 parts of ethanol and preserved at a temperature not exceeding 20°C. The additional amount of water (W) required is calculated according to the formula:

$$W = \frac{4MD}{100} \text{ (kg)}$$

M = Weight of plant-material in kg.

D = Loss on drying in sample, in per cent, and added to the mixture.

The mixture is allowed to stand for not less than 5 days at a temperature not exceeding 20°C and then filtered.

Method 12(d): Liquid external applications

By this method, oils for external use are prepared with 1 part of the dried plants or parts of plants and 10 parts of vegetable oils (e.g., groundnut oil, olive oil or sesame oil).

Mother Tinctures in different methods	Mother Tincture: Alcohol
1. Method 1, 2(a), 19(a)	1. 2 parts mother tincture + 3 parts ethanol (43%)
2. Method 2(b), 19(b)	2. 2 parts mother tincture + 3 parts ethanol (62%)
3. Method 3(a), 19(c)	3. 3 parts mother tincture + 2 parts ethanol (62%)
4. Method 3(b), 19(d)	4. 3 parts mother tincture + 2 parts ethanol (43%)
5. Method 3(c), 19(c)	5. 3 parts mother tincture + 2 parts ethanol (30%)
6. Method 4(a), 4(b), 19(f)	6. 1 part mother tincture + 1 part ethanol

1 part of minced drug mixed with 0.25 parts of ethanol. The mixture is allowed to stand for 12 hours before combining with 10 parts of vegetable oil. The mixture is heated to 60°C–70°C and kept for 3 hours, and then filtered.

Method 12(e): Liquid external applications

By this method, oils for external application, are prepared with 1 part of the dried plants or parts of plants, and 20 parts of vegetable oil (e.g., groundnut oil, olive oil or sesame oil).

1 part of minced drug mixed with 0.25 parts of ethanol. The mixture is allowed to stand for 12 hours before combining with 20 parts of vegetable oil. The mixture is heated to 60°C–70°C, kept for 4 hours, and then filtered.

Method 12(f): Liquid external applications

By this method, oils for external use are prepared with 1 part of the dried plants or parts of plants, and 10 parts of vegetable oil (e.g., ground nut oil, olive oil or sesame oil).

1 part of the minced drug mixed with 10 parts of vegetable oil. The mixture is heated under CO_2, at 37°C, kept for 7 days, and then filtered.

Method 12(g): Liquid external applications

By this method, oils for external use are prepared with 1 part of the dried plants or parts of plants and 20 parts of vegetable oil (e.g., groundnut oil, olive oil or sesame oil).

1 part of the minced drug mixed with 20 parts of vegetable oil. The mixture is heated under CO_2, at 37°C, kept for 7 days, and then filtered.

Method 12(h): Liquid external applications

By this method, oils for external use are prepared with 1 part of an essential oil and 9 parts vegetable oil (e.g. groundnut oil, olive oil or sesame oil).

Method 12(i): Liquid external applications

By this method, oils for external use are prepared by mixing with 1 part of an essential oil and 19 parts of vegetable oil (e.g. groundnut oil, olive oil or sesame oil).

Method 12(j):

By this method, oily preparations for external use are made from liquid dilutions.

Preparation of Oily dilution 3X

1 part of liquid dilution 1X is succussed with 9 parts of anhydrous alcohol (ethanol). 1 part of this dilution is treated in the same way to produce liquid dilution 3X.

1 part of liquid dilution 3X is mixed with 99 parts of vegetable oil.

Preparation of oily dilution 4X and onwards

Same method is followed to produce oily dilution 4X from liquid dilution 2X, and oily dilutions from 5X onwards. Olive oil is normally used; other oils must be declared.

Method 12(k): Liquid external applications

By this method, mother tinctures for external us are made by following process:

1 part of finely minced plant-material is mixed with 3 parts of purified water, and heated to boiling for 30 minutes. Loss of water by evaporation is replaced. After this, 3.76 parts of purified water and 2.24 parts of ethanol (96%) are added. The additional amount of water required (W) is calculated as for method 12C and added to the mixture. The mixture is allowed to stand for not less than 5 days at a temperature not exceeding 20°C, and then filtered.

Method 13: Ointments

Ointments are prepared by using the vehicle wool alcohol. Ointments must comply with the Salben monograph of the G.H.P.

Antioxidants and stabilisers are not permitted.

Decimal scale: Mother tincture and base, ratio 1 : 10.

Centesimal scale: Mother tincture and base, ratio 1 : 100.

Method 14: Suppositories

Suppositories are prepared by using the vehicle hard fat. Suppositories must comply with the suppositorien monograph in the G.H.P.

Excipients used as specified in the G.H.P.

'Uniformity of content' tests are not required.

Decimal scale: Mother tincture and base, ratio 1 : 10.

Centesimal scale: Mother tincture and base, ratio 1 : 100.

Method 15: Eye drops

Eye drops made by sterile aqueous fluids with a residual ethanol content of not more than one per cent.

They are prepared from one or more homoeopathic preparations, and comply with the Augentropfen (eye drops) specified in the monograph in the G.H.P. They contain no additives except for preservatives, and agents used to make it isotonic and adjust the pH.

To manufacture the eye drops, water for injections, or the solutions of the isotonising agent (normally sodium chloride) used to produce the last two decimal dilutions, and the last centesimal dilutions, respectively.

Method 16: Mixtures

Different preparations in this method are:

(a) Liquid and/or solid preparations in which the vehicle has been added in a proportion other than 1 to 10 or 1 to 100.

(b) Mixtures of liquid and/or solid preparations.

(c) Mixtures of liquid and/or solid preparations to which vehicles and/or auxillary substances have been added.

All types of presentations may be produced from the above mixtures. Mixtures containing liqueur wine and/or preparations made by Method 16 must not be processed further. Liquid external applications are manufactured as mixtures of preparations made by Method 12(a).

Method 17: LM potencies

Preparation of LM1 potency: 60 mg of a 3C trituration of the substance is dissolved in 20 ml of ethanol (15%). 1 drop of the solution is transferred to a small vial, and 2.5 ml of ethanol (86%) is added to it and shake vigorously 100 times. 100 gm of size 1 granules (aproximately 50,000 granules) mixed uniformly with the solution. The granules are air-dried in a closed container following impregnation.

Preparation of LM2 potency: 1 granule of the LM1 potency is transferred to a small vial, and dissolved in 4 drop, of water and 2.5 ml of ethanol (86%) is added to it and shake vigorously 100 times. 100 gm of size 1 granules (approximately 50,000 granules) mixed uniformly with the solution. The granules are air-dried in a closed container following impregnation.

All succeeding potencies are prepared in the same way.

To produce liquid LM potencies, 1 granule of the required potency is dissolved in 10 ml of ethanol (15%).

Method 18(a): Heat-treated mother tinctures and liquid dilutions of these

Mother tinctures made by Method 18(a) are produced like mother tinctures made by Method 2(a) and heat-treated.

The mixture containing the total amount of ethanol (86%) required is heated to 37°C in a closed container, and maintained at that temperature for one hour, stirring occasionally. After cooling, the mixture is processed as under Method 2(a).

Potentisation

Decimal scale: 2 parts of mother tinctures and 8 parts of ethanol (43%) are mixed and produce 1X potency. 1 part of 1X potency and 9 parts of ethanol (30%) will produce 2X potency. 1 part of 2X potency and 9 parts of ethanol (15%) will produce 3X potency.

All succeeding potencies are prepared in the same way.

Method 18(b): Heat-treated mother tinctures and liquid dilutions of these

Mother tinctures made by Method 18(b) are prepared like mother tinctures made by Method 2(b) and heat-treated.

The mixture containing the total amount of ethanol (62%) required is heated to 37°C in a closed container and maintained at that temperature for one hour, stirring occasionally. After cooling, the mixture is processed as under Method 2(a).

Ethanol (30%) is used to adjust to any value required by the monograph.

Potentisation

Decimal scale: 2 parts of mother tinctures and 8 parts of ethanol (30%) are mixed and produce 1X potency. 1 part of 1X potency and 9 parts of ethanol (15%) will produce 2X potency.

All succeeding potencies are prepared in the same way.

Method	Preparation		Drug Strength
1	Fresh juice + Ethanol 86%	MACERATION	1 : 1
2 a	Fresh drug + Ethanol 86%		1 : 2
2 b	Fresh drug + Ethanol 30%		1 : 2
3 a	Fresh drug + Ethanol 60%		1 : 2
3 b	Fresh drug + Ethanol 73%		1 : 2
3 c	Fresh drug + Ethanol 43%		1 : 2
4 a	Dry drug: Alcohol 1 : 9		$\frac{1}{10}$
4 b	Dry drug (Animal products): Alcohol 1 : 9		$\frac{1}{10}$
5 a	Solutions—Alcohol, water, or glycerol $\frac{1}{10}$ or $\frac{1}{100}$		$\frac{1}{10}$ or $\frac{1}{100}$
5 b	Aqueous solution, water for injection $\frac{1}{10}$ or $\frac{1}{100}$		$\frac{1}{10}$
6	Trituration $\frac{1}{10}$ or $\frac{1}{100}$		$\frac{1}{10}$
7	Trituration of M.T. or M.S. 1X		
8 a	Liquid from trituration—8X or 4C		
8 b	Liquid from trituration—in water for injection		
9	Tablets—permitted starch up to 10%; Calcium carbonate or Magnesium stearate up to 2%		
10	Globules (Granules)		
11	Parenteral preparations. Liquid dilutions for injection		
12 a	External appliction M.T. (Alcohol: 30–43%)		$\frac{1}{10}$
12 b	External application M.T. (Alcohol: 73%)		$\frac{1}{10}$
12 c	External application M.T. (Alcohol: 20%)		$\frac{1}{10}$
12 d	External application M.T. in oil 60°C–70°C, 4 hours		
12 e–k	External application M.T. in oil under CO_2, 37°C, 7 days		
13	Ointments—Antioxidants, stabilisers are not permitted		
14	Suppositories. Base—hard fat		$\frac{1}{10}$ or $\frac{1}{100}$
15	Eye drops: Sterile aqueous fluids with a residual ethanol content of not more than one per cent		
16	Mixtures of liquid or solid preparations. Liqueur wine—as vehicle		
17	LM potencies		
18 a	Heat-treated mother tinctures, Ethanol 86% as vehicle		
18 b	Heat-treated mother tinctures, Ethanol 62% as vehicle.		

Chapter 19

Potentisation

Definition

It is a mathematico-mechanical process by virtue of which the inherited dormant dynamic curative power of drugs is aroused or increased by modifying drug strength or drug power to dynamic power through simultaneous and successive process of dilution and friction in definite order according to pharmacopoeia.

Hahnemann, in his Preface to the 5th, Volume of **Chronic Diseases** defines: "Homoeopathic Dynamisation are processes by which the medicinal properties, which are latent in natural substances while in their crude state, become aroused and then become enabled to act in an almost spiritual manner in our life, i.e., in our sensible and irritable fibre. This development of properties of crude natural substances (dynamisation) takes place, in the case of dry substances by means of trituration in a mortar, but in the case of fluid substances by means of shaking or succussion, which is also a trituration".

According to **Stuart Close:** "Homoeopathic Dynamisation is a mathematico-mechanical process for the reduction, according to scale, of crude, inert or poisonous medicinal substances to a state of physical solubility, physiological assimilability, therapeutic activity and harmlessness, for use as homoeopathic healing remedies".

The **Doctrine of Drug-dynamisation** was introduced into homoeopathy through the 5th edition of **Organon of Medicine**, published in 1833.

History of Development of the Theory of Dynamisation

(a) **1796:** After the discovery of homoeopathy, in, "*Essay on a New Principle*" published in 1796, Hahnemann gives no information about the drug dynamisation. Since 1796, he selected remedies homoeopathically but used them in the usual form and in ordinary dose. But he came to notice that cure in many cases preceded aggravation of symptoms and consequently more sufferings of the patient; and in more cases definite injury to the patient occurred without bringing eventual recovery of the patient. This led him gradually to decrease the dose.

(b) **1798:** We find him recommending Hufelands journal in an article, "some kinds of continued and remittent fevers," the prescription of *Arnica* root in doses of several grains: *Ignatia* 2 to 3 grains, *Opium* $\frac{1}{5}$ to $\frac{1}{2}$ grain, *Camphor* 30-40 grains, *Ledum* 6-7 grains. In 1798, we find first hints of dilution of drugs.

He used to prescribe *Sabina* and *Hyos* $\frac{1}{16}$ to $\frac{1}{30}$ grain, of the concentrated solution and Stramonium $\frac{1}{100}$ to $\frac{1}{1,000}$ of concentrated juice.

(c) **1799-1801:** He advocated very small doses called infinitestimal doses. In a treatise, "*Treasury of medicine and collection of selected prescription,*" we find increasing number of remarks concerning very small doses. He mentioned the use of *Arsenic* in $\frac{1}{10}$th million part of a grain.

(d) **1802:** We find him using *Verat* $\frac{1}{2,000}$ grain, *Mezereum* $\frac{1}{4,00,000}$ grain, *Stramonium* $\frac{1}{3,00,000}$ grain etc.

(e) **1803:** After obviously making initial experiments with certain medicines of considerable higher dilutions, Hahnemann gradually adapted stronger doses and then later returned to higher degrees of dilution. Thus, we find Hahnemann still growing and experimenting higher and higher without making a final decision regarding the potencies and doses of drugs.

(f) **1804-1811:** Nothing definite was written by Hahnemann. In the "*Medicine of Experience*", published in 1805, there is a good deal about the purely dynamic action of drugs—the incredibly small quantity of them that will suffice for the cure, and the absolute superiority in point of power of the weakest medicine over the severest disease. But all this is insisted upon chiefly in relation to the exalted susceptibility present in disease, for it is stated that the same doses have no effect on the healthy or on those patients for whose disease the drug is not suitable. But there is in this essay no allusion to an increase of power by the increases of trituration and succussion, indeed no particular mention is made of any peculiarity in the homoeopathic pharmaceutical processes. Up to this period, diminution of the doses was advised nominally for the sake of preventing the too violent action of the remedy given according to new therapeutic principle, the sensibility being so much exalted for such medicines in the diseased state. This doctrine is again precisely and explicitly expressed in the short essay published in 1809.

In the first edition of "**Organon of Medicine**", published in 1810, the dynamisation theory is not yet rooted. No change is here spoken of as taking place in the properties of the drug by the processes employed to procure its subdivision, such as we find the subsequently conceived to take place by his pharmaceutical maneuvers. The diminution of the dose has for its only object the prevention of aggravation and of the development of accessory sufferings.

From the above discussion it is evident that Hahnemann's notion at that time was:

(i) by diminishing the size of dose he intended to avoid aggravation and the accessory effects of medicine.

(ii) by the process employed in diminishing the dose, viz. by the intimate mixture of the medicine with a non-medicinal vehicle by means of vigorous shaking, an increase of its activity is alleged to be produced.

(g) **1812-1815:** It was on record that Hahnemann prescribed Arnica in the 18th and Nux. vomica in the 9th centesimal dilution. Definite statements about the use of small quantities of medicines are to be found in his article "*The treatment of Typhus fever at present prevailing*", published in 1814. Experience proved the efficiency of diluted medicines.

(h) **1816-1827:** Hahnemann gradually increased the dilution of medicines with demands for higher and higher dilutions, oppositions from allopaths as well as a section of followers of Hahnemann also grew more and more.

In 1825, violent attacks against Hahnemann and homoeopathy began to be published in various medical journals in Germany. In this year, Hahnemann volunteers, in a literary journal, reply to the question that has been publicly addressed to him in a previous number at the same journal "How can small doses of such very attenuated medicines as homoeopathy employs have any 'effect' on the sick?" With some exceptions, this paper was reprinted in the 2nd edition of Volume Six of **Materia Medica Pura** (1827).

He writes there: "In the preparation of homoeopathic attenuations a small portion of medicine is not merely added to an enormous quantity of non-medicinal fluid, or only slightly mingled with it but by the prolonged succussion and trituration, there ensues not only the most intimate mixture, but at the same time—and this is the most important circumstance—there ensues such a great and hitherto unknown and undreamt of change, by the development and liberation of the dynamic powers of the medicinal substance so treated, so as to excite astonishment".

(i) **1828-1833:** A new chapter in the theory of doses was opened out by the appearance of Hahnemann's **"Chronic Diseases."** In the introduction to Vol. 1, he wrote in unequivocal terms that he began with small doses of one grain in the 2nd or 3rd trituration but experience taught him to give preference to higher dilutions or potencies as he called them. Then began an era of high potencies. But the followers of Hahnemann outdid Hahnemann in using drugs in 60C, 90C, 200C and 1,500C (cf. Gross, Schreter, Korsakoff).

So, Hahnemann came upon the strange idea of setting up a standard dose for all curative remedies used in homoeopathy. This was to be 30C. Hahnemann's final discussion in favour of high potency rested on his conception of dynamisation of drugs after dilution and succussion and was put forth in the 5th edition of "**Organon of Medicine**" (1833).

(j) **1839:** In the 2nd edition of "**Chronic Diseases**" Hahnemann confirmed his dynamisation of drugs in the following words: "Homoeopathic dynamisation of drugs are real awakenings of the medicinal properties that lie dormant in natural bodies during their crude state; which then become capable of acting in almost a spiritual manner upon our life—that is to say, on our persistent (sensitive) and excitable fibres."

As regards preparation of 'potencies', he first recommended that most appropriate number of succussion as two only (5th edition, **Organon**). But he altered his opinion repeatedly within few years. Instructions regarding the latest method of dynamisation of drugs are recorded in Section 270-272 of **Organon**, 6th edition. In this edition, Hahnemann made a tremendous departure from his previous instructions regarding doses and repetitions and preparations of medicines in **Chronic Diseases.** Here, he showed the path of prescribing, "50-Millesimal potency."

Scientific Approach to Homoeopathic Drug Potentisation

Hahnemann believed that substances which are medicinally inert in their crude state are thus rendered active and effective for healing the sick, by the process of *trituration* and *succussion.* For example, *Natrum mur* (or sodium chloride) crystal is an inert substance but it is of immense medicinal value when it is made powerful by increasing its potency through trituration and succussion.

The quantity of the drug in the homoeopathic dose is very very small and of the order of 100^{-30}, 100^{-100}, 100^{-200}, $100^{-10,00,000}$, and cannot be measured by the present scientific instruments and techniques. As homoeopathic medicine is too small in quantity, its chemical interaction with the infecting paracitus is not possible but it shows its medicinal effects.

On the basis of *Avogadro's number,* the presence of material in the Homoeopathic Medicine beyond molecular concentration 10 or 12 becomes negative. This seems to be impractical in a laboratory but it is in accordance with the concept of *relativistic theory.*

In homoeopathy, crude drug substances are potentised by the process of trituration and succussion. Trituration may be considered as successive dilution with vigorous shaking of the medicine with the polar solvent as water or alcohol. The trituration process of the medicine results in micro-emulsion solution of the medicine in the solvent water or alcohol, developing a definite charge. Further trituration of the micro-emulsion solution results in super micro-emulsion solution with less charge density. The charge of the micro-emulsion particles is accelerated with trituration resulting in the emulsion of electromagnetic waves. Thus, in potentisation process, due to absorption of electromagnetic waves, very very light *isotopic molecules* of medicinal materials are created. These very light or weightless isotopic molecules of the medicinal materials retain the properties of the original drug substances. This view is supported by relative kinematics as given below:

The particles of the medicine, the medium vehicle are in motions, so, the relative expression for the medicine particles may be written as:

$E^2 = (PC)^2 + (M_0C^2)^2$, where

E = Total energy of the free particle of the medicine, i.e.,

$E = mC^2 = K + m_0C^2$ = Energy due to external work + Rest energy

P = Relative momentum of the medicine particle

m_0 = Rest mass of medicine particle.

C = Velocity of light

m = Mass of the free particle of the medicine If $m_0 = 0$, the above relativistic relation is reduced to, $E = PC$.

$$P = mu = \frac{m_0 u}{\left\{\sqrt{\left(1-\frac{u^2}{C^2}\right)}\right\}}$$

In order to have non-zero momentum, we have a finite value for the above equation in the limit $m_0 \rightarrow u$, this is only possible if $u \rightarrow C$ as $m_0 \rightarrow 0$.

Hence, massless particles must travel at the speed of light. These massless particles must possess momentum and energy but no rest mass. Thus, in homoeopathic potentised medicine, the medicinal particles may be considered as massless particles which have no mass but only energy. In homoeopathic system, the life force is a dynamic force, which is affected by disease, and can be cured only by dynamic power of medicines, not by its material quantity. Since homoeopathic potentised medicine has massless particles having energy only, this energy is responsible for curing the natural disease.

Objects of Potentisation

1. To avoid unnecessary medicinal aggravation and side-effects by a continued process of reducing the material quantity of a drug.
2. The medicinal properties, which are latent in natural substances while in their crude state, become awakened and developed into activity to an incredible degree.

Examples

(a) In the crude state or in large doses, many poisons and narcotics may bring instantaneous harm, and may be fatal. But they become important and beneficial remedies after potentisation, e.g., Arsenic, Mercury, and some of its salts, Potassium cyanide, Nitroglycerine (Glonoinum), Opium, Strychnine, Lachesis, Naja, Elaps, Crotalus etc

(b) Substances which are medicinally inert in their crude state are thus rendered active and effective for healing the sick, e.g., Natrum mur; Silicea; Charcoal; Lycopodium etc

3. Vital force is dynamic in nature, and the disease force is also dynamic in nature, which attacks the healthy vital force in dynamic plane, causing a diseased state. So, to free the dynamically deranged vital force, the requisite medicine must also be dynamic.
4. The more a drug is potentised, the greater its dynamic medicinal power increased to an incredible degree.
5. Potentisation helps to individualise a drug through its latent pathogenetic power, as is discovered in its homoeopathic drug proving.
6. Potentisation not only preserves the therapeutic potentiality but also increases the pharmacological and therapeutic activity.
7. Abnormal susceptibilities, constitutional abnormalities, miasms can only be cured by the dynamic and deep action of the drug. This is only possible by potentised medicines. The actions of the potentised medicines are deeper, longer and more widespread.
8. The medicinal qualities of other drugs which are more or less active in their natural state are

enhanced and their sphere of action are broadened by this process.

Effects of Potentisation

1. Quantitative reduction but qualitative increase of therapeutic activity.
2. Increase in potential energy—determined by different scales.
3. Elimination of toxic products.
4. Gaining of the maximum potential energy or dynamic power.

Phenomenon of Potentisation

Potentisation includes two phenomena:

(i) Dilution and (ii) Friction.

Factors of Potentisation

(a) Nature of drug, (b) Solvent or vehicle.

Relation between the factors:

1. *Solid vehicle:* Sugar of milk, used for insoluble drugs.
2. *Liquid vehicle:*
   (i) C_2H_5OH—used for drugs soluble in liquid vehicle.
   (ii) Purified water—used in preparing potency.
   (iii) Dispensing alcohol—in some cases.

Processes of Potentisation or Dynamisation

Drugs are potentised principally by two processes:

(i) *Trituration:* In case of insoluble substances.

(ii) *Succussion:* In case of soluble substances.

Scales of Potentisation

1. *For trituration*
   (i) Centesimal scale
   (ii) Decimal scale.
2. *For succussion*
   (i) Centesimal scale
   (ii) Decimal scale
   (iii) 50-Millesimal scale.

Products of Potentisation

'Potency' denotes as

(i) 30, 200, IM., C.M., M.M...... in centesimal scale.

(ii) 1X, 2X, 3X, 6X, 12X ...... in decimal scale.

(iii) 0/1, 0/2, 0/3, 0/4 ...... in 50-millesimal scale.

TRITURATION

Definition: It is an ideal physical, mathematical process of potentisation by which preparation of medicines takes place by the use of solid vehicle, i.e., sugar of milk, by grinding in definite order according to pharmacopoeia.

Vehicle for Trituration

For trituration, sugar of milk is used instead of other solid vehicle because sugar of milk is the best crystalline substance, scentless, gritty to touch, faintly sweet. It has been found by experiment that it is quite competent to ground down to an inconceivably fine powder the particles of such mineral substances which are insoluble either in purified water or in alcohol.

Repeated systematic triturations are quite capable of affecting the system and become very wonderful and most powerful medicines.

Substances taken for Trituration

Hahnemann classified substances into 3 categories as he mentioned in Class VII, Class VIII and Class IX for trituration:

1. Dry insoluble (insoluble in purified water and alcohol) medicinal substances (Class VII)—e.g., Arsenicum album; Alumina; Calcarea carb; Carbo vegetabilis; Graphites; Corallium rubrum.
2. Liquid insoluble medicinal substances (Class VIII)—e.g. Petroleum; Snake venoms such as Lachesis; Elaps; Naja; Crotalus; Vipera etc. Nosodes such as Lyssin, Variolinum, Vaccininum, Malandrinum etc.
3. Fresh vegetable and animal substances (Class IX)—e.g. Anthracinum; Psorinum; Medorrhinum; Syphillinum; Blatta orientalis; Blatta americana; Agaricus; Anacardium etc.

Difference in the process of Trituration in Class VII, Class VIII and Class IX

1. **In Class VII:** For trituration ratio of dry medicinal substance and sugar of milk is 1 : 99 (as per centesimal scale). These 99 parts of sugar of milk are divided into three equal parts (33 + 33 + 33). The trituration process consists of 3 stages, each having 20 minutes. Each part of sugar of milk is to be added at the beginning of each stage.

2. **In Class VIII:** For trituration, ratio of liquid medicinal substance and sugar of milk is 1 : 99 (as per centesimal scale). These 99 parts of sugar of milk should not be divided into 3 equal parts, because, in this case, sugar of milk is very small in quantity. So, whole quantity of sugar of milk should be taken at a time in the mortar at first, and the medicinal substance should be poured over it for preventing sticking of the oily medicinal substance in the surface of mortar.

3. **In Class IX:** Same as the process of Class VIII but the ratio of fresh drug substance and sugar of milk is 2 : 99 (as per centesimal scale). Here, 2 parts are taken because there is always some loss by evaporation during trituration.

Method of Trituration of Dry Insoluble Medicinal Substances

(Class VII, in Hahnemannian method)

Requirements

1. *Ingredients*
   (i) Required amount of crude drug substance.
   (ii) Required amount of sugar of milk.

2. *Appliances*
   (i) One clean unglazed porcelain mortar.
   (ii) One clean unglazed porcelain pestle.
   (iii) One clean horn-made spatula.
   (iv) An empty clean phial of required size.
   (v) A stop-clock or a watch.
   (vi) A freshly marked new velvet cork.
   (vii) Label paper, paste, scissors, pen etc.
   (viii) Balance and weight box.

Procedure in Different Scales

By this process, the potentisation of dry medicinal substance takes place which is insoluble in water and alcohol:

In Centesimal Scale	*In Decimal Scale*
Ratio of drug substance and sugar of milk is 1 : 99 (33 + 33 + 33) (But as per H.P.I, 11 + 33 + 55)	Ratio of drug substance and sugar of milk is 1 : 9 (3 + 3 + 3) (But as per H.P.I, 1 + 3 + 5)

The methods of preparation which are utilised are similar but the only difference is that in centesimal scale, the ratio of drug substance and sugar of milk is 1 : 99 and in the decimal scale, the ratio of drug substance and sugar of milk is 1 : 9.

A. In Centesimal Scale

(a) *Principle:* 1 part of drug substance is triturated with 99 parts of sugar of milk. All subsequent triturations are made by taking 1 part by previous one and 99 parts of sugar of milk.

(b) *Duration:* The whole process is divided into 3 stages, each taking 20 minutes. Each 20 minutes is again divided into (10 + 10) minutes.

Each 10 minute is composed of:

1. 1st Stage: Rubbing with pestle—6 minutes.
2. 2nd Stage: Scraping—3 minutes.
3. 3rd Stage: Mixing (stirring)—1 minute.

(c) ***Procedure***

1. *First stage:* Duration 20 minutes.

1 grain of drug substance is added to 33 grains by weight of sugar of milk in a clean unglazed porcelain mortar. Then it is triturated through the following stages. The first stage is also subdivided by two sub-stages:

(a) First sub-stage: Duration 10 minutes.

(i) Rubbing—6 minutes.

It is grinded with pestle. The grinding should be steady and non-stop with uniform forced strength, in one direction—either clockwise or anti-clockwise.

Mathematical Expression

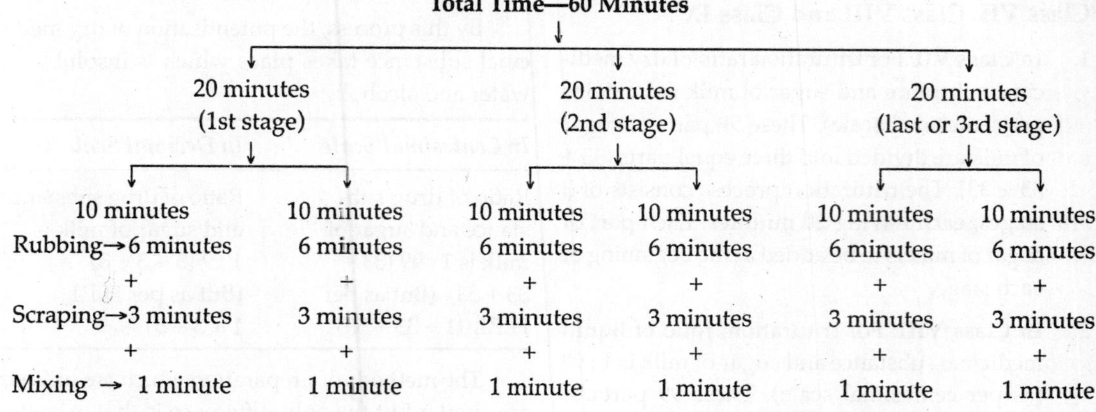

(ii) Scraping—3 minutes.

After rubbing with horn spatula, the particles are scraped off.

(iii) Mixing or stirring—1 minute.

After scraping properly with spatula, the scraped material is mixed and stirred with spatula.

Hence, first sub-stage is completed.

(b) Second sub-stage: Duration 10 minutes. It also consists of three phases:

(i) Rubbing—6 minutes.

(ii) Scraping—3 minutes.

(iii) Mixing or stirring—1 minute.

Procedure in second sub-stage is almost similar to that of the first sub-stage.

Thus, 20 minutes of first stage of trituration is completed.

2. *Second stage:* Duration 20 minutes.

This stage is also sub-divided into two sub-stages:

(a) First sub-stage: Duration 10 minutes. At the beginning of first sub-stage 33 grains of sugar of milk is added to the triturated substance which has been triturated in the first stage. It consists of three phases:

(i) Rubbing—6 minutes.

(ii) Scraping—3 minutes.

(iii) Mixing or stirring—1 minute.

So, first sub-stage is completed.

(b) Second sub-stage: Duration 10 minutes. It also consists of 3 phases:

(i) Rubbing—6 minutes.

(ii) Scraping—3 minutes.

(iii) Mixing or stirring—1 minute.

Now, the 20 minutes of the second stage is completed.

3. *Third stage:* Duration 20 minutes.

Procedure is same as first stage. Here, remaining 33 grains of sugar of milk is added to triturated substance which are triturated in second stage. Now, at the end of one hour, first potency in centesimal scale is produced.

Preparation of 2nd degree trituration:

1 grain of the above product is triturated in a similar way with further 99 grains of sugar of milk. After one hour, it will be the 2nd centesimal potency.

B. In Decimal Scale

The same process, as for potencies under centesimal scale, is carried on, is also applicable for trituration under the decimal scale, excepting that 1 part by weight of the drug substance will be triturated with 9 parts by weight of sugar of milk, for the period of one hour, including three stages, each consuming 20 minutes as in the centesimal scales and dividing the 9 parts of sugar of milk into 3 equal parts (3 + 3 + 3). Thus, in one hour, 1st potency, i.e., IX potency in decimal scale will be produced.

For the 2nd potency, triturate, 1 part of the 1st potency with 9 parts of sugar of milk in the usual way.

Conversion of Trituration into Liquid Potency

We cannot convert every trituration into liquid potency. We can convert only from 6X trituration under decimal scale, and from 3rd under the centesimal scale into liquid potency. Trituration below these degrees of fineness we cannot transform into liquid state, as neither purified water nor alcohol will be able to dissolve them.

The first liquid potency prepared from trituration under centesimal scale is fourth and under decimal scale is 8X.

(a) Conversion in Centesimal Scale—From 3C to 4C

A clean new round phial of one ounce capacity is taken. It is fitted with a new velvet cork. The cork is marked with the name of the drug to be prepared and 4th potency on it. Then the cork is removed and 1 grain of 3rd trituration of the drug is put into the phial. 50 minims of purified water is poured over it. The phial is stirred well to dissolve the drug substance. 50 minims of dilute alcohol is added to it. It is corked.

[The phial must not be filled more than $^2/_3$rd in any case.] The bottom of the phial is placed on the little finger of the right hand. The thumb of the same hand should be placed on the cork. The phial should be tightly held with other fingers. Then ten strokes are given to this phial on the palm of the left hand. Each stroke should end in a jerk. Thus, fourth potency is prepared.

1 minim of the 4th potency, and 99 minims of alcohol after ten successions give the 5th potency. All the following potencies will be prepared by taking 1 minim of the preceding potency to 99 minims of alcohol.

(b) Conversion in Decimal Scale—From 6X to 8X (jumping potency)

A clean new round phial of one ounce capacity is taken. It is fitted with a new velvet cork. The cork is marked with the name of the drug to be prepared and 8X potency written on it. Then the cork removed and 1 grain of 6X trituration of the drug is put into the phial. 50 minims of purified water is poured over it. The phial is stirred well to dissolve the drug substance. 50 minims of dilute alcohol is added to it. It is corked.

[The phial must not be filled more than $^2/_3$rd in any case.] The bottom of the phial is placed on the little finger of the right hand. The thumb of the same hand should be placed on the cork. The phial should be tightly held with other fingers. Then ten strokes are given to this phial on the palm of the left hand. Each stroke should end in a jerk. Thus 8X potency is prepared.

7X potency cannot be prepared according to decimal scale because if 9 minims of alcohol is taken and successed with 1 grain of 6X potency, then it will not be dissolved. For dissolving it fully,

Table 19.1: Differences between Potency and Dilution

Potency	Dilution
1. When the inherent property of the diluted substances are brought into light.	1. It is simply mixing of a liquid with purified water or any other liquid such as alcohol.
2. Dynamic power is increased.	2. Physico-chemical property is reduced.
3. Qualitative power is increased.	3. Quantity of the substance is increased.
4. The term is generally used in homoeopathic scale of potentisation of medicine.	4. The term is generally used in chemistry.
5. There are two types of scales such as—centesimal and decimal scale. In centesimal scale—1st potency should contain $^1/_{100}$th part of the orginal drug. In decimal scale—1st potency should contain $^1/_{10}$th part of the original drug.	5. There is no such scale.

Schematic Representation (in Centesimal Scale)

Preparation of first degree trituration

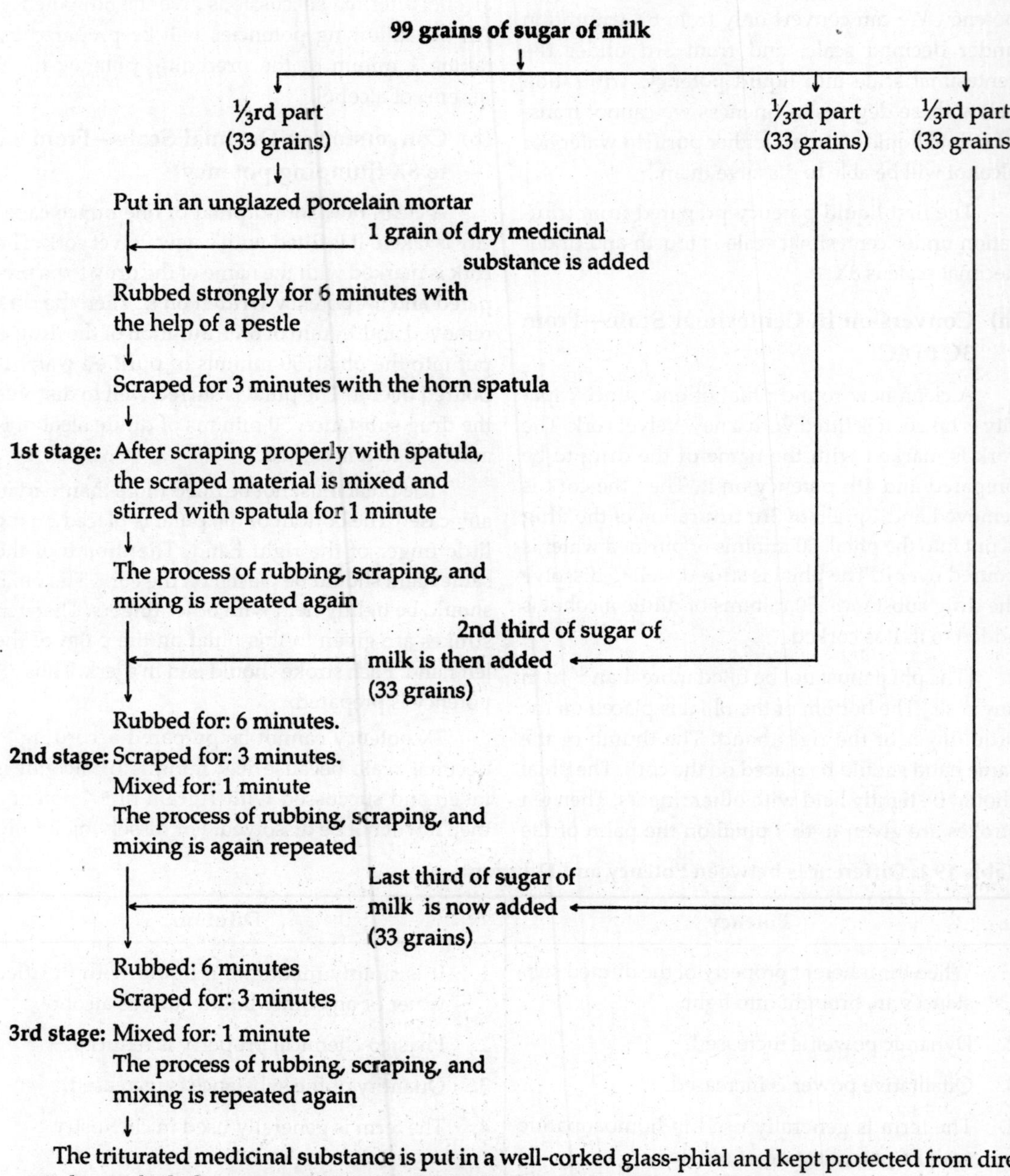

The triturated medicinal substance is put in a well-corked glass-phial and kept protected from direct sunlight to which the name of the drug and designation of first potency is marked.

Time taken for the whole process	= one hour (approx.)
Rubbing—6 × 6 minutes	= 36 minutes
Scraping—3 × 6 minutes	= 18 minutes
Mixing— 1 × 6 minutes	= 6 minutes
	= 60 minutes

50 minims of alcohol and 50 minims of purified water are taken—50 + 50 = 100 minims = 10 × 10. If one part of 6X and 10 minims were to be taken in preparation it would have been 7X, but as we are taking two ten (10) minims, so one more potency will be increased. Thus, it will be 8X.

The preparation of 8X from 6X trituration in this way is known as 'fluxion potency' or 'jumping potency'. Further potencies under decimal scale are prepared by taking 1 part by weight of 8X potency, and succussing it 10 times with 9 parts by weight of alcohol. At least up to 6X potency, we can expect the remedies other than in liquid state, in trituration form because they are not dissolved either in purified water or in alcohol, e.g. Ferrum phos-6X; Natrum phos-6X; Calcarea phos-6X (in trituration).

POTENCY

Definition: Potency (*Potentia* = power in the sense of ability, capacity) denotes power which is derived by the grades of medicinal power as developed by the process of dynamisation are called homoeopathic potencies in different grades. *Potency means dilution plus energy.*

They are the results of a series of successive dilution followed by trituration or succussion.

In other words, homoeopathic potencies are the result of a series of successive reduction in concentration of the basic medicinal substance, whereby each reduction in concentration is followed by vigorous agitation, i.e., dynamisation.

Notes: 1. We hear daily how homoeopathic medicinal potencies are called mere dilutions. But they are the very opposite, i.e. a true opening up of the natural substances bringing to light and revealing the hidden specific powers contained within and brought forth by rubbing and shaking. (Sec. 269, 6th edition of **Organon.**)

2. 'Simple dilution, for instance the solution of a grain of salt will become almost pure water. The grain of salt will disappear in the dilution with much water and will never develop into salt medicine which by means of our well-prepared dynamisation, is raised to most marvellous power.' (Sec. 269, 6th edition of **Organon.**)

Fluxion Potency

Definition: It is a special and peculiar process when the 6X potency obtained by trituration is turned into 8X potency by succussion without having transitional 7X.

Process adapted: Trituration up to 6X followed by succussion. Below 6X, some substances are not soluble in the alcohol or purified water, generally of the metallic origin, e.g., Ars. alb; Ferrum. met; Silver nitrate etc. It is introduced by Hahnemann. It is a noble gift to homoeopathic pharmacy and to colloidal chemistry.

Process: 30 ml phial (clean, rounded, neutral) is taken.

↓

Phial and cork is marked the name of 8X potency of the medicine

↓

1 part by volume of 6X trituration is taken

↓

50 parts by volume of purified water is poured in it

↓

The mixture is fully dissolved by gentle shaking

↓

50 parts by volume of strong alcohol is added. (As per H.P.I. dispensing alcohol)

↓

The phial is corked. The phial must not be filled more than ⅔rd in any case

↓

Typical 10 downward strokes are given

↓

8X is obtained.

High Fluxion Potencies

Liquid attenuations by hand process can be made up to 1M potency. But for making higher than 1M potency such as 10M, 50M, CM, DM, MM etc., required time, labour and alcohol is much more. To combat this problem, some great homoeopaths have invented machines for preparing higher and highest potencies. Such higher potency prepared with the help of machines are known as high fluxion potency.

In this process, purified water is used as vehicle instead of alcohol, for the intermediate step.

The homoeopaths which were in favour of higher and highest potencies in Hahnemannian or post-Hahnemannian age are: Equerry Jenichen of

Wismer, Jahann Ernst Stapf, Gustav Wilhelm Gross, Carl von Boenninghausen, B. Fincke, Swan, Deshere, Boericke, Lehrmann, Skinner, Nash, J. T. Kent etc.

All fluxion potencies are objectionable because, doing away with Hahnemannian procedure, they tend to cause a departure from homoeopathic methods and also because few, if any, correspond to the Hahnemannian scale. It has been demonstrated that the so called M.M. potency of Swan equals about the 10th centesimal potency of Hahnemann.

Straight Potency

(Conversion of trituration into liquid potency)

As per Burt of London, 7X liquid potency can be prepared from its previous 6X trituration.

Method: 1 part of 6X trituration of the requisite drug is taken in a new well-cleansed round phial, and 9 parts of purified water is added to it. Then 10 downward strokes are given, which end in a jerk. Then 1 part of the 7X liquid potency is taken and mixed with 9 parts of alcohol and 10 downward strokes are given. Now, 8X liquid potency is prepared.

Precautions in Trituration

1. Room should be clean, and of moderate tempe-rature and dust-proof, for carrying the process of trituration.
2. The process must be done in a warm and dry atmosphere.
3. Utensils should be perfectly clean and odourless.
4. The mortar and pestle must be unglazed or made rough by rubbing them with moist clean white sand.
5. The mortar and pestle should be washed properly by ether. It should be wiped dry, and then a little amount of alcohol should be burnt inside.
6. After each trituration is completed, all the utensils must be properly cleaned and dried for the next one.
7. It is systematically and symmetrically a rubbing process. So any deviation from this cannot bring success for the process.
8. Must not lift up the pestle or mortar.
9. The pestle must be fully pressed down with the firm grip and thumb on the top, and it is to be moved in anti-clockwise direction (This is convenient for a right-handed person) in a circular fashion, going away from the centre in a spiral, and returning back to centre. This gives chance to practically all the particles to get rubbed uniformly.
10. In trituration Plumbum, the pestle should be used softly.
11. In making the first trituration of Mercury, Graphites, and Plumbum, double time should be taken.
12. In triturating Fer. met, the mortar must be kept warm for removing moisture, while triturating.
13. Burt advises using of a small amount of alcohol for moistening the sugar of milk during trituration, as it will save the troubles of scraping and stirring.

Merits of Trituration

(Why do we triturate drugs?)

1. By the process of trituration, drug-substances can be infinitely divided.
2. Insoluble substances in liquid vehicles become soluble after trituration.
3. The medicinal property of drug which remains latent or dormant, by this process become active (i.e., aroused into activity).
4. Curative powers of drugs are increased by this process, by reducing the quantity of drugs (but the qualitative power is increased).
5. Certain drugs are insoluble in liquid vehicles (purified water or alcohol)—so there is no alternative method but to triturate only.

e.g., (i) Dry medicinal substances (Class VII): Ars. alb; Cal. carb; Ant. cr; Fer. met; Carbo. an; Graph; Arg. nit; Alumina; Carbo. veg; Corralium rubrum; Kali. carb; Zinc. met.

(ii) Liquid medicinal substances (Class VIII): Lachesis; Elaps; Crotalus; Naja; Vipera; Apium virus; Bufo rana; Croton tig; Lyssin; Variolinum; Vaccininum; Malandrinum; Petroleum.

(iii) Fresh vegetable and animal substances (Class IX): Anac; Agaricus; Malandrinum; Medorrhinum; Syphilinum; Anthracinum; Psorinum; Carcinosin; Blatta orientalis; Blatta americanus.

6. By trituration of surface area, surface tension of a drug is increased enormously.
7. By increase of the surface area and finer division, the absorptive qualities, colloidal properties, and catalytic effect will also be increased.

Demerits of Trituration

1. The process is a very long one. The time taken and the labour spent is too much. Some are of the opinion, that there is no necessity of dividing the vehicles into 3 equal parts. With experimental evidence they suggest that by triturating the whole vehicle with the medicine at a stretch gives the same results.
2. If soluble substances are triturated in order to increase the drug power, it is observed that, when they meet some water medium, the molecules will have some ionic changes. (Trituration is really intended to have a maximum distribution of particles in a vehicle and not any other changes).
3. As sugar of milk has got aldehyde ($\frac{R}{H}>C=O$) properties, it is found to reduce some substances, like mercury compounds, during trituration. (In such cases, cane-sugar, which has got less aldehyde properties, will prove to be a greater vehicle).
4. Though sugar of milk is appreciably hard and gritty, it does not cause the communion of substances which are harder than itself like some hard metals. (This is controlled by grinding and sieving the substances before-hand, and changing the vehicle if necessary).

Modern Method of Trituration

In general process of potentisation, the quantity of triturations cannot be increased properly without modifying other conditions, but in doing so, the quality of the resulting triturations may be inferior. But due to increased demand of trituration, and better Homoeopathic Medicines as well as to increase the productivity, and to minimise the cost of production, mechanical devices are being employed nowadays. In this method, all sorts of measures are taken to retain the quality.

In this context, the H.P.I directs that: 'It is not feasible to give strict rules for such mechanical appliances in all their interdependent details'.

Nowadays, trituration is done by machine in which the mortar and pestle are rotated by machines.

SUCCUSSION

Definition: It is a process of potentisation of medicinal substances which are soluble in liquid vehicle (particularly in alcohol) by downward friction.

The term 'succussion' comes from Latin—*succussum succutere*, meaning 'shaking up'.

Vehicle for succussion: Generally, alcohol is used in most of the cases (as in Class I, Class II, Class III, Class IV and Class VI of Hahnemannian old method) except in cases where the medicinal substances are only soluble in water (as in Class V). In such cases, it is only after a certain degree of attenuation has been attained that it is made in alcohol.

Substances taken for succussion: The medicinal substances which are soluble in alcohol or purified water are taken for succussion.

Principle: 1 part by volume of drug or previous potency of medicine is mixed with 9 or 99 parts by volume of vehicle, and 10 downward strokes of uniform strength are applied.

Process: The required amount of drug and vehicle are taken in a new, neutral, well-cleansed rounded and properly labelled glass phial, keeping ⅔rd of the phial empty. This is due to provide effective friction. In old method, the drug is taken according to drug power. The phial is then corked tightly. The bottom of the phial is placed on the little finger of the right hand. The thumb of the same hand should be tightly held with other fingers. Then 10 downward strokes are given.

The strokes should be—(i) forceful, (ii) successive, (iii) each stroke ends in a jerk, (iv) from uniform distance, (v) with uniform strength.

The hand enclosing the phial should go beyond the level of shoulder, but not beyond the level of the upper limit of the pinna. The product is the potency.

Note: Regarding the number of strokes:

(i) Hahnemann's idea: Regarding the number of strokes to be given for each potency, Hahnemann himself has changed his mind several times. In the 5th edition of **Organon of Medicine,** he uses only two strokes but later on uses ten strokes (**Chronic Diseases**).

(ii) A.H.P. and G.H.P.: They still advocate 10 strokes.

Modified Potentisation Techniques

Keeping pace with the scientific and industrial revolution, many followers and students of Hahnemann and homoeopathy started to perceive the principle of potentisation from the view of constructing labour-saving techniques and machines, by which they could prepare high potencies.

Hahnemann always spoke of trituration performed by hand. It was practical and possible to prepare Hahnemannian potencies manually as he mostly used up to the 30th centesimal. Even the modifications suggested in the 6th edition of **Organon of Medicine,** were simple to follow as these required the substance to be triturated up to the 3rd centesimal, and further potencies successed on the 50-Millesimal scale.

But already during his lifetime attempts were made to modify this tiring and long manual labour by mechanical triturators that were able to work more uniformly than the human hand. In their long course of development, they have led to the more efficient triturators and computerised succussion machines.

There existed a small body of overzealous students of Hahnemann, anxious to overstep the Master in potentising. Hahnemann had made use of varied degrees of dilution, from the original tincture up to the 30th centesimal dilution. But the 30th potency was by no means high enough for his students, and so they produced a 60th, 90th, a 200th and finally even a 1500th potency. Among these enthusiasts, Dr. Gross, Dr. N Schreter (1803-1864), and General Korsakoff (1788-1853) of Russia played the principal part. They became the real founders of the theory of high potencies, which later on found an industrious and zealous protagonist in Stapf. After the death of Hahnemann, his followers took up different methods of dynamisation.

Korsakoff of Russia

Count Graf von Korsakoff, nobleman, was fascinated by Hahnemann's dynamisation theory. He was the real originator of high potencies. He claimed that one single medicated globule when placed among many non-medicated globules communicated its medicinal power to the non-medicated globules. He went on to do this with 13,500 unmedicated globules and one single dry globule of Sulphur 30. He warned that, the bottle should not be carried in the pocket for fear of the power being enormously increased because of the shaking of the bottle in the pocket. What Hahnemann did with the fluid potencies, Korsakoff did with the solid dry globule. He believed that the material division of the medicine ceases with the 6th potency and the the medicinal power is communicated by a process analogous to infection of this idea.

Jenichen of Wismar

Caspar Julius Jenichen (1787-1849) was an admirer of Hahnemann, who pursued the idea that further attenuation is not necessary for the potentisation of medicine, but continuous succussion without dilution is sufficient. He advocated that the degree of strength developed through potentisation was directly proportional to the number of strokes given. Thus he suggested that every ten strokes given would increase the dynamic strength of the medicine by one degree.

Carroll Dunham

Carroll Dunham (1828-1877) was one of the early people to mechanise the process of potentisation. He used an abandoned oil-mill for preparing potencies. His potencies were suffixed by letter 'D'.

Bernhardt Fincke

Fincke (1821-1906) was an American physician who devised his own method of dynamisation. He used to take 100 drops of drug substance in a glass jug. He allowed a stream of water to flow into it. For every drachm of water entering in and out of the vessel, he would count it as one potency. Thus 100 drachms of water entering and coming out of the vessel would raise the potency of the containing drug substance to 100. He never believed the value of strokes. He had paid importance only on the water with its exerting force on a medicinal substance in raising the potencies, and not on any strokes applied.

Thomas Skinner

Skinner's potencies were prepared by a process of discontinuous fluxion in contrast to the continuous fluxion of Swan and Fincke. By 1878, Skinner (1825-1906) developed the 'Skinner Fluxion Centesimal Attenuator'. This device was designed to mount above a small sink in the office or home. The motive power was water pressure. The potencies are labeled 'F.C.' (Fluxion Centesimal) to differentiate them from Hahnemannian Centesimal potencies.

Samuel Swan

Samuel Swan (1814-1893) used fractional part of potencies, and attenuated from them. He suggested that if one drop of tincture were used to make 1M potency, then $^1/_{10}$th of a drop of the 1M would be used to make the 10M. This method had more to do with the dilution of the final potency, rather than the serial dilution of each potency along the way.

Multiple or Single Vial Potencies

The method of potentisation given in the German Homoeopathic Pharmacopoeia, requires a new vial to be used for every stage of potentisation, which is the original method developed by Hahnemann. It is known as Hahnemann's Multiple Vial Method.

The French are very accurate in calling potencies produced by this method CH_1, CH_2, CH_3, etc.

Single vial potencies are easier and cheaper to produce. The disadvantage is that they are less accurate. They are called Korsakoff potencies, the method having been developed by the Russian Korsakoff. His method is based on the fact that, when a phial is emptied, some of the fluid remains adhering to the walls.

Hahnemann's Method was and still is more accurate.

Hahnemann mentions that, these potencies should be prepared by hand process. The hand process is suitable for preparing smaller quantities. The question of mechanical devices came up when shaking of large quantities in big vessels became necessary.

Practically, it is too hard to pursue the Hahnemannian hand process in cases of higher and highest potencies that came up after Hahnemann. Hahnemann himself made potencies up to 60C.

Practically, automatic machines now prepare all higher and highest potencies or dilutions.

Mixed Hahnemannian and Korsakovian Method

Begin with Hahnemannian mode of preparation up to 6C or 30C. Then use the single phial method.

Q-Potency

Q-potency is the term used to designate 50-Millesimal potency.

Back Potency

Two to three potencies prior to the frequently used potencies are called back potency.

Examples: For 30CH potency, the back potencies would be 29CH, 28CH or 27CH potency.

For 200CH potency, the back potencies would be 199CH, 198CH or 197CH potency.

Preparation: To prepare 28CH potency—1 part 27CH potency +99 parts vehicle.

To prepare 29CH potency—1 part 28CH potency +99 parts vehicle.

To prepare 30CH potency—1 part 29CH potency +99 parts vehicle.

Utility: It has great advantage for the manufacturer to prepare large quantities of medicines.

Avogadro's Number

The number of molecules in a gram-molecular weight (molecular weight expressed in gram) of any substance, normally represented as NA = 6.023 × 10^{23}. One molecule of a remedy substance in a molecule is considered to be equivalent to the 12C dilution level, i.e., not one molecule of the original substance or material can be found at this dilution level

Chapter 20

External Application

Introduction

From time immemorial, local applications have been used among physicians from Aesculapius down to the present day. This method of treatment was based on the teaching and general belief that if the outward manifestations were removed, the disease was cured. But Hahnemann, after his new discovery of homoeopathy, proclaimed that, external application is nothing but the outward reflexion of the internal derangement of the spiritual dynamic vital force which, when disturbed, expresses itself on the surface as signs.

External applications are not in the strict principle of Homoeopathy. Treatment of diseases by internal medication is the speciality of Homoeopathy. Diseases manifest by signs and symptoms, which are the sole guide of our homoeopathic method of treatment.

No disease is external or local. The immaterial spirit-like vital force throws out the internal malady on the external surface. The nature of external symptoms indicate the nature of internal sickness. By removal of external affections by external application the disease is never cured. On the other hand, they may attack some vital organs of our body, and as a result, we lose the image of the diseases. But for accidental cases, injuries, lacerations, burns etc. we need some local cleansing, and dressing of the part.

Hahnemann gave some arguments against the external applications in his 'Organon of Medicine' (5th edition) in Sec. 196 to Sec. 203. But later on, he saw the necessity of external application, while advocating the administration of medicine per mouth. He felt that, oral route is not the only route for administration of medicine.

So, he clearly explained, in the 6th edition of Organon of Medicine, in Sec. 284 and Sec. 285, about the use of external application. He said that curative remedy should be continued internally while the same remedy is used externally as an ointment, liniment, lotion, cerate etc.

Note: In inveterate and difficult cases of Sycosis (when the Sycosis remains along with the excrescences), *Thuja* may be applied externally. This is the only condition where external application of medicine has been advocated by Hahnemann.

Tenets of Organon towards the employment of External applications

In his **Organon of Medicine**, Hahnemann describes about the external applications.

In the 5th edition of 'Organon of Medicine' we see Hahnemann's arguments against the

external applications, i.e., disadvantages of external applications from Sec. 196 to Sec. 203.

Sec. 196-Sec. 197: *Administration of truly Homoeopathic Medicine both internally, and externally, simultaneously*

It may be argued that, in such topical lesions (so called local diseases), local application of drug, which is curable along with internal application, may be more beneficial. The greatest advantage of this local application is that, the local symptoms will disappear sooner than the internal symptoms. This was often thought as complete cure.

Due to this premature disappearance of the local symptoms, it is difficult and impossible to determine whether the internal disease also has been cured by internal medicine or not.

Sec. 198: *Administration of suitable homoeopathic medicine only externally:*

Only topical application in these local diseases are also inadmissible because of the above reasons, moreover, after removal of the local symptoms by a topical application, we will have to deal with less characteristic, less striking, and more fluctuating indistinct internal symptoms to select our remedy— which will no doubt be very difficult.

Only external applications to local diseases of miasmatic origin.

↓

Removal of local affections, but the too indefinite uncharacteristic and inconstant symptoms are left behind.

↓

No clear picture of the case is available.

↓

Difficult to individualise the case.

↓

Difficult to treat.

Sec. 199: *Removal of local disease by surgery or corroding or drying agent before the selection of a homoeopathic remedy*

Then the case becomes much more difficult as the most characteristic symptoms are removed, and only too indefinite (uncharacteristic), and inconstant symptoms are left out to decide on a remedy. Hence, after the external principal symptom has been removed from our observation, we are deprived of that feature of the case, which would have determined the selection of homoeopathic remedy, the internal use of which could have annihilated the disease completely.

Sec. 200: The persistence of the local affection during its internal treatment would have shown that the cure was not yet completed. If it is removed by internal medicine thus would be a convincing proof that the entire disease has been fully cured— an inestimable, indispensable advantage. But we have to lose this advantage, if we remove the local disease by external applications.

Sec. 201: *Local symptom, enlarged by vital-force, lessens internal disease*

When man's vital-force is encumbered with a chronic disease, which it is unable to overcome by its own powers, it instinctively adopts the plan of developing a local malady on some external part. This is solely for the object that by making, and keeping in a diseased state this part, which is not indispensable to human life, it may thereby silence the internal disease, which otherwise threatens to destroy the vital organs, and to deprive the patient of life. It may thereby, so to speak, transfer the internal disease to the vicarious local affection and, as it were, draw it thither. The presence of the local affection thus silences, for a time, the internal disease though without being able either to cure it or to diminish it materially.

The local affection, however, is never anything else than a part of the general disease. If the internal disease continues gradually to increase, nature is constrained to enlarge and aggravate the local symptom always more and more, in order that it may still suffice as a substitute for the increased internal disease, and may still keep it under.

Sec. 202: When the local symptom is destroyed by the topical application of external remedies, then the dormant internal malady is roused up, which had previously co-existed with the affection.

Sec. 203: Nature tries to protect more vital organs by throwing out everything on the less important organs, and on the external surface. But the application of external medicine alters and reverses the mechanism. As a result the more important vital organs are affected and damaged.

Thus, it becomes the source of thousands of named and unnamed human chronic maladies.

Sec. 203 (Footnote 1): External removal with internal administration of dissimilar medicines cannot cure, but weakens the organism and serves to add artificial chronic disease.

In 6th edition of 'Organon of Medicine', Hahnemann wrote in favour of external application, from Sec. 284 to Sec. 285.

Sec. 284: *Absorption of medicine*

Besides the tongue, mouth, and stomach, which most commonly absorb the medicine, the nose and respiratory organs are receptive of the action of medicine in fluid form by means of olfaction, and inhalation through the mouth.

But the whole remaining skin of the body, clothed with epidermis, is adapted to the action of medicinal solutions, especially if the inunction (i.e., an act of applying oil or ointment) is connected with simultaneous internal administration.

Sec. 285: The cure of very old diseases may be furthered by the physical application externally in the back, arms, extremities by rubbing the same medicine he gives internally, and which showed itself curatively. In doing so, he must but avoid parts subject to pain or spasm or skin eruption.

From this fact may be explained those marvellous cures, however infrequent, where chronic deformed patients, whose skin nevertheless was sound and clean, were cured quickly and permanently after a few baths whose medicinal constituents by chance were homoeopathically related.

N.B. Sec. 285 of the 6th edition of Organon has no corresponding aphorism in its 5th edition.

Sec. 282: If the fig-warts have existed for sometime without treatment, they will need for their perfect cure, the external application of their specific medicines as well as internal use at the same time.

Vehicles as bases for External applications

The vehicles that are used for preparation of external applications:

A. **Liquid vehicles used for External applications**

1. Purified water
2. Glycerine
3. Olive oil
4. Almond oil
5. Rosemary oil
6. Sesame or Teel oil.

B. **Semi-solid vehicles used for External applications**

1. Vaseline (soft-paraffin)
   (a) Yellow soft paraffin
   (b) White soft paraffin
2. Waxes
   (a) Beeswaxes:
      (i) yellow beeswax
      (ii) white beeswax
   (b) Spermaceti
   (c) Lanolin (anhydrous)
3. Prepared lard
4. Isinglass.
5. Soap:
   (a) Soft soap
   (b) Hard soap
   (c) Curd soap
6. Starch.

N.B. *For description of the above vehicles—see Chapter 'Vehicles'.*

List of External applications

1. Glyceroles
2. Ointments
3. Liniments
4. Opodeldocs
5. Lotions
6. Cerates
7. Poultices
8. Fomentations
9. Plasters
10. Oils
    (i) Oil Bouchi (ii) Oil Mullein
    (iii) Oil Olive (iv) Oil Rosemary
    (v) Arnica hair oil (vi) Oil of Winter-green
11. Injections: (i) Rectal
    (ii) Urethral
    (iii) Vaginal
12. Surgical dressings.

GLYCEROLES

Definition

These are the mixtures of solutions of mother tincture in glycerine. Most of them are much viscous with jelly-like consistencies.

Preparation

A. **Principle:** One part by weight or volume of mother tincture is mixed with nine parts by weight or volume of glycerine.
   Or
   One part by weight or volume of mother tincture mixed with four parts by weight or volume of glycerine excepting that of 'starch' (H.P.I.).

B. **Requirements:**

   (a) *Appliances*
   1. A perfectly clean round phial.
   2. A new, non-porous velvet cork.
   3. Balance with weight box.
   4. Weighing bottles.
   5. Pen, paper, gums, scissors etc.

   (b) *Ingredients*
   1. Required quantity of mother tincture.
   2. Required quantity of glycerine.

C. **Procedure:** The proper quantity of glycerine is taken in a clean round phial. The required quantity of mother tincture is poured over it. The cork is fixed and a homogeneous mixture is prepared by vigorous shaking.

Uses

It is anti-fungal, anti-bacterial, anti-pruritic, and is used mostly in the cases of gingivitis and stomatitis.

Precautions

1. Before using the glycerine, its purity test should be done.
2. Cleansing of utensils should be done properly.
3. Mixture should be continued till the colour becomes uniform.
4. A note '**For External use only**' should be pasted on the phial, below the name of the glycerole.

Examples

1. Calendula glycerole
2. Phytolacca glycerole
3. Hydrastis glycerole (Glycerole of Hydrastis)
4. Borax glycerole (Glycerite of Borax)
5. Glycerole of carbolic acid
6. Glycerole of starch.

Glycerole of Starch (Glycero Amyli)

It is a form of ointment prepared in the following manner:

Starch—1 part

Glycerine—8 parts

Mix it in a glass mortar, and rub together till intimately mixed.

↓

Transfer the mixture to a porcelain dish.

↓

Apply heat (gradually raised to 240°F or 115°C) and stir constantly till the starch particles are completely broken and a jelly-like preparation is made.

↓

Add the requisite quantity of medicine in the proportion of one in ten.

OINTMENTS

Etymology

L. unguentum, a salve

Definition

These are semi-solid preparations; they should have the required consistency, so that they may be readily applied on the skin by rubbing. They should be soft, and do not require melting on application. They are also called 'Therapeutic creams'.

Preparation

A. **Principle:** One part by weight or volume of mother tincture is mixed with nine parts by weight or volume of vaseline.

B. **Requirements**

   (a) *Ingredients*
   1. Required quantity of mother tincture.
   2. Required quantity of white vaseline.

(b) *Appliances*

1. Slab; 2. Spatula; 3. Ointment phial; 4. Balance with weight box. 5. Pen, labelling paper, pasting gums, scissors.

C. **Procedure:** The proper quantity of vaseline is weighed, and put on clean slab. The required quantity of mother tincture is poured over it. It is thoroughly mixed with the help of a spatula, till the colour of the whole solution becomes uniform. All ointments other than *Sulphur*, and *Graphites* are prepared as above.

Modern methods of preparation of Ointments

Nowadays, two general methods are adopted for the preparation of ointments:

A. **Mechanical Incorporation or Trituration Method**

This method is applicable when the medicament is in a powdered form. It is made on a glass slab with a spatula. Small portion of the base is used for better results. Slab is usually made of ground glass, and spatula of stainless steel. Spatula should be such that it acts as a roller, to pass over any particle in the ointment mixture. At the end of each operation, slight twist of the wrist is required to reverse the direction of movement of spatula.

B. **Fusion Method**

This method is used when the base of the ointment consists of white-soft paraffin, spermaceti, or wax. They are just melted on a water bath and the required medicine is slowly added and the mixture is properly stirred to make it homogeneous. The mixture is then cooled and becomes ready for use.

Commercially: Ointments are prepared by fusion method in a specially made apparatus, i.e., an ointment mixing vessel with electrical heating and cooling device. The resultant ointments are represented in collapsible tubes. These are mostly made up of aluminium. They (tubes) do not seem to be affecting therapeutic value of the ointment. It is better to use only glass jars to stock the ointments or paper cartons for dispensing them.

For dispensing purpose: Small amount of ointment can be made by rubbing the base with a spatula, and due to friction when it gets slightly thinner in consistency, then the medicine is gradually added drop-wise, and the spatula mixes with the medicine in the same way as is done with the dry powder.

Storage

Should be stored in cool dark place, out of contact with air. Preferably, all ointments can be refrigerated.

Uses

1. For bleeding or non-bleeding piles. In all fissures, ulceration, itchings and bleeding from the rectum.
2. For bruises, contusions and blows, for blackened eyes, bed sores, boils, chilblains, corns, bunions.
3. As a dressing for torn and jagged wounds. As a dressing for indolent ulcers, fistula, lepra, psoriasis, lupus and carbuncles.
   As a dressing for cracked heels.
4. Very useful in burns.

Examples

1. Aesculus ointment
2. Arnica ointment
3. Calendula ointment
4. Cantharis ointment
5. Graphites ointment
6. Hamamelis ointment
7. Hydrastis ointment
8. Thuja ointment
9. Qucabator ointment
10. Sulphur ointment
11. Belladonna ointment
12. Ratanhia ointment
13. Sulphur iod ointment
14. Iodoform ointment
15. Ichthymol ointment
16. Calomel ointment
17. Iodine ointment
18. Menthol ointment
19. Naphthalin ointment
20. Boric acid ointment
21. Mercurial ointment
22. Acetate of lead ointment

23. Rhus tox ointment
24. Symphytum ointment
25. Hypericum ointment
26. Skookum chuck ointment.

Precautions

1. Purity test must be done before using it.
2. Cleansing and mixing should be done very carefully.
3. Labelling must be done and with a note, 'For External Use Only'.

LINIMENTS (EMBROCATIONS)

Definition

Liniments or embrocations are applications of an oily or spirituous consistence. These are mixtures or solutions of different medicines (mainly mother tincture) in oil, alcoholic solutions of soap or emulsions, and are suitable for rubbing or painting over the skin. They also serve as protective coatings. Camphor enters into their composition for its local stimulant action, and also to lessen the risk of these being taken internally as it has characteristic strong smell.

Preparations

A. **Principle**

1 part by weight or volume of mother tincture is mixed with 9 parts by weight or volume of olive oil.

1 part of the required medicine is mixed with 4 parts of olive oil or 'Tincture of soap' (H.P.I. Vol. I).

B. **Requirements**

1. *Ingredients*
   (a) Required quantity of mother tincture.
   (b) Required quantity of olive oil or 'Tincture of soap'.
2. *Appliances*
   (a) A clean round phial.
   (b) A new non-porous velvet cork.
   (c) Balance with weight box.
   (d) Weighing bottles.
   (e) Pen, labelling paper, pasting gums, scissors etc.

C. **Procedure**

Proper quantity of olive oil or 'Tincture of Soap' is taken in a clean glass phial. The required quantity of mother tincture is poured over it. The cork is fixed and a homogeneous mixture is prepared by vigorous shaking.

N.B. Preparation of 'Tincture of Soap':

Soft soap 10 gm.

Strong alcohol 25 ml.

Purified water 16 ml.

Dissolve with gentle heat and strain (H.P.I. Vol. I).

Precautions

A label must be pasted on the body of the phial writing the:

1. Name of the mother tincture.
2. 'For External Use Only'
3. 'Shake Well Before Use'.

Uses

1. Painted over the painful part of the body resulting from falling, blows etc.
2. To reduce the rheumatic pain, to loosen the phlegm accumulated after catching cold.

Examples

1. Arnica liniment
2. Bellis per liniment
3. Phytolacca liniment
4. Rhus tox liniment
5. Ruta liniment
6. Bryonia liniment

OPODELDOCS

Definition

These are semi-solid liniments prepared with the following ingredients

White curd soap: 140 gm (or $4\frac{1}{2}$ ounces)

Purified water: 266 ml (or 9 ounces)

Strong alcohol: 444 ml (or 15 ounces)

Mother tincture: 100 ml (or $3\frac{1}{6}$ ounces)

Method of preparation (Schematic)

White curd soap + purified water

↓←Heated gently

Solutions become transparent
↓ ←Strong alcohol added gradually
←Then mother tincture of drug added
←Stirred well
Strained (while still fluid)
↓
Poured into a suitable phial.

Uses

For sprains, bruises, and rheumatic pains, it is very useful.

LOTIONS

Definition

These are liquid suspensions or dispersions in aqueous media, used as external applications over the affected parts of the body.

Preparation

A. **Principle**

1 part of the requisite mother tincture and 9 parts of purified water are mixed thoroughly.

B. **Requirements**

1. *Ingredients*
   - (a) Required amount of mother tincture.
   - (b) Required quantity of purified water.
2. *Appliances*
   - (a) One clean round phial.
   - (b) One new non-porous velvet cork.
   - (c) Balance with wieght box.
   - (d) Weighing bottle.
   - (e) Pen, labelling paper, pasting gum, scissors etc.

C. **Procedure**

The proper amount of purified water is taken in a clean round phial, and the required amount of mother tincture is poured over it. The phial is corked and shaken well. The mixture is shaken vigorously till its colour become uniform.

Precautions

In the label of the phial containing a lotion, the lines 'Shake Well Before Use', and 'For External Use Only' must be exhibited with the direction of use.

Uses

Used in bruised pain without bloodshed arising from falling, injuries, blows etc.

Examples

1. Arnica lotion
2. Calendula lotion
3. Rhus tox lotion
4. Ruta lotion
5. Cantharis lotion
6. Staphysagria lotion
7. Sabadilla lotion
8. Euphrasia lotion
9. Apis mel lotion
10. Clematis lotion
11. Symphytum lotion
12. Menthol lotion (1%)
13. Ceanothus lotion
14. Carboneum sulph. IX lotion
15. Ilex aquifolium
16. Sanguinaria lotion.

CERATES

Definition

These are unctuous oily substances due to the presence of wax (sera). It gets easily spread over the surface at ordinary temperature, but maintains the solidified state and does not run away as a liquid.

Preparation (by schematic representation)

Spermaceti: 5 parts or Vaseline: 16 parts
+ +
White wax: 2 parts Paraffin: 3 parts
+
Almond oil: 16 parts

These are taken in a well-cleansed porcelain basin.

↓ ← Melted by gentle heat
← Stirred constantly by means of a solid glass rod.
Now, allowed to become cool
↓
When cooled, one part of requisite mother tincture is mixed thoroughly with nine parts by weight of the above mixture.

Uses

Used as poultices on the burns, scalds, boils, carbuncles etc.

Examples

1. Cantharis cerate
2. Urtica urens cerate
3. Arnica cerate
4. Aesculus cerate
5. Hamamelis cerate

6. Calendula cerate 8. Lycopersicum cerate
7. Graphites cerate 9. Chrysarobinum cerate

POULTICES OR CATAPLASMS

Characteristics

1. They are soft, semi-liquid, external applications.
2. They must contain any medicament.
3. They act firmly on a principle so that they either stimulate the body surface or relieve an inflamed area by supplying medicated substances in the presence of heat and moisture.
4. It helps in drawing infective material from the affected area due to its 'hygroscopic' and 'absorptive' characters of its ingredients used, i.e., glycerine, starch etc.
5. They mitigate pain by relaxing tension and promoting perspiration.

Varieties

Poultices may be made as:

1. **Linseed-meal Poultices**

(a) The boiling water should be poured into heated bowl and into this the meal quickly sprinkled with one hand, while the mixture is constantly stirred with a stainless steel knife or spatula with the other, till a thin, smooth paste is formed.

(b) The paste should be quickly spread on the muslin cloth.

(c) A few drops of desired mother tincture (e.g. Ranunculus bulbosus) is added to it.

(d) Then spread it along the cloth with the remaining paste.

Linseed-meal retains heat and moisture for a long time, but is liable to irritate delicate and inflamed skin. Instances of intolerance to Linseed-meal poultice have been reported in which the mere application has brought on almost fatal attacks of asthma.

2. **Bread Poultices**

Put slices of bread into a basin, pour over them boiling water, and place by the fire for a few minutes when the water should be poured off and replaced by fresh boiling water, and this again poured and the bread pressed, beaten with a fork, and made into a poultice.

Bread-poultices are valuable for their bland, non-irritating properties.

3. **Charcoal Poultices**

Uniformly mix charcoal with bread poultice and just before the application of the poultice, sprinkle the surface with a layer of charcoal, and a simple bread-poultice applied over it. Charcoal poultices correct offensive smells from foul sores and favour a healthier action.

4. **Carrot Poultices**

Boiled carrots turn into soft mash with a fork—and apply in the ordinary way.

They are said to make wounds cleaner and healthier.

Uses of Poultices

Poultices are chiefly useful in the following complaints: Pneumonia, Pleurisy, Bronchitis, Pericarditis, Peritonitis, Acute Rheumatism, Lumbago and to mature and facilitate the discharge of matter in abscesses and boils.

To mature abscesses or disperse inflammations, poultices should extend beyond the limits of inflamed tissue; but after the discharge, the poultices should be a little larger than the opening through which the matter is escaping. At no time should they be continued long, or kept applied continuously.

In Pneumonia, and all deep-seated inflammation, they should be renewed as soon as they become cool, and the former one not disturbed till the fresh one is ready to replace it, or else, after the removal of poultice, the part should be rapidly dried with a hot towel and then covered with a sheet of hot cotton wool.

In Acute Lumbago they must be applied thick and hot, large enough to cover the affected part, and be renewed the moment they become cool. After continuing this treatment from one to three hours, the skin should be wiped dry and covered with flannel, and this again with oil-silk.

FOMENTATIONS (FOMENTA)

Fomentations are one of the methods of external applications. They do not contain any medicament. They act firmly on thermal principle.

There are hot and cold fomentations.

Hot Fomentations

By means of flannels, wrung out of hot water, for application to the surface of the body.

The proper way to apply hot fomentations is to take a twofold piece of flannel large enough to cover the affected part. Immerse this folded flannel in a kettle of boiling water or pour boiling water over it in a basin, and lift it by a pair of tongs or a stick, and put it on a wringer—a stout towel or duster with sticks attached to both ends. The water is then squeezed out as much as possible and the flannel is applied to the affected part and covered with a large piece of India-rubber sheeting or oiled-silk, extending about an inch beyond the flannel. Place over this a thick layer of cotton-wool and bandage. The flannel should be changed every 20 or 30 minutes.

Uses

Hot fomentations are useful in relieving pain, arresting inflammation, and checking the formation of matter and are often valuable adjuncts to poultices.

Acne indurata and similar inflamed principles can often be increased or reduced in size by them. Conjoined with poultices, they expedite the passage of matter to the surface, and favour its subsequent expulsion.

Dry Fomentations

When heat alone is required and it is desirable to avoid the relaxation of tissues which moisture would occasion, dry heated substances—flannel, bran, chamomile flowers, salt, sand etc are used. After thoroughly heating the substance it should be placed in a bag made for the purpose and which has also been previously heated.

Hot water bag (made up of rubber) may be used for dry fomentations. The rubber bag is filled up with moderate hot water in its three-fourth part.

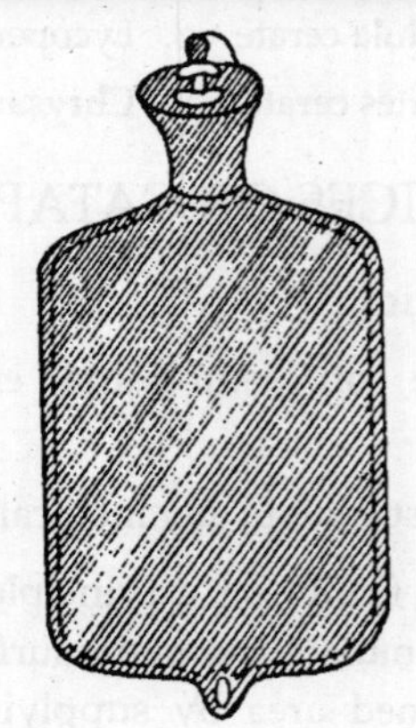

Hot Water Bag

By pressing the mouth of the bag, some amount of vapour is expelled. Then the mouth of the bag is tightly fitted.

Cold Fomentations

It is done to relieve the temperature either by cold water or icebag. It works on the principle of evaporation.

Wet a sterilised clean folded cloth in cold purified water, leave it uncovered to permit evaporation, and apply it to the affected part.

Icebag (Rubber): The ice is broken into small pieces and filled up three-fourth part of the rubber bag, without washing the ice. The mouth of the bag is pressed to expel the air remaining in the bag. Then the mouth of the bag is fitted tightly. The icebag should not be kept on affected area for a long time.

The icebag is put on the head in Meningitis, or concussion, and on the knee-joint for Acute Synovitis.

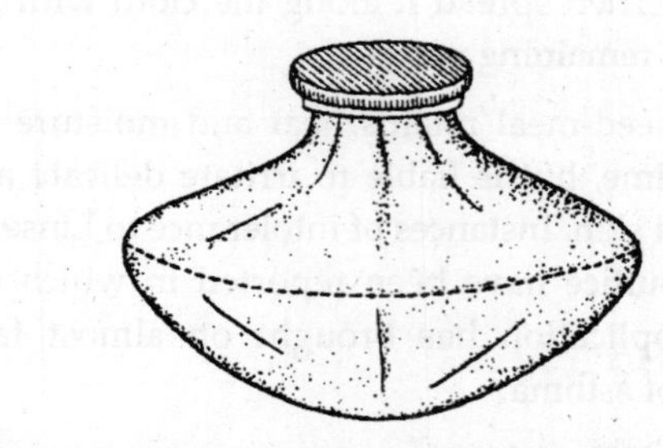

Ice Bag

According to some authorities, cold contracts not only the capillaries of the skin to which it is applied, but by reflex action those of the organs underneath it. Hence, the application of an icebag to the chest to arrest pulmonary haemorrhage.

PLASTERS

Definition

These are sticky and solid compounds, which adhere when applied to some part of the body and produce either general or local effect.

Method of preparation: Base-Isinglass

One ounce (30 gm) isinglass is taken in shreds.

↓

Dissolve it in sufficient quantity of purified water by boiling.

↓

Then the solution is filtered with a clean towel, already moistened with purified water.

↓

The solution is evaporated on a water bath until it is reduced to 10 ounces (or 300 gms).

↓

Half of this spread on a piece of silk, linen, muslin or leather etc.

↓

Remaining half mixed with the mother tincture of the desired drug and with this, spreading is completed.

Uses

It helps in two ways—one to give support and protection to the part and the other to bring the medication in direct contact with the affected parts. In homoeopathy, its use is restricted.

Examples

1. Aconite Plaster
2. Arnica Plaster
3. Belladonna Plaster.
4. Calendula Plaster
5. Rhus tox Plaster

OILS

1. Oil Bouchi

(a) **Source:** The seeds of a common herbaceous weed *Psoralea corylifolia* L (Family—Leguminosae and sub-family papilionaceae). It is known by the name *Babchi* (Hindi).

(b) **Method of preparation**

(i) The seeds are crushed to 20 meshes of fineness.

(ii) Then soaked in *teel oil* (sesame oil). (1 part of seed being soaked in 2 parts of oil).

(iii) Keep it for 10 days, stirring occasionally.

(iv) Oil is then strained and the strength adjusted.

(c) **Uses:** Shows remarkable changes in cases of depigmentation of the skin, psoriasis, boils, tubercles, liver spots and all cases of dirty looking skin. Leucoderma.

2. Oil Mullein

(a) **Source:** The flower extract of *Verbascum thapsus* of family Scrophulariaceae.

(b) **Method of preparation:** Though the preparation is known as Mullein oil, it contains no oil excepting the essential oil present in the flower itself.

Solvents used are: Glycerine, alcohol and other inert substances. 1 part of the flower yields to 10 parts of Mullein essence.

(c) **Uses:** Mullein oil is an extremely beneficial remedy for earache, discharge from the ear, eczema of external ear and its canal, suppurative inflammation of the middle ear. It is a bactericide, recommended in dry, scaly conditions of meatus, otalgia with sense of obstructions, deafness. It softens and facilitates the removal of hardened secretions. Relieves pain quickly.

3. Oil of Wintergreen

(a) **Source:** It is the oil distilled from the fresh plant *Gaultheria fragrantissima.*

(b) **Characters:** Colourless or nearly colourless oil, odour strong, characteristic pungent taste

(c) **Uses:** It is used in rheumatic diseases (e.g. gout, osteoarthritis of knee, lumbar radiculopathy), Pruritus, and Epididymitis.

4. Oil Olive

(a) **Applied externally**

(i) It renders the skin smoother, softer and more flexible.

(ii) It is used for burns and some skin diseases.

(iii) It is recommended to use in nostrils to protect from dusts, cotton fibres, in a patient of allergic shinitis, COPD.

(b) **Applied orally:** As safe purgatives.

5. Arnica Hair Oil

Dry roots of Arnica are coarsely pulverised. One part of its powder form is poured into ten parts of olive oil and kept in well-stoppered bottle for two weeks in a warm room. The content expressed and filtered.

6. Oil Rosemary

Largely used in perfumes and cosmetics. It is medicinally inert.

INJECTIONS

Definition

These are liquids to be introduced into any part of the body by means of a syringe.

Types of Injections

A. **Vaginal injections**

Ludlam's formula:

Desired drug (Q) : 15 ml (or ½ fluid ounce)

Glycerine : 45 ml (or 1½ fluid ounce)

Purified water : 60 ml (or 2 fluid ounces)

These are well-mixed and for each injection, 4 to 5 ml of the mixture is used with sufficient tepid water.

B. **Urethral injections**

Desired drug, say, Hydrastis θ: 30 ml (1 ounce), Purified water: 600 ml (20 ounces) mixed in it.

Urethral injections of other various drugs are prepared by mixing with purified water in the proportion as prescribed by a physician.

C. **Rectal injections**

The prescribed quantity of the drug is mixed with about 60 ml (or 2 ounces) of arrowroot water, or thin starch solution, and injected slowly, so that it may be retained.

SURGICAL DRESSINGS

1. (a) **Absorbent Cotton**

It is prepared from raw cotton fibres by a series of mechanical and chemical cleansing processes to remove the natural wax and other impurities so as to make the property of the cotton more absorbent. Besides roll-form, it can be made into cotton balls. Three sizes are generally available—large, medium and small balls.

Uses: It is used for local medications, for application of antiseptics, cleansing of the skin and before parenteral introduction.

(b) **Non-Absorbent bleached Cotton**

It acts as a water-repellant, the natural wax is retained while cleansing off fibres.

Uses: It is used for packing, padding to give cushioning effect to the bandages over the wound in draining the fluid and in sanitary napkins etc.

2. **Surgical Gauzes**

These give tensile-strength while still maintaining the absorbent quality of the material. The cotton is woven in long threads and then the threads are woven in open mesh cloth. The meshes are measured on the basis of threads per sq. inch.

(a) ***Gauze-pads:*** These are made by folding on one another and cutting into various sizes, taking care that, no loose threads are left behind. During unfolding no cut ends of these gauzes are visible.

The most popular sizes are:

2 × 2 – 12 ply; 3 × 2 – 12 ply;

4 × 4 – 8 and 16 ply.

(b) ***Cotton filmated gauzes:*** These are ecnomically better than simple gauze pads. Thin absorbent cotton is spread evenly in the folds of these gauzes, pads and then folded.

3. **Sanitary Napkins**

These are used in gynaecological and maternity cases. Due to the presence of filler of absorbent cotton cellulose, these are used for better absorption and drainage.

4. **Absorbent Lint**

Has a cotton-fibre jetting out and woven cotton on one another.

Uses:

1. For application of ointment plasters.
2. For better support and protection to the wound.

5. **Bandages**

The different types of bandages are:

(a) ***Common Gauze Roller Bandages***

The commonly used bandages are made of cotton. These are absorbent cotton thread, woven in mesh and prepared in continuous roll of length. They are called 'roller bandage', as the bandaging material is kept rolled. The open end of the bandage is called its 'tail', while the rolled part is called the 'head'. They can be sterilised and used in drainage and bandaging.

(b) ***Electrocrepe (Cotton-crepe) Bandages***

Provides greater compression and support because of its elasticity. It is elastic, but has no rubber. Its elasticity is due to the special weave which allows to stretch practically twice its length. It helps therefore to bandage varicose veins, sprains etc. It allows limited mobility and, therefore, does not impair circulation.

(c) ***Adhesive Bandages***

Made of cotton, these may be inelastic (e.g., leucoplast) or elastic (e.g., elastoplast). These are gaining fast popularity and replacing ordinary bandages widely.

It is used in places where, more support is required, i.e., in fracture of rib or where muscles and ligaments are involved.

(d) ***Plaster of paris Bandages***

These are used in treatment of fractures and dislocations where immobility is required.

These are always kept in waterproof packings as moisture tends to harden the plaster, making it useless.

(e) ***Bandages impregnated with medicament***

e.g., Calendula θ, Bellis perenis θ, are used to protect and soothe the skin as well as to promote healing in chronic conditions, such as varicose veins.

FORMULAE

Glyceroles, Liniments, Ointments, Lotions, Injections, Oils and Cerates

I. Glyceroles

1. GLYCER, ALOES

Rx, Tr. Aloes θ 3i

Glycer 3ix M

Cracked skin, lips, nose, hands, etc. fissured and sore anus.

2. GLYCER. AMYLI

Rx, Pulv. Amyli opt ʒi

Glycer ʒviii

Rubbed together till intimately mixed; then transfer the mixture to a porcelain dish and apply heat, gradually raised to 240°F (115°C), stirring constantly until the starch particles are completely broken, and a translucent jelly is formed.

Broken chilblains; fistula; prolapsus ani; prevention of bed sores; irritation of skin from any cause.

3. GLYCER, AMYLI MEDICAT

Rx, Glycer. Amyli ʒi

Trit. vel. Tinct ʒ M

4. GLYCER BORACIS

Rx, Pulv. Boracis ʒi

Glycer ʒiv solve.

Thrush; pruritus vulvae.

5. GLYCER, EXTRACTI HAMAM

Rx, Extracti Hamam 3i

Glycer
Aq. dest } aa 2iss M

Fistula of anus; prolapsus

6. GLYCER, HYDRAST

Rx, Tr. Hydrastis can 3i

Glycer, ad ʒss M

Inflammation of uterus; sore nipples; fissured anus; cracked lips etc.

7. GLYCER. AC. MUR.

Rx, Ac. hydrochlor. P.B. gtt. v.

Glycer ʒss M

Ulcerated throat; ulcerous thrush etc.

8. GLYCER. AC. MUR. FORT.

Rx, Ac. hydrochlor. P.B. gtt. x

Glycer ℥ss M

Ulcerated throat; thrush etc.

9. GLYCER. PHYTOLACCAE

Rx, Tr. Baccae Phyto decand 3i

Glycer ad ℥iss M

Inflammation of bone; condylomata; excoriation of breast etc.

10. GLYCER. AMYLI C. AC. TANNIC.

Rx, Glycer. amyli 3i

Glycer A. Tannic ℥i M

Itching of anus etc.

11. GLYCER. AC. TANNICI

Rx, Ac. tannic ℥i

Glycer ℥iv

Rub together in a mortar, then transfer the mixture to a porcelain dish and apply a gentle heat until completely dissolved.

12. GLYCER. AC. SULPHUROSI

Rx, Ac. sulphurosi 3ii

Glycer ℥iss M

Chapped hands; chilblains; ringwarm etc.

13. GLYCER. VER.-VIR.

Rx, Tr. Ver.-vir. 3i

Glycer 3ix M

Sore nipples.

II. Liniments

1. LIN. AC. CARBOL.

Rx, Ac. carbol. pur ℥i

Ol. olive. opt ℥iv M

To facilitate desquamation in Scarlet fever, Measles etc.

2. LIN. AC. CARBOL. FORT

Rx, Ac. carbol pur 3ii

Ol. olive, opt. ℥iss M

Burns and scalds; To prevent excoriations etc.

3. LIN ACON.

Rx, Tr. Acon, radix 3 i

Lin. saponia. P.H.B. ad. ℥i M

Neuralgia; local forms of rheumatism.

4. LIN BELL.

Rx, Chlorof. 3 i

Tr. Bell. 3 vi M

Neuralgia; rheumatism

5. LIN. CALCIS

Rx, Gl. Lini ℥ii

Liq. Calcis ℥ii

Tr. Calend, ℥ii M

Burns; chilblains etc.

6. LIN. CAMPHORAE

Rx. Camphorae ℥i

Ol. oliv. opt. ℥iv. solve.

Scarlatina; Chicken pox; Itching.

7. LIN. RHUS TOX

Rx. Tr. Rhus Tox 3iss

Lin. Saponis P.H.B. ad. ℥ISSM

Lumbago and other forms of local rheumatism; Straining.

8. LIN. URTICAE UR.

Rx. Tr. Urt. ur. ℥i

Ol. oliv. opt. ad ℥iii M

Ulcerated burns.

9. LIN. VER.-VIR.

Rx, Tr. Ver.-vir ℥i

Lin. saponis P.H.B. ad. ℥i M

Paralysis; nervous pain over lower part of spine.

III. Ointments

1. UNG. ARNICAE

Rx, Flor. Arnicae ℥iii

Fol. Arnical ℥i

Adipis praeparatae lb ii

Moisten the flowers and powdered leaves with half their weight of purified water, then heat together with the lard in a water bath for three or four hours and strain.

Bruises, contusion and blows where the skin is not broken; blackened eyes; blisters on the feet from chafing of shoes, chafing; bed-sores; boils which do not mature well; itchings; chilblains; corns and bunions; corns; sore from cutting; muscular rheumatism resulting from exposure to cold and dampness.

2. UNG. BALS. PERV

Rx, bals. peru, 3ii

cerat, cetaei, 3iv M

Bed sores.

3. UNG. BISMUTHI

Rx, Bismuth. nit. grs. xxx

Adopis praeparatae ℥i M

Obstinate and intense itching and irritation such as Eczema and other skin diseases.

4. UNG. HEPAR SULPH

Rx, Hep sulph. pur. grs. iii

Adopis praeparatae ℥i M

Ganglion.

5. UNG. HYDRAG. NIT. DUL.

Rx, Hydrarg. nit. P.B. 3i

Cerat. cetacei, ℥i M

Itching of anus.

6. UNG. MERC. BINIOD

Rx,

Biniod. merc. irs. ii

Adipis praeperatae 3iii M

Styes; acne of the beard; ganglion.

7. UNG. PRAECIP. RUB.

Rx, Merc. praecip. rub. grs. iii

ugn. simpl. ℥i M

Tarsal ophthalmia.

IV. Lotions

1. LOTIONES MEDICAT

Rx, Tr. 3i

Aq. dest. ad. ℥vi M

2. LOTIO. AC. BENZ

Rx, Ac. Benz, pur. grs. xv

Aq. dist. 3viii

sp. v. Rect. 3iii

Dissolve the Benzoic acid in the Rec. spirit, add the purified water and shake thoroughly until the precipitate which forms is entirely redissolved.

Sore nipples, itching of the skin etc.—its usefulness has been largely tested.

3. LOTIO AC. CARBOL

Rx, Ac. carbol. pur. qr. x

Aq. dest. ℥v. solve.

Ulcers; Inflammation of mouth; pruritus vulvae.

4. LOTIO AC. CARBOL FORT

Rx, Ac. carbol. pur. 3i ss

Glycer ℥ss.

Aq. dest ad ℥vi

Burns and scalds; To prevent excoriation etc.

5. LOTIO AC. NIT.

Rx, Ac. nit. Fort. gtt xxiv

Aq. dest ℥vi M

6. LOTIO ANT. TART

Rx, Ant. tart. pulv. gr. I

Aq. Calid. ℥ss Glycer ℥ss

Dissolve the antimony in the warm water and add the glycerine.

7. LOTIO ARSENICA

Rx, Tr. Ars. 2x. 3ss–3i

Aq. ℥vi–℥ix M

Ulcers with internal use of Arsenic, pruritus vulvae.

8. LOTIO BORACIS

Rx, Pulv. Boracis gr. xx

Aq. dest. ℥ii solve.

Excoriations; pruritus vulvae.

9. LOTIO BORACIS C. CAMPH.

Rx, pulv. Boracis 3i

Sp. Camph. ℥i

Lin. sapon's ℥ii

Glycer ℥ss

Aq. dest. ℥xii M

Ringworm; Dandruff etc.

10 LOTIO CALC MUR

Rx, Tr. Calc. mur. ix 3i

Aq. dest ad. ℥i M

Boils.

11 LOTIO CARBONICS DETERG

Rx, Liq. Carb. Deterg. ℥ss

Aq. dest. ad. ℥viii M

Prurigo; Eczema; itching of anus.

12. LOTIO HAMAMFORT

Rx, Tr. Hamam θ 3ii

Aq. dest ℥i M

Chilblains; Fistula; Phimosis

13. LOTIO HYDRASTIS MUR

Rx, Hydrast. mur. grs. iii

Aq. dest. ℥iii solve.

Stomatitis.

14. LOTIO KALI HYD

Rx, Kali hyd θ ℥i

Aq. dest ℥viii solve

Glandular swellings.

15. LOTIO SULPHURIS

Rx, Tr. Sulph θ 3i

Aq. dest. ad ℥i M

Ulcers; acne of the beard.

V. Injections

1. INJECTIO GLYCER, HYDRAST

Rs, Hydrast. can. θ 3i

Glycer 3iii M

Aq. dest. ℥ss.

2. INJECTIO MORPHIAE

Rx, Morphia pur. g. ii

Ol. Amyg. dulc. ℥i

Triturate together in a mortar.

3. INJECTIO LIQ. PLUMBI

Rx, Liq. Plumbi diacet, 3ss

Aq. dest ℥ii M

4. INJECTIO POT. PERMANG

Rx, Pot. permang. cryst. grs

v. vel. x

Aq. dest. ℥i solve

5. INJECTIO GLYCER. AC. TANN

Rx, Glycer AC. tann. ℥iii

Ol. oliv. ℥i

Mucilage ℥i M

6. INJECTIO ZINC. CHLOR.

Rx, Zinci chlor. grs. viii

Aq. dest. ℥viii solve

VI. Oils

Extract of the fresh plants in olive and linseed oil.

1. OL. ARNICAE

For external applications in all cases where Arnica is indicated.

2. OL. HYPERICI

For application to bed-sores, to painful effects, and broken limbs.

VII. Cerates

1. ARNICA CERATE

Tr. Arn. 3i

Simple cerate 1b

Melt in a sand-bath and stir till cold.

2. AESCULUS CERATE

Tr. Aesc. hip. ℥i

Simple cerate lb.

Glycerine ℥i

White wax ℥i

Mix the Tr. with the glycerine, but all in the melted cerate, stir till cold.

Chapter 21

Preservation of Drugs and Potentised Medicines

General Rules

1. **Labelling:** It must be done on required vessels while preserving drugs.
2. **Containers:** All substances should be preserved in neutral glass, earthenware jar, or bottles, being well-corked or stoppered.

   Exceptions

   (a) Hard glass (potash) bottles with glass stoppers for preserving corrosive substances, such as acids or alkalis.

   (b) Actinic glass bottles (coloured) covered outside with a solution of asphaltum, or black varnish for preserving drugs which may be affected by light or sunlight.

   (c) Gutta-purcha bottle—for preserving Fluoric acid.

   (d) Avoid: (i) Blue-coloured bottles—as blue colour has some dynamic effects injurious to drugs (as per Burt) (ii) yellow or amber coloured bottles—as these acquire some medicinal virtue, after exposed to sunlight (H.P.U.S.).
3. **Place and method of preservation**

   (a) Plants and their parts: should be kept in a cool dark place or a little quantity of water should be sprinkled over them from time to time.

   (b) Pulverised drugs: should be perfectly dried before storing, otherwise their moisture content may mould. This drying is done by spreading out the pulverised drugs on a water-bath (F.N. Sec. 268) or for bigger quantities, in a temperature-adjustable drying chamber.

   (c) Animals and animal products: As they decompose very quickly, should be used immediately after collections. If necessary, may be preserved in refrigerator. Venoms can be preserved in deep-freeze, being kept in glycerine.
4. **Separate arrangement**

   (a) For strong smelling substances: Such as *Asafoetida, Camphor, Kreosote, Iodine, Moschus, Oleum* etc. should be kept separately in tightly closed bottles, so that the peculiar odours of such drugs may not contaminate other drugs.

   (b) Drugs possessing the power of reaction should be preserved separately.
5. Fresh drugs which cannot be used immediately should be kept in refrigerator.

6. Fresh drugs which are to be collected from a distant place, should be packed loosely, and carefully in ordinary cases or botanical boxes and kept cool.
7. Drugs which need drying before transportation, should be dried by tying in loose bundles, and hanging in a shade away from direct sunlight, dust, rain, insects, worms etc.
8. Drugs which are to be preserved for a long time are to be dried in an especially constructed chamber (where temperature can be adjusted), allowing hot air to flow for drying the drug-substances.
9. **Avoid:** Strong light, direct sunlight, smoke, dust, strong odour etc.

Preservation of Mother preparations

1. **Labelling:** All containers should be properly labelled in proper pharmaceutical names mentioning their strength and alcohol content by % v/v, date of manufacturing, name of manufacturer, as far as possible, while storing.

   The sign 'Q' is affixed after the name of each mother tincture, e.g., *Chelidoneum* Q. The Q solution and O is affixed for mother solutions and mother substances.
2. **Containers:** Mother tinctures or solutions should be stored in new, well-cleansed, colourless, neutral flint glass bottles, in dry and cool place.

   Exceptions

   (a) Hard glass bottles with glass stoppers: for preserving acid or caustic preparations.

   (b) Actinic glass bottles (coloured) covered with a solution of asphaltum or black varnish: for preserving tinctures or solutions which may be affected by light or sunlight.

   (c) Gutta-purcha bottles: for preserving *Fluoric acid* and Q solution.

   (d) Glycerine in phial: for preserving *Lachesis* mother substnaces.

   (e) Avoid: (i) Blue-coloured bottles—as these have some dynamic effects injurious to drugs (as per Burt), (ii) yellow or amber coloured bottles—as these acquire some medicinal virtue, after exposed to sunlight (H.P.U.S.).
3. **Avoid:** (i) Too much heat or cold—on exposed to great cold, some tincture or solution may become turbid with muddy sediment, or even form crystals, (ii) Strong light, direct sunlight, smoke, dust, damp, strong odours etc.
4. **Temperature:** Tinctures or solutions should be kept at even temperature of about 60°F (15.6°C).
5. **Filtration:** Tinctures or solution should be filtered before storing.
6. **Separate arrangement:** Strong smelling durgs e.g., *Asafoetida, Camphor, Iodine, Moschus, Terebinth, Oleum* etc., should be kept separately in air-tight, well-closed glass-bottles.

Directions for preservation of drugs

	Name of drug (mother tincture/ solution/substance)	How to preserve
1.	Argentum nitricum solution.	Amberic glass bottles
2.	Causticum θ	Alembic glass bottles
3.	Hepar sulphur O	Actinic glass bottles covered outside with a solution of asphaltum
4.	Fluoric acid θ solution	Gutta-purcha bottle
5.	Lachesis O	Glycerine in sealed vial
6.	Phosphorus θ	preserved under water, in which it is insoluble, because it is inflammable in the air.

Preservation of Potentised medicines

1. **Labelling:** Name of the potentised medicine with the respective number of potency and the scale should be distinctly marked both on the cork and on the container's label, e.g. *Aconite* 6x, *Aconite* 6 and *Aconite* 0/6 etc. Date of manufacturing and name of the manufacturer should also be stated in the container. Original manufacturer should also write down the—(i) Batch no; (ii) p.c. by alcohol content, by volume and (iii) Date of expiry (if possible).

2. **Containers:** All potentised medicines should be preserved in well-stoppered bottles, which are kept in boxes, or drawers—in cool, dry place, protected from light.

   Exceptions

   (a) Hard glass (Potash) bottles with glass-stoppered—for preserving acids and caustic preparations.

   (b) Actinic glass bottles (coloured), covered with a solution of asphaltum or black varnish—for preserving potentised medicines which may be affected by light or sunlight.

   (c) Gutta-purcha bottles: for preservation of Acid fluor.

   (d) Glycerine in phial: for preservation of Lachesis.

   (e) Avoid: (i) Blue-coloured bottles—as the blue colour has some dynamic effect injurious to potentised medicines (as per Burt), (ii) yellow or amber coloured bottles—as they acquire some medicinal virtue, after exposure to sunlight.

3. **Avoid:** Dust, odours, smoke, damp, strong light etc., which affect the purity of the potentised medicines.

4. **Separate arrangement**

   (a) Potentised medicines should be kept separately from the crude drugs.

   (b) Preparation of Camphor should always be kept separate, otherwise they may antidote almost all medicines of vegetable origin.

   (c) Separate arrangement should be kept for potentised medicines and other odorous or non-odorous evaporating substances.

5. Bottles should not be filled entirely, as the potentised medicines shall come in contact with the corks.

6. Reject potentised medicines immediately, if they change their normal colour.

Notes: 1. Phials used for keeping one medicine should never be used for any other medicine nor for the same medicine in any other potency.

2. Two phials containing different potencies or remedies should never be opened at the same time in close proximity.

Specific directions for preservation of some potentised medicines as laid down in the monograph of H.P.I.

Name of medicine	How to preserve
Acid mur	Preserve HCl in well-closed container.
Acid nit	Preserve in well-closed container with glass-stopper up to 3X potency.
Acid sulph.	Potencies prepared in purified water should be freshly prepared and all preparations of this acid should be kept in round stoppered bottle.
Alumina	Kept in tight container and stored in cool place.
Ammon. carb	Preserve in well-closed light resistant containers preferably and a temperature not above 30°C.
Arg. nit	Arg. nit and its preparation up to 6X potency are to be kept in well-closed container, protected from light.
Benzoic acid	Kept in well-closed container.
Borax	Kept in well-closed container.
Cal. carb	Kept in well-closed container.
Camphora	Kept in well-closed container.
Carbo veg	Kept in well-closed container.
Croton tig	Kept in well-closed glass-stoppered bottle.
Carbo. acid	Kept in well-closed glass-stoppered bottle.
Hep. sulph	Kept in well-closed glass-stoppered bottle.
Ferrum met	Preserve in tightly closed containers.
Iodum	Preserve iodine in an amber glass-stoppered bottle or in earthenware container with a well-waxed bung.
Hydrofluoric acid	Kept in well-closed bottles, interior of which is coated with paraffin, or well-closed containers of paraffin, lead or wax.

Name of medicine	How to preserve
Kali bichromicum	Below 3X fresh preparation of this salt should be used, and should be discarded if there is discoloration, sedimentation or visible particles.
Kreosotum	Kept in well-closed container, protected from light.
Lachesis	It should be stored in glycerine.
Merc. iod	Preserve in tight, light resistant containers.
Merc. sol	Kept in well-stoppered bottles protected from light.

Name of medicine	How to preserve
Nat. mur	Kept in well-closed container.
Nat. sulph	Preserve in tight container and kept in cool place.
Petroleum	Preserve in well-stoppered bottle.
Phosphorus	Kept under water, in strong, well-closed containers, in cool dark place and protected from light. Handle carefully with forceps.
Picric acid	Kept in well-closed containers, in cool place away from fire.
Salicylic acid	In well-closed container protected from light.

Chapter 22

Pharmacology

Definition

The word "Pharmacology" is derived from the Greek words *'pharmakon'* meaning, 'drug', and *'logos'* meaning 'knowledge'.

Pharmacology is that branch of medical science, which deals with the drugs, their sources, appearance, chemistry, preparations, actions, and therapeutic uses. It may be called Allopathic Materia Medica.

It describes the action of drugs on the general system, or on the individual parts of the body, in health.

Fundamentals of Homoeopathic Pharmacology

The fundamentals of homoeopathic pharmacology is to explore the peculiar, characteristic pharmacological language and therapeutic potentiality of the drugs. The homoeopathic pharmacology is based on 'Theory of Dynamisation'.

Branches of Pharmacology

Two branches: 1. Pharmacognosy,
2. Pharmacodynamics.

PHARMACOGNOSY

The term originates from the *'gnosia'* (Latin) which means, 'the knowledge of drugs'.

It is a branch of pharmacology that deals with the physical characteristics and botanical sources of crude drugs.

It is the science which deals with the history, source, cultivation, collection, preparation, distribution, identification, composition, purity, preservation and commerce of crude drugs of vegetable and animal origin.

PHARMACODYNAMICS

Definition

It is one of the branches of homoeopathic pharmacology, which helps us to acquire knowledge about the dynamic actions and effects of drugs on healthy organisms. It constitutes the fundamental aspects of homoeotherapeutics.

Prover

Healthy human beings.

Doses

May be large, moderate, small or infinitesimal doses.

Objects

To study the individual action of a drug over and above its general actions, produced due to specific 'dynamic action of drug' that was lying latent and which constitutes the fundamental aspects of homoeotherapeutics.

Result

Contains subjective, objective, both of common and determinate value and uncommon peculiar symptoms of physical and mental spheres and, by careful and methodical observations of those symptoms, one proceeds for proper 'individualisation' for search of a good similimum.

Procedures for ascertaining disease-producing power

1. **Homoeopathic drug-proving** (For details, see 'The Technique of Homoeopathic Drug-provings' chapter)
2. **Toxicological findings** (Poisonings and overdosing)

These findings reveal the gross effect of those poisonous drugs, indicating changes in anatomical and pathological tissue changes. The 'chemical' and 'physical'—local effects must be eliminated. These changes which are noticed from homoeopathic therapeutic angle are not useful but those produced by their absorption, either in large or small infinitesimal doses, are important.

3. **Laboratory investigation or experiments**

In laboratory, before administering the drugs in varying doses, it is experimented on lower animals to assess their effects in different organ or organs. Then the actual quantitative and qualitative changes that have taken place in the organs, tissue functions and metabolism are carefully observed. This mostly helps to correlate the date with the actual disease state. It has no such value in determining the drug action.

The data and information collected by 'Homoeopathic drug proving', 'Toxicological findings' and 'Laboratory investigation or experiments' constitute what is known as Materia Medica and the sum total data of the powers of drug is pharmacodynamics.

Drug-action on Healthy Human Beings

Drug has threefold action on human beings:

1. **Chemical action:** Depending on the chemical affinity which exists between drug and body tissue. This is independent of the vitality.
2. **Mechanical action:** This is exhibited by the effort of the body to throw away the offending substance. Due to mechanical action of Ipecacuanha, the offending substance is thrown away by vomiting from stomach.
3. **Dynamic action:** Dynamic actions are those actions whose technical know-how cannot be explained but the effects are perceived. These actions are observed by their effects.

These dynamic effects may be:

(a) Generic—Common to all the members of a certain class of drug. e.g. vomiting, diarrhoea, cold sweat and cramp of extremities are the symptoms produced by dynamic effects of Arsenic, Cuprum, Veratrum, Antimony.

(b) Specific—Related to particulars. It is related to the susceptibility of the patient and the condition of application and also the doses.

Hahnemann had recognised these actions by primary and secondary action. The chemical and mechanical action of drug belongs to primary action and dynamic action belongs to secondary action.

Primary action: 'Every agent that acts upon the vitality, every medicine, deranges more or less the vital force, and causes a certain alteration in the health of the individual for a longer or a shorter period. This is termed as primary action. Although a product of the medicinals and vital powers conjointly, it is principally due to the former power' (Sec. 63).

Secondary action: The automatic, defensive reaction of the vital force against the primary action of the drug is called secondary action. It may be of two types:

(a) Secondary counter-action: When an exact opposite condition of primary action is possible—the vital force reacts equally and opposite to the primary action. It depends upon the principle of *'contraria contraris curantur'*—opposite cures opposite.

(b) Secondary curative action: When an exact opposite condition of primary action is not possible—the vital force indifferentiates itself and employs its increased energy to extinct the medicinal disease which gradually decreases and thus ultimately regains health. It depends upon the principle of *'similia similibus curantur'*—like cures like.

The following facts are observed as regards drug action to the specificity and varying doses in which they are administered in healthy human beings:

1. **Drugs administered in excessively large doses:** Produce certain symptoms during initial stages of their drug action which are followed by the symptoms exactly opposite in nature to those symptoms produced in initial stages. First series of symptoms due to primary action and the latter series of symptoms due to secondary action. So in large doses drug produces secondary action, in addition to primary action.
2. **Drugs administered in moderate doses:** Rarely produce secondary action, they only produce primary action with the exceptions in cases of 'Narcotic Drugs'. In moderate doses even, narcotic drugs produce secondary action (Sec. 113).
3. **Drugs administered in infinitesimal doses:** Never produce secondary action except in idio-syncratic persons.

From Sec. 116, we know that, symptoms produced by the medicine varies:

(a) Some symptoms produced more frequently in many individuals,

(b) Others, more rarely or in few persons,

(c) Some only in very few healthy bodies. To the latter category being the so-called idio-syncracies.

Modern medicine classified all these drugs depending on their action on individuals such as Diuretics, Cathartics, Cardio-toxin, Emetics, Febrifuge etc. But Homoeopathy does not deal with such classification. In Homoeopathy, drug action is the sum total of the action on the organism, and the total reaction that it can induce in the vital force. As each individual is different from each other—react differently—the Materia Medica produced by the provings on an individual must be 'individualistic'.

Difference between homoeopathic pharmacodynamics and pharmacology of old school

Points	Homoeopathic Pharmaco-dynamics	Pharmacology of old School
1. Prover	Healthy human beings.	Lower animals (Guinea-pig, rat, mice, monkey).
2. Doses	May be large, moderate, small or infinitesimal doses.	Physiological or massive doses.
3. Objects	To study the individual action of drugs over and above its general actions, produced due to specific 'dynamic action of drugs' that was lying latent, and which constitutes the fundamental aspects of homoeotherapeutics.	To study the physiological, and toxicological effects produced due to the chemical or biological properties of drugs.
4. Result	Contains subjective, objective, both of common and determinate value, and uncommon peculiar symptoms of physical and mental spheres and by careful and methodical observations of those symptoms thus one proceeds for proper 'individualisation' for search of a good similimum.	It contains only objective, of common symptoms.

DRUG STRENGTH

Drug strength means the power or strength of the drug in proportion to its solvent.

All pharmacopoeia should follow a standardised process for preparation of medicines whether in solution or in trituration, i.e., all trituration and all alcoholic medicinal solutions (e.g., tinctures, extracts, etc.) and their dilutions might be made of uniform drug-strength to be represented by the dry crude drug as the unit of strength in the case of θ made from dried substances and the plant juice as the unit when made from fresh green drugs. For this purpose Hahnemann introduced centesimal scale based on the principle that the 1st potency should contain $\frac{1}{100}$th part of the original drug and each succeeding potency should contain $\frac{1}{100}$th part of the one preceding it. This principle worked well so far as mother trituration and potency trituration of dry drug substances were concerned.

But difficulty arises in standardising the drug strength in alcoholic solution (which was overlooked by Hahnemann) of dry substances and plant juice when collected from fresh green drugs were noticed by the compilers of B.H.P. in 1876.

The lack of uniformity in drug-strength was due to different degrees of solvency of different kinds of drug substances in alcohol or water and varying quantities of plant moistures, in differnt varietes of plants used in homoeopathy.

It is observed that water in the form of moisture present in plant is a solvent and a part of the vehicle or menstrum forms no part of its total medicinal substance. Hahnemann's view was that the plant moisture is part of the drug substance but A.H.P. claims that it is only a solvent.

Previous editions of A.H.P. divided all vegetable and animal substances into four classes for preparation of θ of which the first three classes treat fresh plants and the fourth animals and dried plants. The amount of drug substance was $\frac{1}{2}$, $\frac{1}{3}$, $\frac{1}{6}$ and $\frac{1}{10}$ in each of the respective classes accordingly as, the plants contain a large quantity of juice, a small quantity of juice, or the plants are dry and animal products, fresh or dried.

Accordingly, nine different classes of formulae were adopted in the preparation of θ, dilutions and triturations of medicines used in homoeopathic practice. To obviate these diversities and to bring out an uniformity in strength (drug-strength) of all homoeopathic medicinal preparations, whether in tinctures or in triturations, the American Institute of Homoeopathy set up a special committee in 1888 on whose recommendations the Pharmacopoeia Committee followed the directions of the B.H.P. to take in every instance of the drug crude substances as the starting point from which to calculate its strength and the θ containing all the soluble matter of one gram of the dry plant in 10 cubic centimetres of the θ. The tincture (θ), therefore, containing $\frac{1}{10}$th part medicinal substance, should represent the 1X ($\frac{1}{10}$), thereby corresponding its strength with 1X trituration.

In short, the dry crude drug has been made the unit from which to estimate the drug strength in all tinctures and triturations.

With the exception of a few drug H.P.U.S. (official) in 1941 prescribed the uniform standard of 10% drug strength in all cases of medicinal preparations. This standard eliminates the double standard of Hahnemann (in cases of alcoholic solutions or dry drugs and fresh plant juice) the centesimal scale or potency, the previously adopted classification of medicinal materials and different formulae in connection with the preparation of Homoeopathic Medicine and a uniformity of standard is thus secured.

As much can be argued on either side, H.P.I., therefore, recognises both the methods of preparation of mother tincture viz. old Hahnemannian method and new or modern method.

Drug strength as per old Hahnemannian method:

1. Class I: $\frac{1}{2}$
2. Class II: $\frac{1}{2}$
3. Class III: $\frac{1}{6}$
4. Class IV: $\frac{1}{10}$

Drug strength as per modern method:

Uniform drug strength: $\frac{1}{10}$, with the exception of few drugs.

Tinctures or Solutions other than 10 percent Drug Strength

Remedies	*Drug Strength*
Acidum butyricum θ solution in dilute alcohol	$\frac{1}{100}$
Acidium hydrocyanicum θ using the acid in a 2% solution with equal volume of strong alcohol	$\frac{1}{100}$
Acidum picricum θ solution, in strong alcohol	$\frac{1}{100}$
Ambra grisea θ	$\frac{1}{100}$
Ammonium aceticum θ solution in purified water	$\frac{1}{100}$
Arsenicum album θ solution	$\frac{1}{100}$
Bromium θ solution	$\frac{1}{100}$
Cactus grandiflorus θ solution	$\frac{1}{20}$
Calcarea caustica θ solution, in purified water	$\frac{1}{1000}$
Causticum θ { 500 c.c. Causticum / 500 cc. strong alcohol } to make 1,000 cc of θ	
Crotalus horridus θ solution, in glycerine	$\frac{1}{100}$
Croton tiglium θ	$\frac{1}{100}$
Cuprum aceticum θ solution, in purified water	$\frac{1}{100}$
Elaps corrallinus θ solution, in glycerine	$\frac{1}{100}$
Glonoinum θ solution	$\frac{1}{100}$
Kali arsenicosum θ solution	$\frac{1}{100}$
Kali chloricum θ solution, in purified water	$\frac{1}{100}$
Kali parmanganicum θ solution, in purified water	$\frac{1}{100}$
Mephitis mephitica θ	$\frac{1}{100}$
Moschus θ	$\frac{1}{20}$
Phosphorus θ	$\frac{1}{667}$
Sulphur θ, in strong alcohol	$\frac{1}{5000}$

DYNAMIC POWER

The dynamic power is that quality of the substance whose mechanism of action (i.e., modus operandi) cannot be explained.

Examples:

1. The earth, by virtue of hidden energy, carries the moon around her in twenty-eight days and several hours, and the moon alternately, in definite fixed hours, raises the seas to flood tide and again correspondingly lowers them to ebb. Apparently this takes place not through material agencies, not through mechanical contrivances.

   Likewise, we see numerous other events about us as results of the action of one substance on another substance without being able to recognise a sensible connection between cause and effect. Hahnemann calls such effects dynamic, or virtual, that is, such as results from absolute, specific pure energy and action of the one substance upon the other substance.

   (Sec. 11, F.N.—6th edition)

2. One sees that the piece of iron is attracted by one pole of magnet, but how it is done is not seen. This invisible energy of the magnet does not require mechanical (material) auxiliary means, hook or lever, to attract the iron. The magnet draws to itself and this acts upon the piece of iron or upon a steel needle by means of a purely immaterial, invisible, conceptual, inherent energy, i.e. dynamically.

   (Sec. 11, F.N.—6th edition)

3. If one looks upon something nauseous and becomes inclined to vomit, did a material emetic come into his stomach which compels

him to this anti-peristaltic movement? No, it is solely due to the dynamic effect of the nauseating substance.

(Sec. 11, F.N.—6th edition)

In a similar way, the effects of medicines on human beings is to be judged. Substances, which are used as medicines, possess each its own specific energy to alter the state of health of man through dynamic influence by means of the living sensory fibre, upon the conceptual, controlling principle of life. These medicines act upon healthy body without communication of material parts of the medicinal substances, thus dynamically. There lies invisible in the moistened globule or in its solution, an unveiled, liberated, specific medicinal force contained in the medicinal substance which acts dynamically by contact with the living animal fibre upon the whole organism and acts more strongly the more free and more immaterial the energy has become through the dynamisation.

(Sec. 11, F.N.—6th edition)

In short, dynamic action implies a process whereby one substance is acted on by another substance without communication or actual interchange of the material parts of the substances concerned but rather qualitatively through the qualities inherent in them. This quality of exerting the dynamic action of a substance is known as the dynamic influence or power of that substance.

Exceptional Drug Strength of tinctures or solutions in Homoeopathic Pharmacy

Drug Strength	Drugs
$\frac{1}{2}$	Causticum
$\frac{1}{20}$	Cactus grandiflorus, Moschus
$\frac{1}{100}$	(i) Vegetable kingdom: Croton tiglium. (ii) Animal kingdom: Mephitis mephitica and snake venoms such as Crotalus horridus, Elaps corllinus, Naja tripudians, Vipera torva (iii) Chemicals and Minerals: Ammonium aceticum, Arsenicum album, Arsenicum iodata, Ars sulph flavum, Ars sulph rubrum, Bromium, Butyric acid, Cuprum aceticum, Glonoinum, Hydrocyanic acid, Kali arsenicosum, Kali chloricum, Kali permanganicum, Mercurius cyanatus, Picric acid (iv) Nosodes: Diphtherinum, Medorrhinum, Tuberculinum
$\frac{1}{667}$	Phosphorus
$\frac{1}{1000}$	Bufo rana, Calcarea caustica, Chlorinum, Hippuric acid
$\frac{1}{5000}$	Sulphur

Chapter 23

Identification of Some Homoeopathic Drugs

THE ROOT

The root is the underground non-green part of the vascular plants. It grows into the soil forming the descending axis of the plant. It is negativelly phototropic, and absorbs water and minerals from soil. It has nodes and internodes, and does not bear leaves or buds. The root apex can be differentiated into four distinct regions: root cap, zone of cell division, zone of elongation, and zone of maturation.

Root System

The root system is the descending (growing downwards) portion of the plant axis. When a seed germinates, radicle is the first organ to come out. It elongates to form primary or the tap root. It gives off lateral branches (secondary and tertiary roots) and thus forms the root system.

Two types of root system are recognised:

Characteristics of Roots

Main features of roots by which you can recognise them are:

1. Non-green due to absence of chlorophyll;
2. Not divided into nodes and internodes;
3. Absence of leaves and buds;
4. Positively geotropic (**grow towards gravity);**
5. Positively hydrotropic (**grow towards water);**
6. Negatively phototropic (**grow away from light).**

Types of Root Systems

Root systems are mainly of two types:

1. **Tap root system:** It is the root system that develops from the radicle and continues as the primary root (tap root) which gives off lateral roots. They provide very strong anchorage as they are able to reach very deep into the soil. It is the main root system of dicots e.g., gram, china rose, neem.
2. **Fibrous root system:** In this root system, the primary root is short lived. A cluster of slender, fiber-like roots arises from the base of the radicle and plumule which constitute the fibrous root system. They do not branch profusely, are shallow and spread horizontally, hence cannot provide strong anchorage. Fibrous root system is the main root system of monocots, e.g., maize, grasses, wheat.

Types of Roots

1. **Tap root:** It is the primary and the main root that develops from the radicle, bears many branches and remains underground. It is

usually found in dicots e.g., sunflower, mustard, carrot, mango.

2. **Adventitious root:** These are roots that develop from any part of the plant except the radicle. They may be aerial or underground. They may grow from node (money plant, bamboo), stem cutting (rose), tree branch (banyan) or stem base (fibrous roots in monocots).

Regions of Root

Apical region of roots of any root system shows the same zones or regions. A longitudinal section of root apex shows the following structure:

1. **Root cap region:** It is a thimble-like structure produced by meristematic (rapidly dividing) zone and protects the tender apex (apical meristem) from harsh soil particles. As the root grows further down in soil, root cap wears out but it is constantly renewed . In aquatic plants (*Pistia* and water hyacinth) root cap is like a loose thimble called **root *pocket*.**

2. **Region of meristematic cells:** It is a small region of actively dividing cells called the apical meristem. It consists of:

   (i) Dermatogen (outermost layer whose cells mature into epiblema and root cap);

   (ii) Periblem (inner to dermatogen whose cells mature into cortex);

   (iii) Plerome (central region whose cells mature into stele). In monocots, cap is formed by independent group of cells known as Calyptrogen.

3. **Region of elongation:** Lies next to the meristematic region, the cells elongate and enlarge to make the root grow in length.

4. **Region of maturation:** Lies next to the region of elongation. The cells mature and differentiate into various tissues constituting:

   (i) *Root hair or piliferous region* having unicellular hairs which absorb water and mineral salts from soil and

   (ii) *Permanent region* which lies behind the root hair zone and is without hairs. It roduces lateral roots, anchors the plant in soil and conducts water and minerals upwards.

Modification of Roots

Tap roots and adventitious roots can get modified into a variety of forms to perform various functions.

Tap roots modification

1. Conical root
2. Fusiform root
3. Napiform root
4. Tuberous root

Adventitious roots modification

1. Tuberous root
2. Fasciculated root
3. Nodulose roots
4. Moniliform
5. Annulated roots
6. Assimilatory roots
7. Epiphytic roots
8. Pneumatophores
9. Sucking roots or haustoria
10. Prop roots
11. Stilt roots
12. Climbing roots
13. Clinging roots
14. Floating roots

A. Tap roots modification

In general, the secondary and tertiary roots of tap root system are thin, and are known as fibrous. But, in some plants tap root does not branch and becomes swollen to store food; however, if it branches, then the branches also become swollen or tuberous to store the food material.

The different forms of modified tap roots are:

1. **Conical root:** Base is broad and tapers gradually towards apex, e.g., Carrot

2. **Fusiform root:** Swollen in middle tapering towards both ends, e.g., Radish

3. **Napiform root:** Spherical at base tapering sharply towards the tip, e.g., Turnip, beet.

4. **Tuberous root:** Thick and fleshy with no definite shape, e.g., 4 o'clock plant.

B. Adventitious roots modification

Adventitious roots get modified for various functions:

1. ***Modification for food storage***

   (a) *Tuberous root:* A portion of a root swells for food or water storage, e.g. sweet potato. A type of storage root distinct from taproot.

   (b) *Fasciculated root:* Swollen roots developing in a cluster from the stem, e.g, Dahlia, Asparagus.

(c) *Nodulose root:* Only apices of roots become swollen like single beads, e.g., Mango-ginger.

(d) *Moniliform root:* Roots alternately swollen and constricted presenting a beaded or moniliform appearance, e.g., Grasses, Sedges.

(e) *Annulated root:* Looks as if formed by a number of discs placed one above the other, e.g., Ipecac

2. ***Modification for photosynthesis***

Assimilatory roots: Roots which when exposed to sun develop chlorophyll, turn green and manufacture food e.g., *Tinospora* (aerial root), orchid.

3. ***Modification for absorbing atmospheric moisture***

Epiphytic roots: Aerial roots of epiphytes are greenish and covered with spongy tissue (Velamen) with which they absorb atmospheric moisture, e.g., orchids (*Vanda*).

4. ***Modification for better gaseous exchange***

Pneumatophores or respiratory roots: Some roots grow vertically up (negatively geotropic) into air. Exposed root tips possess minute pores through which roots respire, appear like conical spikes coming out of water, e.g., Mangroves (marshy plants) *Rhizophora*.

5. ***Modification for sucking nutrition from host***

Sucking roots or haustoria: Parasitic plants give out sucking roots or haustoria which penetrate living host plant and suck food, e.g., *Cuscuta*.

6. ***Modification for strong support***

(a) *Prop or pillar roots:* Roots develop from tree branches, hang downwards and ultimately penetrate the ground, thus support heavy branches, e.g., Banyan tree.

(b) *Stilt roots:* Extra roots developing from nodes near the base of stem, grow obliquely and penetrate the soil giving strong anchorage, e.g., Sugarcane, maize.

(c) *Climbing roots:* Weak climbers twine around and clasp the support with the help of climbing roots arising from their nodes, e.g., money plant, betel.

(d) *Clinging roots:* Special clinging roots arise, enter the crevices of support and fix the epiphyte, e.g. Epiphytes, orchids.

7. ***Modification for buoyancy and respiration***

Floating roots: Spongy, floating roots filled with air, arise from nodes of some aquatic plants, and help in floating and respiration, e.g, *Jussiaea*.

Functions of Roots

1. **Anchorage:** Roots anchor the plant firmly to the soil (mechanical function).
2. **Absorption:** Roots absorb water and mineral salts and conduct them upwards (physiological function).
3. **Special functions:** By undergoing modifications in their structure, roots perform special physiological functions like food storage, assimilation, absorption of atmospheric moisture, sucking food from host, better gaseous exchange and mechanical functions like floating (buoyancy), stronger anchorage and climbing. Some important examples are:

In banyan, the aerial branches produce the **prop roots** to provide mechanical support to the foliage.

In maize, *Pandanus* and sugar-cane, the **stilt roots** from the nodes just above the ground provide additional support to the stems.

In Ivy and betel, the roots serve as organs of **climbing** and **clinging** to their natural habitats.

In carrot, radish, turnip, *Dahlia, Asparagus* and sweet potato, the roots store the food material.

In *Rhizophora* and *Sonneratia*, the roots come out of the soil to help in aeration and respiration.

In banyan and orchids, the aerial roots are modified to absorb moisture from the atmosphere.

In parasites such as *Cuscuta* and *Orobanche*, the **haustorial roots** absorb food form their respective hosts.

In legumes, the roots containing *Rhizobium* help in the fixation of atmospheric nitrogen.

In *Asparagus* and sweet potato, the roots are employed for vegetative propagation.

In *Tinosora* and *Trapa* roots act as additional assimilatory organs and in *Jussiaea*, as floating organs.

In some aquatic plants e.g., *Utricularia, Wolffia, Lemna, ceratophyllum* and *Myriophyllum* roots may be lacking.

SHOOT SYSTEM

Shoot system is an aerial and erect part of plant body which grows upwards. It is usually above the soil and develops from plumule of the embryo. It consists of stem, branches, leaves, flowers, fruits and seeds.

Characteristics of Stem

1. Arises as a prolongation of plumule (one end of an embryo).
2. Grows and bends towards light (**positively phototropic**) and away from gravity (**negatively geotropic**).
3. Divided into **nodes** (point of attachment of leaf) and **internodes** (regions between two nodes).
4. Bears leaves, branches and flowers on nodes.
5. Bears **vegetative buds** which could be terminal (apical bud) for plant to grow upwards, or axillary (bud in the axil of leaf), which gives rise to lateral branches.
6. Bears **floral buds** (terminal or axillary) that grow into flowers.

The Shoot Apex

Shoot apex is the terminal, dome shaped part of shoot and is formed of meristem called **apical shoot meristem** is responsible for the development and differentiation of primary permanent tissue and mainly causes growth in length. It is divided into two regions: **Tunica** and **Corpus**.

1. **Tunica** (covering): An outer zone of shoot apex, 1-3 layers in thickness. It gives rise to epidermis and is responsible for surface growth.
2. **Corpus** (body): Inner multi-layered zone of cells which divide in all directions. These finally give rise to *procambium* (forms vascular tissue) and *ground meristem* (forms ground tissue). These cells also form leaf primordia (a newly developing leaf).

Origin of Lateral branches

Branches arise from axillary buds present in the axil of leaves. Each axillary bud is a small, compact, underdeveloped shoot covered with a large number of overlapping leaf primordia. Internodes of this bud enlarge and develop into a branch. Therefore the development of branches is **exogenous** (exo = outside).

Types of Stem

The stem may be

1. **aerial** (erect, rigid, strong and upright as in herbs, shrubs and trees)
2. **subaerial** (weak, unable to stay upright and trail on ground as **creepers** or climb up as **climbers**) or
3. **underground** (buried in soil and produce aerial branches under favourable conditions only).

Table 23.1: Morphological differences between Stem and Root

STEM	ROOT
1. Develop from plumule	Develop from radicle
2. Young stem is green coloured because of chlorophyll	Non green because chlorophyll is absent
3. Divided into nodes and internodes	Not divided into nodes and internodes
4. Bears leaves, vegetative and floral buds	Absent
5. No cap present at the apex	Root cap is present at the apex
6. Positively phototropic and negatively geotropic	Negatively phototropic, but positively geotropic
7. Origin of lateral branches is exogenous (originating from outer layers)	Origin of lateral roots is endogenous (originating from inner layers).

Modification of Stem

Stems are variously modified into underground, subaerial and aerial stems for performing functions like manufacturing and storing food, perennation (overcoming unfavourable climatic conditions), providing mechanical support and protection and for propagating vegetatively.

Types of Stem and Modifications

Underground	Subaerial	Aerial
Rhizome	Runner	Tendrils
Corm	Stolon	Thorns
Bulb	Offset	Phylloclade
Tuber	Sucker	Cladode

A. **Underground modified stems:** Since underground, they may seem like roots but can be recognised them as stem due to the presence of: (i) Nodes and internodes, (ii) Scaly non green leaves, (iii) Buds.

They serve two functions:

(a) Act as perennating structures by remaining leafless and dormant in winter but giving off aerial shoots under favourable conditions (next season).

(b) Store food and become thick and fleshy.

1. **Rhizome:** Thick, fleshy, flattened, horizontally growing stem near the soil surface. Bears scale leaves on nodes, terminal and axillary buds, adventitious roots e.g., Ginger (*Adrak*), Turmeric (*'haldi'*).

2. **Corm:** Fleshy, spherical stem with flattened base, grows vertically; bears many scale leaves, distinct nodes and internodes, buds and adventitious roots e.g., Saffron (*'kesar'*), Yam (*'zimikand'*), Gladiolus.

3. **Bulb:** Reduced, flattened discoid stem with crowded nodes bearing overlapping fleshy (inner) and dry (outer) scale leaves. Terminal bud (in centre) forms foliage (green) leaves. Adventitious roots grow from discoid base. e.g., Onion.

4. **Tuber:** Swollen tips of underground lateral branches of stem, store food as starch, bear "eyes". Each eye is a node which bears bud and scar of scale leaves. e.g., Potato.

B. **Subaerial modifications of Stem:** Stems are weak, therefore, lie prostrate on the ground or may get partially buried in the top soil. The plants bearing such stems are called creepers. Their stems serve the function of vegetative propagation.

1. **Runner:** Long, weak, slender branch with long internodes. Runs horizontally on soil surface giving off adventitious roots at nodes. e.g., Grass, Oxalis.

2. **Stolon:** Weak lateral branch, which grows upwards, then arches down to meet the soil, strike roots and produce daughter plants. e.g., Mint (*'Pudina'*), Jasmine.

3. **Offset:** Like runner but thicker and shorter, grow for a short distance then produce cluster (rosette) of leaves above and adventitious roots below; generally in aquatic plants. e.g., Water hyacinth, Water lettuce.

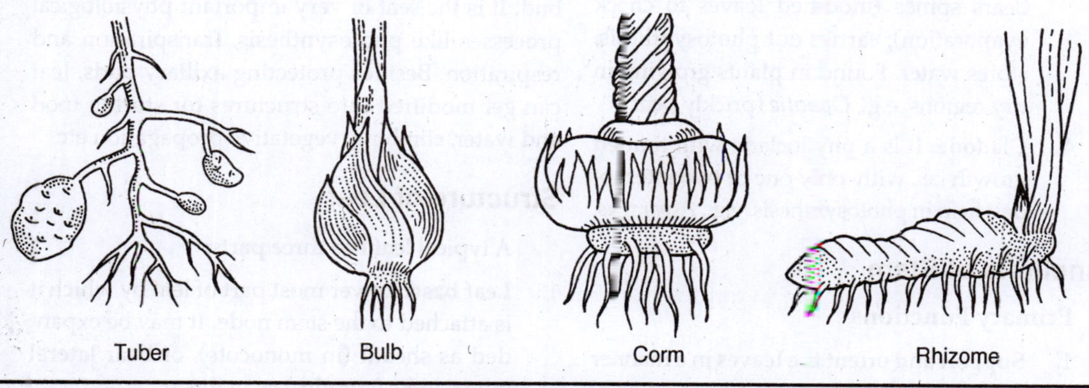

Root Storage System Diagram

4. **Sucker:** Underground runner, which grows horizontally for a distance under soil, then emerges obliquely upwards, strikes roots and forms daughter plants. e.g., Chrysanthemum.

C. **Aerial stem modifications:** Whole stem or its part (axillary or terminal bud) gets modified to perform definite functions. You can recognise them as stems by following features: (i) Arise in the axil of leaf (ii) Bear nodes and internodes (iii) May bear leaves, buds, flowers.

1. **Stem tendrils:** Threadlike, spirally coiled, leafless structures (tendrils), which twine around neighbouring objects and help weak plants to climb. e.g., Grape vine (Vitis vinifera).

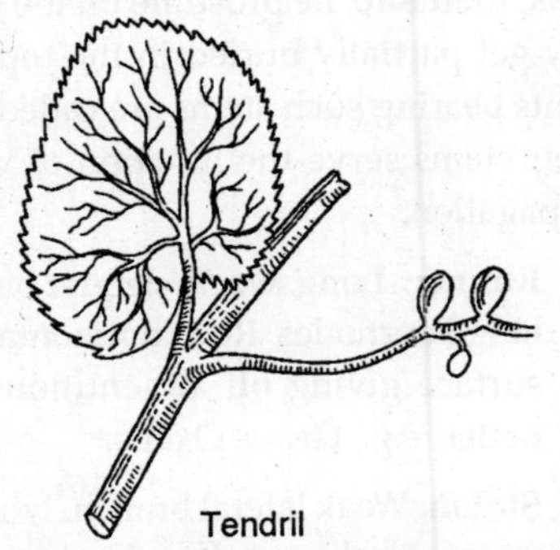

Tendril Diagram

2. **Thorns:** Straight, pointed, hard structures; modifications of axillary (*Citrus*), or terminal (*Carissa*) bud; act as defence organs, or as climbing organs. e.g., *Citrus, Duranta Carissa ('Karonda')*.

3. **Phylloclade:** Green, flattened or cylindrical fleshy stem, with nodes and internodes; bears spines (modified leaves to check evaporation); carries out photosynthesis, stores water. Found in plants growing in dry regions. e.g., *Opuntia* (prickly pear).

4. **Cladode:** It is a phylloclade with limited growth i.e., with only one or two internodes; help in photosynthesis. e.g., *Asparagus*.

Functions of Stem

A. Primary Functions

1. **Support and orient the leaves** in a manner that they are exposed to maximum sunlight, and for efficient gaseous exchange during photosynthesis and respiration.
2. **Conduct water and minerals** from roots to leaves and manufactured **food** from leaves to different parts of the plant.
3. **Bear flowers and fruits.**

B. Secondary Functions

1. **Storage:** Stems store food and water in plants e.g., Potato.
2. **Perennation:** The underground stems help tide over the unfavourable growing periods e.g., Ginger.
3. **Vegetative propagation:** Stem can be a means of vegetative propagation e.g., rose, sugarcane.
4. **Photosynthesis:** In certain plants like xerophytes (desert plants), where leaves are reduced, the stem takes up the function of photosynthesis. These stems possess chlorophyll e.g., *Opuntia.*
5. **Protection:** In some plants, the axillary bud modifies into thorn and protects the plants from animals e.g., Citrus, *Duranta.*
6. **Climbing:** Tendrils or hooks are modified branches or buds. They coil around the support and help the plant to climb e.g., Grape vine.

LEAF

Leaf is a flattened and expanded lateral appendage of stem, or branch developing from its node. It originates from leaf primordium formed by the shoot meristem and bears a bud in its axil called axillary bud. It is the seat of very important physiological processes like photosynthesis, transpiration and respiration. Besides protecting axillary buds, leaf can get modified into structures for storing food and water, climbing, vegetative propagation etc.

Structure of Leaf

A typical leaf has three parts:

1. **Leaf base:** Lower most part of leaf by which it is attached to the stem node. It may be expanded as sheath (in monocots), or bear lateral outgrowths (stipules) as in dicots.

2. **Petiole:** Is the stalk of leaf. Leaf can be **petiolate** (with petiole) as in many dicots or sessile (without petiole) as in most monocots. Petiole may get modified and swell (e.g., Water Hyacinth) or develop wings (e.g., Orange) or become flat like a leaf (e.g., Australian Acacia).

3. **Lamina or leaf blade:** It is a green, thin, flattened and expanded part of leaf with veins and veinlets traversing through its surface. The most prominent vein running from base to apex and present in the middle of leaf blade is called **midrib**. Veins provide support and conduct water, minerals and prepared food.

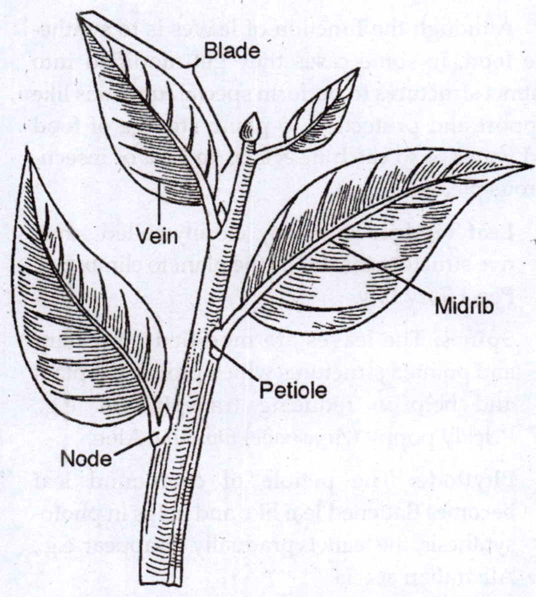

Parts of a Leaf Diagram

Leaf shows a lot of variation in

(i) Shapes of lamina.

(ii) Leaf apices.

(iii) Leaf margins.

Venation in Leaves

Arrangement of veins and veinlets in the lamina is known as **Venation**. It is of two types:

Reticulate venation: veins forming a network e.g., dicots.

Parallel venation: veins arranged in parallel rows e.g. monocots.

Reticulate and parallel venation may be **unicostate**, giving out secondary veins like in feather, hence **pinnate** or **multicostate**.

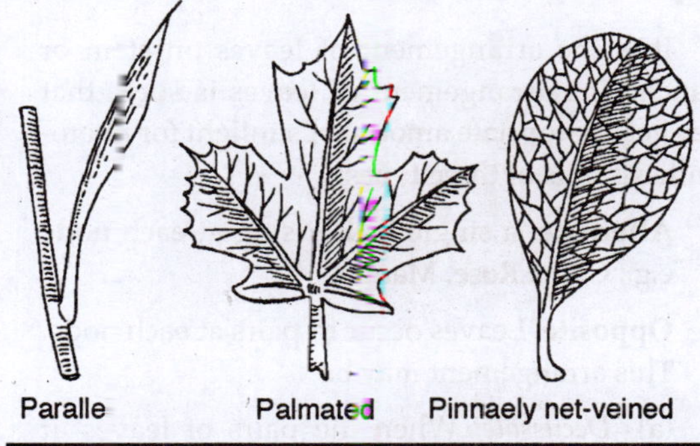

Venation Diagram

Types of Leaves

There are two types of leaves **Simple** and **Compound**. Since a leaf bears a bud in its axil, you can recognise a compound leaf from a simple one by locating the axillary bud. A bud is present in the

Table 23.2: Differences between Simple and Compound Leaf

	Simple leaf	Compound leaf
1.	The leaf has a single undivided lamina.	The lamina is divided into many segments called **leaflets**.
2.	If divided, the incision does not touch the midrib.	Incisions touch the midrib.

Table 23.3: Types of Compound Leaf

	Pinnate	Palmate
1.	Leaflets are attached to midrib or rachis and are arranged laterally.	Leaflets radiate from the end of petiole like fingers of a palm.
2.	Leaflets and midrib may get further divided to form compound leaves that are unipinnate, bipinnate, tripinnate and decompound.	Depending upon the number of leaflets compound leaves are bifoliate, trifoliate, quadrifoliate and multifoliate.

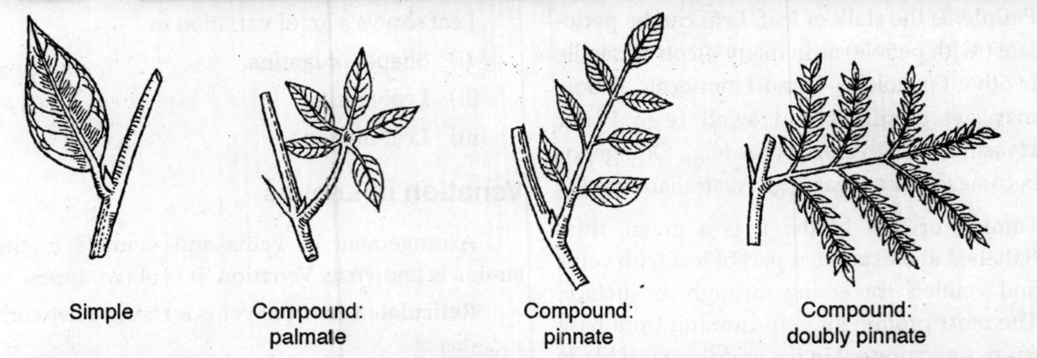

Leaf Arrangements Diagram

axil of both simple and a compound leaf, but not in the axil of leaflets.

Phyllotaxy

It is the arrangement of leaves on stem or branch. The arrangement of leaves is such, that they get appropriate amount of sunlight for photosynthesis. It is of three types:

1. **Alternate:** a single leaf arising at each node e.g., China Rose, Mango.
2. **Opposite:** Leaves occur in pairs at each node. This arrangement may be
   (a) *Decussate:* When the pairs of leaves at upper and lower nodes are at right angles e.g .,"Tulsi", *Calotropis.*
   (b) *Superposed:* when the leaf pairs at upper and lower nodes are exactly in the same plane e.g., Guava.
3. **Whorled:** There are more than two leaves at each node arranged in a circle or whorl e.g., *Nerium.*

Modifications of Leaves

Although the function of leaves is to synthesise food, in some cases they get modified into distinct structures to perform special functions like support and protection to plant, storage of food and water or to catch insects as in case of insectivorous plants.

1. **Leaf Tendril:** Thin wiry, closely coiled sensitive structure that helps the plant to climb. e.g., Pea, Glory Lily.
2. **Spines:** The leaves are modified into sharp and pointed structures which protect the plant and help in reducing transpiration. e.g., Prickly poppy (*Argemone*) *Opuntia,* Aloe.
3. **Phyllode:** The petiole of compound leaf becomes flattened leaf like and helps in photosynthesis; the leaflets gradually disappear. e.g., Australian acacia.
4. **Leaves of Insectivorous plants:** In pitcher plant the whole leaf gets modified into pitcher while in bladderwort some segmented leaves

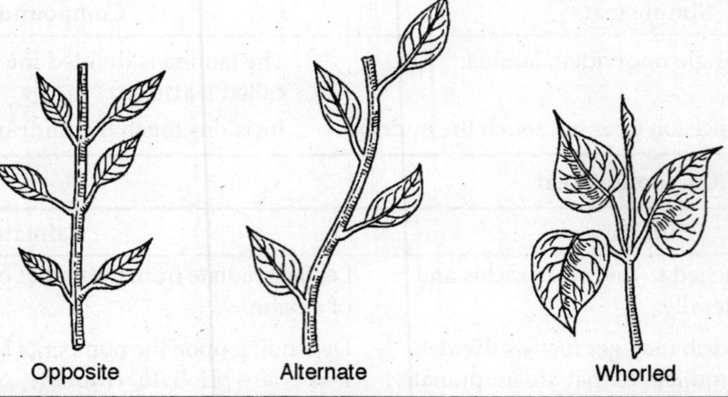

Stem Arrangement Diagram

get modified into bladders. They help in trapping insects. e.g., Pitcher plant (*Nepenthes*), Bladderwort (*Utricularia*).

Heterophylly (heteros = different): Some plants show more than one type of leaves in the same plant, this phenomenon is called heterophylly. It is found in some plants which remain partly submerged in water e.g., Water chestnut, *Limnophila.*

Functions of Leaf

Leaf performs following functions:

1. **Photosynthesis:** Leaves manufacture food in the presence of sunlight.
2. **Exchange of gases:** Stomata help in exchange of gases, which are important for respiration and photosynthesis.
3. **Transpiration:** Evaporation of excess of water in vapour form takes place through stomata which helps in ascent of sap and cooling of leaf surface.
4. **Guttation:** Exudation of excess of water containing salts takes place in liquid form from leaf margins in plants, growing in humid climate.
5. **Modifications for special functions:** In certain plants, leaves perform functions like manufacturing and storing food, providing support and protection, vegetative propagation and trapping insects.

FLOWER

Flowers are a thing of beauty for us, but for the plants, these are vital as they are the seat of sexual reproduction. They produce fruits and seeds.

A flower is a modified shoot because, it has (i) Nodes very close to one another and (ii) Floral leaves arranged in successive whorls.

Parts of a Typical Flower

Take a flower of any colour or size growing in your area, you'll find its basic plan to be the same i.e., the flower is a borne on a stalk called **pedicel.** The pedicel has a swollen tip known as **thalamus** or **receptacle** on which are borne four whorls successively in definite order as given below:

Accessory whorls

1. **Calyx** (collection of sepals): The outer most whorl of green sepals whose main function is protection.
2. **Corolla** (collection of petals): The next whorl of variously coloured petals.

They help in attracting insects for pollination.

Reproductive whorls

3. **Androecium** (male reproductive part): It consists of collection of stamens. Each stamen has a long slender **filament** with a bilobed **anther** at its tip with a **connective.** Anthers produce pollen grains for pollination.
4. **Gynoecium** (female reproductive part): It is centrally located. It consists of a collection of **carpels or pistils.** Each carpel has three parts:

(a) *Ovary:* It is the swollen basal part, one to many chambered (called **locules**) containing ovules which get fertilised to form seeds and the ovary forms the fruit.

(b) *Style:* It is the elongated tube connecting ovary and stigma.

(c) *Stigma:* It is the receptive surface for pollen.

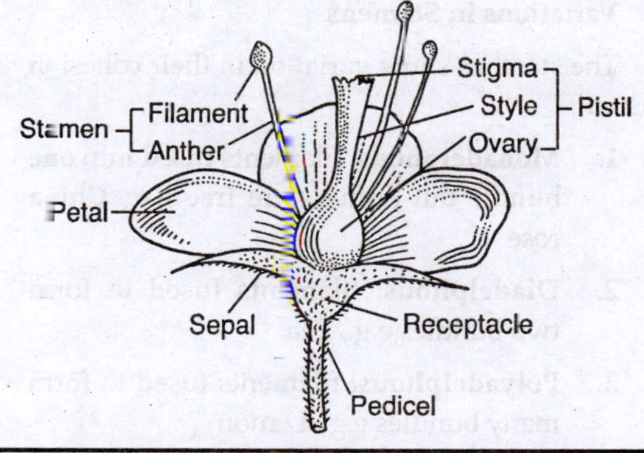

Parts of a Flower

Common variations in Flower and its Floral parts

Flowers show a lot of variations.

A. Variations in Sepals and Petals

1. **Polysepalous** and **Polypetalous** (poly-free): sepals or petals are free, respectively.

Table 23.4: Variations in Flower

Variation	Characters
1. **Complete/Perfect** flower	All 4 floral whorls present
2. **Incomplete/Imperfect** flower	Any one or more of floral whorl is absent
3. **Bisexual** (Hermaphrodite)	Both reproductive organs i.e., stamens and Carpels present
4. **Unisexual**	Only one reproductive organ present
(a) ***Staminate*** or male flower	Only stamens present
(b) ***Pistillate*** or female flower	Only carpel present
(c) On the basis of occurrence of unisexual flowers, plant is	
(i) *Monoecious*	Both male and female flower occur on same plant e.g., Cucumber
(ii) *Dioecious*	Male and female flower occur on different plants e.g., Papaya
5. **Neuter** flower	Both stamens and carpels are absent
6. **Actinomorphic** (Regular) flower	If it can be divided into two equal halves through any vertical plane e.g., Mustard
7. **Zygomorphic** (Irregular bilateral)	If it can be divided into two similar halves only through one particular plane e.g., Pea
8. **Asymmetrical** (Irregular)	It cannot be divided into two similar halves in any vertical plane e.g., Canna

2. **Gamosepalous and Gamopetalous** (gamo-united): all sepals or petals are fused.
3. **Perianth:** Sepals and petals not distinguishable e.g., Onion.

B. Variations in Stamens

The stamens show variation in their cohesion (fusion):

1. **Monadelphous:** filaments fused into one bundle but anthers are free e.g., China rose
2. **Diadelphous:** filaments fused to form two bundles e.g., Pea
3. **Polyadelphous:** filaments fused to form many bundles e.g., Lemon
4. **Syngenesious:** filaments are free but anthers are fused e.g., Sunflower
5. **Synandrous:** stamens are fused throughout the length e.g., Cocks-comb

Other variations in stamens are as follows

6. **Epipetalous:** stamens are attached to petals but anthers are free e.g., Brinjal
7. **Didynamous:** four stamens, two short and two long e.g., Tulsi
8. **Tetradynamous:** six stamens, inner four are long and outer two are short e.g., Mustard.

C. Variation in Carpel

On the basis of number of carpels, flowers may be

1. ***Monocarpellary:*** hynoecium having one carpel e.g., Pea.
2. ***Polycarpellary:*** many carpels (e.g., China rose). It may be
   (a) *Syncarpous:* carpels are fused e.g., Tomato, Mustard
   (b) *Apocarpous:* carpels are free e.g., Ranun-culus, Lotus.

Position of Floral whorls on thalamus with respect to ovary

Flower could be of three kinds

1. **Hypogynous:** ovary occupies the highest position on thalamus, other three whorls are successively below it. Ovary is said to be superior e.g., China rose, Mustard.
2. **Perigynous:** The thalamus is disc-like on which the carpels are borne in the centre and

rest of floral whorls are located on rim of thalamus. Ovary is said to be half inferior e.g., Peach, Plum, Pea.

3. **Epigynous:** thalamus forms a cup-shaped structure; and encloses the ovary completely and fuses with it. The other whorls are positioned above the ovary.

The position of ovary is now inferior e.g., Sunflower, Cucumber.

Placentation

It is the manner in which placentae are distributed in the ovary. Placenta is the point of attachment of ovules (or future seed) to the ovary.

Types of Placentation

1. **Marginal:** The ovary is one chambered and ovules are arranged along the margin of the ovary. e.g., Pea, Gram.
2. **Axile:** Ovary is many chambered and ovules present on the placenta develop from the central axis of ovary e.g., China rose, Tomato, Bhindi,
3. **Parietal:** Ovary is one chambered and ovules are attached in its inner wall where margin of adjoining carpels meet e.g., Mustard, Cucumber,
4. **Basal:** Ovary is one chambered and placenta develops at the base of ovary and bears a single ovule e.g., Sunflower.
5. **Free central:** gynoecuum is syncarpous and polycarpellary but unilocular as septae are absent. In the central part the placenta bears many ovules e.g., *Dianthus, Primula*.
6. **Superficial:** Ovary is polycarpellary syncarpous and multilocular in which entire inner walls of chambers are lined with placental tissue so that ovules develop all around e.g., Water lily (*Nymphaea*).

Inflorescence

Inflorescence is the arrangement of flowers on the floral axis called peduncle. Inflorescence could be terminal or axillary.

Types of Inflorescence

The various types depend upon the type of branching of peduncle and arrangement of flowers. There are two major types of inflorescence.

1. **Racemose.** The main axis does not end in a flower but continues to grow.
2. **Cymose.** The main axis ends in a flower and the growth is limited.

Types of Racemose Inflorescence

A. **With main axis elongated**

1. **Raceme:** Flowers present on the floral axis are stalked. e.g., Mustard.
2. **Spike:** Like raceme but the flowers are sessile. e.g., Achyranthes ('Latzira').
3. **Spikelet:** Cluster of one or more flowers (florets' and their associated bracts). e.g., Wheat.
4. **Catkin:** Like spike but the axis is pendulous bearing unisexual flowers. e.g., Mulberry.
5. **Spadix:** Like spike but the axis is fleshy and enclosed by a large showy bract (Spathe). e.g., Colocasia, Banana.

B. **With main axis shortened**

6. **Corymb:** Lower (older) flowers have longer stalks than the younger ones, thus all flowers come at same level. e.g., Candy-tuft.
7. **Umbel:** Flower with stalks of equal length arising from the same, point. e.g., Coriander.

Table 23.5: Differences between Racemose and Cymose Inflorescence

Racemose	Cymose
1. Main axis shows unlimited growth	Growth is limited
2. Axis does not terminate in a flower	Axis ends in a flower
3. Flowers occur in acropetal order (oldest flower below and youngest near the apex)	Flowers in basipetal order (terminal flower is older)

C. **With main axis flattened**

8. **Head or capitulum:** Main axis is flattened into convex receptacle on which sessile flowers (florets) are arranged in centripetal order (older towards periphery). Whole inflorescence is surrounded by involucre of bracts. e.g., Sunflower.

Types of Cymose Inflorescence

1. **Monochasial cyme:** Main axis ends in a flower. A lateral branch comes from one side and ends in a flower. e.g., Cotton.
2. **Dichasial cyme:** Two lateral branches develop form either side of terminal flower and each branch ends in a flower. e.g., *Dianthus, Jasmine.*
3. **Multichasial cyme:** Number of lateral branches come from the sides of terminal flower, each lateral branch ends in a flower. e.g., *Calotropis.*

Special types of Inflorescence

1. **Hypanthodium:** The fleshy receptacle forms a cup like cavity and has an apical opening. The male and female flowers are borne on the inner wall of the cavity e.g., Fig. Peepal.
2. **Cyathium:** A type of inflorescence characteristic of Euphorbia, in which a cup shaped involucre encloses a single flower surrounded by a number of male flowers. A nectary is present at the rim of involucre.
3. **Verticillaster:** It is a series of condensed dichasial cyme at each node with a cluster of sessile flowers in the axil of leaves e.g., *Ocimum* (Tulsa), *Salvia.*

FRUIT

A true fruit is a ripened ovary, that develops after fertilisation. Ovules develop into seeds and the ovary wall matures into fruit wall which is now called pericarp. The pericarp may be thick or thin. In fleshy fruits like Mango, pericarp is thick and differentiated into three regions: (a) **Epicarp** forms the skin of the fruit, (b) **Mesocarp,** middle pulpy, (c) **Endocarp** inner hard and stony (Coconut, Mango) or often thin membranes (Orange). In **dry fruits** pericarp, is thin, dry, papery or thick, woody and but not divided into three regions.

Sometimes along with ovary, other floral parts like thalamus, receptacle or calyx may develop as part of fruit, such fruits are called false fruits. e.g., Apple, Pear (thalamus), Fig (receptacle).

Parthenocarpic fruit: It is a fruit that develops without fertilisation. It is seedless, or has non-viable seeds e.g., Banana, Grapes. Horticulturists are producing such fruits artificially.

Kinds of Fruits

There are three basic types:

1. **Simple fruit:** Develops from single monotopolycarpellary, syncarpous (fused) ovary e.g., Pea, Tomato.
2. **Aggregate fruit:** Collection (etaerio) of simple fruits, or fruitlets on same thalamus developing from polycarpellary, apocarpous (free carpels) ovary e.g. *Calotropis.*
3. **Composite or multiple fruit:** Fruit develops from a number of flowers juxtaposed together or from inflorescence, e.g., Mulberry, Pineapple.

Major categories of Fruits

1. **Simple:**

(a) *Dry:*

Dehiscent: (i) Legume—Pea, Bean, Groundnut, (ii) Siliqua—Mustard, (iii) Follicle—Calotropis, (iv) Capsule—Cotton, Poppy, *'Bhindi'*.

Indehiscent: (i) Caryopsis—Wheat, Rice, (ii) Nut—Almond, Cashew nut, (iii) Cypsella—Sunflower, Marigold, (iv) Samara—Yam, Hiptage.

(b) *Fleshy:*

(i) Drupe—Mango, Coconut.
(ii) Berry—Tomato, Banana, Date palm.
(iii) Pepo—Cucumber, Watermelon.
(iv) Hesperidium—Lemon, Orange.
(v) Pome—Apple, Pear.

2. **Aggregate:**

(i) Etaerio (cluster) of drupes—Raspberry.
(ii) Etaerio of achenes—Strawbery, rose.
(iii) Etaerio of berries—Custard apple.
(iv) Etaerio of follicles—Periwinkle, Larkspur.

Table 23.6: Common Fruits and their Edible Parts

	Name	Type	Edible Part
1.	Banana	Berry—simple, fleshy	Mesocarp and endocarp
2.	Apple	Pome—simple, fleshy	Fleshy thalamus
3.	Coconut	Fibrous drupe—simple, fleshy	Endosperm
4.	Custard apple	Etaerio of berries—aggregate	Pericarp
5.	Date palm	Berry—simple, fleshy	Pericarp
6.	Cashew nut	Nut—simple, dry indehiscent	Peduncle and cotyledons
7.	Mango	Drupe—simple, fleshy	Mesocarp
8.	Orange	Hesperidium—simple, fleshy	Juicy hairs from endocarp,
9.	Tomato	Berry—simple, fleshy	Pericarp and placentae
10.	Pear	Pome—simple, fleshy	Fleshy thalamus
11.	Pineapple	Sorosis—composite	Outer portion of receptacle, bracts and perianth
12.	Fig	Syconus—composite	Fleshy receptacle
13.	Litchi	Nut—simple	Juicy aril
14.	Wheat	Caryopsis—simple dry indehiscent	Starchy endosperm
15.	Strawberry	Etaerio of achenes—aggregate	Succulent thalamus

3. **Multiple or composite:**
   (i) Sorosis—Pineapple, Mulberry, Jackfruit.
   (ii) Syconus—Fig.

A. VEGETABLE KINGDOM

Aconitum napellus

Botanical name : Aconitum napellus Linn.

Family : Ranunculaceae

Synonyms : Monk's hood; Wolf's-bane; Helmet flower.
Beng. Kathbish.

Description

1. It is a perennial herb.
2. **Leaves:** The leaves are alternate long stalked, hairy on the under surface. They are palmately lobed, the lower more deeply than the upper into three or five segments, which are again divided.
3. **Stem:** The stem is upright, 3 to 6 ft (1-2 metres) high, round, green and slightly hairy above.
4. **Flower:** The flowers are of dark-violet colour and appear from May to July. They are stalked and racemose. Petaloid sepals five, the upper helmet-shaped and beaked nearly hemispherical, the two lateral are roundish and hairy internally, the lower two are oblong oval.
5. **Root:** Perpendicular, tapering and tuberous.

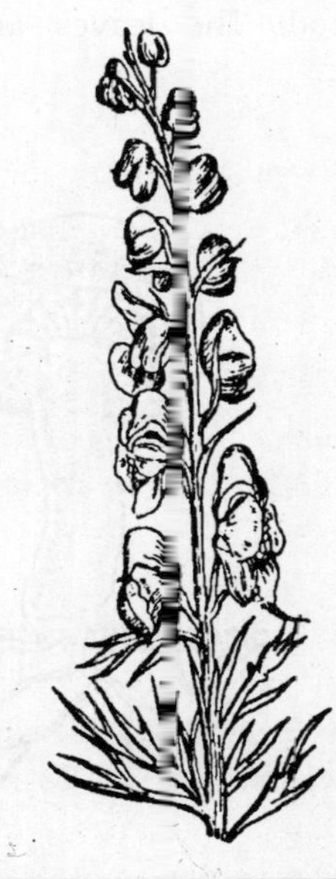

Aconitum napellus

Habitat: It grows on damp, shady fields, at high altitudes of mountains. It is found in the Alpine and sub-Alpine regions of Himalayas in India, from Nepal to Kashmir in Central Asia, Central and Southern Europe and Siberia.

Part used: The whole plant (H.P.I.).

Aegle folia

Botanical name : Aegle folia.

Family : Rutaceae.

Synonyms : Bael or Bela

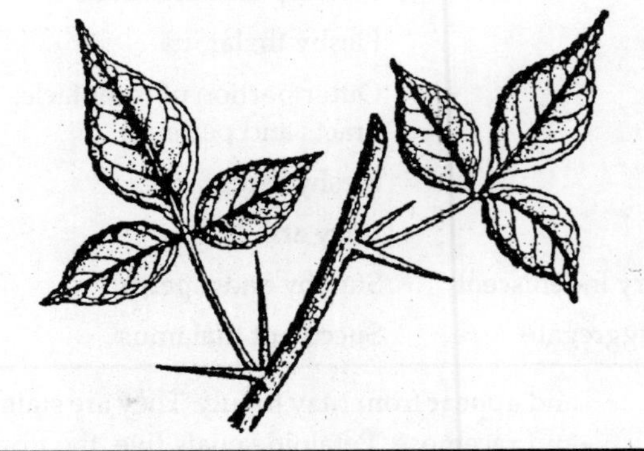

Aegle folia

Description

It is a slow-growing tree attaining a height of 30 ft to 40 ft in many years, having a rough bark and hard wood. The leaves are peculiarly arranged—three leaves being fixed to a petiole, like a trident. The fresh leaf has an aromatic odour which comes out when slightly crushed in hand. The juice of the leaf is bitter.

Habitat: Throughout the world.

Part used: Fresh, full-grown leaves.

Agaricus muscarius

Botanical name : Amanita muscarius Linn.

Family : Agaricaceae.

Synonyms : Amanita muscaria Linn; Bug or fly agaric.

Description

1. *Pileus:* 7-13 cm broad, globose at first, then dumb-bell in shape, convex, then expanded nearly flat with age; margin slightly striate. The surface of the cap is covered with white floccose scales.
2. *Gills:* The gills are pure white, very symmetrical, various in length, the shorter one terminating under the cap very abruptly.
3. The stem is white, often yellowish with age, pithy and often hollow, becoming rough and shaggy, finally scaly.

Habitat: Northern Europe, Asia and America.

Part used: The whole young fungus except the outer skin (H.P.I.).

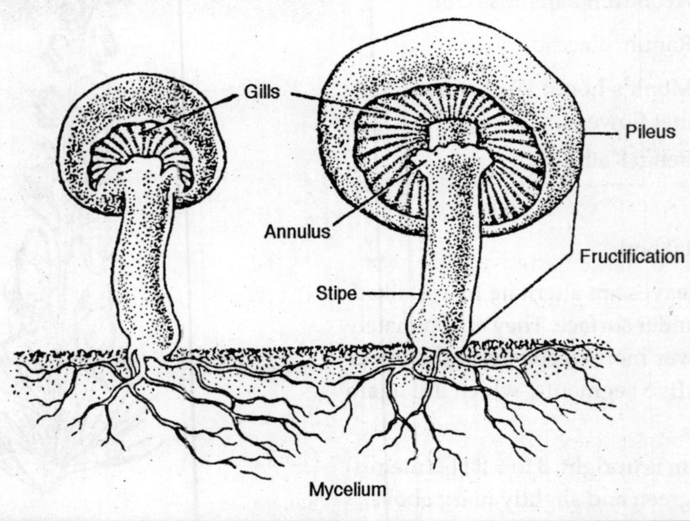

Agaricus muscarius

Allium cepa

Botanical name : Allium cepa Linn.

Family : Liliaceae

Synonyms : Piyaz; Onion.

Description

1. A bulbous plant, with a fistulous scape, swelling towards the base. The scape appears in the second year, approximately 1 meter high, and is surmounted by a large globular umbel of greenish-white flowers.
2. The fresh onion consists of a pear-shaped bulb, bearing fibrous roots from its base. The bulb consists of a compressed stem at the base covered by dry membranous scales on extreme outside and fleshy-scale leaves on upper side.
3. The leaves are terete, fistulous, pointed.

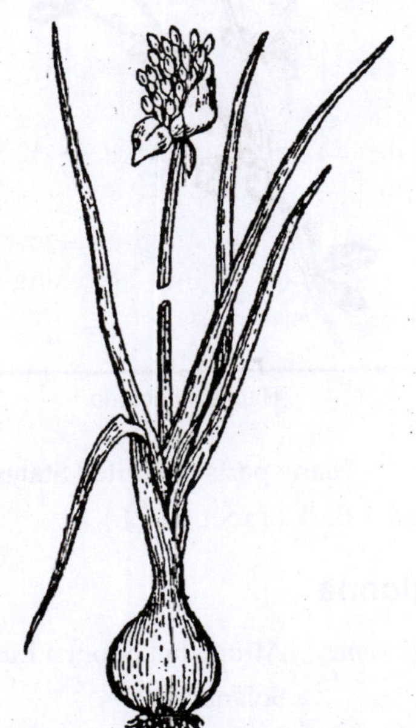

Allium Cepa

Habitat: It is very commonly cultivated in India.

Part used: The red, mature bulbs (H.P.I.).

Arnica montana

Botanical name : Arnica montana Linn.

Family : Compositae

Synonyms : Crysanthemum latifolium; Leopard's bane; Mountain arnica; Mountain tobacco.

Description

1. A perennial herb with a creeping, slender, blackish rhizome, 2-5 cm long and 5 mm in thickness, giving from its sides and undersurface numerous dark brittle, wiry, curved and twisted roots, about 8 cm in length.
2. *Stem:* 25-30 cm high, is erect, pubescent, rough, striated, either simple or with one pair of opposite branches.
3. *Leaves:* 10-20 cm long, are few, entire, sessile opposite, abovate; radical ones crowded at the base, the upper smaller than the rest.
4. *Flowers:* Yellow and numerous with tubular corolla with five spreading teeth and appear in July and August.

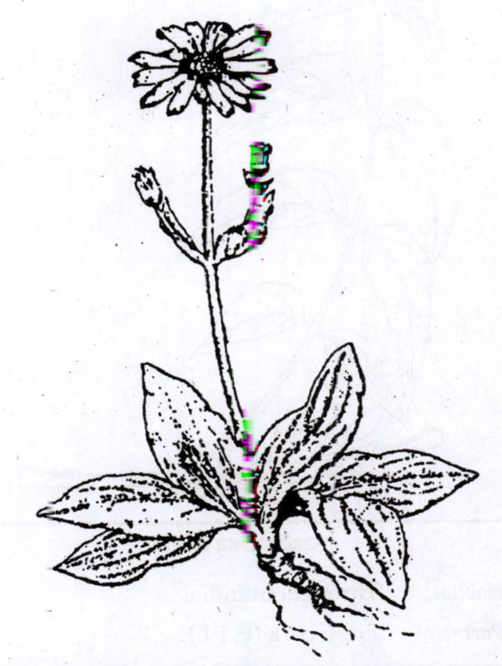

Arnica montana

Habitat: Central Europe; Russia and Siberia.

Part used: Whole plant (H.P.I.).

Azadirachta indica

Botanical name : Azadirachta indica A. Juss.

Family : Meliaceae.

Synonyms : Melia azadirachta; Neem; Indian lilac; Margosa.

Description

1. A large evergreen tree, up to 50 ft (15 m) in height, with a straight trunk.
2. *Leaves:* Simply pinnate, 20-38 cm long, crowded near the end of the branches. Leaflets 9-12, sub-opposite, obliquely lanceolate, sometimes felcate, acuminate, serrate, glabrous on both suraces.
3. The bark has a dark grey to a greyish black colour, rough, feebly fissured and exfoliating.

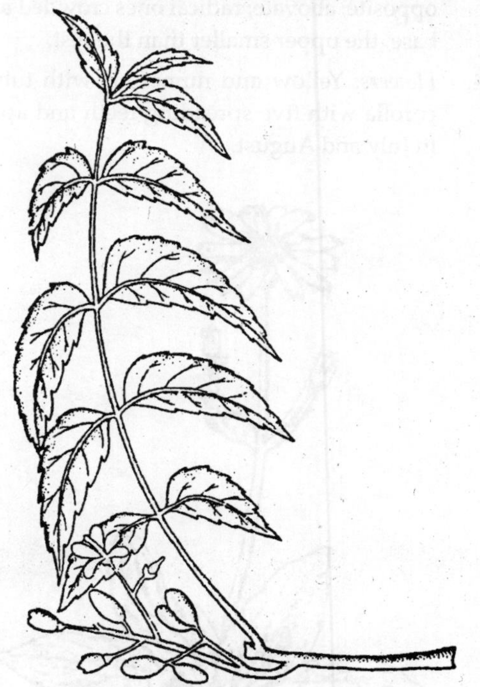

Azadirachta indica

Habitat: Throughout India.

Part used: Fresh bark (H.P.I.).

Baptisia tinctoria

Botanical name : Baptisia tinctoria Vent.

Family : Leguminosae.

Synonyms : Sophora tinctoria Linn; Wild indigo.

Description

1. It is an erect, perennial herb.
2. *Stem:* 2 to 3 feet (0.6–.9 m) high, round, smooth, branched.
3. *Leaves:* Palmately compound, small, three foliate, wedge obovate, bluish green, almost sessile.
4. *Flowers:* Bright-yellow about 1.25 cm long, few in numerous racemes. Each flower has an erect petal not much larger than the straight lateral petals and keel.
5. *Root:* Fleshy, up to 4 cm in thickness, more or less worthy, and marked by stem scales. Outer surface dark-brown and inner surface yellow.

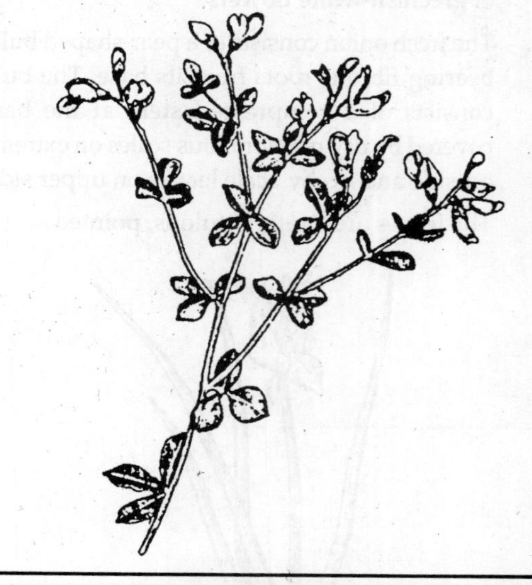

Baptisia tinctoria

Habitat: Many parts of United States.

Part used: Bark of root (H.P.I.).

Belladonna

Botanical name : Atropa belladonna Linn.

Family : Solanaceae.

Synonyms : A. lethalis; Belladonna baccifera; Solanum fluriosum; Deadly night-shade.

Description

1. It is a herbaceous perennial plant with thick, fleshy branched stem, 3-5 feet (.9–1.5 m) high.
2. *Leaves:* Alternate, green or brownish-green, short-stalked, mostly 3-9 inch (7.5–22.5 cm) long and ovate.
3. *Stems:* Hollow, flattened, finely hairy when young.

4. *Flowers:* Axillary, stalked, solitary, drooping.
5. *Root:* Thick; juicy; branched spreading.

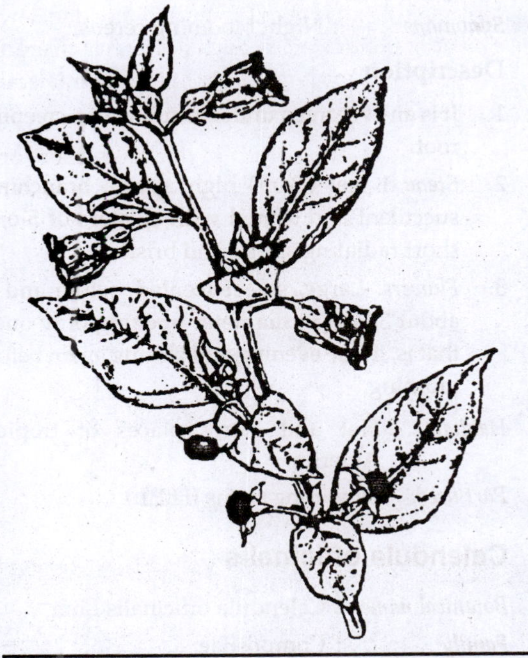

Belladonna

Habitat: Common in Europe. Cultivated in Kashmir and Simla.

Part used: Whole plant (H.P.I.).

Berberis vulgaris

Botanical name : Berberis vulgaris Linn.

Family : Berberidaceae.

Synonyms : Berberis canadensis, B. sinensis; B. scrrulata, Pipperidge bush.

Description

1. A deciduous shrub having roots of pale yellow colour.
2. *Leaves:* In tufts, somewhat obovate, more or less pointed, serrated and fringed and with three clefts spreading, sharp thorns at the base of each leaf bud.
3. *Flowers:* In drooping, many-flowered racemes; golden-yellow with red glands.

Habitat: India; Europe; North of Assam.

Part used: Bark of the root (H.P.I.).

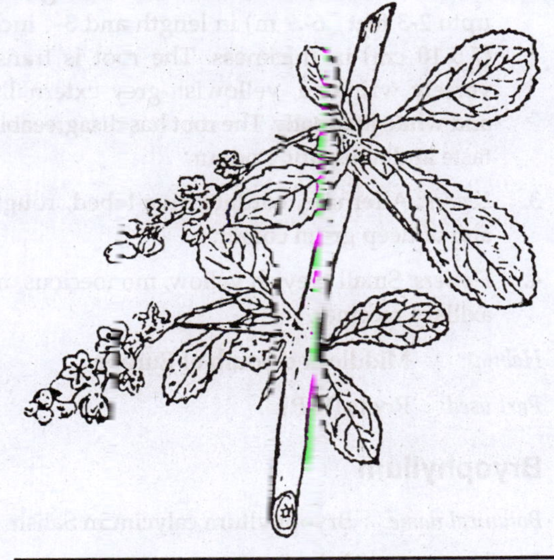

Berberis vulgaris

Bryonia alba

Botanical name : Bryonia alba Linn.

Family : Cucurbitaceae.

Synonyms : Bryonia vera; Uva angina; Vitis alba wild hops.

Description

1. A perennial climbing herbaceous vine growing in hedges.

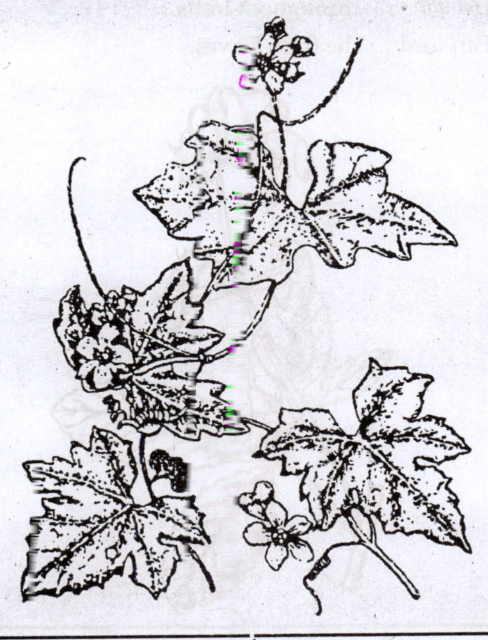

Bryonia alba

2. *Roots:* Fusiform, branched. The root grows upto 2-3 feet (.6-.9 m) in length and 3-4 inch (7.5-10 cm) in thickness. The root is transversely wrinkled, yellowish-grey externally and white internally. The root has disagreeable taste and nauseating odour.
3. *Leaves:* Alternate, cordate, five-lobed, rough and of deep green colour.
4. *Flowers:* Small greyish yellow, monoecious, in axillary racemes.

Habitat: Middle and South of Europe.

Part used: Roots (H.P.I.).

Bryophyllum

Botanical name : Bryophyllum calycinum Salish.

Family : Labiatae.

Synonyms : Coleus aromaticus; Himsagar; Patharkuchi; Amroda.

Description

1. It grows to a height of 1-3 feet (.3–.9 m) having numerous soft stems.
2. *Leaves:* Sessile, smooth and somewhat serrate. When pressed between fingers, leaves yield aromatic juice. Young shoots grow from ripe leaves.

Habitat: Throughout India.

Part used: The fresh leaves.

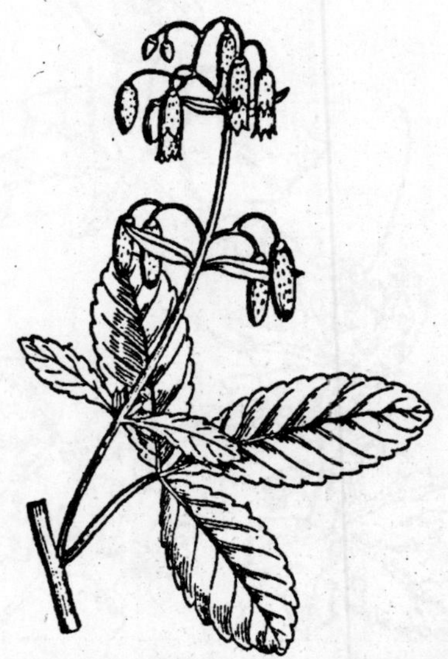

Bryophyllum

Cactus grandiflorus

Botanical name : Cereus grandiflorus Mill.

Family : Cactaceae.

Synonyms : Night blooming cereus.

Description

1. It is an evergreen under-shrub with a creeping root.
2. *Stem:* 1 feet (.3 m) high, green, branching, succulent and armed with clusters of 5 or 6 short radiating spines and bristles.
3. *Flowers:* Large, sweet-scented, white and is about 30 cm in diameter opening only once, that is, in the evening and closing again before morning.

Habitat: Hot and stony places of tropical America.

Part used: Flowering stems (H.P.I.).

Calendula officinalis

Botanical name : Calendula officinalis Linn.

Family : Compositae.

Synonyms : Marigold.

Description

1. It is an annual herb, 30-60 cm high.

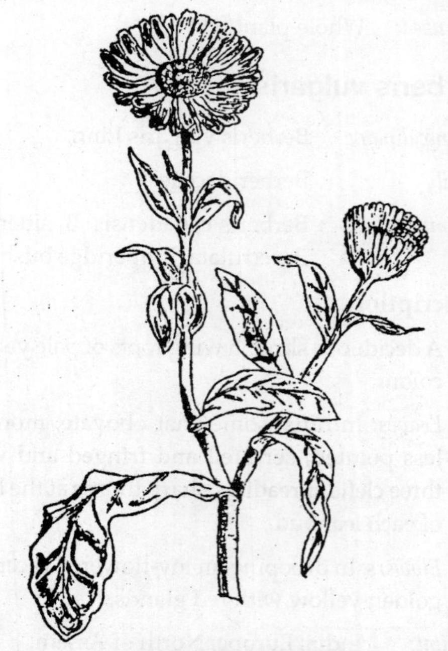

Calendula officinalis

2. *Leaves:* Thickish, oblong and acute somewhat broad and little cordate at the base, the upper lanceolate, the margins entire, often hispid with short hairs.
3. *Stem:* The stem is staggering, 6" (15 cm) to 18" (45 cm) high with numerous bushy branches, striated, green, succulent, pubescent.
4. *Flowers:* Flower heads are large terminal, solitary upon each branch, yellow or orange. Flowers generally appear during March to May.
5. *Root:* Fibrous, hairy, pale-yellow.

Habitat: It is cultivated in India.

Part used: Fresh flowering tops and leaves (H.P.I.).

Calotropis gigantia

Botanical name : Calotropis gigantia R. Br.

Family : Asclepiadaceae.

Synonyms : Asclepias gigantia; A. procera; Akanda, Madar.

Description

1. It is an evergreen plant with long, woody branching root.
2. *Stem:* Large, erect and grows to the height of 6–8 feet (1.8–2.4 m) with numerous downy branches.
3. *Leaves:* Sub-sessile, thick glaucous, green, opposite and cordate.
4. *Roots:* The roots are woody but light, greyish white or greyish yellow, cylindrical and often curved, with the surface, considerably fissure longitudinally.

Habitat: Throughout India.

Part used: Roots (H.P.I.).

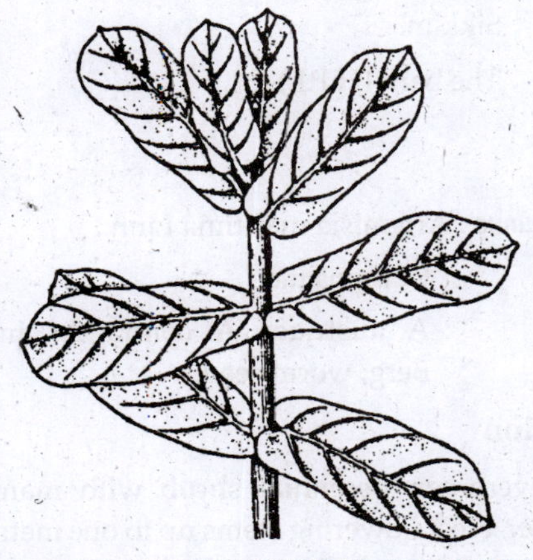

Calotropis gigentia

Chamomilla

Botanical name : Anthemis nobilis Linn.

Family : Compositae.

Synonyms : Chameanelum vulgare; Chamomille nostras; C. officinalis; C. vulgaris; Bitter chamomile.

Description

1. It is an annual herb growing in sandy regions.
2. *Root:* Large, woody, fibrous.
3. *Stem:* Erect, 30 to 60 cm high, solid, smooth, shining, strongly striated with long, slender branches.
4. *Leaves:* Numerous; alternate, sessile, amplexicaul, upper simple, the other bi- or tripinnatifid, the segments star shaped, narrow and minutely pointed.
5. *Flowers:* Numerous, terminal, solitary on striated naked peduncles, flowers are yellow and white and bloom from May to August.

Habitat: India, Asia; Europe.

Part used The whole fresh plant (H.P.I.).

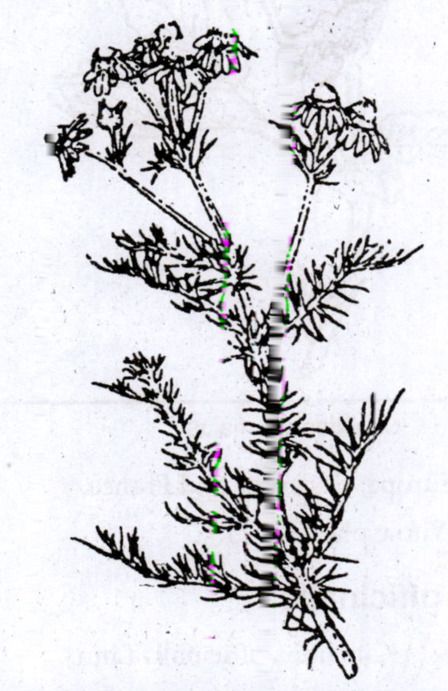

Chamomilla

Chelidonium majus

Botanical name : Chelidonium majus Linn.

Family : Papaveraceae.

Synonyms : Calandine; Tetterwort.

Description

1. An erect perennial herb, 30 to 120 cm in height.
2. *Root:* Fusiform, several headed, reddish-brown, yields an acrid juice.
3. *Stem:* Erect, branching, very brittle.
4. *Leaves:* Large, alternate, petiolate, glaucous.
5. *Flowers:* Small, yellow, pedunculated and umbilated in axillary cluster. They bloom from May to October.
6. *Fruit:* The fruit is two-valved linear capsule containing numerous seeds.

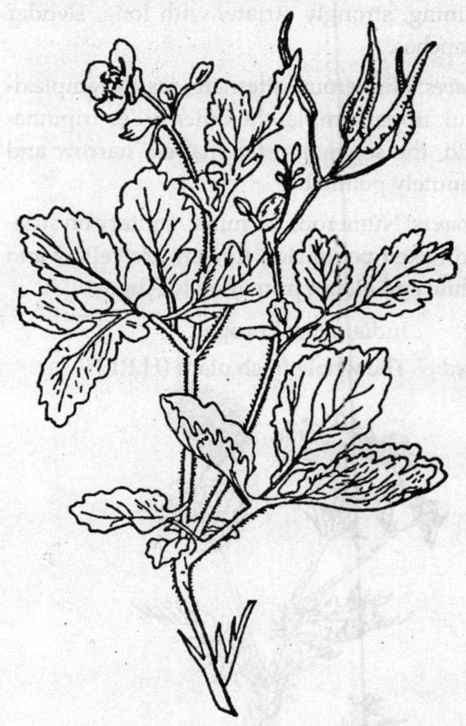

Chelidonium majus

Habitat: Europe, Germany and France.

Part used: Whole plant (H.P.I.).

Cinchona officinalis

Botanical name : Cinchona officinalis Linn.

Family : Rubiaceae

Synonyms : C. calisaya; C. succirubra; C. condaminea; Peruvian bark.

Description

1. Cinchona bark is obtained from the branches, trunk and root of the tree. There are several species of the shrubs or trees. The bark of the different species differs in its appearance.
2. Stem bark quilled, 5.5 to 10.5 feet long, 2 inches in diameter, and 0.13 to 0.25 inch thick. Outer surface dull brown-grey or grey, rough, being marked with transverse fissures. Inner surface striated and varying in colour, from pale yellowish brown to deep reddish brown.

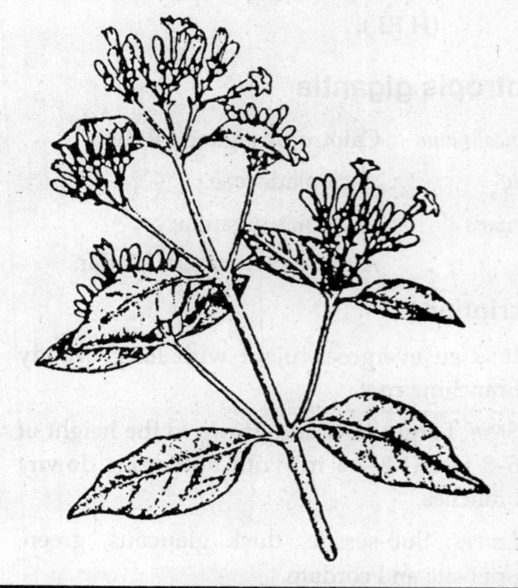

Cinchona officinalis

Habitat: India (Nilgiris, Asom, Khasia hills) and Sikkim.

Part used: The bark (H.P.I.).

Cina

Botanical name : Artemisia maritima Linn.

Family : Compositae.

Synonyms : A. austriaca, A. contra; A. cina Berg; worm seed.

Description

1. An evergreen perennial shrub with many slender, erect flowering stems up to one metre high, much branched.

2. *Flower heads:* greenish-yellow—1.5 to 4 mm long, elongated, ovoid in shape and somewhat angular. Surface is shining and only slightly hairy. The flower heads are very dense at the top portion of the branches.The flower appears in September.

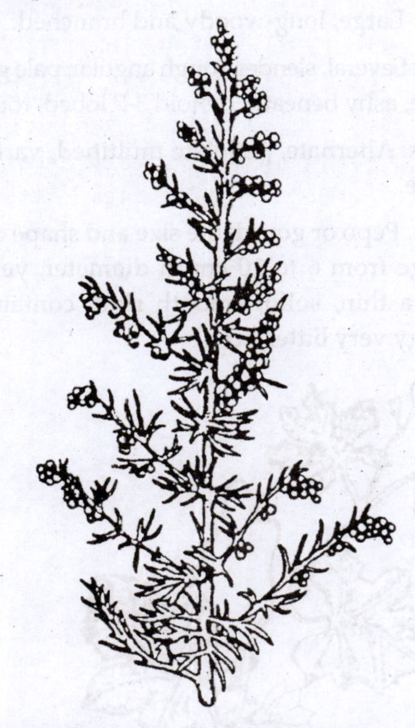

Cina

Habitat:	In temperate region, Western Himalayas.
Part used:	Flower heads (H.P.I.).

Cocculus indicus

Botanical name	: Anamirta cocculus W & A.
Family	: Menispermaceae.
Synonyms	: Anamirta paniculata; Indian cockle; Kakamari.

Description

1. A large woody climber with corky bark.
2. *Leaves:* 10 to 20 cm long, broadly ovate, acute or obtuse, rounded or sub-cordate at the base, thinly coriaceous, glabrous above, paler and with small tufts of hairs in the axils of the veins beneath.
3. *Flowers:* Small, greenish-white,, pendulous, compound racemose.
4. *Fruits.* The dried fruits are known as coculus indicus. The fruit is in clusters. Drupe dusky reddish-brown to moderate brown, kidney-shaped and wrinkled 8-13.5 mm in length and 7–11 mm, in breadth. The base marked by a circular stems scar. Pericarp tough, enclosing a single seed. Seeds yellowish-grey, urn-shaped.

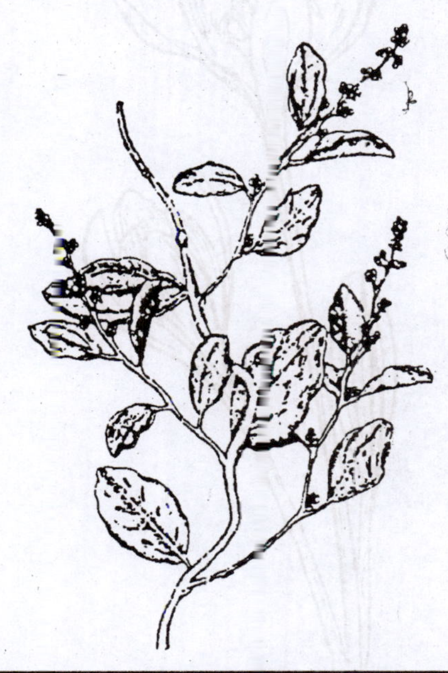

Cocculus indicus

Habitat	India (Malabar, Asom), Bangladesh, Sri Lanka, Burma (Myanmar).
Part used:	Seeds (H.P.I.)

Colchicum autumnale

Botanical name	: Colchicum autumnale Linn.
Family	: Liliaceae.
Synonyms	: Meadow saffron; Naked lady; Tuber root; Wild saffron.

Description

1. It is a bulbous perennial herb.
2. The underground stem (corm) tunicate. Corm in slices up to 2-5 mm thick and sub-reniform to ovate in outlines, with yellowish edges; a few pieces are sub-conical or plano-convex. The slices are hard and break readily with a short, mealy fracture; the cut surfaces are white and starchy.

3. *Flowers:* 1-4 cm or 6 cm, 7-10 cm across when expanded, appearing in autumn, with slender tube.
4. *Leaves:* Lanceolate, 25 cm or less long or 5 cm or less wide.

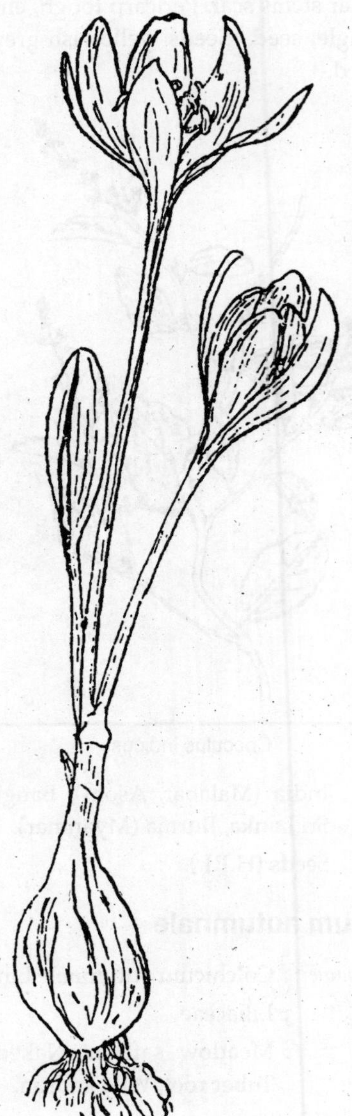

Colchicum autumnale

Habitat: Cultivated in India.

Part used: Bulbs (H.P.I.).

Colocynthis

Botanical name : Citrullus colocynthis Linn.

Family : Cucurbitaceae.

Synonyms : Colocynthis vulgaris; cucumis colocynthis; Bitter gourd; Indra varuni; Makal Phal.

Description

1. It is an annual, deciduous climber.
2. *Roots:* Large, long-woody and branched.
3. *Stems:* Several, slender, rough angular, pale green above, ashy beneath, deltoid 3-7 lobed, tough.
4. *Leaves:* Alternate, petiolate multified, variable in size.
5. *Fruits:* Pepo or gourd, the size and shape of an orange from 6 to 10 cm in diameter, yellow with a thin, solid, smooth rind, containing spongy very bitter pulp.

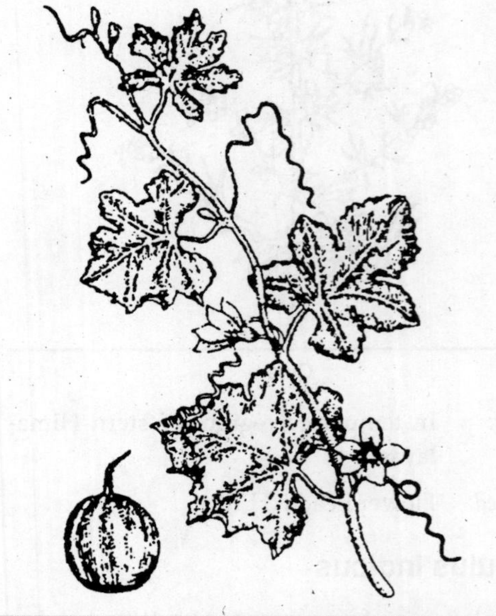

Colocynthis

Habitat: India, Sri Lanka, Arabia, North Africa, France, Spain.

Part used: Pulp of the fruit rejecting the seeds (H.P.I.).

Conium maculatum

Botanical name : Conium maculatum Linn.

Family : Umbelliferae.

Synonyms : Poison hemlock; Cicuta vulgaris; Conium major; Spotted hemlock.

Description

1. It is a deciduous herb.
2. *Root:* Biennial, whitish.
3. *Stem:* Round, hollow, erect, branching, smooth, marked with reddish-brown spots and growing to the height of 4 to 8 feet (1.2-2.4m).

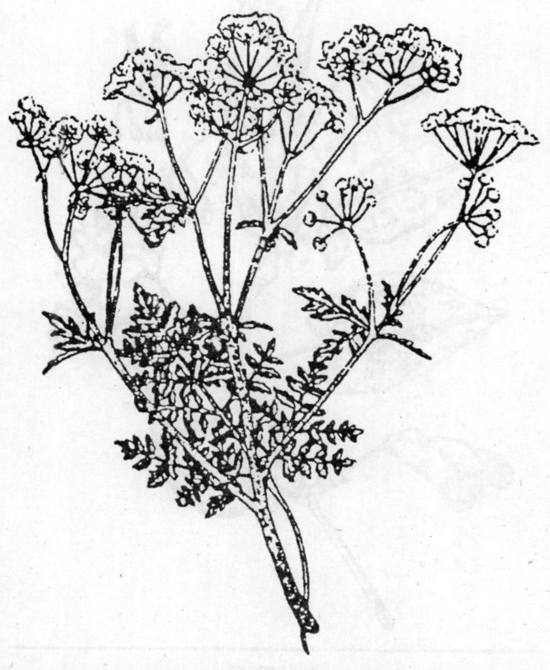

Conium maculatum

4. *Leaves:* Pinnately decompound, large, alternate, having long furrowed petioled, dark-green above, pale beneath emitting a foetid odour when bruised.

Habitat: Asia, Europe and N. Africa.

Part used: The whole plant (H.P.I.).

Digitalis purpurea

Botanical name : Digitalis purpurea Linn.

Family : Scrophulariacea.

Synonyms : Common fox-glove; Digitalis; Finger-hut; Purple glove.

Description

1. This is a biennial or perennial deciduous plant up to 2 metres high.
2. *Leaves:* Alternate, ovate or oblong, pubescent, greenish above and whitish underneath. The radial leaves are long stalked often growing up to 1 foot long. The stem leaves are short stalked becoming smaller towards the top of the stem.
3. *Flowers:* Purple, at times white inside sprinkled with black spots: they are numerous, bell-shaped and grow in terminal racemes. They appear from June to August.

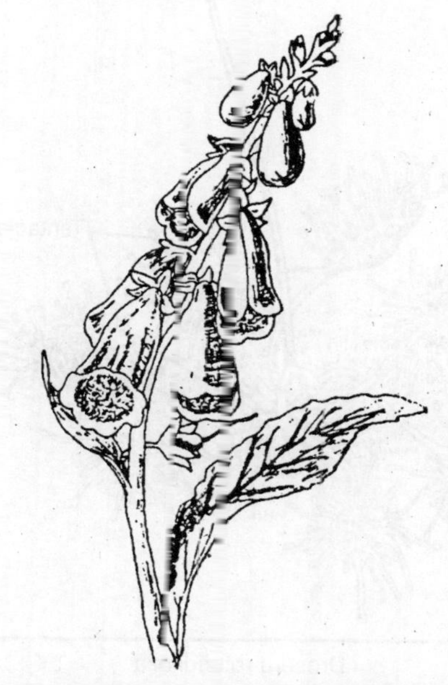

Digitalis purpurea

Habitat: Cultivated in India, Southern and Central Europe, England, Norway etc.

Part used: Leaves of the second year's growth (H.P.I.).

Drosera rotundifolia

Botanical name : Drosera rotundifolia Linn.

Family : Droseraceae.

Synonyms : Round leaved sundew; Red rot.

Description

1. It is an aquatic, carnivorous, perennial herb.
2. *Root:* Thin; fibrous with deep brown colour.
3. The plant is almost stemless.
4. *Leaves:* The leaves spreading on the ground. Leaves are radicle, clustered circular having

hairy petioles. Leaves are also covered with long reddish viscid hair on the upper surface. Each hair bears a small gland at the tip, which when exposed to sun exudes a clear shining juice. These hair are irritable.

5. *Flowers:* Small, white, opening in sunshine, appear in July and August.

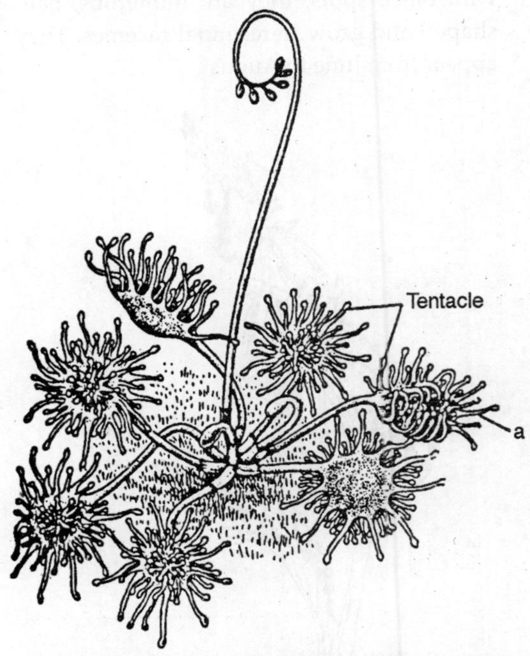

Drosera rotundifolia

Habitat: Europe, N. America, Asia.

Part used: Whole plant (H.P.I.).

Dulcamara

Botanical name : Amara dulcis; Dulcis amara; Bitter sweet; Garden night shade; Scarlet berry.

Description

1. A deciduous climbing shrub.
2. *Root:* Woody, irregularly branched, creeping, yellowish-green, smelling like potato.
3. *Stem:* Woody at base, pubescent above, alternately branched.
4. *Leaves:* Alternate, petiolate, entire, the lower ones cordate, the upper hastate, or with two ear-like lobes at the base, pubescent beneath.
5. *Flowers:* Purple, small, lateral, extra axillary, drooping cymes.
6. *Berries:* Berries scarlet, oval and poisonous.

Habitat: Europe, Asia, Africa, North America.

Part used: The whole plant (H.P.I.).

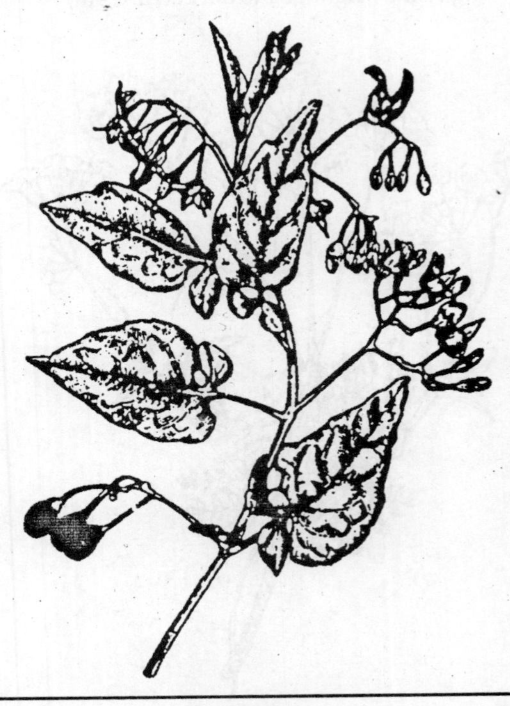

Dulcamara

Ficus indica

Botanical name : Ficus indica Linn.

Family : Urticaceae.

Synonyms : Banyan tree; Ficus benghalensis; Bata.

Description

1. It grows to a height of about 100 feet (30 m).
2. The woody trunk grows to an enormous size.
3. Aerial roots in raceme descend from branches and penetrate into the ground.
4. The bark is thick and glabrous.

Habitat: Throughout India by the roadside and also in lower Himalayas.

Part used: Hanging aerial roots issuing from the branches.

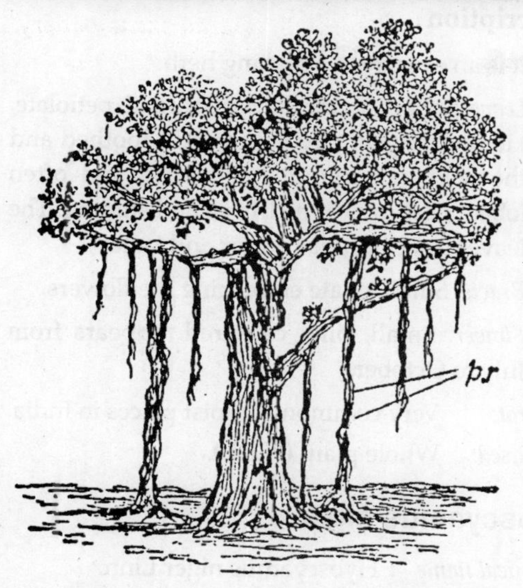

Ficus indica

Ficus religiosa

Botanical name : Ficus religiosa Linn.
Family : Moraceae.
Synonyms : Peepul tree; Ashwath.

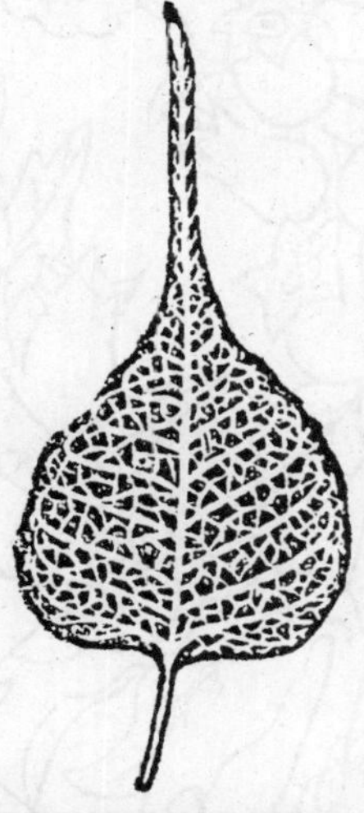

Ficus religiosa

Description

1. *Leaves:* Deciduous, cordate, petiolate, shining, drooping, 10 to 18 cm long, narrowed upwards and with the apex produced into a linear lanceolate tail $\frac{1}{3}$ the whole length of the blade base broad, rounded or truncate.
2. *Bark:* Grey, exfoliating in roundish irregular flakes.

3. *Fruits:* Looks like figs, small size.

Habitat: India.
Part used: Tender leaves (H.P.I.).

Granatum

Botanical name : Punica granatum Linn.
Family : Granateae.
Synonyms : Pomegranate; Dalim.

Description

1. It is a large perennial shrub or tree.
2. *Stem:* Well-branched, slender, 18 to 20 feet (5-6 m) high.
3. *Leaves:* Opposite, lanceolate, pointed, entire, oblong or obovate, glabrous and short-petioled.
4. *Flowers:* Red sessile, appear solitary or in clusters of two or three.
5. Bark is light brownish grey.

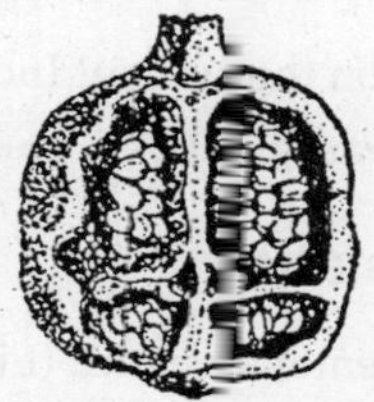

Granatum

Habitat: Many parts of India, Persia and other warmer places of the world.
Part used: Dried bark of the root.

Holarrhena antidysenterica

Botanical name : Holarrhena antidysenterica wall.
Family : Apocynaceae.
Synonyms : Kurchi.

Description

1. A small deciduous tree, with brown bark exfoliating in irregular flakes.
2. *Leaves:* Sessile or nearly so, rather thin glabrous or more or less tomentose.
3. *Flowers:* White, arranged in terminal cymes, pedicles slender.
4. The wood is lustrous, straight and close-grained, fine and even-textured, moderately soft and light.

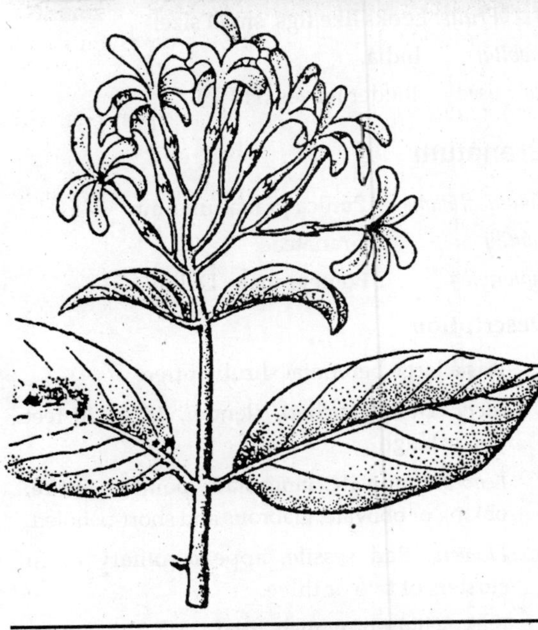

Holarrhena antidysenterica

Habitat: Common throughout India.

Part used: Dried bark (H.P.I.).

Hydrocotyle asiatica

Botanical name : Centella asiatica (Linn) urb.

Family : Umbelliferae.

Synonyms : Hydrocotyle asiatica Linn; Thick-leaved penny-wort.

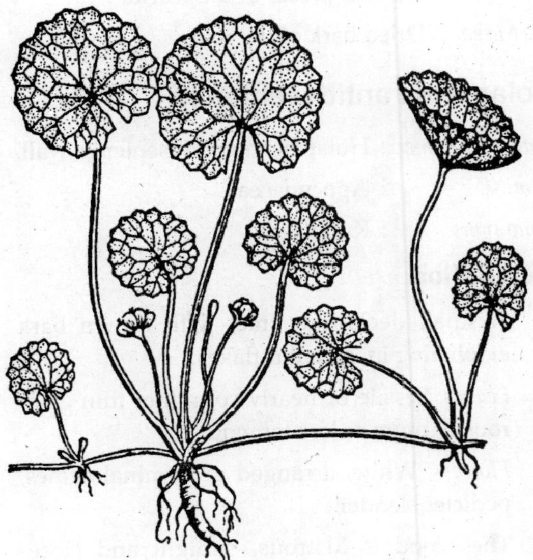

Hydrocotyle asiatica

Description

1. It is an evergreen, creeping herb.
2. *Leaves:* About an inch (2.5 cm) broad, petiolate, kidney-shaped, circular, margin toothed and the teeth are rounded (crenate), and often lobed. Glabrous or nearly so and shining. The leaves have peculiar odour and taste.
3. *Bracts:* Small, ovate embracing the flowers.
4. *Flower:* Small, pink coloured, appears from July to October.

Habitat: Very common at moist places in India.

Part used: Whole plant (H.P.I.).

Hyoscyamus niger

Botanical name : Hyoscyamus niger Linn.

Family : Solanaceae.

Synonyms : Henbane; Poison tobacco.

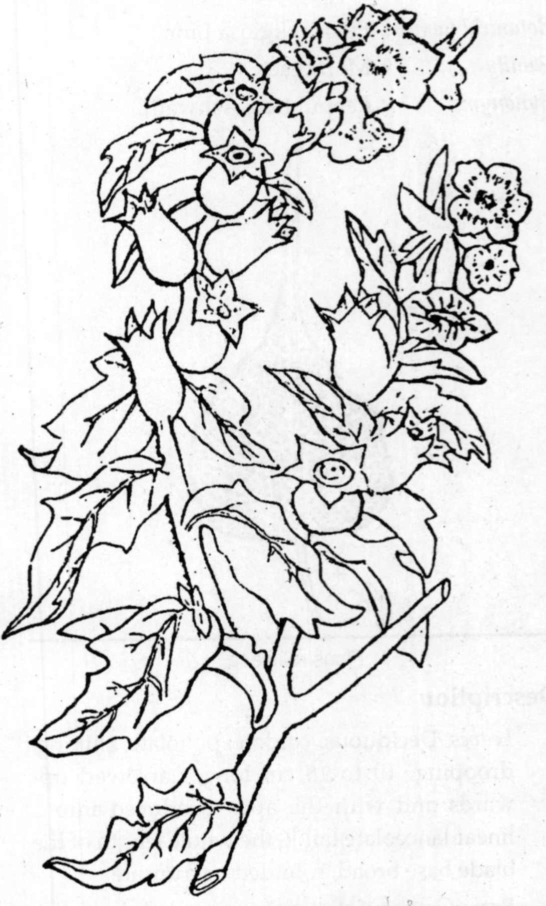

Hyoscyamus niger

Description

1. A biannual deciduous plant.
2. *Stem:* Tapering, thick, cylindrical, growing up to 2 feet (.6 m) in height. Stem is covered with long, soft, pointed, glandular white hairs.
3. *Leaves:* Large, pale-green, hairy, alternate, sessile, oblong and irregularly lobed.
4. *Flowers:* Dull-yellow, appear from July to August.

Habitat: India; Europe.

Part used: Plant of second year's growth (H.P.I.).

Hypericum perforatum

Botanical name : Hypericum perforatum Linn.

Family : Hypericaceae.

Synonyms : Fuga daemonum; H. umbelicalis; H. officinale; H. pseudoperforatum; H. virginicum; St. John's wort.

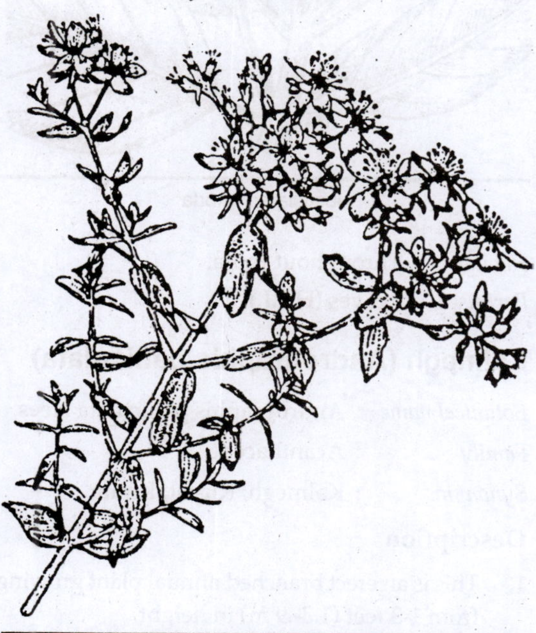

Hypericum perforatum

Description

1. A deciduous perennial herb, with woody branches.
2. *Root:* Dark brown.
3. *Stem:* 30 cm or more in height, much branched, producing runners from the base, somewhat 2-edged and smooth.
4. *Leaves:* Opposite, entire, oblong, punctate, with numerous scattered pellucid dots.
5. *Flowers:* Deep yellow, in terminal, open, leafy, cymes.
6. The herb has a characteristic balsamic odour and a bitter, resinous, somewhat astringent taste.

Habitat: India, Asia, Europe, North Africa and North America.

Part used: Whole plant (H.P.I.).

Ignatia amara

Botanical name : Strychnos ignatia Berg.

Family : Loganiaceae.

Synonyms : St. Ignatius bean.

Description

1. A small tree, stem erect, branches opposite, glabrous.
2. *Leaves:* Petiolate, ovate, opposite, acute, 12.5-15 cm long.
3. *Flowers:* numerous, white, long, in small axillary panicles having the odour of jasmine.

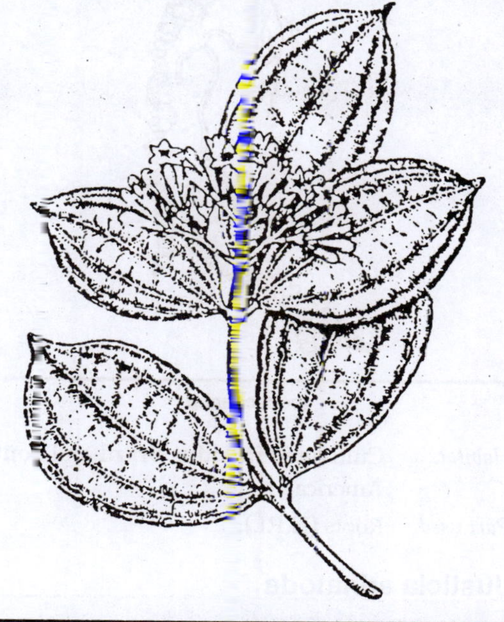

Ignatia amara

4. *Fruit:* Pear-shaped, having seeds 20-24 in numbers, embedded in a bitter pulp. The seeds are about an inch (2.5 cm) long, oblong or ovate in shape, obscurely angular, with one side flat, another convex. It is almond-like, grey or clear-brown in colour, having a brownish, translucent hard shell.

Habitat: Philippine Islands and China.

Part used: The bean (H.P.I.).

Ipecacuanha

Botanical name : Caphaelis ipecacuanha (Brot) A. Rich.

Family : Rubiaceae.

Synonyms : Ipecac; C. ametica.

Description

The roots are tortuous, seldom more than 15 cm long, 0.6 mm thick, from dark brick-red to very dark brown. Closely annulated external ridges rounded and completely encircling the root. Rhizome short length attached to roots, cylindrical, up to 1 mm in diameter, finely wrinkled longitudinally and with pith approximately one-sixth of the whole diameter.

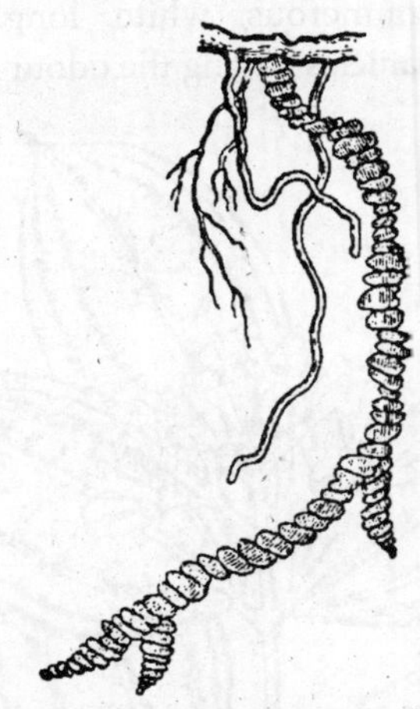

Ipecacuanha

Habitat: Cultivated in India, Brazil and South America.

Part used: Roots (H.P.I.).

Justicia adhatoda

Botanical name : Adhatoda vesica Nees.

Family : Acanthaceae.

Synonyms : Justicia adhatoda; Vasaka.

Description

1. A dense evergreen shrub 1-2.5 metre high.
2. *Leaves:* 12-20 cm long, elliptic, lanceolate, acuminate, acute at both the ends, petiolate, thin, smoth on both sides with very fine hair both on the blade and on the petiole.

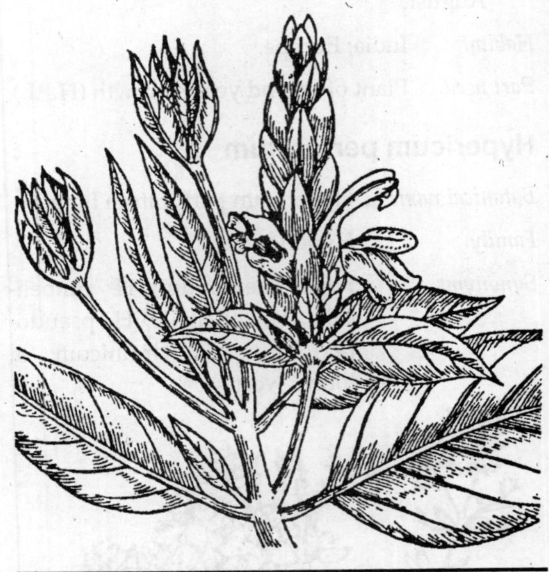

Justicia adhatoda

Habitat: Throughout India.

Part used: Leaves (H.P.I.).

Kalmegh (Andrographis paniculata)

Botanical name : Andrographis paniculata Nees.

Family : Acanthaceae.

Synonyms : Kalmegh; Kiryat; Kirata.

Description

1. This is an erect branched annual plant growing from 1-3 feet (1.3-.9 m) in height.
2. *Leaves:* About 3 inches (7.5 cm) in length, lanceolate, acute, tapering at the base, petioled, glabrous, pale beneath, main lateral nerves 4–6 pairs, petioles none or up to 0.6 mm long.
3. *Flowers:* Small, solitary, arranged in lax spreading axillary and terminal racemes or panicles.

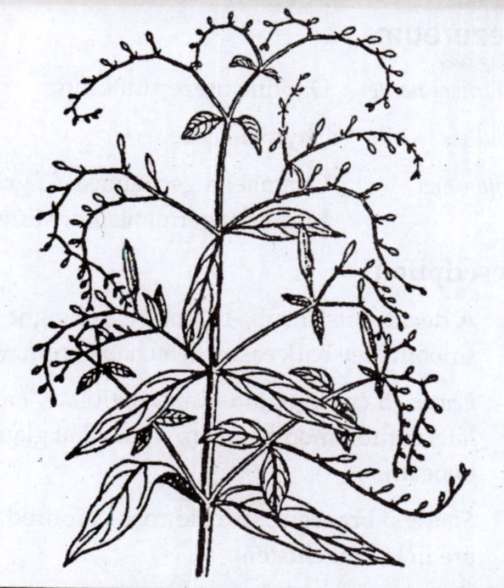

Andrographis paniculata (Kalmegh)

Habitat: In the plains, throughout India.

Parts used: Whole plant (H.P.I.).

Nux vomica

Botanical name : Strychnos nux-vomica Linn.

Family : Loganiaceae.

Synonyms : Poison-nut; Kuchila.

Description

1. A deciduous tree, having short, thick trunk and ash-coloured bark.

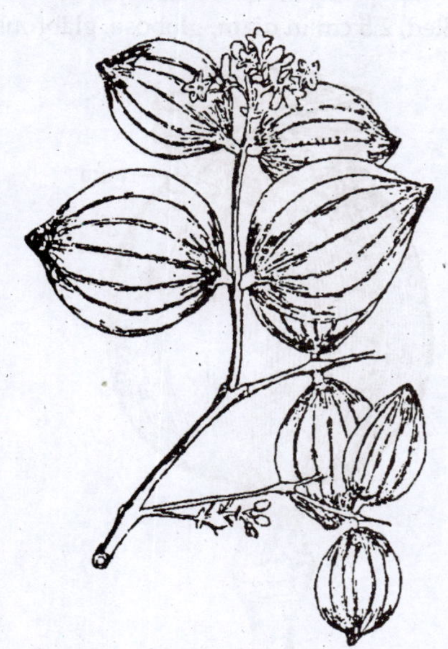

Nux vomica

2. *Leaves:* 7–15 cm long, short-petioled, oval, 3–5 veined, opposite, smooth on both sides.
3. *Flowers:* Many, greenish-white, appear in cold season.
4. *Berry:* globose, 2.5-7.5 cm in diameter, rough and shining, clothed on both sides with fine silky hair radiating from the centre. Each berry contains 1-2 seeds.
5. *Seeds:* Disc-shaped, 10-30 mm in diameter and 4–6 mm thick. Flat or concavo-convex. Margin rounded, surface ash-grey, covered with short satiny hair. No odour. Taste extremely bitter.

Habitat: Forests of Western Ghats and Himalayas.

Part used: Seeds (H.P.I.).

Ocimum sanctum

Botanical name : Ocimum sanctum Linn.

Family : Labiatae.

Synonyms : Tulsi

Description

1. It is an under-shrub, 2-4 feet (0.6-1.2 m) high with much branched twigs.
2. *Leaves:* 2-5 cm long, oblong or elliptic oblong, obtuse or acute, entire or subserrate, hairy on

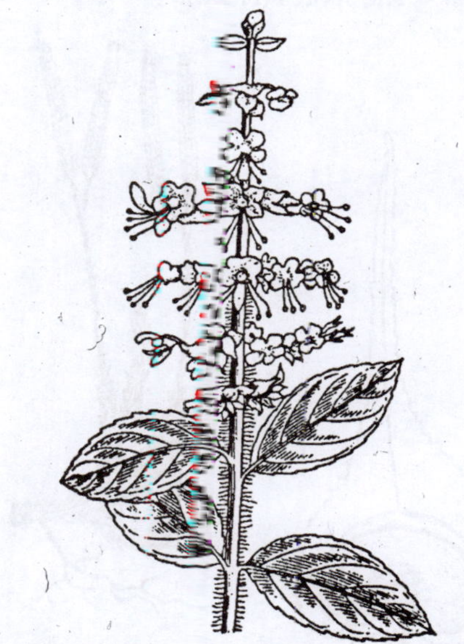

Ocimum sanctum

both surfaces and minutely dotted. Petioles 1.25 to 2.5 cm long.

Habitat: It is cultivated and planted throughout India.

Part used: Whole plant excluding roots (H.P.I.).

Lycopodium clavatum

Botanical name : Lycopodium clavatum Linn.

Family : Lycopodiaceae.

Synonyms : Club moss; witch meal; Stag's horn; vegetable sulphur.

Description

1. *Roots:* Consists of strong-spreading fibres which look like wolf's feet.
2. *Stem:* Trailing branching, several metres long.
3. *Leaves:* Linear-oval shaped, flat, ribless, smooth, tipped with fine bristle, curved upward, and of a light green colour.
4. The fructification is in terminal spikes, single or in pairs, with crowded, ovate, entire pointed scales, bearing in the axil a transversely oval sporangium which splits nearly to the base and contains a spore. Spores are pale yellow and form mobile powder.

Habitat: Bengal, Sikkim, Asom, Khasi, Manipur.

Part used: The spores (H.P.I.).

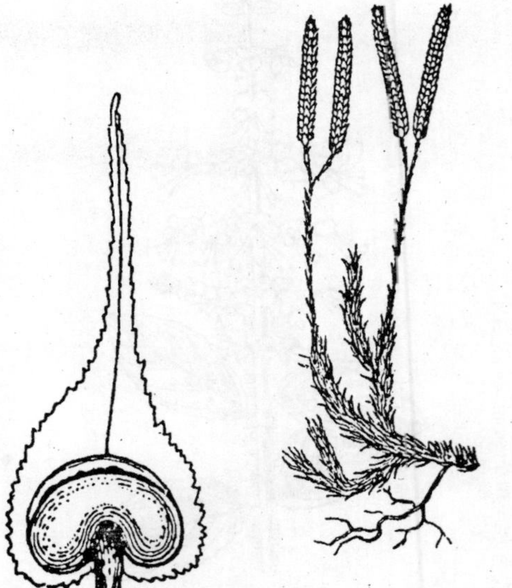

Lycopodium clavatum

Mezereum

Botanical name : Daphne mezerum Linn.

Family : Thymeliaceae.

Synonyms : Chamaelia germanica; C. gridus; Mezerum germanicum; Mezereon

Description

1. A deciduous shrub, 1.3 metre in height with smooth grey bark easily detachable from wood.
2. *Leaves:* 5 cm long alternate, petiolate, lanceolate, entire, smooth, green, somewhat glaucous beneath.
3. *Flowers:* Fragrant, purple rose-coloured, and are in lateral clusters.
4. The fruit is in a berry.

Habitat: Europe, especially in central countries.

Part used: The bark (H.P.I.).

Opium

Botanical name : Papaver somniferum Linn.

Family : Papaveraceae.

Synonyms : Poppy; Afim; Meconium; Opium; Crudum.

Description

1. The capsule 3 or 4 on each plant, smooth, stalked, 2.5 cm in diam, globose, glabrous.

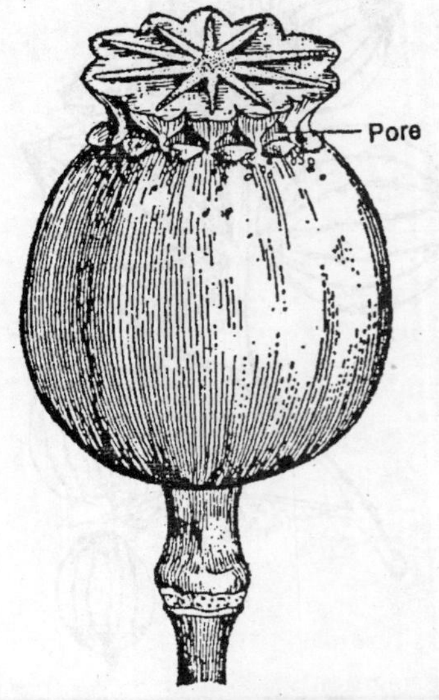

Opium

2. The capsule contains numerous seeds known as poppy seeds (posta dana) which are edible. All parts of the plant contain a white milky juice, which is most abundant in the capsules. This is obtained by first incising the capsule and some hours later scraping upon leaves, the juice will have attained different degrees of consistency.

Habitat: India.

Part used: Gummy juice (H.P.I.).

Pulsatilla nigricans

Botanical name : Pulsatilla nigricans Linn.

Family : Ranunculaceae.

Synonyms : Anemone pratensis; Pulsatilla pratensis; Wind flower.

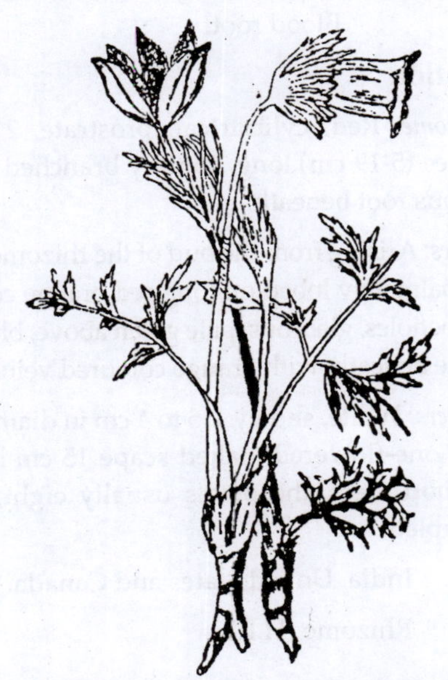

Pulsatilla nigricans

Description

1. A deciduous, perennial herb.
2. *Root:* Spindle-shaped, thick ligeneous dark-brown, oblique, several-headed root.
3. *Stem:* Stem up to 1.5 meter high, simple erect, rounded.
4. *Leaves:* Radical, petiolate, bipinnatifid, with linear segments, at the base surrounded by several ovate, lanceolate sheaths.
5. *Flowers:* Varying in colour from dark violet to light blue, bell-shaped pendulous, terminal reflexed at the open.

Habitat: Europe, Russia, Asia.

Part used: Whole plant (H.P.I.).

Rhus toxicodendron

Botanical name : Rhus toxicodendron Mitch.

Family : Anacardiaceae.

Synonyms : R. radicans; R. humile; R. pubescens; Poison ivy; poison oak; poison ash.

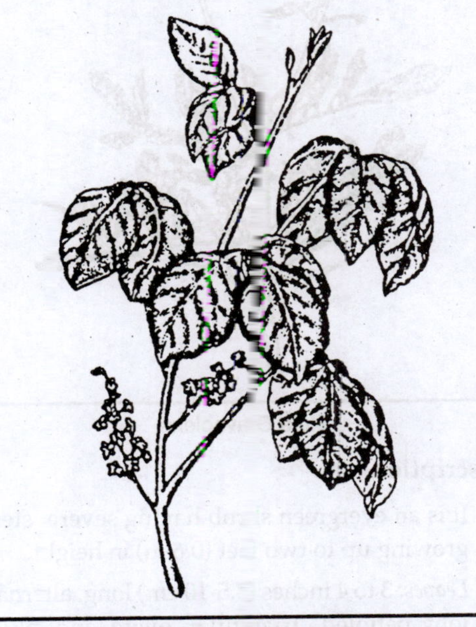

Rhus toxicodendron

Description

1. A deciduous shrub growing from 1–3 feet (0.9 m) in height.
2. *Leaves:* Alternate, ternate, the lateral leaflets unequal at the base and sessile, the terminal one larger at the end of prolongation of the common petiole, rhombic-ovate, pointed.
3. *Flowers:* Small, greenish-white, polygamous; and in loose and slender axillary panicles.
4. *Fruits:* Globular, glabrous, greyish, drupe.

Habitat: Found in thickets and low grounds of United States.

Part used: Leaves (H.P.I.).

Ruta graveolens

Botanical name : Ruta graveolens Linn.

Family : Rutaceae.

Synonyms : Common rue; Ruta; R. latifolia; Bitter herb.

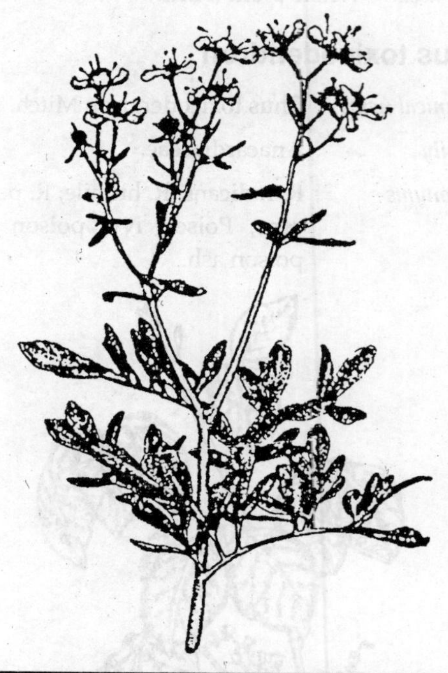

Ruta Graveolens

Description

1. It is an evergreen shrub having several stems growing up to two feet (0.6 m) in height.
2. *Leaves:* 3 to 4 inches (7.5-10 cm) long, alternate, long-petioled, triangular ovate and bluish green in colour.
3. *Flowers:* Yellow in divaricately spreading corymbs; pedicles longer than the capsule.

Habitat: Cultivated in gardens throughout India.

Part used: The whole plant (H.P.I.).

Sambucus nigra

Botanical name : Sambucus nigra Linn.

Family : Caprifoliaceae.

Synonyms : Black berried European elder.

Description

1. Deciduous tree, 4 to 9 metres high with deeply furrowed whitish bark; branches greyish and strongly leaticellate.
2. *Leaves:* Petiolate, opposite, odd-pinnate, leaflets 3-7 short-stalked, elliptic, acuminate sharply serrate, shining.
3. *Flowers:* Creamy-white, in five-parted cymes.
4. *Fruits:* Black, lustrous, globose, three celled, and 50 to 65 mm in diameter.

Habitat: Europe, West Africa, Great Britain, Japan and Siberia.

Part used: Leaves and flowers.

Sanguinaria canadensis

Botanical name : Sanguinaria canadensis Linn.

Family : Papaveraceae.

Synonyms : S. acaulis; S. grandiflora; S. minor; Blood root.

Description

1. *Rhizome:* Red, cylindrical, prostrate, 2 to 4 inches (5-19 cm) long, slightly branched with fibrous root beneath.
2. *Leaves:* Arising from the bud of the rhizome, are 5-9 palmately lobed on long red orange coloured petioles, glabrous, pale green above, bluish-white beneath, with orange coloured veins.
3. *Flowers:* White, showy, 2.5 to 4 cm in diameter, on a one-flowered, naked scape 15 cm high, the bud erect, the petals usually eight; not crampled.

Habitat: India, United States and Canada.

Part used: Rhizome (H.P.I.).

Secale cornutum

Botanical name : Claviceps purpurea Tul.

Family : Hypocreaceae (Fungi).

Synonyms : Acinula clavus; Clavaria clavus; Ergot of Rye.

Description

1. A fungus growing upon the seed of the secale cornutum.
2. The grains, or ergots, are 8–12 mm long, 3–6 mm in diameter, sub-cylindrical, or obtusely-

triangular, tapering towards the ends, transversely cracked with three longitudinal furrows. Internally it is purplish-black, internally whitish. It has a peculiar, offensive odour, a rancid taste.

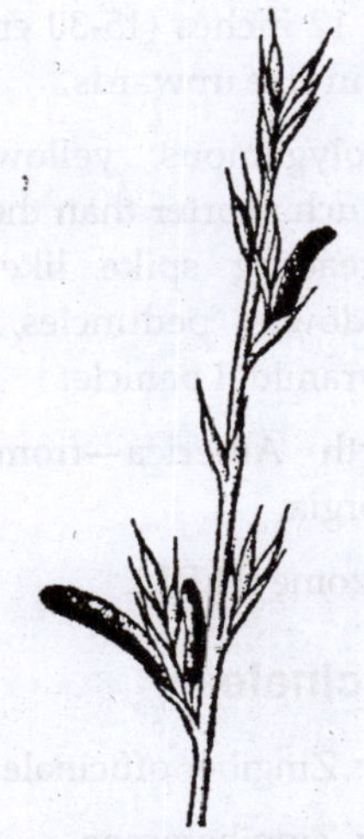

Secale cornutum

Habitat: Found in fields on the rye plant.

Part used: Whole fungus freshly dried in coarse powder (H.P.I.).

Spigelia marilandica

Botanical name : Spigelia marilandica Linn.

Family : Loganiaceae.

Synonyms : Pink-root.

Description

1. A perennial herb, 30-40 cm high, small, twisted, knotty horizontal rhizome, 5 cm long, 2-3 mm in diameter, giving numerous long, slender fibrous yellow roots beneath.
2. *Stems:* Several, erect, purplish, smooth, quadrangular above and rounded below.
3. *Leaves:* Opposite, sessile, existipulate, ovate, lanceolate, acute, smooth.
4. *Flowers:* 4 to 12, brilliant red, large, sessile or very short-stalked, tubular, funnel shaped.
5. *Fruit:* Loculicidally dehiscent capsule, compressed laterally, two-celled, smooth, yellow or greenish-yellow.

Habitat: West Indies, East North America to Florida and Texas.

Part used: Whole plant (H.P.I.).

Thuja occidentalis

Botanical name : Thuja occidentalis Linn.

Family : Cupressaceae.

Synonyms : American arborvitae; Tree of life.

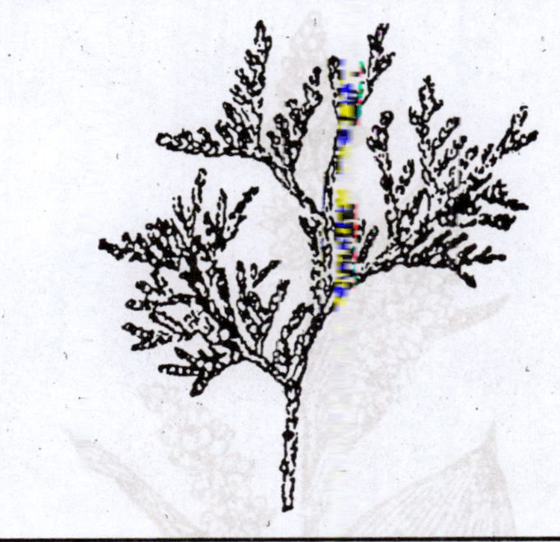

Thuja occidentalis

Description

1. A tall tree up to 20 metres in height.
2. *Leaves:* Acute, apiculate, usually conspicuously glandular, bright green above and yellowish green beneath. Twigs entire or broken, fanshaped, flattened, bearing 4 rows of appressed, scale-like leaves, all bearing glands on back. The leaves, when rubbed between the palms of hands, give off a pungent aromatic resinous odour.
3. *Flowers:* Minute, solitary, terminal, appear in May and June.

Habitat: United States.

Part used: Leaves and Twigs (H.P.I.).

Veratrum album

Botanical name : Veratrum album Linn.

Family : Liliaceae.

Synonyms : European hellebore.

Description

1. A perennial deciduous herb with an erect rhizome, frequently dividing into 2-3 branches.

2. *Rhizome:* 5 cm long, 2 cm in diameter, dull black, rough and wrinkled externally with the remains of numerous concentrically arranged leaf base at the upper part and root-scars containing a distinct slender xylem in the centre. Rootlets numerous, completely enveloping the rhizome, dull-grey or yellowish, and shrivelled longitudinally. Lower extremity of the rhizome, bluntly conical or truncate.

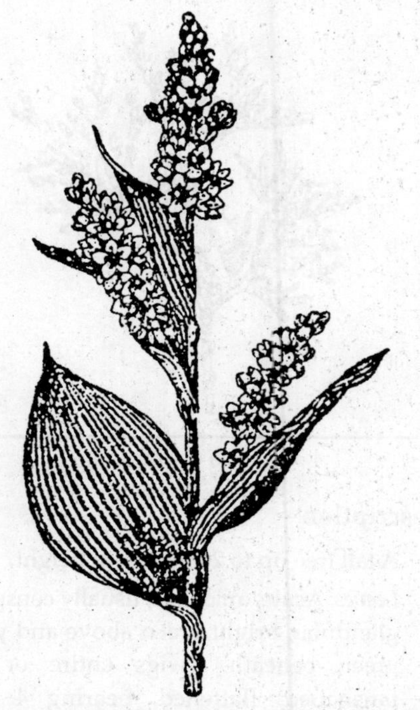

Veratrum album

Habitat: Middle and Southern Europe, Russia, China and Japan.

Part used: Rhizome (H.P.I.).

Veratrum viride

Botanical name : Veratrum viride Ait.

Family : Liliaceae.

Synonyms : Hellonias viridis; American white hellebore.

Description

1. *Rhizome:* Coarse, thick, fleshy, more or less horizontal, with numerous white rootlets upon the lower part having a strong, unpleasant odour when fresh, nearly odourless when dried. It is about 5 to 8 cm long, 2 to 3.5 cm wide, sub-cylindrical and obconical below.
2. *Stem:* About 1.33 m high, stout, erect, simple, leafy to the top, striated and pubescent.
3. *Leaves:* 3-ranked, broadly-oval, the lower leaves 6 to 12 inches (15-30 cm) long, curly, decreasing in size upwards.
4. *Flowers:* Polygamous, yellowish-green on pedicles, much shorter than the bracts, are in dense, spreading spike like racemes on roundish, downy peduncles, composing a terminal pyramidal panicle.

Habitat: North America—from Canada to Georgia.

Part used: Rhizome (H.P.I.).

Zingiber officinale

Botanical name : Zingiber officinale Ros-coe.

Family : Zingiberaceae.

Synonyms : Ginger; Amonum zingiber, Zingiber albus; Ada; Adrak.

Description

1. A perennial, deciduous shurb.
2. *Rhizome:* Large, horizontal, solid, tough rhizome, roundly jointed, fleshy, cylindrical flat and covered with brown thin skin.

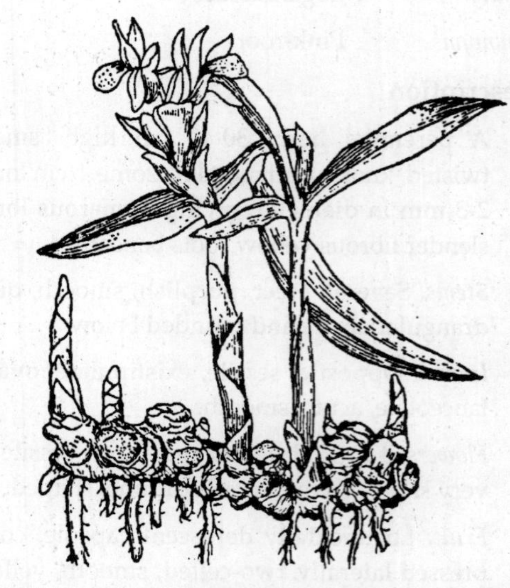

Zingiber officinalis

3. The stem is 2–4 feet (0.6–1.2 m) high and is erect, oblique invested by the smooth sheaths of the leaves. The leaves are alternate.
4. The flowers are greenish with a small dark purple, or purplish black lip.

Habitat: Throughout India and many other parts of Asia.

Part used: The fresh roots.

Syzygium jambolanum

Botanical name : Syzygium cumini (Linn).

Family : Myrtaceae.

Synonyms : Eugenia jambolana; Jam; Jambool seeds.

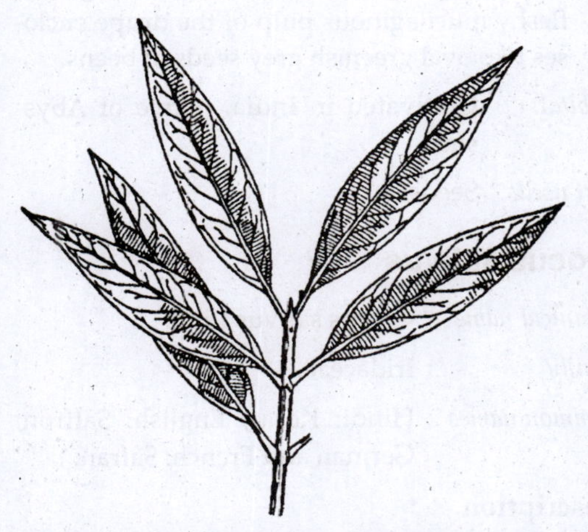

Syzygium jambolanum

Description

1. A large tree, bark light-coloured, thick, rough, exfoliating.
2. *Leaves:* Coriaceous, Lanceolate, elliptic oblong or broadly, ovate-elliptic, acute, sub-obtuse or shortly acuminate.
3. *Fruits:* The shape of an olive, subglobose, varying in size from a pea to a pigeon egg, dark purple, smooth, juicy, one-seeded.
4. *Seeds:* Are stony. Seeds exalbuminous with straight, curved or twisted embryo.

Habitat: Throughout India.

Part used: Seeds (H.P.I.).

Cephalandra indica

Botanical name : Cephalandra indica Naud.

Family : Cucurbitaceae.

Synonyms : Coccinia cordifolia; Telakucha; Kanduri.

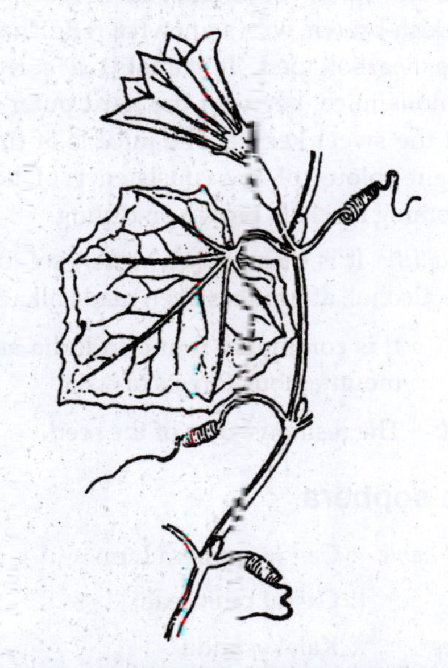

Cephalandra indica

Description

1. It is a perennial creeping herb.
2. *Leaves:* Deep green leaves, alternate, palmately lobed, palmi-veined, exstipulate.
3. *Flowers:* White, appear in July.
4. *Fruit:* A smooth cylindric berry.
5. *Root:* Long, tapering, tuberous.

Habitat: Throughout India.

Part used: The fresh green leaves.

Anacardium orientale

Botanical name : Semecarpus anacardium Linn. f.

Family : Anacardiaceae

Synonyms : Marking nut.

Description

1. It is an evergreen tree up to 7 metre in height with rough and ash-coloured bark and numerous spreading branches.

2. *Leaves:* The leaves are petiolate, alterate, about 45 cm long and 10 or 13 cm broad.
3. *Flower:* The flowers are small and of a green-yellow colour.
4. *Fruit:* The fruit is borne on a pear shaped receptacle and ripens in January or February. It is blackish-brown, with somewhat reddish tinge. It is heart-shaped. It contains a corrosive resinous juice, between the hard outer shell and the sweet kernel. The juice is at first of a light colour, of the consistency of honey, becoming blackish brown on drying.
5. *Solubility:* It is insoluble in water; soluble in 90% alcohol, after it has been made alkaline.

Habitat: It is commonly found in India and in mountainous forests of Asia.

Part used: The resinous juice of the seed.

Cassia sophera

Botanical name : Cassia sophera Linn

Family : Cassal piniaceae

Synonyms : Kalakasunda.

Description

1. A diffuse shrub with yellow flowers, 1.3 to 3.4 metre high.
2. *Leaves:* 18–23 cm long, rachis grooved, glabrous or nearly so, with a solitary conical gland near the base. Leaflets 6–12 pairs acute or acuminate mostly 2.5–7.5 cm long, cuneate at the base.
3. *Flowers:* The flowers are in short axillary and terminal panicles. Pods 7.5 to 10 cm long, slightly falcate somewhat turgid, transversely septate between the seeds.
4. *Seed:* The seeds are 30 to 40 in number, broadly ovoid, compressed dark brown.

Habitat: The plant is found throughout India and in most tropical countries. It is common in wastelands, on roadsides and in the forests.

Part used: Root bark.

Coffea cruda

Botanical name : Coffea arabica Linn.

Family : Rubiaceae.

Synonyms : Coffee; French: Cafe; German: Kaffee.

Description

1. An evergreen shrub or small tree attaining a height of 5–10 metres.
2. *Stem:* It has main stem with lateral branches which grow in pairs opposite each other, or in whorls around the stem.
3. *Leaves:* Opposite, thin coraceous or bright green in colour.
4. *Flowers:* White fragrant, borne, in clusteres in the axils of leaves.
5. *Fruits:* The fruits are small, fleshy drupes, bright green when young, changing to yellow and later to scarlet red with ripening. The fleshy mucilaginous pulp of the drupe encloses two oval greenish grey seeds of beens.

Habitat: Cultivated in India, native of Abyssinia.

Part used: Seeds.

Crocus sativus

Botanical name : Crocus sativus Linn.

Family : Iridaceae.

Common names : Hindi: Kesar; English: Saffron; German and French: Safran.

Description

1. A perennial, low growing, bulbous plant.
2. *Corm:* Globular producing 6 to 9 sessile leaves surrounded in lower part by 4 or 5 broad membranous scales.
3. *Flowers:* Flowers terminal on scape. Perianth pale reddish-purple forming cylindrical tube about 10 cm long terminating in 6 oblong oval segments; stemens 3, and carpels 3. Oyary interior, 3-celled. Style slender, elongated, pale-yellow in perianth tube and divided in upper region into 3 drooping, deep red stigmas. Stigmas 3, united or separate, attached to styles; usually about 25 mm in length, cornucopia-shaped, of dark-red colour, margin fimbriate or dentale; styles about 10 mm in length, more or less cylindrical solid, moderate yelowish-brown to yellowish-orange.

Odour strong, characteristically aromatic; taste bitter, aromatic. Upon chewing the saliva is coloured bright orange-yellow.

Habitat: India (Kashmir), Southern Europe and Asia.

Part used: Dried stigma.

Croton tiglium

Botanical name : Croton tiglium Linn.

Family : Euphorbiaceae

Synonyms : Jamal ghota; English: Croton oil plant, purging nut; French: Huite de croton; Germann: Crotonol.

Description

1. A small evergreen tree 5–7 metres high.
2. *Leaves:* The leaves are 5–10 cm long, thinly membranous, glabrous ovate, acuminate.
3. *Capsule:* The capsule 18 mm long, white, turbinately ovoid, obtusely trigamous, 3 seeds, the seeds resemble castor beans in general structure.
4. *Seeds:* The seeds are albuminous, ovate-oblong, slightly quadrangular, convex on the dorsal and somewhat flattened on the ventral surface; 10–15 mm in length, externally dull greyish brown, often mottled with black, due to abrasion in the testa. The oil is viscid with nauseous odour, when extracted from the seeds is a transparent, cherry coloured, viscid liquid, has a faint rancid smell.

Habitat: Bengal, Asom, South India.

Part used: Oil from seeds.

Cynodon dactylon

Botanical name : Cynodon dactylon Pers.

Family : Graminae

Synonyms : Durba; Bernuda grass.

Description

1. *Leaves:* The leaves are 2 to 10 cm by 1.25 to 3 mm, narrowly linear or lanciolate, finely acute to macronate more or less glancons, smooth, soft, usually conspicuously distichous in the barren shoots and at the base of stems sheath tight, glabrous or hairy.
2. *Stem:* The stem is about 7.5 to 30 cm high, slender, widely creeping forming matted tufts with slender, erect or ascending flowering branches.

Habitat: Throughout India.

Part used: Whole plant.

Lobelia inflata

Botanical name : Lobelia inflata Linn.

Family : Lobeliaceae

Common name : Red Indian tobacco.

Description

1. An annual or biennual herb up to 60 cm in height.
2. *Stem:* The stem is yellowish-green, pubescent, branched.
3. *Leaves:* The leaves are alternate, ovate or oblong with serrate denticulate margin.
4. *Fruit:* The fruit is bladdery, ovoid or ellipsoical.

Habitat: U.S.A. and Canada.

Part used: Whole plant excluding roots.

Rauwolfia serpentina

Botanical name : Rauwolfia serpentina Benth ex kurze.

Family : Apocynaceae

Synonyms : Sarpagandha, Chotachand.

Description

1. A small erect shrub up to 1 metre high with pale coloured bark.
2. *Leaves:* The leaves are whorled, 7–18 cm long by 1.25–5 cm wide, lanceolate, acute or acuminate, tapering gradually into the petiole, thin, pale, beneath.
3. *Flowers:* The flowers are white or pinkish, arranged in terminal or lateral corymbose cymes.
4. *Root:* The roots are stout, thick, about 10 cm long and 2 to 22 mm in diameter, tortuous,

slightly wrinkled surface, rough with course longitudinal markings, rarely branched, fracture, short irregular, root bark greyish yellow to brownish; wood pale yellow.

Habitat: Sub-Himalayan ranges and Western Ghats of India.

Part used: Root.

Rheum

Botanical name : Rheum officinalis Boillon

Family : Polygonaceae

Common name : Revandchini.

Description

1. A herbaceous perennial plant, which is about 2 metre high.
2. *Rhizome:* It has a bulky rhizome with a great many fibrous roots.
3. *Leaves:* The leaves are numerous, long petioled, arising from upper part of the vertical rhizome.
4. *Flowers:* The flowers are arranged in penicles, each flower having 6 pale yellow petals and 9 stamens.
5. *Fruits:* The fruits are pendulous achenes enclosed in a thin membrane.

Habitat: India, China and Tibet.

Part used: Rhizome.

Saraca indica

Botanical name : Saraca asoka

Family : Caesalpiniaceae

Synonyms : Hemapushpa, Gandhapushpa, Anganapriya, Asok, Asoka.

Description

1. It is a small evergreen tree, 6–8 metre high.
2. *Leaves:* They are paripinnate; leaflets 4–6 pairs, oblong or oblong-lanceolate.
3. *Flowers:* They are orange or orange-yelow, eventually turning vermillion, fragrant, in dense auxillary corymbs.
4. *Pods:* They are flat, linear-oblong, leathery, 10 to 25 cm long.
5. *Seeds:* Are 4 to 8, ellipsoid-oblong, compressed.

Habitat: The plant is found throughout India up to an altitude of 750 metre in the central and in the Eastern Himalayas and Khasi, Garo and Lushai hills, Wild in Chittagong, Bihar, Orissa, Konkan, Deccan, Mysore.

Part used: Bark of trees.

Senna

Botanical name : Cassia acutifolia Delile.

Family : Fabaceae

Common name : Alexandrian senna.

Description

1. It is a low branching shurb, growing to about 3 feet in height.
2. *Leaves:* The leaves are paripinnately compound, the leaflets opposite. The inflorescence is a raceme, or some arrangement or racemes.
3. *Flowers:* The flowers produce no nectar. The petals are 5 in numbers, similar to each other, yellow, or rarely white.
4. *Fruits:* The fruit is a legume, indehiscent or tardily dehiscent.

Habitat: This plant is native throughout the tropics, with a small number of species reaching into temperate regions.

Part used: Leaves (or pods).

Stramonium

Botanical name : Datura stramonium Linn.

Family : Solanaceae

Common name : Sada dhutura; Thorn apple.

Description

1. A coarse bushy annual, 0.6 to 1.2 metre high.
2. *Leaves:* The leaves are dark, greyish-green. The petiole is short and twisted. Young leaves bear numerous trichomes but older ones are almost glabrous.
3. *Stem:* The stems dichotomously branched.

Habitat: Occurs abundantly in the Temperate Himalayas from Kashmir to Sikkim up to 3,000 metres, hilly tracts of Madhya Pradesh and South India.

Part used: Whole plant.

Vinca minor

Botanical name : Vinca minor, Linn.

Family : Apocynaceae – Dogbane family.

Synonyms : *Pervinca heterophyla, Vinca acutiflora, Vinca ellipticifolia, Vinca humilis.*

Common name : Common periwinkle, Myrtle, Ground myrtle, Running myrtle, Lesser myrtle.

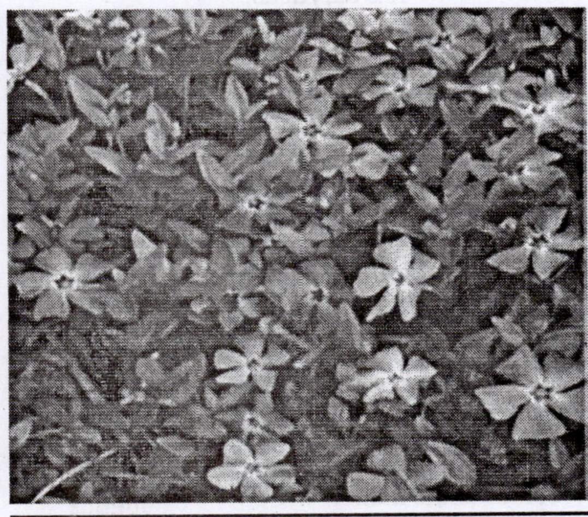

Vinca minor

Description

1. A low, trailing groundcover, evergreen, only 3 inch to 6 inch tall, spreads many feet.
2. *Stem*: The stems are smooth, green, round, sometimes pubescent, and often hollow, although it does produce woody rhizomes. The plant forms thick sprawling mats with the flowering stems more or less erect.
3. *Leaves*: Its leaves are simple and arranged oppositely on the stem, though sometimes the nodes are so close together that two pairs of leaves seem to form a whorl. The leaves are oblong-ovate to elliptical, approximately 2-5 cm long and 1-2.5 cm wide, with petioles 1-3 mm long.
4. *Flowers*: It is showy, purple to blue and occasionally white, borne singly in an axillary position on a 1-1.5 cm pedicel.

Habitat: Native to southern and central Europe. Also widely naturalised overseas in the British Isles, northern Europe, southern Africa, New Zealand, North America and southern South America (e.g. Chile). Commonly grown in gardens in cooler places in India.

Part used: Whole plant with roots and fruits.

E. MINERAL KINGDOM

Antimonium tartaricum

Chemical symbol : $K(SbO)C_4H_4O_6 \cdot \frac{1}{2} H_2O$

Mol. Wt. : 333.932

Synonyms : Tartarate of Antimony and Potassium; Tartar emetic.

Description

1. A colourless, transparent crystals or a white, granular, odourless powder, having a sweet metallic taste. The crystals effloresce upon exposure to air.
2. It is soluble in 12 parts of water and in 3 parts of boiling water; insoluble in alcohol.
3. It may be prepared by boiling a mixture of Antimony trioxide (Sb_2O_3) and cream of tartar (Potassium bitartarate):

$$KHC_4H_4O_6 + \frac{1}{2}Sb_2O_3 = K(SbO)C_4H_4O_6 \cdot \frac{1}{2}H_2O$$

Argentum nitricum

Chemical symbol : $AgNO_3$

Mol. Wt. : 169.875

Synonyms : Silver nitrate; Argenti nitras; Lunar caustic.

Description

1. A colourless white crystal; odourless, having a bitter caustic, metallic taste.
2. Soluble in 0.4 part of water, in slightly more than 0.1 part of boiling water.
3. Its specific gravity is 4.3 and melting point 212°C.
4. It is prepared in transparent rhombic plates by dissolving silver in hot dilute HNO_3 and concentrating the solution to crystalisation:

$$Ag + 2HNO_3 = AgNO_3 + NO_2 + H_2O.$$

Arsenicum album

Chemical symbol: AS_2O_3

Mol. Wt. : 197.841

Synonyms : Acidum arsenicum; White arsenic; Arsenious acid; Arsenious trioxide; Arsenious anhydride.

Description

1. A white or transparent amorphous lump or crystalline powder; odourless; stable in air.
2. It is slowly soluble in water. The amorphous variety is more soluble than the crystalline variety. It is sparingly soluble in alcohol. It is completely soluble in glycerine.
3. It is made by roasting arsenical ores, such as pyrites and condensing the volatile arsenious oxide in flues as a white matter.
4. A small quantity warmed with about 5 ml of HCl gives a brown coloured, or white precipitate on the addition of few drops of solution of Stannous chloride.
5. An acidified solution gives a yellow precipitate with H_2S.

Aurum metallicum

Chemical symbol: Au

Mol. Wt. : 196.967

Synonyms : Aurum precipitatum; Aurum foliatum; precipitated gold; Gold leaf; Metallic gold.

Description

1. A bright yellow metal; most malleable and ductile; in powdered form it is brown. It is not attacked by air or by hydrogen sulphide, ordinary acids do not attack.
2. Soluble in *aqua regia*. (1 part conc. nitric acid + 3 parts conc. hydrochloric acid). Its specific gravity is 19.3. It melts at 1,063°C and boils at about 2,600°C. Gold generally occurs in the free state and its commercial purification is commonly effected electrolytically.
3. With NaOH, solutions of gold salts give a brown precipitate which is soluble in excess of the reagent.
4. When treated with stannous chloride, solution of salt in aqua regia slowly forms a purple precipitate.

Baryta carbonica

Chemical symbol: $BaCO_3$

Mol. Wt. : 197.349

Synonyms : Barium carbonicum; Carbonate of barium; Barii carbonas; Carbonas baryticus.

Description

1. A white, heavy powder with no taste and odour; it is almost insoluble in water; readily decomposed by acids with the evolution of CO_2.
2. Soluble in dilute HCl, HNO_3 and CH_3COOH. Its specific gravity is 4.43. It occurs in nature as mineral witherite and is purified by precipitation. Contains not less than 98 per cent of $BaCO_3$.
3. Moistened with HCl and heated on a platinum wire in a Bunsen flame; it imparts a green colour to the flame.
4. Heat 1 gm with 5 ml of HNO_3, cool, dilute with three times its volume of H_2O and filter; the filtrate gives a precipitate with H_2SO_4.

Calcarea carbonica

Described in Chapter 15, 'Hahnemannian Method of Preparation of Drugs."

Calcarea phosphorica

Chemical symbol: $Ca_3(PO_4)_2$

Mol. Wt. : 310.183

Synonyms : Calcii phosphas precipitatus; Calcium phosphoricum; Precipitated phosphate of calcium; Tribasic calcium phosphate; Calcarea phosphate

Description

1. A white, amorphous or micro-crystalline powder; odourless and tasteless.
2. It is almost insoluble in water and is decomposed slightly by boiling water; insoluble in

alcohol. It is readily soluble in dilute HNO_3 or HCl. Its specific gravity is 3.14.

3. It is formed as a white precipitate on adding ammonium phosphate and excess of ammonia to calcium chloride solution:

$$3Ca^{++} + 2HPO_4^- + 2OH = Ca_3(PO_4)_2 + 2H_2O$$

Camphora

Chemical symbol : $C_{10}H_{16}O$

Mol. Wt. : 152.238

Synonyms : Camphor officinarum; Camphor; Karpur; Kapur.

Description

1. A colourles or white crystalline powder, granules or crystalline masses; or pressed blocks of crystalline structure, easily cut with a knife. It has a strong characteristic odour and pungent, bitter taste followed by a cooling sensation.
2. Tough but readily pulverisable in presence of little alcohol (90%), solvent ether and chloroform.
3. It is soluble in 840 parts of water, 1 part of alcohol and 1 part of ether. Its specific gravity is about 0.99. It melts between 174°C and 179°C and slowly volatilises at ordinary temperature.

Carbo vegetabilis

Synonyms : Wood charcoal; Vegetable charcoal; *Angara*.

Description

1. A bluish-black porous substance, having a peculiar glistening aspect and retaining minutely both the form and texture of the wood from which it was made.
2. It is odourless and tasteless; insoluble and infusible. Its specific gravity is 1.7.
3. When heated in air, it is converted into CO_2.
4. When burnt, it should give no smoke, or unpleasant odour.
5. Absence of flame shows freedom from organic compounds.

Causticum

Described in Chapter 15.

Cuprum metallicum

Chemical symbol : Cu.

At. Wt. : 63.54

Synonyms : Copper; Cuprum; Metallic copper; Cupreum filum; Copper wire.

Indian name: Beng. Tama; Hindi and Oriya: Tamba; Telegu: Ragi.

Description

1. A rose-red, lustrous, malleable and ductile metal. It may be in the form of a very fine powder. Becomes gradually coated with a green basic carbonate when gradually exposed to air.
2. Next to silver, it is the best conductor of electricity. Its specific gravity is 8.9. It melts at 1,083°C.
3. It is very slowly attacked by HCl or dilute H_2SO_4 but is readily dissolved by dilute HNO_3:

$$2Cu + 4HCl + O_2 = 2CuCl_2 + 2H_2O$$

$$2Cu + 2H_2SO_4 + O_2 = 2CuSO_4 + 2H_2O$$

4. It slowly dissolves in ammonia water.
5. An addition of excess of ammonia to a solution in HCl produces ultimately a deep-blue coloured solution.
6. When a solution in HCl is treated with a solution of Potassium ferrocyanide, a reddish-brown precipitate is formed.

Glonoinum

Chemical formula : $C_3H_5N_3O_9$

Mol. Wt. : 227.09

Synonyms : Glonoine; Nitroglycerine, Glyceryl trinitrate.

Description

1. A colourless, odourless liquid, with a sweet burning taste. Almost insoluble in water, readily soluble in alcohol, explodes on concession or rapid heating.
2. Begins to decompose at 50°C to 60°C, appreciably volatile at 100°C, evolves nitrous yellow vapours at 135°C and explodes at 218°C.
3. It is prepared by nitrating glycerine with a mixture of HNO_3 and H_2SO_4, called nitration acid.

Graphites

Synonyms : Plumbago; Black lead; Carbo minerals.

Indian name: Beng: Kalo-sisa; Hindi: Kala-sisa.

Description

1. Blackish-grey, soft, unctuous, lustrous solid, composed of hexagonal crystalline scales; odourless.
2. Its specific gravity is 2.0 to 2.5 and is a good conductor of electricity.

Hepar sulphur

Described in Chapter 15.

Kali carbonica

Described in Chapter 15.

Mercurius corrosivus

Chemical symbol: $HgCl_2$

Mol. Wt. : 271.496

Synonyms : Mercuric chloride; Corrosive sublimate; perchloride of mercury; Corrosive mercuric chloride; Hydrargyri chloridum corrosivum.

Description

1. A heavy, white, crystalline mass, or rhombic prisms; odourless and of a strong metallic taste. It is soluble in 13.5 parts of water, in 2.1 parts of boiling water; soluble in 3.8 parts of alcohol. When heated to 277°C, it changes to a colourless liquid.
2. Its boiling point : 32°C, its specific gravity is about 5.4.
3. It is commonly prepared by the direct combination of mercury and chlorine. Contains not less than 99.5 per cent of $HgCl_2$.

Mercurius solubilis

Described in Chapter 15.

Natrum muriaticum

Chemical symbol: NaCl

Mol. Wt. : 58.443

Synonyms : Common salt; Sodium chloride; Table salt; Sodii chloridum; Natrum chloratum; Chloride of sodium.

Description

1. Colourless, odourless, transparent cubical crystals, or a white crystalline powder with a saline taste. It is stable in air.
2. It is soluble in 2.8 parts of water; slightly soluble in alcohol and insoluble in HCl. Its aqueous solution is practically neutral.
3. Its specific gravity is 2.163. It fuses at about 804°C. It is obtained by passing HCl gas into a saturated solution of the salt, thus separating the crystals.

Nitric acid

Chemical symbol: HNO_3

Mol. Wt. : 63.013

Synonyms : Aqua fortis; Hydrogen nitrate; Acidum nitri.

Description

1. A fuming liquid, very caustic, and has a characteristic irritating odour. It is miscible with water and dilute alcohol in all proportions.
2. Its specific gravity is 1.41; it boils at 120°C.
3. It is prepared by oxidation of ammonia, with air in the presence of platinum as catalyst. It attacks most metals evolving brown fumes. It contains not less than 69% and not more than 71% w/w of HNO_3.

Phosphorus

Chemical symbol: P

At. Wt. : 30.974

Synonyms : Phosphore.

Description

1. White or pale yellow, semi-translucent, or transparent waxy solid with garlic-like smell and tasteless.
2. It is brittle and crystalline at low temperatures but soft and pliable at ordinary temperature. When exposed to air, it emits white fumes

which are luminous in the dark and have garlicky odour.

3. It is almost insoluble in water; soluble in 400 parts of absolute alcohol. Its specific gravity is 1.82. Melts at about 44°C.

4. When heated at about 50°C, it ignites spontaneously with brilliant white flame.

Phosphoric acid

Chemical symbol : H_3PO_4

Mol. Wt. : 97.995

Synonyms : Orthophosphoric acid; Acidum ossium; Acidum phosphoricum.

Description

1. A colourless, odourless liquid with a syrupy consistency.
2. Soluble in water and alcohol in all proportions. It contains not less than 89.0% w/w of the absolute acid.
3. Its specific gravity is 1.71.
4. It may be obtained by the oxidation of phosphorus in contact with water. It contains not less than 88% and not more than 90% w/w of H_3PO_4.
5. It is strongly acidic even when freely diluted with water.
6. When carefully neutralised with Potassium hydroxide test solution and a solution of $AgNO_3$ added, a characteristic yellow precipitate, soluble in NH_4OH, is formed.

Platinum metallicum

Chemical symbol : Pt

Synonyms : Platina, Metallic platinum; Platine.

Description

1. A lustrous, greyish-white, malleable and ductile metal; good conductor of heat and electricity.
2. It is stable in air and does not tarnish on exposure to air. It is insoluble in single acid but is soluble in hot aqua regia with the formation of Chloroplatinic acid.
3. Its specific gravity is 21.45. It melts at 1,773°C.

Plumbum metallicum

Chemical symbol : Pb

At. Wt. : 207.19

Synonyms : Plumbum; Lead; Metallic lead.

Description

1. A heavy, bluish-grey, soft, feebly lustrous metal; tarnishes on exposure to air. Pure water does not attack it in the absence of air. It is attacked by all acids when heated.
2. Insoluble in dilute HCl; slowly soluble in hot conc. HCl but readily in dil. HNO_3; scarcely attacked by conc. HNO_3.

Silicea

Chemical symbol : SiO_2

Mol Wt. : 60.06

Synonyms : Silica; Silicon dioxide; Quartz; Pure Flint.

Description

1. It is a white, odourless, tasteless, amorphous powder.
2. It is insoluble in water and in dilute acids, excepting only hydrofluoric acid:

$$SiO_2 + 4HF = SiF_4 + 2H_2O$$

3. It is made from sand or silicate mineral by fusing with excess sodium carbonate, in a platinum crucible when sodium silicate is formed—the fused mass is extracted with boiling water; the aqueous extract of sodium silicate on acidification with HCl yields a gelatinous precipitate of silicic acid, which is washed with water, dried and ignited:

$$MgSiO_3 + Na_2CO_3 = MgCO_3 + Na_2SiO_3$$
$$Na_2SiO_3 + 2HCl = 2NaCl + H_2SiO_3$$
$$H_2SiO_3 + H_2O = SiO_2$$

Stannum metallicum

Chemical symbol : Sn

At. Wt. : 1[illegible]9.09

Synonyms : Tin, Metallic tin.

Description

1. A silver white, lustrous, soft, easily fusible (m.p. 232°C), very malleable and ductile metal.

Only slightly tenacious, easily powdered, conductor of electricity.

2. At. Wt. : 118.7; B.P. : 2,260°C; M.P. : 232°C; Sp. Gr : 7.5.
3. Insoluble in water and alcohol but soluble slowly in cold dilute HCl, dilute HNO_3 and in hot H_2SO4; readily dissolved by conc. HCl.

Sulphur

Chemical symbol : S

At. Wt. : 32.07

Synonyms : Brimstone; Flowers of sulphur; Sublimed sulphur.

Description

1. A fine yellow, slightly gritty powder; odour faint and not unpleasant, tasteless. Burns with a blue flame with the production of SO_2.
2. It is almost insoluble in water, and in alcohol; incompletely soluble in carbon disulphide.
3. M.P. : 113°C; B.P. : 444.6°C; it has very poor conductivity of heat and electricity.

Zincum metallicum

Chemical symbol : Zn

Synonyms : Zinc; Metallic zinc.

Description

1. A bluish white metal having a crystalline structure, or a fine grey powder, free from all but small aggregates.
2. Soluble in dil. HCl or dil. H_2SO_4.
3. It burns in air with a green flame; if strongly heated, forming white clouds of zinc oxide, which settles in woolly flocks (Philosopher's wool).

$$2Zn + O_2 = 2ZnO$$

Alumina

Chemical symbol : $Al(HO)_3$

Mol. Wt. : 78.120

Synonyms : Aluminium trihydrate, Aluminium hydroxide.

Description

1. The gel is a white, viscous suspension, translucent in thin layers, from which small amounts of water may separate on standing.
2. The dried gel is a white, odourless, tasteless, amorphous powder. It is insoluble in water and in alcohol but soluble in dilute mineral acids and fixed alkali.
3. It is prepared by treating a hot solution of potassium alum with a hot solution of sodium carbonate. The precipitated aluminium hydroxide is then washed thoroughly to make it free of sulphates.

Borax

Chemical symbol : $Na_2B_4O_7{\cdot}10H_2O$

Mol. Wt. : 381.373

Synonyms : Sodii boras, Natrum boracicum, Borate of sodium, Sodic pyroborate.

Description

1. A colourless, odourless, transparent crystal, or a white crystalline powder; taste sweetish, an alkaline.
2. It is soluble in 16 parts of water and in 1 part of boiling water; insoluble in alcohol; Sp. gr is 1.694.
3. It is mainly prepared from borax minerals and is also found native.

Carbo animalis

Synonyms : Leather charcoal.

Description

1. It occurs as an odourless, tasteless powder.
2. Crude animal charcoal is the material, prepared by heating bones with a limited access of air and consists chiefly of calcium phosphate and other inorganic constituents of bone, with about one-tenth of its weight of carbon; it occurs in dull black, granular fragments, or as a dull black, odourless powder.
3. It may be prepared by the following process: Place a thick piece of Oxhide on red hot coal, and leave it there so long as it burns with a flame. As soon as the flame ceases, lift off the

red-hot mass and press it between two flat stones. Boil it with HCl, washing thoroughly, drying and reheating. It may yield as much as 10 percent of ash.

Iodium

Chemical symbol : I

At. Wt. : 126.904

Synonyms : Iodum, Iodinum.

Description

1. Heavy, greyish-black, brittle, rhombic prisms, or granules with a metallic lustre; odour characteristic.
2. Volatile at ordinary temperatures. It is slightly soluble in water and in 12.5 parts of alcohol. Its Sp. gr. is 4.93.
3. It is chiefly obtained from the ashes of the sea-weeds. Contains not less than 99.5% of I.

Aceticum acidum

Chemical symbol : CH_3COOH

Mol. Wt. : 60.053

Synonyms : Acidum aceticum glacial, Aceti acidum, Glacial acetic acid.

Description

1. A clear, colourless liquid having a very strong odour of vinegar and a sharp acid reaction.
2. It is miscible with water and alcohol in all proportions.
3. Its specific gravity is 1.0471. It boils at about 118° and congeals at a temperature not lower than 15.6°. Contains not less than 99.4 percent of $C_2H_4O_2$.
4. It is prepared from alcohol or by synthesis.

Argentum metallicum

Chemical symbol : Ag

At. Wt. : 107.87

Synonyms : Silver; French: Argent; German: Silber.

Description

1. A white, brilliant, tenacious, ductile metal; tasteless and odourless. Next to gold, it is the most malleable and ductile of all metals.
2. It is insoluble in water, alcohol and in most acids; readily soluble in dilute nitric acid and in hot sulphuric acid.
3. Its specific gravity is 10.49. It melts at 960.5° and boils at 1950°. It does not oxidise in air, but is tarnished quickly by hydrogen sulphide.
4. It is prepared from native silver ores.

Magnesium phosphoricum

Chemical symbol : $MgHPO_4.7H_2O$

Mol. Wt. : 174.34

Synonyms : Magnesii phosphas, Magnesia phosphorica, Magnesium phosphate (Diabasic), Magnesium hydrogen phosphate.

Description

1. A white crystalline powder, slightly soluble in water, insoluble in alcohol; readily soluble in dilute acids.
2. Prepared by dissolving two parts of sulphate of magnesia in thirty-two parts of distilled water and mixing with a solution of three parts of phosphate of soda in thirty-two parts of distilled water and setting aside to crystallise. The salt separates in the course of twenty-four hours in tufts of prisms or needles.

C. ANIMAL KINGDOM

Apis mellifica

Zoological name : Apis mellifica

Phylum : Arthropoda

Class : Insecta

Synonyms : Hindi: Madhu-makkhee; English: Honey bee; common live bee.

Description

1. A swarm of bees consist of—Queen bee, several hundred drones (males) and ten thousand or more workers (female). The queen bees are the only perfectly developed females.
2. The bees have three parts of body, separated by constrictions. The head carries the eyes, antennae and mouth parts; the thorax, the wings and legs; the abdomen, the wax glands and sting.

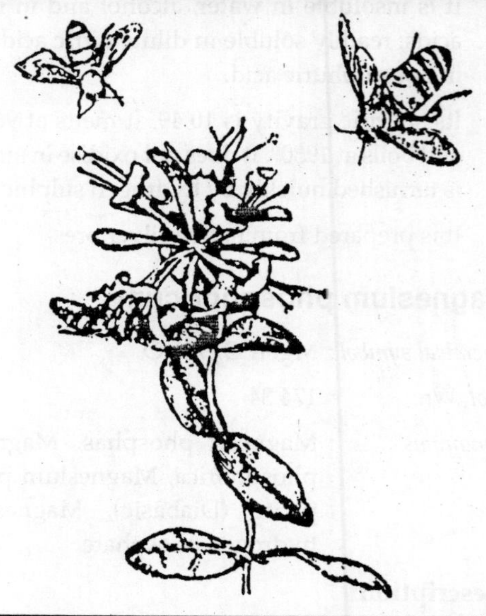

Apis mellifica

3. The shorter abdomen of the female marks the external difference from the male.
4. Only queens and workers have poisonous apparatus, commonly called the sting.

Parts used: The live bees.

Habitat: India and also other parts of the world.

Cantharis

Zoological name : Lytta vesicatoria febricus

Phyllum : Arthropoda

Class : Insecta

Synonyms : Cantharis vesicatoria; Spanish fly; Cantharides; Blister beetle; Fabricus.

Description

1. The insect is about half an inch (1.25 cm) long; of a golden-yellow green colour.
2. Head inclined, almost cordiform; antennae filiform, of twelve joints, black; anternulae equally filiform, the posterior swollen at the extremity; eyes large, of a deep brown colour; mouth with an upper lip and two bifid jaws; body marked with longitudinal streaks; head and foot full of whitish hair; the odour is sweetish, nauseous; taste very acrid, almost caustic.

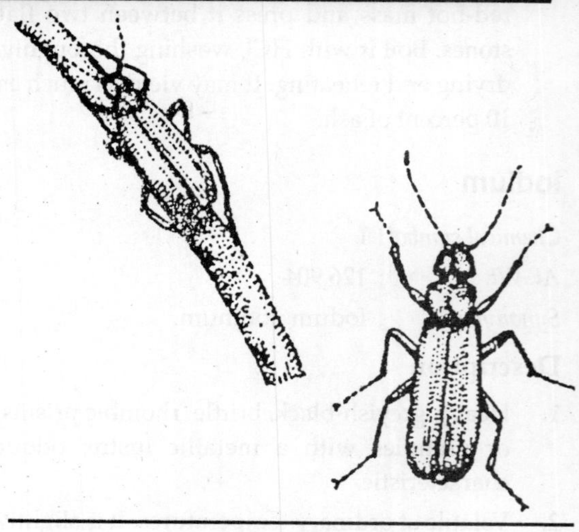

Cantharis

3. It has a strong disagreeable odour. Its blistering property is due to the substance called cantharidin ($C_{10}H_{12}O_4$) which may be extracted from the beetles with ether or chloroform. It is separated and purified by crystallisation.

Parts used: The whole dried fly.

Habitat: Southern France and Spain.

Lachesis

Zoological name : Crotalus mutus

Phyllum : Chordata

Class : Reptillia

Synonyms : Lachesis mutus; Surukuku-snake-poison; Deadly bush-master.

Description

1. It is about seven feet (2.1 m) in length and its poison fangs are nearly one inch (2.5 cm) long. The skin is reddish-brown, marked along the back with large rhomboidal spots of blackish brown colour.
2. The poison resembles saliva, is less viscous, limpid, inodorous, without any marked taste.
3. The venom is obtained by stunning it with a blow and then collecting the poison on sugar of milk by pressing the fangs upwards against the poison sac.

Part used: Venom.

Habitat: Hot countries of South America.

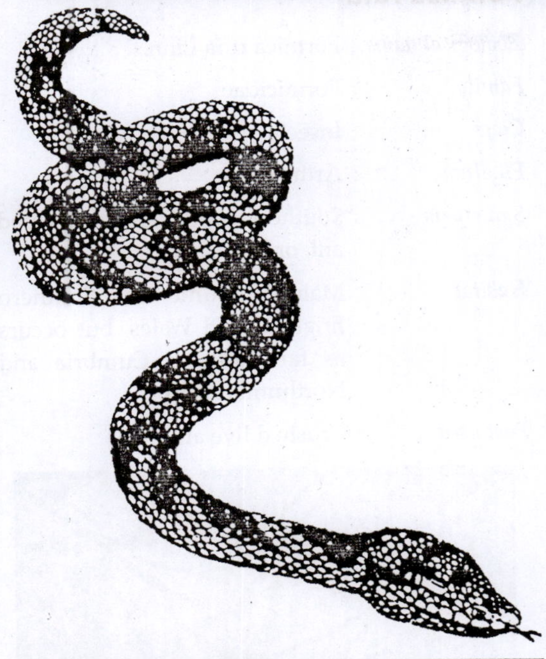

Lachesis

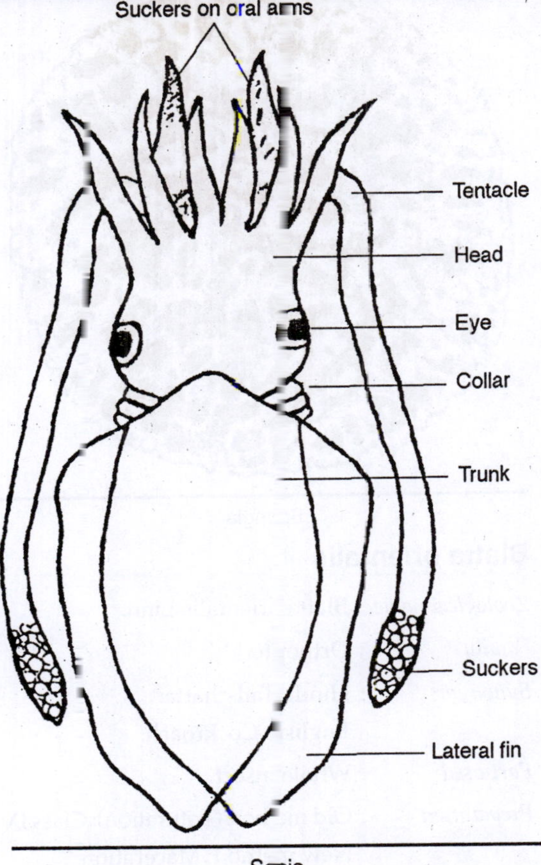

Sepia

Sepia

Zoological name : Sepia officinalis Linn.

Phyllum : Mollusca

Class : Cephalopoda

Synonyms : Inky juice of cuttle fish.

Description

1. The cuttle-fish ink is an excretory liquid contained in a bag about the size and shape of a grape within the abdomen of a sepia; it is blackish-brown, and issued by these animals to darken the water when they wish to catch their prey or escape from their pursuers.
2. Sepia in a dry state, as it occurs in trade, appears to be a dark blackish-brown solid mass of shining, conchoidal, very brittle structure, having a faint smell of sea fish, nearly without taste and scarcely dyeing the saliva.

Parts used: Inky juice found in bag-like structure in the abdomen of the cuttle-fish.

Habitat: Indian Ocean and other seas of Europe and the Mediterranean.

Spongia

Zoological name : Sycon gelatinosum.

Phyllum : Porifera

Class : Calcarea or calcispongiae.

Synonyms : Sponge; Spongia tosta; S. officinalis.

Description

1. The horny skeleton, from which the desired substance is prepared, consists mostly of siliceous or calcareous matter, while the spongy portion is soft, elastic and compressible and traversed by many lacunae, with circular openings on the surface.
2. The selected sponge must be free from foreign substances and then cut into small pieces and roasted until brown and friable.

Parts used: Whole body including skeleton.

Habitat: The Mediterranean, near Syria and Greece.

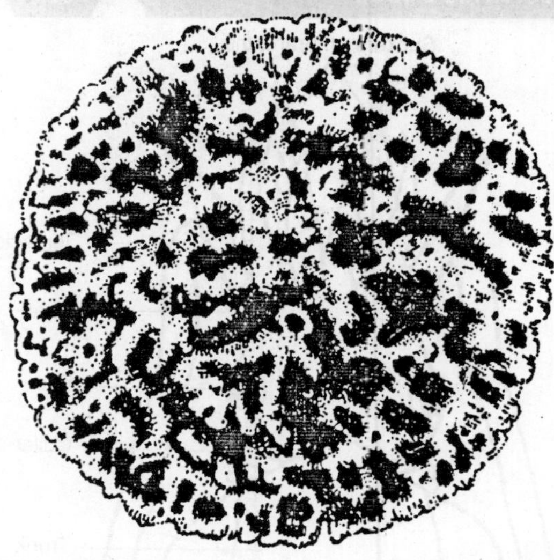

Spongia

Blatta orientalis

Zoological name : Blatta orientalis Linn.

Family : Orthoptera.

Synonyms : Hindi: Tail-chatta; English: Cockroach.

Part used : Whole insect.

Preparation : Old method (Trituration): Class IX New method: Maceration.

Description

1. It is an orthopterous insect, with an elongated oval, rather flat body, from 12 to 16 lines in length, of a red or brown-red colour, which becomes paler under belly.
2. The wings are striate and reticular, of the length of elytra.
3. The antennae, which are longer than the body, exhibit at their base a small yellowish point.
4. The feet are provided with black prickles and terminate in the tarsus, with 5 articulations.

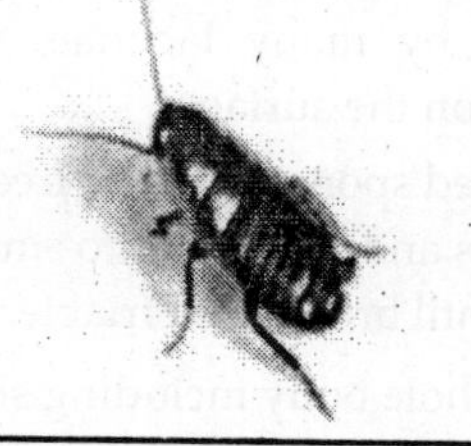

Blatta orientalis

Formica rufa

Zoological name : Formica rufa Linn.

Family : Formicidae

Class : Insecta

Phyllum : Arthropoda

Synonyms : Southern wood ant, red wood ant, or horse ant.

Habitat : Mainly found in Southern England and Wales, but occurs as far north as Cumbria and Northumberland.

Part used : Crushed live ants.

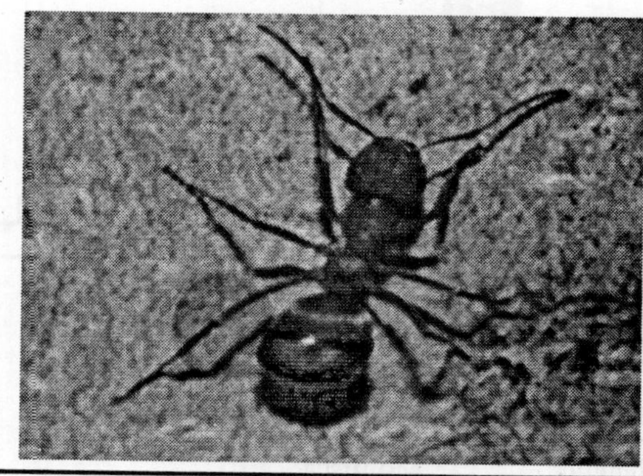

Formica rufa

Description

1. It is a large ant with workers reaching 10 mm in length and queens 12mm in length.
2. This ant has an orange-and-black body, dark head and large mandibles.
3. The lack of a fringe of hairs on the eyes and around the margin of the head (when viewed head on) distinguishes the southern wood from similar wood ants.

Tarentula cubensis

Zoological name : Tarentula cubensis

Family : Lycosidae

Class : Arachnida

Phyllum : Arthropoda

Synonyms : Mygale cubensis, Cuban spider, Lycosa cubensis. English: Cuban spider. German: Tarentel.

Habitat : Mexico and Cuba

Part used : The entire living spider.

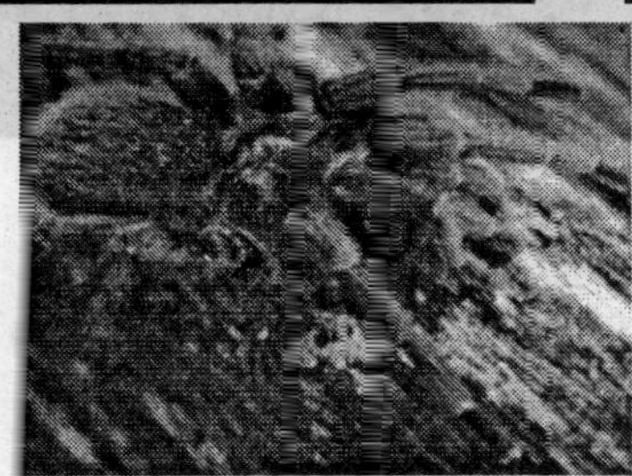

Tarentula

Description

It is a larger spider, of a dark brown colour, less poisonous, and covered with more hairs than the *Tarentula hispanica*. They have short glands and ducts and their fangs move vertically. They have two pairs of lungs.

Chapter 24

Various Constituents in Plant Substances (Phyto-constituents)

Plants form the major source for many of the drugs. The chemical substances obtained from plants are called *'phyto-constituents'*. Phytochemistry is the chemistry of plants, plant products and natural substances. The medicinal value of a plant depends upon the nature of the chemical constituents present. The chemical constitutent which is responsible for the therapeutic effect is called the *active principle.*

A plant or vegetable substance consists of cellulose and lignin which form the basic frame material of the roots, stem, leaves and other parts of the plant, apart from water which forms the major constituent. The constituents in plant depend upon the species of the plant, its habitat, the height at which these grow, the soil on which these thrive and the various seasons of the year. Often there is variation in composition of these constituents in the different parts of the plant. These constituents reach a peak level at a certain time in certain parts. Therefore, the pharmacopoeias recommend the use of different parts of the different plants accordingly.

The quality of drug means the amount of medicinal principles contained in the drug. These principles or constituents of drugs are classified into groups, e.g. 1. Carbohydrates, 2. Lipids, 3. Alkaloids. 4. Glycosides, 5. Tannins and Tannic acid, 6. Oils, 7. Resins, 8. Gums, 9. Vitamins.

A short summary of the various constituents normally found in plant substances are given next.

CARBOHYDRATES

Characteristics

1. Carbohydrates are polyhydroxyaldehydes and polyhydroxyketones and their condensation products.
2. These contain carbon, hydrogen and oxygen, the ratio of hydrogen and oxygen being generally 2: 1.
3. The general chemical formula is $C_n(H_2O)_n$, but there are many exceptions.
4. On heating they lose water and a black mass is left behind, which is nothing but Carbon.
5. Present more abundantly in the storage regions of plants.

Classifications

These are classified into:

(a) Sugars, (b) Non-sugars.

A. *Sugars*

These are soluble carbohydrate food matters, usually sweet to taste. These occur as reserve materials in many monocotyledons and also in some dicotyledons like Beet and Carrot.

(a) **Monosaccharides:** These are the simplest carbohydrates, i.e., these cannot be hydrolysed further into simpler ones.

These may be:

1. *Pentoses:* Sugars with 5 carbon atoms are not common in plants.
   Examples: (i) Arabinose, (ii) Ribose.
2. *Hexoses:* Sugars with 6 carbon atoms.
   Examples:
   (i) *Glucose:* Present in all green plants.
   (ii) *Fructose:* Occurs in the fruits.
   (iii) *Others:* Mannose and Galactose.

(b) **Oligosccharides:**

1. ***Disaccharides:***
   (i) *Sucrose:* It is widely distributed in some plant tissues, often reaching very high concentration in storage organs. It is extracted mainly from Sugarcane stems and Beet roots.
   (ii) *Maltose:* Commonly found in germinating seeds during digestion of starch.
2. ***Trisaccharides:***
   Raffinose: It occurs in very small quantities.

B. ***Non-Sugars***

(a) **Polysaccharides:**

1. ***Inulin:*** Occurs in colloidal condition in the cell sap of the vacuoles of plants like Dahlia.
2. ***Starch grains:*** These are universal occurrence in the green plants with the exception of some algae.
   Starch grains may occur in all parts of the plants, but these are more abundant in the storage organs, cereals, fruits and seeds.
3. ***Glycogen:*** It occurs in blue green algae, some moulds, fungi and bacteria and serves as reserve food.

(b) **Compound Carbohydrates:** These are complex carbohydrate molecules, e.g., Gums and mucilages; Tannins; Glycosides.

ORGANIC ACIDS, FATTY ACIDS AND LIPIDS

Organic acids metabolised in plants are mainly the tricarboxylic acids of the Krebs cycle and other less common ones such as formic, tartaric and oxalic acids; these are classified according to the carboxylic or other functional groups these possess. The **Fatty acids** in plants are usually bound as esters of glycerol thus fats or lipids. There are three major classes of lipids: the triglycerides, phospholipids and glycolipids. The Fatty acids are normally long chains of carbon and can be saturated such as myristic and stearic, and unsaturated such as the oleic acid group. The organic acids are soluble in water and are colourless while the lipids can be taken in isopropanol followed by chloroform and methanol (2 : 1).

ALKALOIDS

Alkaloids means "alkali-like". The alkaloids are classified according to its therapeutic property and chemical structure.

Characteristics

1. It is a secondary metabolite of a plant, basic in nature and a nitrogen-containing heterocycle in structure.
2. The alkaloids are mostly active in its pharmacological behaviour and most of those have an amino acid as its biosynthetic precursor.
3. Some alkaloids occur in plants as free bases, but a great majority of them are present in the form of soluble salts.
4. Some alkaloids may be present as insoluble tannates in which case they have, first of all, to be brought into free form before commencing the extraction procedure.
5. Alkaloids bases are generally soluble in organic solvents and are insoluble in water but its salts are soluble in aqueous solvents while insoluble in organic liquids.
6. These are extremely bitter, but some, like 'Piperine', are tasteless.
7. Most are odourless but Nicotine etc. have strong odour.

8. Many are deadly poisons, but in minute doses, act as valuable therapeutic agents.
9. These are generally colourless, but a few are yellow, e.g., Berberine.
10. Names of the alkaloids terminate in English-in-ine (Quinine), in Latin, *in-ina* (Quinina).

Identification of alkaloids

The identification is based on melting point, specific rotation, crystalline form, and solubility.

Infra-red spectrography is used in the present-day laboratory technology.

The alkaloids are precipitated by one or more of the given reagents. The process also helps in identifying some of them:

(i) Mayer's reagent (Mercuric potassium iodide): Alkaloids give white to buff ppt.

(ii) Wagner's reagent (Iodine in potassium iodide): Alkaloids give brown ppt.

(iii) Dragendorff's reagent (Potassium bismuth iodide): Alkaloids give orange ppt.

Examples:

Name of the Drug	Alkaloids
Aconitum napellus	Aconitine ($C_{34}H_{45}NO_{11}$)
Belladonna	Atropine ($C_{17}H_{23}NO_3$)
China	1. Quinine ($C_{20}H_{24}O_2N_2$) and its salts 2. Cinchonine ($C_{19}H_{22}N_2O$) 3. Quinidine ($C_{20}H_{24}N_2O_2$)
Coca	Cocaine ($C_{17}H_{21}NO_4$)
Coffea cruda	Caffeine ($C_8H_{10}N_4O_2$, H_2O)
Colchicum autumnale	Colchicine ($C_{22}H_{25}O_6N$)
Conium maculatum	Conine ($C_8H_{17}N$)
Hydrastis canadensis	Hydrastine ($C_{21}H_{21}NO_6$)
Hyoscyamus niger	Hyoscyamine ($C_{17}H_{23}NO_3$)
Ipecacuanha	Emitine ($C_{20}H_{40}N_2O_4$)
Nux vomica	Strychnine ($C_{21}H_{22}N_2O_2$)
Physostigma	Physostigmine ($C_{15}H_{21}O_2N_3$, $C_7H_6O_3$)
Piper nigrum	Piperine ($C_{17}H_{19}O_3N$)
Secale cornutum	Ergotine ($C_{35}H_{41}O_6N_5$)
Tabacum	Nicotine ($C_{10}H_{14}N_2$)

GLYCOSIDES

It is a non-reducing compound which on hydrolysis yields two components:

(i) An aglycone, sometimes called a genin, and (ii) One or more reducing sugars. The physical or chemical nature of a glycoside depends on:

1. The chemical structure of the aglycone which may be derivative of some known systems such as steroids, anthracenes etc.
2. The kind of linkage existing between the aglycone and the glycone, for example C—O—C, C—N—C, C—S—C and C—C—C etc.
3. The number and kind of sugar residues (usually the number of sugar residues is directly proportional to the solubility of the glycoside in water).

The glycosides are soluble in water and alcohol, but are insoluble in organic solvents. But once these are hydrolysed into the fundamental components, it has been found that the aglycone is soluble in organic solvents while the sugar part is not.

The term 'Glucoside' is applied only to those glycosides in which the sugar component is glucose.

The names of all glycosides end in "in".

Examples:

Name of Glycosides	Source
Adonidin	Adonis vernalis
Agaricin	Agaricus muscarius
Aloin	Aloe socotrina
Arbutin	Uva ursi
Colocynthin	Colocynthis
Digitalin	Digitalis
Phloridzin	Pyrus malus
Saponinum	Quillaia saponaria

TANNINS

These are heterogeneous group of complex compounds found in many plants especially in the leaves and bark. These are non-nitrogenous. Tannins are phenolic matter soluble in water and alcohol and have an astringent or bitter taste.

These are precipitated by heavy metals, albumin and alkaloids. All vegetable astringents contain tannin.

Examples:

Rhus toxicodendron;

Hamamelis virginica;

Millefolium;

Acacia germanica.

OILS

Oils are chemical compounds of C, H and O (but the ratio of Hydrogen to Oxygen is not 2 : 1) which remain liquid at ordinary temperature (10°C-20°C). The solid state of oils is termed as fats. Oils obtained from various parts of plants fall under two main categories, viz.

A. Volatile or essential oils and

B. Fixed or fatty oils.

A. Volatile oils

As plants often owe its characteristic odour to these oils, they are often spoken to as essential oils.

These are obtained from the plants, from either of the following methods:

(i) Distillation with steam (most of the oils are obtained by this process).

(ii) Expression (e.g., lemon oil).

(iii) Extraction.

Characteristics

(i) These are volatile (i.e., readily evaporating substances) can be distilled and do not leave a permanent grease spot on paper.

(ii) These do not form soaps with alkalis as these do not contain any fatty acid.

(iii) These do not become rancid, but tend to resinify on exposure to light and air.

(iv) Mostly inflammable.

(v) Cannot be saponified and emulsified with difficulty.

Examples:

Common name	Botanical name	Parts
Anise oil	Pimpinella anisum	Dried ripe fruit
Caraway oil	Carum carvi	Dried ripe fruit
Cajuput oil	Melaleuca leuca-dendron	Leaves
Cinnamon oil	Cinnamomum cassia	Leaves and twigs
Clove oil	Eugenia caryo-phyllus	Dried flower buds
Coriander oil	Coriandrum sativum	Dried ripe fruit
Eucalyptus oil	Eucalyptus spp	Fresh leaves
Fennel oil	Foeniculum vulgare	Dried ripe fruit
Lavender oil	Lavendula officinalis	Fresh flowering top
Lemon oil	Citrus limon	Fresh peel of fruit
Myristica oil (Nutmeg oil)	Myristica fragrans	Dried kernels of ripe seeds
Orange oil	Citrus sinensis	Fresh peel of ripe fruit
Peppermint oil	Mentha piperita	Fresh over-ground parts of flowering plant
Rosemary oil	Rosemarinus officinalis	Flowering Tops
Rose oil	Rosa gallica	Fresh flowers
Sandalwood oil	Santalam album	Wood
Spearmint oil	Mentha spicata	Fresh parts of flowering plant
Turpentine oil	Pinus spp	Oleo-resin

Many other drugs contain volatile oils, such as:

Arnica montana (flowers 0.1%; roots 0.5% to 1.5%); Asafoetida (6.17%); Azadirachta indica (blossoms 0.5%); Cheiranthus (flowers 0.06%); Zingiber officinale (rhizome 1% to 3%).

B. Fixed oils

These are mixtures of olein (liquid), palmitin (semi-solid), and stearin (solid), with a small amount of other bodies in addition. These are mostly found in seeds, occurring within the cytoplasm as drops or crystals. These are insoluble in water, sparingly soluble in alcohol, freely in ether, chloroform, carbon di-sulphide and turpentine. With alkalis these form soap and glycerine.

Characters of fixed oils

1. These are non-volatile so leave a permanent grease spot on paper.
2. These cannot be extracted by simple distillation but may be obtained by mere pressure.
3. These decompose under the influence of heat and become rancid.
4. These are almost bland non-irritating substances (except croton oil) with nutrient and emollient properties.
5. They form soap with alkalis.

Examples:

Common name	Botanical name	Parts
Almond oil	Prunus amygdalus	Seeds
Arachis oil	Arachis hypogaea	Seeds
Castor oil	Ricinus communis	Seeds
Chaulmoogra oil	Hydnocarpus kurzii	Seeds
Cottonseed oil	Gossypium arboreum	Seeds
Croton oil	Croton tiglium	Dried ripe seeds
Linseed oil	Linum usitatissimum	Seeds
Olive oil	Olea europaea	Fruits
Sesame oil	Sesamum indicum	Seeds
Hydnocarpus oil	Hydnocarpus wightianus	Seeds

PLANT EXUDATES

1. Resin

These are natural or induced exudates from plants, solids and semi-solids in nature. These are insoluble in water but are readily dissolved in alcohol, ether and volatile oil. These are usually oxidised turpins or volatile states of plants. When pure these are transparent, when these contain water these are opaque.

Examples:

Asafoetida (40%-64%); Croton tig; Dioscorea; Gelsemium; Hypericum; Podophyllum; Zingiber officinale.

2. Oleo-resin

When resins are found dissolved in volatile oils, these are known as Oleo-resins. These are obtained by incising the trunk of a tree.

Examples:

Copaiva officinalis; Terebinthina; Rhus tox.

3. Gums

These are colloidal carbohydrates which—on swelling or dissolving in water—form viscid adhesive fluid known as mucilage. These are exudations from the stems or branches, or both, of plants.

Examples:

Ammoniacum gummi; Asafoetida (25%).

4. Gum-resins

These are natural mixtures of gums and resins obtained as an exudate from the plants.

Examples:

Asafoetida; Gambogia; Podophyllum.

5. Balsams

A semi-fluid fragrant, resinous vegetable juice. Balsams are resins with a high proportion of aromatic acids.

Examples:

Tolu balsam; Peru balsam; Gurjun balsam.

VITAMINS

These are not generally synthesised by plants. But few of it which do—viz. (i) Alfalfa and Spinach contains Vitamin K; (ii) Oranges contain Vitamin C; (iii) Wheat germ oil—contains Vitamin E. But many do not synthesise vitamins but these have their precursors as: (i) Carotene in carrots is a precursor of Vitamin A; (ii) Plant sterol, ergosterol in yeast, moulds and fungi is the precursor of Vitamin D.

Chapter 25

Eclectic Preparations of Medicinal Plants

Resinoids or Active Principles

Resinoids are the precipitates in powder form obtained by mixing a strong alcoholic tincture of any given plant or part thereof, with 3 to 4 times its bulk of purified water. In these processes, all alcohol-soluble substances are precipitated. The precipitates are then collected, dried and pulverised and are known as 'resinoids'. It is said that these precipitates (i.e., resinoids) represent the 'active-principles' of the respective plants.

No definite directions or rules for the preparation of these products are published. So, the manufacturers seem to be guided by their individual experiences. These resinoids were used at a time by the eclectic physicians.

Nowadays, mother-tinctures are extensively used for their better result than these resinoids. So, the application of these resinoids in the field of Homoeopathy are greatly diminished.

Examples of some resinoids are:

Active Principles	From which they are derived
Aconitin	Aconitum napellus
Aletrin	Aletris farinosa
Alnuin	Alnus rubra
Aloin	Aloe socotrina
Ampelopsin	Ampelopsis quinquefolia
Apocynin	Apocynum cannabinum
Asclepin	Asclepias tuberosa
Atropin	Belladonna
Baptisin	Baptisia tinctoria
Barosmin	Barosma crenata
Bryonin	Bryonia alba
Caulophyllin	Caulophyllum thalictroides
Cerasin	Cerasus virginiana
Chelonin	Chelone glabra
Chimaphillin	Chimaphila umbellata
Chionanthin	Chionanthus virginica
Collinsonin	Collinsonia canadensis
Colocynthin	Colocynthis
Cornin	Cornus florida
Corydalin	Corydalis formosa
Cypripedin	Cypripedium pubescens
Digitalin	Digitalis purpurea
Dioscorin	Dioscorea villosa
Emetin	Ipecacuanha
Ergotin	Secale cornutum

Contd.

Contd.

Active Principles	From which they are derived
Euonymin	Euonymus atropurpureus
Eupatorin	Eupatorium perfoliatum
Euphorbin	Euphorbium officinarum
Fraserin	Frasera caroliniensis
Gelsemin	Gelsemium sempervirens
Geranin	Geranium maculatum
Gossypin	Gossypium herbaceum
Hamamelin	Hamamelis virginica
Helonin	Helonias dioica
Hydrastin	Hydrastis canadensis
Hyocyamin	Hyocyamus niger
Irisin	Iris versicolor
Juglandin	Juglans cinerea
Leptandrin	Leptandra virginica
Lobelin	Lobelia inflata
Lycopin	Lycopus virginicus
Macrotin	Actaea racemosa
Menispermin	Menispermum canadense
Morphin	Opium
Myricin	Myrica cerifera
Phytolaccin	Phytolacca decandra
Populin	Populus tremuloides
Podophyllin	Podophyllum peltatum
Ptelein	Ptelea trifoliata
Rumin	Rumex crispus
Sanguinarin	Sanguinaria canadensis
Scutellarin	Scutellaria laterifolia
Senecin	Senecio aureus
Stillingin	Stillingia sylvatica
Trillin	Trillium pendulum
Veratrin	Veratrum album
Viburnin	Viburnum opulus
Xanthoxylin	Xanthoxylum fraxineum

Chapter 26

Drug Action: Characteristics of Some Important Drug Substances

Definition of Drug Action

Drug action is the sum-total of the action imparted on an individual living human being and the sum-total of the reaction that it can induce in the vital force of the same.

Drug action depends upon the dose and the general receptive capacity of the body mechanism.

Principle of Drug Action

1. Drug may stimulate or depress the function.
2. Pharmacological agents may replace the secretion absent or present in insufficient quantity in man.
3. Drugs may alternate or kill the invading organism (e.g., bacteria, virus or fungus), thus affecting the process of cure.

Physiological Action

Physiological action is the action of a drug in physiological dose. **Stuart Close**, defines physiological dose as "A dose of a drug, empirically selected, of sufficient quantity and strength to produce a definite predetermined effect or group of symptoms. Practically it amounts to the *maximum dose* consistent with safety."

The physiological doses stimulate the normal physiology or functions of different organs or systems of our body and, hence, the symptoms thus appearing are known as *physiological symptoms.* A medicine thus acts on different systems, may act on different nerves, may produce alteration in the functions of circulation, digestion, respiration etc.

The "Physiological action" of a drug is not its therapeutic or curative action. It is exactly the opposite of a curative action, and is never employed in homoeopathic practice for therapeutic purposes. The use of the word "Physiological" in connection with 'Durg action' and drug dosage tends to mislead the unwary and justify the use of measures, which would otherwise be regarded as illegitimate. So, in Homoeopathy, for healing purposes, no medicine or remedy is administered in physiological or massive doses. The 'modus operandi' of a dose of homoeopathic medicine takes place only in dynamic plane.

The homoeopathic medicines should not be used in physiological doses, as these are toxic in nature and injurious to the health of the patient. The symptoms produced by large doses or by crude drugs are pathogenetic, not curative.

Various thoughts are present regarding the action of drugs. Those who believe in the physiological actions and depend upon them have ideas different from the homoeopaths.

Classification according to Drug Action

A. According to Centre of Action

Burt. classified drugs into two groups:

(a) Those which have their centre of action in the animal (cerebro-spinal) nervous system, are the true remedies for acute and sub-acute diseases; and (b) Those which have their centre of action in the organic (ganglionic) nervous system, are the true remedies for sub-acute and chronic disseases.

Animal group (Cerebro-spinants)

Aconite	Digitalis pur
Ammonium carb	Dulcamara
Antimonium crud	Gelsemium sem
Antimonium tart	Helleborus niger
Arnica montana	Hyoscyamus niger
Baptisia	Ignatia amara
Belladonna	Ipecacuanha
Bryonia alba	Lachesis
Cactus grand	Nux. vomica
Cannabis sativa	Opium
Cantharides	Pulsatilla nigricans
Capsicum	Rhus tox
Causticum	Spigelia
Chamomilla	Stramonium
Cinchona	Tabacum
Coffea cruda	Tarentula cuben
Colocynthis	Tarentula hispa
Conium mac	Veratrum album
Crotalus hor.	

Organic group (Ganglionics)

Aloe soc	Natrum mur
Apis mellifica	Nitric acid
Argentum nit	Petroleum
Arsenicum alb	Phosphorus
Aurum met	Podophyllum pelt
Calcarea carb	Secale cor
Carbo vegetabilis	Sepia
Croton tiglium	Silicea
Graphites	Sulphur
Hepar sulphur	Sulphuric acid
Kali carbonicum	Thuja
Lycopodium	
Mercurius	

B. According to the Nature of Drug

(a) *Corrosives*

1.	Strong acids	(i)	Inorganic acid: Acid sulph; Acid nitric.
		(ii)	Organic acid: Acid acetic; Acid carbolic; Acid oxalic.
2.	Strong alkalies		Potash group

(b) *Irritants*

1.	Inorganic	(i)	Non-metallic: Bromium; Iodium; Phosphorus.
		(ii)	Metallic: Ars. alb; Mercurius, Antimony; Copper; Lead; Silver etc.
2.	Organic	(i)	Vegetable: Aloe soc; Capsicum; Coloc; Crot. tig.
		(ii)	Animal: Apis mel; Cantharides; Lachesis; Naja; Crotalus; Sepia.

(c) *Neurotics*

1.	Cerebral	(i)	Somniferus: Opium
		(ii)	Deliriant: Can. ind; Bell; Hyos.
2.	Spinal		Nux vom; Gelsemium
3.	Cardiac		Aconite nap.

Definition of some terms:

Anesthetics: Drugs which diminish sensibility by depressing the terminations of sensory nerves (local) or lead to a total loss of consciousness (general) e.g., Acidum carbolicum; Belladonna; Bromium; Chloral; Chloroformum; Cocaine; Ether; Iodoform; Kali brom; Opium; Platina; Valeriana; Veratrum viridi.

Anhydrotic, Antihydrotic, Antisudorific:

Drugs which prevent, reduce perspiration that is opposite to diaphoretic, e.g., Agaricin; Atropinum; Hyoscyamus niger; Stramonium; Belladonna; Opium.

Anthelmintics: Drugs which are used to kill or expel the worms. It may be vermicide (which kill the worms) or vermifuge (which expels the worms without killing), e.g., Carbon tetrachloride; Chelone; Oil of chenopodium; Cina; Spigelia; Stannum; Teucrium marum varum; Thymol; Kausso brayera.

Antipyretics: Drugs which lower the temperature of the body in pyrexia, e.g., Acetanilidum (antifebrin); Aconitum napellus; Arnica montana; Belladonna; Bryonia alba; Micromeria.

Antiseptics: Drugs which prevent or retard the growth of micro-organisms as long as those remain in contact with those but do not destroy those, e.g., Acidum carbolicum; Acidum boracic; Arbutin; Canchalagua; Chloral; Borax; Kreosotum; Myristica sebifera; Myrtus communis; Pyrogen; Cinchona; Sulphur.

Antispasmodics: Drugs which relax the spasm of the muscular coat of the bronchial tubes, e.g., Belladonna; Chloroformum; Mag. phos; Passiflora.

Aphrodisiacs: Drugs which increase sexual desire, e.g., Cantharides; Camphora; China; Coffea; Ether; Moschus; Nux vomica; Phosphorus; Stramonium; Nasturtium aquaticum; Valeriana; Vanilla; Yohimbinum.

Astringents: Drugs which cause contraction or shrinkage of the tissues or diminished exudations or secretions, e.g., Adrenaline; Hamamelis; Hypericum; Sanicula; Zinc oxidatum; Tannic acid.

Carminatives: Drugs which help in expulsion of gases, e.g., Chamomilla.

Caustics or Escharotics: Drugs which destroy the vitality of the part on which they are applied, e.g., Ars. alb; Mercurius; Sulph ac.

Cholagogues or Hepatic stimulants: Drugs which increase the amount of bile actually secreted, e.g., Aloe. soc; Colchicum; Croton tig; Euonymus; Eupetorium per; Iris versicolor; Leptandra; Manganum; Merc; Podo; Rheum; Sanguinaria; Verat. alb.

Deodorants: Drugs which destroy offensive or disagreeable odours, e.g., Formalin.

Diaphoretics or Sudorifics: Drugs which increase the secretion of sweat. When a diaphoretic acts very powerfully, it is called sudorific, e.g., Aconite nap; Achyranthes aspera; Apocyanum; Aurum met; Belladonna; Chamomilla; Colchicum; Ether; Eucalyptus glob; Eup. per; Gelsemium; Ipecac; Jaborandi; Opium; Pulsatilla; Muscarine; Samb. nigra; Sec. cor; Sulphur; Verat. alb; Antipyrine.

Disinfectants: Drugs which destroy the pathogenic microbes, e.g.,

(a) *Oxidising disinfectants:* Chlorine and its preparations; Bromine and its preparations; Iodine and its preparations; Permanganate of Potassium; Ozone.

(b) *Antizymotic disinfectants:* Benz ac; Borax; Carbo ac; Caustic lime; Chloride of zinc; Cinchona; Eucalyptus; Kreosote; Salicylic ac; Sulphate of Iron; Sulphur. Sulphurus ac; Thymol.

(c) *Desulphurating disinfectants:* Metallic salts; Lime; Zinc salts.

(d) *Absorbing disinfectants:* Charcoal; Coffea; Chloride of lime; Aluminium.

Diuretics: Drugs which increase the flow of urine, e.g., Acon. ferox; Acidum salicylic; Adonidine; Amyl. nitrosum; Apocynum; Aralia hisp; Arg. phos; Arbutin; Arnica montana; Asparagus; Caffeine; Coffea; Collinsonia; Chelidonium majus; Cicera arist; Digitalis; Eucalyptus; Eup. per; Fabiana imbricata; Gelsemium; Gummi guttae; Hyoscyamus niger; Hypericum; Juncus effusus; Juniperus communis; Kreosotum; Liatris spic; Millepedes; Nat. sulph; Ononis spinosa; Pulsatilla; Senega, Strophanthus; Thuja; Urotropin; Valeriana; Verbena; Verat. viride.

Ecbolics: Drugs which cause expulsion of the contents of the uterus by contracting the uterine muscle, e.g., Borax; Secale. cor; Ustilago; Jonosia asoka.

Emetics: Drugs which produce vomiting, e.g., Acon. nap; Alumen; Ant. tart; Cheld; Cocculus; Colch; Crot. hor; Cup. sulph; Digit; Eup. per; Helonias; Ipecac; Iris versicolor; Kreos; Lach; Nat. mur; Opium; Phyto; Robinia; Sec. cor; Sanguinaria; Tabacum; Verat viride; Zinc. sulph.

Emmenagogues: Drugs which increase or restore menstrual flow when deficient or absent, e.g., Aloe; Borax; Gossypium; Hell; Ign; Kreos; Opium; Sec. cor; Ustilago.

Expectorants: Drugs which increase bronchial secretion and help its expulsion, e.g., Adrenaline; Ammon mur; Antim. tart; Apomorphinum; Balsum peru; Belladonna; Camphora; Guaiacol; Grindelia; Ipecac; Kali iod; Kreos; Lobelia; Oleoresin; Senega; Squilla; Volatile oils.

Galactogogues: Drugs which increase the secretion of milk, e.g., Jaborandi; Lactuca virosa; Spiranthes; Urtica urens.

Hemostatic: Drugs which constrict the blood vessels, e.g., Adrenaline; Calendula; Calcar-sulph-stibiata; Ceanothus; Hydr. mur; Hypericum; Ipecac; Matico, Millefolium; Tannic acid.

Hypnotics: Drugs which are employed to induce or maintain sleep, e.g., Aspirin; Acetanilidum; Bromide of Lithium; Bromide of Sodium; Bromide of Potassium; Chloral hydrate; Codeine; Morphinum; Opium; Passiflora; Sulphonal; Rauwalfia serpentina.

Mydriatics: Drugs which dilate the pupils, e.g., Acidum salicylic; Belladonna; Chloroformum; Cina; Cinchona; Conium mac; Digit; Hyos; Sec. cor; Spig; Stramo; Valeriana; Verat viride.

Myotics: Drugs which contract the pupils, e.g., Gels; Jaborandi; Nux vom; Opium; Tabacum.

Parasiticides: Drugs which kill the parasite, e.g., Cina; Filix mas; Plantago major.

Purgatives: Drugs which cause evacuation of the bowels.

(a) **Cathartic (drastic):** Drugs which excite greatly increased secretion and peristaltic movements.

(i) *Hydragogue (because of the large amount of secretion they excite):* Aloe soc; Coloc; crot. tig; Euonymus; Gummi guttae; Hell; Podo; Jalapa.

(ii) *Others:* Colch; Elaterium; Helonias; Iris ver; Kreos; Leptandra; Momordica charant; Merc. dulc; Pinus lamb; Rheum; Tabacum.

(b) **Laxatives:** Drugs which slightly increase the action of bowels by stimulating their muscular coat, e.g., Mag carb; Nat. sulph; Sulph.

(c) **Saline purgatives:** Mag. sulph.

Rubefacients: Drugs which produce congestion and redness of the skin, e.g., *Chaulmoogra oil*; Crot. tig.

Sialogogues: Drugs which increase the amount of saliva, e.g., Arum triph; Calcarea carb; Digit; Hell; Iodine; Iris ver; Jaborandi; Ipecac; Kali chlor; Kreos; Mercurius; Muscarine; Nat. mur; Mur. ac; Podo; Sanguinaria; Sulph ac.

Stomachics: Drugs which increase the activity of gastric juice secreted, e.g., Cham; Aloe; Jaborandi; Tabacum.

Vesicants: Drugs which produce vesicles over the skin, e.g., Crot. tig; Mez; Rhus tox.

Physiological Action of some important Drugs

Aconitum napellus (Acon. nap.)

Centre of action: Cerebro-spinal nervous system.

Analgesic; Sedative; Anti-neuralgic; Antipyretic; Antiphlogistic; Irritant; Emetics; Paralysant; Diaphoretic; Diuretic; Vasodilator.

1. **Heart:** Inhibitory paralysis; Blood pressure lessened.
2. **Circulation:** Vaso-motor paralysis.
3. **Temperature:** Depressed with diaphoresis.
4. **Cerebro-spinal nervous system:** Paralysis, first paralyses the sensory and then the motor part of the cord.
5. **Mucous membranes:** Sthenic inflammation.
6. **Stomach:** Emesis; Congestion; Neuralgia.
7. **Lungs:** Centric vagi paralysis; Congestion; Inflammation.
8. **Tendons and Fibrous tissue:** Rheumatoid inflammation.
9. **Serous membranes (especially the capillaries of serous membranes):** Plastic inflammation.

Adonis vernalis (Adonis v.)

Centre of action: Cerebro-spinal nervous system.

1. **Heart**: It acts distinctively on the heart. It is a *heart tonic*. It regulates the pulse and increases the cardiac contractions. By its action on heart and circulation it slows down the pulse and acts calming on the fear and restlessness which accompany the heart disease.
2. **Kidney**: Diuresis is increased by its action on heart as well as kidneys.

Allium cepa (All. cepa)

Centre of action: Cerebro-spinal nervous system.

1. **Mucous membranes (nose):** It causes acute catarrhal inflammation of ***mucous membranes of nose*** producing acrid, profuse, watery discharge.
2. **Eyes:** It causes irritation of ***conjunctiva*** producing profuse, bland lachrymation.
3. **Venous system:** It causes inflammation of veins (phlebitis) especially in puerperal period.
4. **Nerves:** Due to its affection of nerves produces inflammation of nerves (neuritis).

Aloe socotrina (Alo. soc.)

Centre of action: Organic (ganglionic) nervous system.

Abortificient; Cholagogue and Hepatic stimulant; Emmenagogue; Hydragogue cathartic; Stomachic.

1. **Liver (Cholagogue and hepatic stimulant):** Causes portal congestion and increased biliary secretion.
2. **Stomach (Stomachic):** In small doses, causes increased secretion of gastric juice.
3. **Large intestine (Muscular coat):** Hydragogue cathartic. It not only excites the secretion but also increases the muscular contraction, i.e., increases peristalsis.
4. **Female sexual organs (Emmenagogue; Abortificient):** It causes uterine irritation, increases the menstrual flow. Abortion may be produced with large doses.
5. **Skin:** Producing eczema and, on the scalp, the hair turns gray and falls out in spots.
6. **Blood:** Corpuscles increased; Fibrin decreased.

Antimonium crudum (Ant. cr.)

Centre of action: Cerebro-spinal nervous system.

1. **Mucous membranes:** All mucous membranes of gastro-intestinal tract are affected but especially the stomach, producing slow digestion. Mucous membranes become loaded with mucus.
   In large doses, produces severe nausea and vomiting. Slow digestion produces fermentation; Flatulence.
2. **Skin:** Corns, Callosities, and pustules.
3. **Female sexual organs:** Prolapse of uterus.

Antimonium tartaricum (Ant. tart.)

Centre of action: Cerebro-spinal nervous system

Irritant; Depressant; Emetic.

1. **Mucous membranes:** Catarrh, and pustular inflammation.
2. **Stomach (emetic):** As an emetic, it produces depression, with a nausea in a much greater degree than most other emetics; and the repeated vomiting accompanied by great straining.
3. **Respiratory organs:** The drug directly depresses the medullary respiratory centers. Through the vagus nerves, it produces intense catarrhal inflammation of larynx, trachea and bronchi.
4. **Spinal cord:** Motor and sensory paralysis.
5. **Kidneys:** The urine is first increased, but, in severe poisoning, scanty and blood, even suppressed.
6. **Skin:** Pustular inflammation.
7. **Circulation and blood:** Heart depressant, Blood liquefied.
8. **Muscular system:** Paralysis; Loss of reflex action.

Apis mellifica (Apis mel.)

Centre of action: Organic (ganglionic) nervous system

1. **Cellular tissue:** Oedema and dropsy.
2. **Skin:** Urticaria; Exanthema; Erysipelas.
3. **Serous membranes (heart, brain, abdomen):** Hydropericardium; Hydrocephalus and ascites.
4. **Mucous membranes (eyes, mouth, fauces, throat, gastro-intestinal tract, kidney, bladder):** Oedematous inflammation.
5. **Glandular system (ovaries, testicles):** Congestion, mild inflammation and hypertrophy.

Argentum nitricum (Arg. nit.)

Centre of action: Organic (ganglionic) nervous system.

1. **Mucous membranes (stomach, intestine):** Atony with great flatulence. In large doses, nausea, vomiting and violent gastro-intestinal inflammation, especially destructive type.
2. **Cartilaginous system (ears, nose, false ribs, tendons, ligaments):** Destructive inflammation.
3. **Glandular system (salivary glands, testicles, liver, kidney):** Induration and fatty-degeneration.
4. **Blood:** Destruction of R.B.C.; anaemia; depressed temperature.
5. **Skin:** Nodular and vesicular inflammation.
6. **Cerebro-spinal system (Motor tract):** Convulsions.

Arnica montana (Arn. mont.)

Centre of action: Cerebro-spinal nervous system.

Irritant; Stimulant; Depressant; Antipyretic; Vulnerary; Diuretic.

1. **Skin:** Vesicular and erysipelatous inflammation.
2. **Venous system:** Stimulating absorption.
3. **Muscular system:** Paresis and myalgia.
4. **Digestive organs:** Produces heat in the fauces, increases the flow of saliva; irritates the stomach, causes nausea and vomiting.
5. **Serous membrances:** It acts upon the venous capillaries of secretions in the serous membranes, causing stagnation and inflammation, which soon passes on to effusion in the cavities.
6. **Circulation:** Accelerated, with high temperature.

Arsenicum album (Ars. alb.)

Centre of action: Ganglionic nervous system.

Caustic.

1. **Mucous membranes (G.I. tract):** Congestion, destructive inflammation, with a thin, ichorous discharge, tending to malignant ulceration, and accompanied with a low fever of a typhoid form.
2. **Serous membranes (pleura, pericardium, peritoneum):** Oedematous inflammation; Copious serous effusion.
3. **Kidneys:** Fatty degeneration; albuminuria.
4. **Skin:** Eczema; Gangrene; General anasarca.
5. **Blood:** Disintegration; Hemorrhages; Serous effusions.
6. **Heart:** Fatty degeneration; Motor paralysis.
7. **Circulation:** Vaso-motor paralysis; Asthenia.
8. **Liver:** Fatty degeneration; Disorganisation.
9. **Lungs:** Congestion; Asthma; Malignant catarrh.
10. **Cerebro-spinal nervous system:** Motor and sensory paralysis; Neuralgia.

Aurum metallicum (Aur. met.)

Centre of action: Autonomic nervous system.

1. **Lymphatic glandular system (particularly liver and testicles):** Congestion; induration.
2. **Bones (palatine bones):** Caries and exostosis.
3. **Digestive organs:** Gastro-intestinal inflammation.
4. **Vascular system:** Excited and raised temperature.
5. **Skin:** Copious diaphoresis.
6. **Sexual organs:** Greatly excited and increased sexual desire in both sexes.
7. **Mind:** It causes profound mental depression. It may even lead to suicide.

Baptisia (Bapt.)

Centre of action: Cerebro-spinal nervous system.

1. **Blood:** Disorganisation and decomposition; Typhoid condition.
2. **Mucous membranes (Mouth, Throat, Intestinals):** It produces fetid breath, catarrhal inflammation and ulceration, with watery, putrid, sanious discharges.
3. **Lymphatic system:** Putrid secretions.
4. **Cerebrospinal nervous system:** Motor and sensory paralysis.

Belladonna (Bell.)

Centre of action: Cerebro-spinal nervous system.

Mydriatic; Antispasmodic; Irritant; Narcotic; Anesthetic; Anodyne; Antipyretic; Diaphoretic; Vasodilator; Anti-asthmatic; Analgesic.

1. **Cerebrospinal system:** Motor and sensory paralysis.
2. **Circulation:** Cardiac inhibitory centers stimulated; Capillaries contracted.
3. **Temperature:** Rises from 1°F or 3°F.
4. **Vagus nerve:** Respiratory centre stimulated.
5. **Muscles of hollow viscera (Abdomen etc.):** Paralysis.
6. **Kidneys:** Congested; Bladder; Sphincter paralysed.
7. **Sexual organs:** Congestion; Arrested secretion.
8. **Glandular system (Mucous and salivary glands):** Inflammation; Arrested secretion leading to dryness of mouth and fauces.
9. **Skin:** Erysipelatous inflammation; Copious perspiration.
10. **Eye:** Mydriasis; Congestion, inflammation.
11. **Mucous membranes:** Secretions entirely arrested.

Bryonia alba (Bry. alb.)

Centre of action: Cerebro-spinal nervous system.

Antipyretic.

1. **Serous membranes (Pleura; arachnoid; synovial membranes; liver; peritoneum):** Rheumatoid inflammation; effusions.
2. **Mucous membranes (Large intestine; respiratory):**
   (i) It affects the large intestines, producing an atonic, dry mucous surface, with constipation.
   (ii) It affects the respiratory mucous membranes causing nasal catarrh which is dry, the cough has little expectoration, and is continuous, irritating, and violent, often causing retching, and pains in the walls of the chest.
3. **Muscular system:** Rheumatoid inflammation.
4. **Circulation:** Accelerated; Temperature raised.

Cactus grandiflorus (Cact. grn.):

Centre of action: Cerebro-spinal nervous system.

1. **Heart and Arteries:** Cactus is a special irritant of the heart, and controls its action through the ganglia of that organ It affects the circular fibers of the heart and arteries; causing irritability, hyperesthesia, neuralgia, spasm, and palpitation of the heart.
2. **Vagus nerve:** By its action upon the vagus nerve Cactus affects the heart, lungs, and stomach; producing, in the stomach, indigestion and excessive acidity; in the lungs constriction and asthma.
3. **Muscular System:** Rheumatoid Inflammation.
4. **Skin:** By its action on skin causes irritations with pruritus and pustules.

Calcarea carbonica (Cal. carb.)

Centre of action: Vegetative (ganglionic) nervous system.

1. **Osseous system including cartilages:** Non-ossification, rachitis and caries.
2. **Lymphatic glandular system:** Atony and hypertrophy.
3. **Skin:** Pale, atonic, flabby; copious perspiration.
4. **Mucous membranes:** Catarrhal mucorrhoea.
5. **Blood:** Hydraemia; anaemia; water increased.

Cannabis indica (Can. ind.)

Centre of action: Cerebro-spinal nervous system.

1. **Cerebro-spinal nervous system (Brain):** It has a great soothing influence in many nervous disorders like epilepsy, mania, dementia and irritable reflexes.
2. **Mental sphere:** It produces a state of exaltation with sublime visions, delusions and hallucinations in a great variety. Due to its intoxication it produces an exaggeration of all the perceptions and conceptions.

Cannabis sativa (Can. sat.)

Centre of action Cerebro-spinal nervous system.

Sedative; Narcotic; Hypnotic; Diuretic.

1. **Mucous membranes (Urethra):** It affects all mucous membranes, especially that of bladder,

urethra and *prepuce*; producing acute inflammation, with painful, difficult micturition; severe chordae; burning in urethra; the prepuce is dark, red, hot and inflamed, with mucous discharges from the urethra.

2. **Cerebro-spinal nervous system (Brain):** It produces intoxication and arrest of function, congestive headache; violent throbbing, with heat in the head; drowsy and much lassitude; vomiting of bile, and constipation.

Cantharides (Canth.)

Centre of action: Cerebro-spinal nervous system.

Aphrodisiac; irritant.

1. **Mucous membranes (Genito-urinary organs, gastro-intestinal tract, respiratory organs):** Violent inflammation.
2. **Sexual organs (Aphrodisiac):** Excessive sexual desire: Acute inflammation.
3. **Gastro-intestinal canal (Mouth to anus):** Congestion, burning heat, inflammation and vesication of the gastro-intestinal mucous membranes.
4. **Serous membranes (especially pleura, peritoneum):** Congestion, inflammation, followed by plastic fibrinous effusions.
5. **Skin:** Violent, acute vesicular inflammation.
6. **Glandular system (Salivary, Testicles, Ovaries):** Inflammation.
7. **Cerebro-spinal system:** Spasms; inflammations.

Capsicum annum (Cap. a.)

Centre of action: Cerebro-spinal nervous system.

1. **Mucous membranes:** Acrid, irritant; Congestion; Inflammation followed by a relaxed, atonic mucous membranes.
2. **Spinal cord (Posterior portion):** Excessive amount of chilliness.

Causticum (Caust.)

Centre of action: Cerebro-spinal (epecially spinal) nervous system

1. **Spinal cord (Motor tract):** It acts on medulla oblongata, and inferior recurrent branch of vagus causing congestion and inflammation of mucous membrane of the larynx and trachea, with paresis, or complete paralysis, of the vocal organs.
2. **Mucous membranes:** Atony; Catarrhal inflammation.
3. **Facial nerve (Motor part):** Paralysis of facial muscles.
4. **Digestive organs:** Atony; Congestion; Tympanitis.
5. **Urinary organs:** Paralysis or paresis of the sphincter of the bladder; Increased urinary solids.

Chamomilla (Cham.)

Centre of action: Cerebro-spinal nervous system.

Diaphoretic; Emmenagogue; Carminative; Stomachic; Anthelminthic.

1. **Spinal cord (posterior part):** Produces a state of excessive hyperesthesia, which extends to the emotional nerve centers, producing excessive anger and vexation. It probably has some specific action on the pulp of the teeth.
2. **Digestive organs**

   (a) *Stomach:* It produces excessive acidity, nausea and vomiting.

   (b) *Liver:* Portal congestion.

Cinchona officinalis (Cinch. of.)

Centre of action: Cerebro-spinal nervous system.

Mydriatic; Antiseptic; Aphrodisiac; Disinfectant.

1. **Brain:** Intense hyperaemia; bursting headache; coma.
2. **Auditory nerve:** Paralysis; various sounds in the ears, as singing, roaring, hissing, buzzing etc.; hardness of hearing and deafness.
3. **Eye (Mydriatic):** Dilatation of pupil; sometimes complete blindness.
4. **Trigeminus:** Hyperaesthesia; Neuralgia.
5. **Spine (Motor portion):** Convulsions; paralysis.
6. **Vagi:** Tonic; paresis; slow digestion.

7. **Lungs:** Venous congestion; Dyspnea; Anaemia.
8. **Spleen:** Venous hyperaemia; Hypertrophy; Hydraemia.
9. **Liver:** Paresis; Chronic congestion; Jaundice.
10. **Kidney:** Diminished urea and uric acid.
11. **Male sexual organ:** Debilitating nocturnal emissions. Impotence from long-continued seminal losses, with sexual dreams and complete prostration from undue sexual excitement.
12. **Female sexual organ:** Sexual excitement; Profuse haemorrhage.
13. **Muscular system:** Anemia; Paresis; Intermittent myalgia.
14. **Skin:** Acne-like eruption; Hydraemia; Anasarca.
15. **Blood:** Anaemia; Destroyed W.B.C. Fibrin increased.
16. **Circulation:** Tonic; Cardiac and vasomotor paralysis.
17. **Temperature:** Febrile temperature greatly lowered.
18. **Antiseptic:** Arrests fermentation with great rapidity.

Coffea cruda (Coff. Cr.)

Centre of action: Cerebro-spinal nervous system.

1. **Cerebral cortex**: It stimulates the mental centres and produces obstinate insomnia.
2. **Spinal cord**: Through posterior white column of spinal cord it paralyses the sensory nerve fibres.
3. **Vagus nerves**: It actively stimulates the respiratory centre of medulla oblongata through vagus nerve.
4. **Circulation**: It stimulates vasomotor nerves and increases blood pressure.
5. **Digestive system**: It initially stimulates and later on retards the function of digestive organs.
6. **Reproductive organs**: It initially excites and later on paralyses the reproductive organs.
7. **Kidneys**: It increases the renal arterial blood pressure and produces diuresis and diminishes the urine.

Colocynthis (Coloc.)

Centre of action: Cerebro-spinal and abdominal sympathetic nervous system.

Hydragogue cathartic.

1. **Gastro-intestinal canal:** Violent hydragogue cathartic.
2. **Mucous membranes (Intestines):** Violent inflammation.
3. **Serous membranes (peritoneum):** Inflammation.
4. **Spinal cord (posterior):** Hyperaesthesia; Violent neuralgia.

Crataegus oxyacantha (Crat. Oxy.):

Centre of action: Cerebro-spinal nervous system.

Cardiotonic; Hypotensive; Vasodilator; Sedative; Diuretic; Antioxidants; Anticoagulant; Antispasmodic.

1. **Heart (Myocardium):** Acts on muscle of heart and is considered a ***heart tonic*** recommended for myocarditis. No influence on the endocardium. Crataegus has cardio-protective qualities, "cleans up" the arteries removing the crustaceous matter stuck to their lining.
2. **Circulation**: Crataegus may improve coronary artery blood flow and the contractions of the heart muscle, hence used widely in cardiovascular disorders like arrhythmia, myocardial infarction, congestive heart failure. Crataegus also helps to reduce total cholesterol, triglycerides, LDL and increases HDL in blood.

Crotalus horridus (Crot. Hor.)

Centre of action: Cerebro-spinal nervous system.

1. **Central nervous system**: It acts on ***central nervous system*** affecting nerve centres producing rapid depression of sensorium and affecting the medulla oblongata producing disturbance in both nutrition and circulation.
2. **Blood**: It acts on ***blood*** causing rapid decomposition and produces slow, oozing haemorrhages from every orifices of the body.

3. **Liver**: It acts strongly on the ***liver*** and corresponds to jaundice and yellow fever (Malignant jaundice).
4. **Skin**: Ecchymosis, gangrene, severe local suppuration, malignant oedema.

Croton tiglium (Crot. tig.)

Centre of action: Abdominal sympathetic nervous system.

Hydragogue Cathartic; Cholagogue; Rubefacient; Vesicant.

1. **Gastro-intestinal Canal:** Most violent hydragogue cathartic.
2. **Mucous membranes (Intestinal):** Violent inflammation.
3. **Vagus nerve:** Nausea and violent vomiting.
4. **Liver:** Hepatic stimulant; Bile increased.
5. **Skin (Locally):** Eczema; Vesicular and pustular.

Gelsemium (Gels.)

Centre of action: Cerebro-spinal nervous system.

Myotic; Diuretic; Motor depressant; Diaphoretic.

1. **Cerebro-spinal system:** Centric motor and sensory paralysis; Congestion.
2. **Lungs:** Paralysis of respiratory centre; Asphyxia.
3. **Eyes (Myotic):** Diplopia; Pupil contracted; Muscle paralysed; Ptosis.
4. **Heart:** Paralysis; Blood-pressure lowered.
5. **Temperature:** Lowered in disease (especially in malaria).
6. **Male sexual organ:** Muscle paralysis; Emissions; Impotence.
7. **Female sexual organ:** Paralysis; Motor spasm; Neuralgia.
8. **Urinary organs:** Diuresis; Sphincter paralysis; Enuresis.

Glonoine (Glon.)

Centre of action: Cerebro-spinal nervous system.

1. **Brain and Spinal cord:** Through its action upon medula oblongata, vagus nerve, and vasomotor nerves, it produces active cerebral hyperaemia, palpitation of heart, severe headache resembling sunstroke.
2. **Gastro-intestinal canal**: Glonoine acts upon the digestive apparatus, as shown by the burning in the throat; nausea, vomiting, hiccough; pain in the epigastrium, and sometimes severe colicky pains with diarrhoea.
3. **Blood circulation**: It causes violent and sudden disturbance in blood circulation resulting violent pulsations, bursting and throbbing.

Helleborus niger (Hell. nig.)

Centre of action: Cerebro-spinal nervous system.

Hydragogue cathartic; Emmenagogue; Sialogogue.

1. **Glands (Salivary, Pancreas, Liver):** Increased secretion.
2. **Stomach (Vagi):** Nausea and violent vomiting.
3. **Intestinal canal:** Gastro-enteritis; Hydragogue cathartic.
4. **Kidneys:** Congestion; Inflammation; Albuminuria.
5. **Circulation:** Increased blood pressure; Heart slowed.
6. **Brain:** Congestion; Inflammation; Effusion.
7. **Spinal cord:** Congestion; Inflammation; Effusion; Paralysis.
8. **Serous membranes:** Inflammation; Dropsical effusion.
9. **Generative organs:** Emmenagogue.

Hydrastis canadensis (Hydr. can.)

Centre of action: Organic nervous system.

1. **Mucous membranes**: It acts on mucous membranes causing catarrhal inflammation, with a tendency to haemorrhage and ulceration, catarrh may be anywhere such as nose, eyes, throat, stomach, uterus, urethra which is characterised by profuse, thick, sticky, stringy, yellow, tenacious discharge.
2. **Digestive organs**: Tonic; Increased secretions; Constipation.
3. **Glandular System**: (Lymphatics): Hydrastis not only acts upon the gastric and intestinal

glands, but also affects the larger glands, as the liver, salivary, and lymphatics, producing increased secretions.

Hyoscyamus niger (Hyos. nig.)

Centre of action: Cerebro-spinal nervous system.

Analgesic; Narcotic; Mydriatic; Diuretic; Vasoconstrictor; Anhydrotic.

1. **Brain:** Violent, Loquacious, Quarrelsome, Delirium; Insomnia.
2. **Cord (Motor tract):** Convulsions; Paralysis.
3. **Eyes:** Powerful mydriatic.
4. **Ears:** Paresis of the auditory nerve; Deafness.
5. **Digestive organs:** Paralysis of all sphincter muscles.
6. **Intestines:** Involuntary diarrhoea.
7. **Urinary organs:** Diuresis; Sphincter paralysis.
8. **Circulation:** Slowed with increased blood pressure.
9. **Temperature:** (i) Increased, (ii) Diminished.

Ignatia amara (Ign.)

Centre of action: Cerebro-spinal nervous system (especially spinal).

Emmenagogue.

1. **Spinal cord:** It has a special action upon the medulla oblongata and spinal cord, producing tetanic convulsions, dyspnoea, asphyxia and death.
2. **Eyes:** Hysterical asthenopia.
3. **Throat:** Globus hystericus.
4. **Stomach:** Atony; Goneness or great emptiness.
5. **Intestines:** Diarrhoea; Prolapsus ani.
6. **Kidneys:** Nervous diuresis.
7. **Female sexual organ:** Profuse menstruation; Hysteria.

Kali bichromicum (Kali. bich.)

Centre of action: Organic nervous system.

1. **Mucous membranes**: It acts prominently on mucous membranes - eyes, nose, mouth, throat, bronchi, gastro-intestinal and genitourinary tracts producing catarrhal inflammations characterised by excessive secretion of mucus which is viscid and tough in character. Its action sometimes goes on to ulceration and superficial loss of tissue or formation of false membranes in respiratory tract.
2. **Glandular system**: It acts on the glandular system especially liver and kidney. It corrects the action of the liver so that healthy bile is formed and the gall stones are dissolved. It causes acute inflammation of kidney with albuminuria.
3. **Fibrous and periosteal tissues**: It works on fibrous tissues and periosteum causing active inflammation, congestion, disorganisation and destruction of the parts.
4. **Skin**: Pustular Inflammation.

Lachesis (Lach.)

Centre of action: Cerebro-spinal nervous system.

1. **Brain:** Congestion; Coma; Sensory nerve life destroyed.
2. **Spinal cord:** Spasms, Convulsions; Sudden prostration.
3. **Vagus nerve:**
   (i) *Bronchi:* Spasm of throat,
   (ii) *Stomach:* Emesis.
4. **Blood:** Rapid decomposition; Hemorrhage; Asthenic fever.
5. **Circulation:** Vaso-motor paralysis; Asthenia.
6. **Heart:** Paralysis.
7. **Skin:** Ecchymosis; Gangrene; Haemorrhages; Jaundice.
8. **Glandular system:** All glands congested; Fatty degeneration.
9. **Female sexual organ:** Ovarian atony; Delayed, scanty menses.

Lithium carbonicum (Lith. carb.)

Centre of action: Cerebro-spinal nervous system.

1. **Mind:** The action of Lithium carb is marked on the mind. It is a wonderful medicine that helps manage cases of depression, claustrophobia and bipolar disorder.

2. **Heart:** Due to its action on heart it produces symptoms of rheumatic heart disease associated with cystitis.
3. **Urinary organs:** It acts on urinary organs causing pain and soreness in urinary bladder with red-brown sediment in urine. There may be uric acid crystals in urine.
4. **Skin:** Dry skin with a rough rash all over the body with itching.
5. **Joints:** It acts on joints producing inflammatory changes with deposition of uric acid crystals.

Lycopodium clavatum (Lyco.)

Centre of action: Autonomic nervous system.

Decongestant; Antipruritic.

1. **Mucous membranes (Lungs; Kidneys):** Atony; Congestion; Catarrhal inflammation; profuse mucous discharges.
2. **Kidneys:** Frequent painful micturition and cloudy, sedimentous urine like brick-dust and sometimes with mucus and blood.
3. **Skin:** Brown liver spots; Papules; Eczema.
4. **Digestive organs:** Slow, irregular digestion; Flatulence; Constipation.
5. **Liver:** Congestion; Hypertrophy.
6. **Lymphatic glandular system (Neck):** Atony; Congestion; Induration.

Mercurius (Merc.)

Centre of action: Autonomic nervous system.

Cholagogue; Sialogogue; Cathartic; Caustic

1. **Lymphatic glandular system:** Paralysis; Congestion; Inflammation; Ulcer.
2. **Salivary glands:** Salivation; Excessive offensive secretion.
3. Pancreas: Salivation; Congestion; Inflammation; Hypertrophy.
4. **Liver:** Increased secretion of bile; Jaundice.
5. **Kidneys:** Congestion; Inflammation; Albuminuria; Diabetes.
6. **Mucous membranes (Intestinal):** Congestion; Inflammation; Haemorrhage.
7. **Intestinal canal:** Increased peristalsis; Cathartic.
8. **Mucous membranes (Air-passage):** Catarrhal inflammation.
9. **Eyes:** Congestion; Inflammation; Ulceration; Iritis.
10. **Serous membranes:** Inflammation; Effusion.
11. **Peritoneum (Fibrous tissue):** Congestion; Inflammation; Rheumatism.
12. **Bones:** Inflammation; Caries; Nightly bone-pains.
13. **Blood:** Decomposed; Fibrin, Albumin, R.B.C. decreased.
14. **Skin:** Vesicular and Pustular eczema; Jaundice.
15. **Female sexual organ:** Menorrhagia; Amenorrhoea; Miscarriage.
16. **Cerebro-spinal system:** Shaking palsy; Neuroses.

Mercurius corrosivus (Merc. Cor.)

Centre of action: Autonomic nervous system.

1. **Mucous membranes (Rectum and urinary bladder):** It especially acts on mucous membranes of rectum and urinary bladder causing inflammation and irritation producing intense tenesmus of rectum and urinary bladder.
2. **Eyes:** Due to its action on eyes it produces hypopyon, corneal ulcer, syphilitic iritis.
3. **Skin:** Phagedenic ulcers which burn intensely.
4. **Sexual organs:** Acts on male sexual organs causing manifestations of primary and tertiary syphilis, in the form of hard chancre and necrosis of bones.

Naja tripudians (Naja t.)

Centre of action: Cerebro-spinal nervous system.

1. **Nervous system:** It acts on ***nervous system*** especially cerebellum and medulla oblongata producing features of typical bulbar paralysis and feeling of intoxication, followed by gradual loss of power of lower limbs, loss of power to speech (blurred speech), loss of power in breathing, loss of power in deglutition and loss of power to control.
2. **Heart:** It has a strong action on ***heart*** causing different heart diseases such as chronic hyper-

trophy of heart, rheumatic heart disease, angina pectoris, chronic palpitation, cardiac asthma, low blood pressure, slow pulse etc.

3. It causes no haemorrhage or septic conditions like Lachesis and Crotalus but produces only oedema.

Natrum muriaticum (Nat. mur.)

Centre of action: Autonomic nervous system.

1. **Blood:** Anaemia; Great loss of R.B.C.
2. **Lymphatics:** Secretions excessively excoriating.
3. **Liver:** Hypertrophy; Anaemia; Jaundice; Despondency.
4. **Spleen:** Hypertrophy, with great anaemia.
5. **Salivary glands:** Increased and perverted secretions.
6. **Mucous membranes:** Congestion; Inflammation.
7. **Digestive organs:** Increased secretions; Constipation.
8. **Skin:** Eczema; Boils; Urticaria; Fissures; Loss of hair.
9. **Female sexual organ:** Delayed menses; Diminished sex desire.
10. **Eyes:** Excoriating secretions.
11. **Spinal cord (Posterior):** Great chilliness from anaemia.

Nitric acid (Nit. ac.)

Centre of action: Organic nervous system.

1. **Mucous membranes (Mouth, Anus):** Inflammation; Destructive ulceration.
2. **Glandular system (Lymphatic):** Congestion; Inflammation; Offensive discharge.
3. **Liver:** Congestion; Hypertrophy; Jaundice.
4. **Skin:** Pustular ulceration; Fungoid growths; Perspiration.
5. **Blood:** Broken-down; Septic condition.

Nux vomica (Nux vom.)

Centre of action: Cerebro-spinal nervous system.

Aphrodisiac

1. **Cord (Gray portion):** Tetanic convulsion; Death from asphyxia.
2. **Motor nerve:** Exhaustion; Paralysis.
3. **Sensory nerves:** Hyperaesthesia.
4. **Eyes** Pupils contracted; Hyperaesthesia; Vision increased.
5. **Ears:** Hearing augmented.
6. **Nose:** Sense of smell increased.
7. **Circulation:** Vaso-motor spasm; Increased arterial blood pressure.
8. **Heart:** Paresis of inhibitory nerves.
9. **Stomach:** Increased appetite; Acid vomiting; Gastralgia.
10. **Intestinal canal:** Constipation; Haemorrhoids.
11. **Bladder:** Paralysis of muscular coat; Incontinence.
12. **Male sexual organ:** Increased sexual desire; Impotence.
13. **Female sexual organ:** Menses too soon; lasts too long.
14. **Lungs:** Dry cough; Flatulent asthma.
15. **Blood:** Oxidation arrested.

Opium

Centre of action: Cerebro-spinal nervous system.

Anaesthetic; Diaphoretic; Emetic; Emmenagogue; Hypnotic; Myotic.

1. **Brain:** Intense congestion; profound coma.
2. **Spinal cord (Posterior):** Complete anaesthesia.
3. **Vagus nerve:** Paralysis of respiratory centre; Asphyxia.
4. **Eyes:** Oculo-motor paralysis; Pupils greatly dilated.
5. **Heart:** Pulsations lessened, from vagus paralysis.
6. **Vaso-motor spasm:** Small doses excite; large doses paralyse.
7. **Digestive organs:** Appetite destroyed with great thirst.
8. **Mucous membrane:** Secretions completely arrested.
9. **Stomach:** Nausea and vomiting (centric).

10. **Intestinal canal:** Constipation.
11. **Kidneys:** Secretion diminished; Solids increased; Renal stones.
12. **Male sexual organs:** (i) Sexual excitement; (ii) Impotence.
13. **Female sexual organs:** (i) Menses increased; (ii) Suspended.
14. **Skin:** Copper coloured; Diaphoretic; Prurigo; Eczema.
15. **Nutrition destroyed:** Emaciation; imbecile; Chronic liars.

Passiflora incarnatea (Passi in.):

Centre of action: Cerebro-spinal nervous system.

Anti-anxiety; Analgesic; Anti-convulsant; Aphrodisiac; Anti-asthmatic.

1. **Nervous system:** CNS depressant. It induces sleep, inhibits convulsions and hyperactivity. It is helpful for generalised anxiety disorder (GAD).
2. **Stomach:** It prevents chemotherapy induced nausea and vomiting.

Phosphorus (Phos.)

Centre of action: Autonomic nervous system.

Aphrodisiac

1. **Stomach:** Gastritis; Gastralgia; Haematemesis; Hypertrophy.
2. **Small intestine:** Congestion; Inflammation; Watery diarrhoea.
3. **Liver:** Congestion; Inflammation; Jaundice; Hypertrophy; Fatty degeneration.
4. **Spleen:** Congestion; Hypertrophy; Fatty degeneration.
5. **Kidneys:** Inflammation; Albuminuria; Haemorrhage; Fatty degeneration,
6. **Heart:** Fatty degeneration; Venous stagnation.
7. **Lungs:** Congestion; Inflammation; Hepatisation.
8. **Arteries:** Fatty degeneration; Haemorrhage.
9. **Blood:** Haemolysis; Hydraemia; Ecchymoses.
10. **Cerebro-spinal system:** Stimulate; Nutrition destroyed; Paralysis; Neural.
11. **Male sexual organ:** Aphrodisiac; Paralysis; Impotence.
12. **Female sexual organ:** Small doses stimulate; Large doses paralyse.
13. **Bones (Maxillae):** Periostitis; Caries; Necrosis.

Podophyllum (Podo.)

Centre of action: Abdominal sympathetic nervous system.

Cathartic; Cholagogue; Sialogogues.

1. **Mucous membranes (Stomach; Small intestine):** Inflammation.
2. **Intestinal canal:** Drastic cathartic; Duodenitis.
3. **Salivary glands:** Copious salivation.
4. **Liver:** Hepatic stimulant; Bile greatly increased.

Pulsatilla (Puls.)

Centre of action: Cerebro-spinal nervous system.

Diuretic; Diaphoretic; Emmenagogue.

1. **Mucous membranes:** Catarrhal inflammation; Unnatural dryness of the surface, followed by copious and profuse mucus discharges.
2. **Eyes:** Catarrhal inflammation; Profuse mucus discharge.
3. **Ears:** Sub-acute inflammation of middle ear; Recent catarrhal deafness; Otalgia.
4. **Stomach:** Indigestion of fat and other rich food; Acidity; Yellow-coated tongue.
5. **Intestines:** Flatulence; Passive mucus diarrhoea.
6. **Urinary organs:** Catarrhal inflammation; Mucus in urine.
7. **Male sexual organ:** Orchitis; Varicocele; Neuralgia.
8. **Female sexual organ:** Ovaritis; Scanty, late menses.
9. **Venous system:** Acute varicosis.
10. **Synovial membranes:** Rheumatico-gouty inflammation.
11. **Skin:** Urticaria; Miliary eruption.
12. **Spinal Cord (Posterior):** Chilliness; Hyperaesthesia; Neuralgia.

Rhus toxicodendron (Rhus tox.)

Centre of action: Cerebro-spinal nervous system.

1. **Skin:** Irritation; Vesicular erysipelas; Pemphigus; Sour sweat; Herpes (especially herpes zoster)
2. **Mucous membrane (Conjunctiva; Fauces; G. I. tract):** Catarrhal inflammation.
3. **Eyes:** Acute rheumatic conjunctivitis; Strumous ophthalmia.
4. **Lungs:** Congestion; Infiltration; Typhoid pneumonia.
5. **Mouth:** Acute inflammation; Sordes.
6. **Stomach:** Loss of appetite; Nausea; Vomiting; Gastritis.
7. **Abdomen:** Typhoid enteritis; Tympanitis; Involuntary stools.
8. **Sero-fibrous tissue (Tendons, Fasciae):** Rheumatoid inflammation.
9. **Lymphatics:** Secretions acrid; Congestion; Inflammation.
10. **Blood:** Septic fever; Fibrin increased.
11. **Cerebro-spinal system:** Profound depression; Rheumatic paralysis.

Secale cornutum (Sec. cor.)

Centre of action: Cerebro-spinal nervous system.

Abortificient; Emetic; Mydriatic; Diaphoretic; Ecbolic; Emmenagogue.

1. **Heart:** Inhibitory paralysis; Diminished pulsations.
2. **Circulation:** Tonic arterial contraction; Dilated veins.
3. **Temperature:** Greatly lowered, sometimes 5 degrees.
4. **Uterus:** Abortificient; Violent tetanic contractions from arterial anaemia and venous hyperaemia. Death of foetus from uterine tetanus.
5. **Stomach:** Violent emesis; Haematemesis.
6. **Small intestines:** Increased peristalsis; Watery diarrhoea.
7. **Sphincter muscles:** All paralysed.
8. **Cerebro-Spinal system:** Formication; Muscular cramp; Epilepsy.
9. **Eyes:** Pupils dilated; Amaurosis from arterial anaemia.
10. **Skin:** Diaphoresis; Furuncles; Eczema; Gangrene; Purpura.

Sepia (Sep.)

Centre of action: Autonomic nervous system.

Laxative; Diaphoretic; Disinfectant.

1. **Venous system:** Venous congestion of the portal system.
2. **Ovaries:** Venous congestion; Atony; Scanty menses.
3. **Uterus:** Venous congestion; Leucorrhoea; Ulceration; Prolapsus.
4. **Gastro-intestinal canal:** Portal congestion; Torpidity; Constipation.
5. **Liver:** Congestion; Torpidity; Acid secretions.
6. **Kidneys:** Scanty urine; Increased uric acid; Lithiasis.
7. **Skin:** Cachectic, yellow, earthy, waxy, chloasma; Eczema.

Silicea (Sil.)

Centre of action: Organic nervous system.

1. **Bones and fibrous tissue:** Suppuration and complete destruction of bones. Periosteum and fibrous tissue. Caries of the shafts of epiphyses of any of the bones, with excessive nightly bone pains.
2. **Lymphatics:** Congestion; Hypertrophy; Suppuration.
3. **Skin:** Pustular inflammation; Cold extremities; Offensive sweat.
4. **Mucous membranes:** Catarrhal inflammation; Ulceration.
5. **Cerebro-spinal nervous system:** Loss of nutrition; Neurasthenia; Spasms.

Stannum metallicum (Stan. met.)

Centre of action: Cerebro-spinal nervous system.

1. **Cerebro spinal system:** It chiefly affects on *cerebrospinal nervous system* especially the

spinal cord causing slows down the activity and develops the prostration, paralysis, convulsions along with neuralgic pains.

2. **Sexual organs**: It influences the ***uterus and vagina*** develops paralytic weakness of the uterus and vagina. Profound debility and neurasthenia. Even there is complete inability to sit down on the chair.

3. **Lungs (Bronchioles)**: Acts upon the mucous membrane of the lungs, especially that of the bronchioles, producing catarrhal inflammation, and profuse muco-purulent expectoration, with dilatation of the bronchi, and complete exhaustion of the nerves of the lungs.

4. **Larynx**: It causes an inflammation of the vocal cord and develops the complete loss of voice.

5. **Gastro-intestinal tract**: Due to its action on ***gastro-intestinal tract***, especially rectum causing paralysis of the rectal muscles. There is complete inability to pass stool with constipation due to inactivity of muscles.

6. **Blood**: It attacks ***blood*** and reduces the oxygen carrying capacity of haemoglobin resulting changes of colour of blood from red to yellow.

Stramonium (Stram.)

Centre of action: Cerebro-spinal nervous system.

1 **Peripheral and sympathetic nervous system**: Its action is more or less similar to Belladonna except on sympathetic nerves. Stramonium has more powerful action on sympathetic nervous system than Belladonna. It produces marked and persistent disorder of the mental faculties; hallucinations; fixed notions, violent delirium, etc. It increases the mobility of the muscles of expression and of locomotion; the motions may be graceful, rhythmic or disorderly, of head and arms.

2. **Eyes**: It causes dilatation of pupils and inflammation; acts as a mydriatic.

3. **Sexual organs**: Due to its action on sexual organs it produces complete indecent and voluptuous sexual excitement followed by complete prostration of sexual desire and temporary impotency.

4. **Heart and circulation**: It acts on circulation, especially of heart and capillaries producing tonic capillary contractions and increased circulation.

5. **Lungs**: It acts on respiratory organs causing diminished secretion and producing a dry, spasmodic cough.

6. **Intestines**: Due to its action on intestinal tract produces diarrhoea as well as obstinate constipation.

7. **Skin**: It affects the skin producing fiery redness of skin and vesicular erysipelas.

Sulphur (Sulph.)

Centre of action: Organic nervous system. Laxative; Diaphoretic; Disinfectant.

1. **Venous system:** Chronic capillary congestion; Exudation; Suppuration.

2. **Portal system:** Chronic congestion; Constipation; Piles.

3. **Lymphatic system:** Profuse acrid secretions, excoriating all parts.

4. **Serous membranes:** Serous effusions; Exudative inflammation.

5. **Mucous membranes:** Profuse excoriating mucus discharge.

6. **Skin:** Vesicular and pustular inflammation; Alopecia.

7. **Sympathetic nervous system:** Defective assimilation; Hot flushes.

8. **Blood:** Fibrin increased; Rheumatoid affections.

9. **Sulphur fumes:** Disinfectant; Deodorising.

Symphytum officinalis (Symph. of.)

Centre of action: Cerebro-spinal nervous system.

1. **Bones and periosteum**: It acts on ***bones and periosteum*** and helps in healing of non-union of broken bones. It reduces soreness and pricking pain at the point of fracture and in areas after amputation. Acts on joints generally.

2. Eyes: It acts on ***eyes*** and reduces soreness of eyes following injury.

Tabacum (Tabac.)

Centre of action: Cerebro spinal nervous system.

1. **Brain and vagus nerve**: It acts on ***medulla oblongata and motor fibres of vagus nerve*** causing their irritation producing complete prostration and relaxation of muscular system, with free secretions, vomiting, profuse sweat, lachrymation, salivation etc.
2. **Mucous membranes (Stomach, small intestines)**: Profuse secretions.
3. **Heart**: Due to its action on ***heart*** causing contraction of coronary arteries resulting symptoms of angina pectoris or may even precipitate acute myocardial infarction, in persons addicted to tobacco chewing or smoking.
4. **Stomach**: Powerful emetic; Gastritis: Gastrodynia.
5. **Intestines (Small)**: Violent tetanic contractions; Cathartic.
6. **Circulation**: Greatly lowered; Vaso-motor paralysis.
7. **Eyes**: Myosis; Amaurosis; Atrophy of the retina.
8. **Sexual organs**: Sexual appetite destroyed; Menses delayed.
9. **Lungs**: Respiration lessened; Laryngismus.
10. **Skin**: Gray (sweat glands); Profuse sweats.

Thuja occidentalis (Thuja)

Centre of action: Organic nervous system.

Diuretic; Insecticidal; Anthelminthic.

1. **Skin:** Fig-warts; Condylomata; Tubercles; Sycosis.
2. **Mucous membranes:** Acrid secretions; Corroding ulcers; Polypi.
3. **Male sexual organ:** Chronic blennorrhoea; Prostatitis.
4. **Female sexual organ:** Delayed menses; Leucorrhoea; Ovaritis.
5. **Blood and serum:** Dissolution; Acridity.
6. **Urinary organs:** Diuretic; Sphincter paralysed.

Chapter 27

Experimental Pharmacology (E.P.)

Introduction

Samuel Hahnemann was the founder of Homoeopathy. He established the fundamental principles of the science and art of Homoeopathy.

He is called the Father of Experimental Pharma-cology because he was the first physician to prepare medicines in a specialised way; proving them on healthy human beings, to determine how the medicines acted to cure diseases. Before Hahnemann, medicines were given on speculative indications, mainly on the basis of authority without experimental verification.

The term pharmacology is often confused with the term pharmacy, but they are not synonymous. Pharmacy is the profession dealing with the effective use of medication, while pharmacology is more closely linked to chemistry—a study, not a practice.

Pharmacology is the study of drugs and their effects. Experimental pharmacology is study through experimental use in controlled situations. Human and animal drug testing falls into the category of experimental pharmacology. Scientists design drugs as well as they can without experimental evidence and then test them on humans or on animals in an experimental setting to gather more information and to perfect their drugs.

Research involving experimental pharmacology is generally conducted long before pharmacists or consumers have access to the drugs being tested.

The basis of Homoeopathic Medicine is experimental pharmacology (drug proving or homoeopathic pathogenetic trial-HPT, as known in homoeopathy). This essentially calls for that the raw material should be one used in the proving.

Definition

It is that branch of pharmacology which deals with the effect of drugs on living system.

It can be studied on healthy human beings as well as on animals.

Thus it helps in under studying the nature of drug action and the un-alterability of the living systems to the attract by chemicals that serves as the basis on which:

(a) New therapeutic agents are developed and

(b) Toxic consequences of chemical exposure may be activated.

The experiment can be carried out in whole animal (in vivo) or in isolated organs (in vitro).

Aims of Experimental Pharmacology

The main aims of Experimental Pharmacology in Homoeopathy are:

(a) To study the mechanism of action of potentised homoeopathic drugs in animal models.

(b) To study the site of action of homoeopathic drugs.

(c) To study the toxicity of crude drugs.

(d) To find out a therapeutic agent suitable for human use.

(e) To add new and better drug in therapeutics.

(f) To discover new, simple and better techniques for experimental.

(g) For bioassay and standardisation of drug.

Experimental studies on Animal models

In the field of Homoeopathy animal models are used both for testing the principle of dilution/ potentisation and for studying the possible mechanism of action of Homoeopathic Medicines in a thorough and repeatable manner, as well as for discovering medicines to be used in the veterinary context. The aim of this type of experimental work is to provide a rational approach to the investigation of the various aspect of the '*similia similibus curantur*' principle and of the use of high dilutions, in order to construct a plausible framework of ideas capable of facilitating further basic and clinical research into these historical yet also modern medical principles. Acceptance of the homoeopathic claims requires supporting evidence of plausible mechanisms and high quality studies exploring its effectiveness in experimental settings.

Animal studies in Homoeopathy refer to three important goals:

1. **Preclinical research to test in animals, the medicines before their employed in human beings:** The preclinical research in Homoeopathy has virtually never pursued and the situation is inverted with respect to conventional pharmacological research. In fact, Homoeopathy is based on human 'provings' and medicines have been employed in humans for two centuries without verification of their effects in animal models. Only in the recent decades some researchers have begun testing in animal models some already commercially available Homoeopathic Medicines, especially low-dose complex formulations. The main studies in immunological and immuno-pharmacological fields have been here reported and gave, in general, positive results. Even if these medicines are already in the human use, pursuing this line of research in animals could be useful to better identify new fields of pathologies where those medicines could be potentially employed and to improve formulations as regards their constituents and/or their grade of dilution.

2. **Finding new, non-toxic therapies for animals in veterinary research:** As the veterinary research is concerned, only few research articles are published regarding immuno-stimulating effects of Homoeopathy and/or protection from infectious diseases. So, to the best of our knowledge, the question of the potential utilisation of Homoeopathy in the infectious diseases of domestic animals or in natural farming is still largely unexplored, or unpublished.

3. **Exploring in controlled and reproducible settings specific aspects and mechanisms of action of homoeopathic approach:** The study of the mechanisms of therapeutic action would be the main goal of basic research in Homoeopathy. Here, two major themes are under investigation:

   (i) the 'high dilution' effects, i.e., the question whether and how substances diluted (and potentised) in away that few or no molecules of active principle may have pharmacological effects; and

   (ii) the mode of action of the 'simile' effect, i.e., how a substance known to have pathogenetic effects in healthy organisms (cells, animals and humans) may turn to become a therapeutic agent in diseased organisms.

These two themes may be, in turn, split in a number of minor questions regarding the methods of dilution, the most useful model to show the effect, the type of solvent used (distilled water, saline solutions, water/ethanol mixtures) and other technical details that may often affect the final outcomes.

Different Research works on Animals

1. At a veterinary college, scientists have showed that homoeopathic remedy *Chelidonium majus* had lowered serum cholesterol when given twice a day to **rabbits** on a cholesterol rich diet. [v. Baumans, C. J. Bol, W. M. T. Owe Lutti-khuis, and A. C. Beynen. "Does Chelidonium 3x lower serum cholesterol?" British Homoeopathic Journal, 76 (January 1987): 14-15.]
2. It has been found that out of the 77 **mice** that received a transplant in fibrosarcoma, 52% survived more than one year with homoeopathic remedies. The 77 mice that were untreated died within 10-15 days. [H. Choudhury, "Cure of cancer in experimental mice with certain biochemic salts," British Homoeopathic Journal, 69 (1980): 168-170.]
3. It has been shown that homoeopathic remedy *Silicea* had a significant effect on stimulating macrophages in **mice**, which destroy foreign particles, bacteria, and old cells. [Elizabeth Davenas, Bernard Poitevin, and Jacques Benveniste, effect on mouse peritoneal macrophages of orally administered very high dilutions of Silica, "European Journal of Pharmacology." 135 (April 1987): 313-319.]
4. A study showed that homoeopathic doses of *Arsenic* eliminated crude doses of trapped Arsenic that had been previously fed to **rats**. [J.C. Cazin et al. "A study of the effect of decimal and centesimal dilution of Arsenic on retention and mobilisation of Arsenic in the rat," Human toxicology, July 1987.]
5. Karen Nieber, a professor of Pharmacology, put a **rat's** intestine in a fluid culture medium and used organic threads to fix it to a sensor so that she could measure any shortening of the intestine caused by cramps. Then she added a stimulant (Atropine) to the fluid culture medium to produce severe cramps in the rat's intestine. The intestine shrank and the scales showed a strong traction. When she added *Belladonna* X 90 to the culture medium, the intestine relaxed and the scales showed less traction. This proved that homoeopathy is effective in the absence of any material substances—and in 2003 she won the € 10,000 Hans Heinrich Reckeweg award. [ECH GENERAL ASSEMBLY-XVIII Symposium of GIRI 12 to 14th of November 2004 Scientific Report- Chang FY, Lee SD, et al. Rat Gastro-intestinal Motor Responses mediated via activation of Neurokinin Receptors. J Gastro-enterol Hepatol 1999;14:39-45. Cristea A, Nicula S, Darie V. Pharmacodynamic effects of very high dilutions of Belladonna on the isolated rat duodenum. In: Bastide M(ed), Signals and Images. Kluwer Academic Publishers 1997: 161-170].
6. Scientists have found that **rodents** given *Hypericum* were able to inhibit pain responses. Rodents were able to remain on a hot plate longer than the control group. When given Naloxone, which inhibits pain killing Endorphins, the protective effects of Hypericum was reduced, showing that homoeopathic *Hypericum* activates Endorphins when needed. Those rodents were free to walk off the hot plate whenever discomfort was noticed. [G.R. Keysall, K.L. Williamson, and B.D. Tolman. "The testing of some Homoeopathic preparations in rodents," proceedings of the 40th International Homoeopathic Congress (Lyon. France, 1985). Pp. 228-231]
7. In one very intriguing study, *Thyroxine* 30x (Thyroid hormone) was placed in the water of **tadpoles**. When compared to tadpoles who were given a placebo, the study showed, morphogenesis of the tadpoles into frogs was slowed for those, who were exposed to the homoeopathic doses. Because Thyroid hormone in crude doses is known to speed up morphogenesis, it makes sense from a homoeopathic perspective that homoeopathic doses would slow it down.
8. Specifically, several researchers administered (usually to **rats**) crude doses of *arsenic, bismuth, cadmium, mercury chloride, or lead.* The research showed that animals who were pre-treated with homoeopathic doses of these substances

and then given repeated homoeopathic doses after exposure to the crude substance, excreted more of these toxic substances through urine, feces, and sweat than did those animals given a placebo.

Further, nine studies on mice which tested homoeopathic doses beyond 15c demonstrated a 40% decrease in mortality compared to mice in the control group.

9. Several studies noted that pre-treatment and treatment with potentised doses of substances different from those to which the animal was being exposed did not provide any benefit. The research suggests that Homoeopathic Medicine may play a significant role in the treatment of toxicological exposure. Homoeopathic research has also explored the benefits of Homoeopathic Medicines to protect against radiation (Khuda-Bukhsh, and Banik, 1991a, 1991b).

10. **Albino mice** were exposed to 100 to 200 rad of X-rays (sublethal doses) and then evaluated after 24, 48, and 72 hours. *Ginseng* 6x, 30x, and 200x and *Ruta graveolens* 30x and 200x were administered before and after exposure. When compared with mice given a placebo as treatment, mice given any of the above Homoeopathic Medicines experienced significantly less chromosomal or cellular damage.

11. In another study, **Albino Guinea-pigs** were exposed to small doses of *X-ray* that cause reddening of the skin. Studies showed that *Apis mellifica* 7c or 9c had a protective effect and a roughly 50% curative effect on X-ray-induced redness of the skin (Bildet, Guyot, Bonini, et al., 1990). *Apis mellifica* (honey-bee) is a Homoeopathic Medicine for redness, swelling, and itching, common symptoms of bee-venom.

12. A 3x potency of *Chelidonium* lowered cholesterol in **rabbits** by 25 percent.

13. Microdoses of *Arsenicum* (10x up to 30x; and 5c up to 15c) helped **rats** eliminate toxic doses of Arsenic from their systems, a study that has important implications for humans who are increasingly exposed to many heavy metals in the environment.

And pigs given *Caulophyllum* had half as many still-births as those who received a placebo.

Different Laboratory Animals and Their Applications in Experimental Pharmacology

Common Laboratory Animals

These are those animals which can be used and reared (maintain) in the laboratory under suitable conditions. The common laboratory animals are rat, mice, guinea pig, rabbit, frog and hamster. Other animals used for experimental purpose are cat, dog, monkey, pigeon etc. Since long animal experiments have been a milestone in advanced medical research. Any or every animal is not suitable for experimental work. Their selection is based on the following criteria:

1. **Size:** Smaller animals are prefered because they are easy to handle and less quantity of drug is required.
2. **Availability:** Animals which are commonly available should be selected, e.g., frogs, rats, rabbits and dogs.
3. **Sensitivity:** Animals which are sensitive to drugs under trial, e.g., guinea pig is sensitive to effect of Histamine.
4. **Species:** In rabbits intra-cerebro ventricular injection of 5-HT induces a lowering of temperature, but in cats, it induces fever.

Characteristics and Advantages of Different Animals

A. RAT (*Rattus norvegicus*)

Albino rat is one of the commonest laboratory animals suitable for experimental work because of its small size and greater sensitivity to most drugs. It is also the most standardised of all laboratory animals. It can be used to obtain pure and uniform strains and is found to be very sturdy to withstand long periods of experimentation under anaesthesia. It is small in size compared to other animals so drugs are required in small quantity. Vomiting centre is absent and so drug can be administered orally. Gall bladder and tonsils are absent. Because of the absence of gall bladder in rat there is continuous flow of bile into the intestine. This facilitates the study of drugs acting on bile, cholesterol reabsorption. Pancreas is diffused, therefore difficult to produce Pancreactomy. In stomach, fundus and pyloric parts have clear lining between them. The Gastric acid secretion is continuous.

Experimental uses:

(Adult wt. 180-200 gm, age suitable for most of the experiment—1.5 months)

1. Psycho-pharmacological studies.
2. Study of analysis of anticonvulsants.
3. Bioassay of various hormones, such as insulin, oxytocin, vasopressin etc.
4. Study of oestrus cycle, mating behaviour and lactation.
5. Studies on isolated tissue preparation like uterus, stomach, vas deferens, anococcygeus fundus strip, heart, etc.
6. Chronic study on blood pressure.
7. Gastric acid secretion studies.
8. Study of hepatotoxic and antihepatotoxic compound.
9. Acute and chronic toxicity studies.

B. Guinea-pig (*Cavia porcellus*)

It is docile animal, highly susceptible to TB and anaphylaxis and also highly sensitive to histamine and penicillin. It requires exogenous vitamin C in diet.

Experimental uses:

(Adult Wt. 400-600 gms, age suitable for experiments—3 months)

1. Evaluation of bronchodilators.
2. Anaphylaclic and immunological studies.
3. Study of histamine and antihistamincs.
4. Bioassay of digitalis.
5. Hearing experiments because of sensitive cochlea.
6. Studies on isolated tissues specially, ileum tracheal chain, vas deferens, etc.
7. Study of tuberculosis and ascorbic acid metabolism.

C. Mouse (*Mus musculus*)

Swiss albino mice are commonly used. They are smallest cheap and easy to handle.

Experimental uses:

(Adult weight: 20-25 gm, age suitable for experiment—2 month)

1. Toxicological studies, specially acute and subacute toxicities. They are also used in teratogenicity (foetal abnormalities).
2. Bioassay of insulin.
3. Screening of analgesics and anticonvulsants.
4. Screening of chemotherapeutic agents.
5. Studies related to genetics and cancer research.
6. Study of drugs acts on CNS.

D. Rabbit (*Oryctolagus cuniculus*)

Rabbit are also docile animals with large ears. Usually New Zealand white rabbits are used. It has huge caecum and large appendix. The enzyme atropine esterase is present in rabbit liver and plasma, so it can tolerate large doses of Belladonna (atropine). Cardioaortic nerve forms a separate depressive nerve. Vaso dilator nerves are absent and so vasomotor reversal phenomenon cannot be demonstrated. Histamine causes increase in blood pressure. Ovulation is related to the release of luteinising hormone and occurs 10 hours after coitus.

Experimental uses:

(Adult weight: 1.5–3.0 kg, age suitable for experiment—5-6 months).

1. Pyrogen testing.
2. Bioassay of antidiabetics, curareform drugs and sex hormones.
3. Screening of agents affecting capillary permeability.
4. Irritancy tests.
5. Screening of antitoxic agents and teratogens.
6. Studies related to reproduction (antifertility agents).
7. Isolated preparation like heart, dudenum, ileum, Finkleman preparation.
8. Study of local anesthetics (surface anaesthesia).
9. Study of miotics and mydriatics.

E. Hamster (*Mesocricetus auratus* and *Cricetulus griseus*)

They have short body with short legs and tail. The skin is loose and covered with dense short soft fur. The cheeks pouches are prominent and extend up to the shoulder region.

Experimental uses:

(adult weight 80–90 gm, average age suitable for experiments, 1 month)

1. Chinese hamsters have low chromosome number—making them useful for cytological genetics tissue culture and radiation research.
2. Research on diabetes mellitus
3. Research related to virology, immunology and implantation studies.
4. Bioassay of prostaglandins.

F. Frog (*Rana tigrina*)

One of the most commonly used experimental animals in physiology, pharmacology and toxicology. It has been used in experiment for 200 years. It is easily available during rainy reason. It is an amphibian animal and safe to handle. It cannot be used in laboratory.

Adrenaline is neurotransmitter in the sympathetic system.

Experimental uses:

1. Study of isolated tissue such as rectus abdominis muscle and heart preparation.
2. Study of drugs acting on CNS.
3. Study of retinal toxicity of drugs, light blea-ches rhodopsin in eye within one hour and is regenerated within one hour in dark.
4. Study of drugs acting on neuromuscular junctions (using gastrocnemius, sciatic muscle nerve preparation.)

G. Cat

It is a carnivorous animal relatively easy to obtain and to use for experimental purpose. The physiology of circulatory and neuromuscler system is very much similar to that of man. It has highly developed nictitating membrane which is contracted by sympathetic nerves. Morphine produces excitation of central neruous system in cat.

Experimental uses:

1. Acute experiments for the drugs affecting BP.
2. Bioassay of NA (using spinal cat).
3. Studies on ganglions blockers (using nictitating membrane in vivo).
4. Studies on neuromuscular system (using gastrocnemius, sciatic muscle nerve preparation.)
5. Toxicity studies of compound like acetanilide.

H. Dog

Experimental uses:

1. Gastric acid secretion studies (Pavlov pouch).
2. Acute experiments for drug affecting BP and intestinal movements etc.
3. Studies on antidiabetic agents.

I. Monkey and Apes

These are the primates belonging to the highest order of the mammals. The anatomy and physiology of these animals are closely related to that of man. The studies done in monkeys are directly translated to man. Considering the human respects, tests in primates should be done only in last stage of evaluation of drugs before clinical trials. They are used in the fields of psychopharmacology, urology, immunology, nutrition, reproduction, parasitology, etc.

J. Leech

The dorsal muscle of leech is used for bioassay of acetylcholine.

Procurement of Animals

It will be economical to procure animals from reliable sources rather than breeding them if the requirement of animals is minimal The various species of animals required for medical colleges should be procured from recognised sources. Local procurement sources should be identified by the medical colleges for the supply of non-laboratory bred animals. Medical colleges with breeding facilities should procure the breeding stock from a reliable source for initiating a colony ensuring that genetic makeup and health status of animals is known. Additionally the following aspects has to be taken care of:

1. Healthy animals should be obtained from a recognised source.
2. Acceptable methods and norms of transportation should be followed, considering the distance, seasonal and climatic conditions and the species of animals.

3. The animals should be given a reasonable period for physiological, psychological and nutritional stabilisation before their use.

Food and Water

1. Animals should be fed palatable, non-contaminated, and nutritionally adequate food.
2. Feeds should be procured from reliable source.
3. Good quality feeds and water should be provided ad libitum.
4. Areas in which feeds are processed or stored, should be kept clean and enclosed to prevent entry of insects and wild rodents.
5. Watering devices, such as drinking tubes, should be examined routinely to ensure their proper operation.
6. Feeders should allow easy access to food and watery while minimising contaminating by urine and faeces.

Sanitation and Cleanlines

Animal rooms, corridors, storage spaces, and other areas should be cleaned with appropriate detergents and disinfectants. Animals should be kept dry except for those species whose natural habitation need water. Where larger animals and non-human primates are housed, soiled litter material should be removed routinely. Cages should be cleaned each time before animals are placed in them. Animal cages, racks and accessory equipment, such as feeders and watering devices, should be washed and cleaned frequently to keep them free from contamination. Cages, water bottles, sipper tubes, stoppers and other watering equipment should be washed and disinfected regularly. Deodorisers or chemical agents other than germicides should not be used to mask animal odours.

Veterinary Care

Wherever required, adequate veterinary care must be provided under the supervision and gui-dance of a registered veterinarian or a person trained and experienced in laboratory animal sciences. Animals should be observed regularly and problems of animal health and behaviour, recorded and addressed. For animals kept for experiments of longer duration, the steps should be adopted as:

1. All animals should be observed for signs of illness, injury or abnormal behaviour by the animal house staff and reported to the attending veterinarian.
2. Diseased animals should be isolated from healthy ones.

Personnel Hygiene and Training of Staff

Initial in-house training should be imparted to the staff associated with animals facility. Appropriate and protective gears (gloves, masks, head cover, coat,shoes, etc.) be used by the personnel in the animal facility as per requirement. Personnel should have periodic medical check-ups to ensure there health status.

Surgical Procedures and Duration of Experiment

Multiple surgical procedures on an animal for any experiment are not to be practiced unless specified in a protocol.

Restraint

Devices, wherever required, suitable in size and design for holding animals for examination and collection of samples should be made available to minimise stress and avoid injury to the animals and handlers.

Records keeping

Animal facilities should have the following records:

1. Animal House plan
2. Name and addresses of the staff including the facility incharge and their contact telephone nos.
3. Health records of staff
4. Training record of staff involved in animal care and procedures
5. Records pertaining to the items in stock
6. Animal stock procurement and supply register
7. Records of experiments or procedures conducted with the number of animals used in each experiment
8. Clinical record of sick animals and any treatment administered
9. Mortality and ailing record.

Animal House

Animal houses should be made of durable and preferably moisture-proof material equipment. The doors should be rust- and vermin-proof with provision for door closure. Rodent barriers should be provided at all entry points of animal houses. The walls and ceilings should be free of cracks. The floors should be smooth, non-absorbent and skid proof.

The temperature and humidity in animal facilities should be controlled for the comfort of the laboratory animals. As far as possible the usage of smaller animal during the extreme weather conditions should be avoided. Proper lighting system with adequate illumination at cage level should be maintained in the animal room.

The animal cages should provide adequate space to permit freedom of movement and normal postural adjustments, and have a resting place appropriate to the species; provide a comfortable environment; have an escape-proof enclosure that confines animal safely; have easy access to food and water; provide adequate ventilation; meet the biological needs of the animals; keep the animals dry and clean, be consistent with species requirements.

However, aquatic animals like frogs and toads need to be kept in clean water free from chlorine and copper, preferably in containers attached to running tap water to prevent the accumulation of waste products. Houses, pens, boxes, shelves, perches, and other furnishings should be constructed in a manner and made of materials that allow cleaning or replacement in accordance with generally accepted husbandry practices. Physical separation of animals by species, wherever possible, is recommended to prevent inter-species disease transmission, eliminate anxiety, and possible physiological and behavioural changes due to inter-species conflict. Population density and group composition should be maintained as stable as possible, particularly for canines, non-human primates, and other social mammals. Animal facilities should be maintained free from pests and vermins.

Anaesthesia

The scientists should ensure that the procedures which are considered painful are conducted under appropriate anaesthesia as recommended for each species of animals. It must also be ensured that the anaesthesia is administered to sustain for the full duration of experiment, and at no stage the animal is conscious to perceive pain during the experiment.

Laboratory Anaesthetic Agents

Object: Choice of laboratory anaesthetic agents.

General anaesthetic agents bring about loss of all sensation particularly pain along with reversible loss of consciousness. Consciousness is regained after the agent is metabolised or excreted.

A general anaesthetic fulfills the following requirements:

(a) Induction of anaesthesia should be quick and pleasant.

(b) It must have longer duration of action.

(c) There should be adequate muscle relaxation.

(d) It should not interfere with effect of drug under study.

(e) It should be cheap and non-inflammable.

General anaesthesia of two types:

1. **Volatile general anaesthetics:** These could be liquid like ether, halothane, ethyl chloride, trichlorethylene, gases as N_2, O, ethylene and cyclopropane. They are not used commonly in experimental animals, because they require constant monitoring and costly instrument set up. Ethyl chloride is rarely used in experiments of rats and cats.

2. **Non-volatile anaesthetics:** These agents are more commonly used for producing anaesthesia in various animals, because it is easy to administer these agents and no complicated technique is required. Commonly used agents are: chloralose, urethane, barbiturates, $MgSO_4$, paraldehyde etc.

   (a) *Chloralose:* It is the compound of chloral and glucose prepared by heating equal parts of anhydrous glucose and chloral when both A chloralose (active form) and B chloralose (inactive form) are formed. Chloralose is the active form (A-chloralose) freely soluble in hot water, in alcohol and in ether and slightly soluble in cold water.

Dose: 80-100 mg/kg body weight 1% solute used given I.V routes.

Advantages:

1. It produces surgical anaesthesia lasting for 3-4 hrs.
2. Respiration and BP are not depressed so can be used in conditions where they have to be recorded.
3. Reflexes are not depressed.

Disadvantages:

1. Poor water solubility, so solution is prepared in lukewarm water or 10% propylene glycol or ether.
2. Large volume is needed.
3. Jerky movement are seen.
4. Unsuitable for rabbits where it produces narcosis instead of anaesthesia.

(b) ***Urethane (Ethyl carbamate):*** It is readily soluble in water giving a neutral solution. Usually 25% solution is used I.M. This is also suitable for acute non recovery type of experiments in dog, cat, rabbit and rats. Duration of action is 3–4 hrs. Frogs can be anaesthetised by keeping them covered in beaker containing 5–10% solution.

Advantages:

1. It does not affect reflexs, CNS, and respiration.
2. It is readily soluble in water.
3. Anaesthesia remains for 3–4 hrs.

Disadvantage:

1. Induction is slow so, injection of morphine 2mg/kg body weight is given, IM 30 mins before giving Urethane as pre-anaesthetic agent so induction is quick and smooth.
2. It has irritant nature, so animal feels pain.
3. Amount of solution injected to be large, so has to be given at various sites.
4. It has delayed toxic effect on liver and may also cause agranoulocytosis and pulmonary adenomas. Mice develop high incidence of lung tumours regardless of route of administration.

(c) ***Barbiturates:*** These are most commonly used agents.

Advantages:

1. Induction is very rapid and smooth with minimal excitation.
2. No pre-anaesthetic medication is required.

Disadvantages:

1. It produces depression of cardiovascular and spinal reflex, by interfering with nerve impulse transmission both in CNS and ganglia.
2. Muscle relaxation is inadequate therefore, mucle relaxants have to be given simultaneously.
3. Anaesthesia produced is of short duration, therefore small doses of these agents are to be injected at regular intervals.

They can be classified as:

(i) *Long acting barbiturates:* e.g., Phenobarbitone 10% aqueous solution is used. Dose 120–180 mg/kg. of body weight intraperitoneally.

(ii) *Short acting barbiturates:* e.g., Thiopentone sodium 2.5% aqueous solution in dose of 15-25 mg/kg. body weight is given I.V. duration of action is 20-30 minutes.

(d) ***Paraldehyde:*** It has wide margin of safety as it depresses only the cerebrum and not medullary centres. Dose 1 mg/kg. body weight I.P. or 2 mg/kg. body weight I.M. in dogs and cats.

(e) ***Magnesium sulphate:*** 20% solution in a dose of 5 ml/kg. intravenously produces anaesthesia for one hour, Calcium gluconate is used I.V. to counteract the depressant effect immediately. Its principle use is in producing euthanasia (mercy-killing).

Euthanasia (Painless killing)

When animals are killed at the end of the experiment it should be done by a humane method. The procedure should be carried out quickly and painlessly in an atmosphere free from fear or anxiety. The choice of a method will depend on the nature of study, the species of animal and number of animals to be sacrificed. The method should in all cases meet the requirements as:

(i) Death, without causing anxiety, pain or distress with minimum time lag phase.

(ii) Minimum physiological and psychological disturbances.

(iii) Compatibility with the purpose of study and minimum emotional effect on the operator.

(iv) Location should be separate from animal rooms, method should be reliable, safe to the personnel, simple and economical.

Methods of Euthanasia

1. **Chemical Method:** It is the painless death produced by administration of chemical poisons. Certain chemicals are injected and there are:

   (i) Magnesium sulphate I.V./intra cardiac (15gm/kg. body weight)

   (ii) Chloroform.

   (iii) A large volume of air (/kg. body weight)

   (iv) Sodium citrate in large quantity (anticoagulant).

   (v) Paraldehyde and $MgCl_2$ can also be used.

   (vi) In open chest operations, adrenaline can be touched at the apex of ventricles—arrythmias will be started—death.

2. **Mechanical Method:** The quickest and commonest method for killing mice, rats, guineapigs and rabbits is stunning which is carried out by striking the dorsal part of head against the edge of table or sink. This leads to stiffening of all muscles followed by a series of convulsions and then gradual relaxatation of the limbs and the body. As a result of stunning, animals get sudden shock and temporarily becomes semiconscious—one should have practice to stun by a single hard stroke only. Multiple strokes do not comply with the principle of euthanasia.

Physiological Salt Solutions (PSS)

Object: To study the physiological salt solutions used in experimental pharmacology and various drug dilutions.

As animal experiments have to be done with isolated organs, it is necessary to use a certain number of physiological solution of different ionic concentration, which almost act as a substitute to the tissue fluid. Those provide isotonicity, nutrition and acts as a buffer when drugs are added. It was "Ringer" who first introduced the idea that tissue could be kept alive by providing proper nutrition, O_2 and temperature.

PSS can be defined as artificially prepared solution to keep isolated tissue alive under experimental conditions. The content of these solutions carries according to tissues and animals taken. These solution provide food material, i.e., energy, O_2, electrolytes as in the same proportion as that present in tissue fluid. They exert same osmotic pressure as that of interstitial fluid, i.e., isotonic with body fluids. Any variant from the principle will lead to shrinkage or blotting depending on hypertonicity and loss of physiological function.

For these, two points should the kept in mind:

(a) Solution should be prepared carefully with pure materials.

(b) These can be kept for about 24 hrs. As these are good media for the growth of microorganisms these must be refrigerated and should be freshly prepared after 24 hrs.

Some points should be carefully noted at the time of preparation of solution:

1. **Balance of cations:** Absolute quantity of each ion and prepartion among each other especially with Ca^{+2} and K^+ must be maintained. The common cations and their significance are:

   (a) Na^+ ions: responsible for maintenance of excitability, contractivility and rhythmicity of muscles and nerves.

   (b) K^+ ions: responsible for increased relaxation of heart, increased neuromuscular transmission and excitability of nerves.

   (c) Ca^{++} ions: increase force of contraction and tone of heart and decrease excitability of nervous tissues.

   (c) Mg^{+2} ions: responsible for contraction of smooth muscles

2. **pH of solution/reaction of solution:** pH of various PSS varying from 7.3-7.8 depending upon organ. At lower pH value, tone of preparations tend to decrease and effect of drug is also altered. pH affects tissue directly and by

ionisation. At higher pH, ionisation is less and leads to alkalinity and thus improves cardiac and smooth muscle activity. During experiment there can be accumulation of metabolite which may change the pH. Buffering agents like HCO_3 and PO_4 are added in saline solution and solutions are changed frequently.

3. **Glucose:** Introduced by "Locke" and serves as an energy-source, increases contractility of tissue. It is not essential constituent for amphibians tissue but indispensable for mammalian tissues.
4. **Distilled Water:** It acts as a vehicle to dissolve various ingredients.
5. **Control of temperature:** In order to get consistent effect, it is important to maintain the temperature of PSS, particularly for mammalian tissue. For instance, when temperature of solution is below 370°C tone of intestine is decreased, increased—the contracts become smaller and contracts and relaxation time increases. Whereas, amphibaian tissues survive for longer time at room temperature only.
6. **Areation:** Air, O_2 or O_2 + 5% CO_2 is needed for the proper functioning of the tissues. Besides providing O_2 for the tissues, the stream of gas bubbles also stirs the solutions in the bath—thereby facilitating diffusion of the drugs.

The solution in the bath should be changed frequently because prolonged areation tends to alter pH.

Different physiological salt solutions and their uses:

(i) Ringer lock's solution: It is used in isolated rabbit heart perfusion.

(ii) Frog's Ringer's solution: Used in frog's rectus abdominis muscle and leech dorsalis muscle preparation.

(iii) Tyrode's solution: It is used in experiment of rabbit intestine and guinea-pig ileum.

(iv) De-jalon's solution: Used in rat uterus, duodenum-colon experiment.

(v) Kreb's Henseleit solution: Used in guinea-pig tracheal chain preparation and rabbits aortic strip preparation.

Commonly used Instruments in Experimental Pharmacology

1. Dale's organ bath
2. Sherrington's research kymograph
3. Levers
4. Onchometer
5. Jackson's enterograph
6. Marey's tambour
7. Piston recorder
8. Mercury manometer
9. Arterial cannula
10. Venous cannula
11. Tracheal cannula
12. Murphy's drip
13. Bulldog clamp
14. Von Frey's hair asthesiometer
15. Syringes
    (i) Simple glass syringe
    (ii) Tuberculin syringe
16. Rat holder

Effective dose

An effective dose in pharmacology is the amount of drug that produces a therapeutic response in 50% of the subjects taking it; sometimes also called ED-50.

In Pharmacology, effective dose is the median dose that produces the desired effect of a drug. The effective dose is often determined based on analysing the dose-response relationship specific to the drug. The dosage that produces a desired effect in half the test population is referred to as the ED–50, for "Effective dose, 50%".

Lethal dose or LD_{50}

The median lethal dose, or LD_{50} (originally abbreviated as DL_{50} for *Dosis letalis*, 50%) is a test used in animal experiments. It was designed by the British pharmacologist J W Trevan in 1927. LD_{50} is the dose of any substance tested required to kill half the number (50%) of test animals. The animals are usually rats or mice, although rabbits, guinea-pigs, hamsters, and so on are sometimes used.

The test shows how much of a substance must be taken before it becomes deadly. For example, a rat must be fed 50 mg of nicotine per kilo of body-weight before it dies.

Various forms of LD_{50} test include feeding the substance by mouth, applying it on the skin, and injecting it into veins, muscle tissues or the body cavity.

Animal rights activists oppose LD_{50} animal testing because the death from poisoning is slow and painful. The LD_{50} test is also controversial among scientists because of doubts about the usefulness and reliability of the results it gives. Some types of LD_{50} test, especially oral, have been phased out or banned in the UK.

Biotransformation and Excretion of Drugs

The term biotransformation of drugs can be defined as the chemical conversion of drugs to other compounds in the body. These conversions are usually mediated by enzymes in the body's organs, tissues, or biofluids, but occasionally they may occur by non-enzymic reactions and even by a combination of both enzymic and non-enzymic processes. Synonymous with biotransformation in this context is the word metabolism, and indeed the terms drug biotransformation and drug metabolism are used to describe the same events and are often interchanged, seemingly somewhat randomly. If anything, the latter is the more popular term.

Compared to the established scientific disciplines, the study of the biotransformation of drugs constitutes a relatively new subject area: the earliest scientific papers are little more than a century old. Regarded by many as a branch of pharmacology, drug biotransformation more properly belongs to biochemistry. However, knowledge of the biotransformation of drugs often contributes, in no small way, to a better understanding of pharmacologic, toxicologic, and clinical phenomena, and papers on drug biotransformation are to be found in journals specialising in these other subjects as well as those of biochemistry and chemical analysis.

A leading pioneer in drug biotransformation research was the late R. T. Williams, who wrote Detoxication Mechanisms, the first major text on the subject published in 1963, and a classic to this day. Subsequently, the literature on drug biotransformation grew steadily until recent years, when it seems to have expanded almost exponentially. The major driving forces for this proliferation include the realisation of the importance of drug biotransformation knowledge in promoting a better understanding of certain pharmacologic, toxicologic, and/or clinical findings; governmental legislation requiring drug biotransformation studies as part of new chemical entity safety evaluation programs; major advances in the necessary scientific instrumentation; and the commercial availability of isotopically labeled compounds, whose use can greatly facilitate drug biotransformation studies.

Bioavailability of Drugs

In pharmacology, bioavailability is a measurement of the extent to which a drug reaches the systemic circulation. It is denoted by the letter F.

Bioavailability refers to the extent to and rate at which the active moiety (drug or metabolite) enters systemic circulation, thereby accessing the site of action.

In Pharmacology bioavailability is used to describe the fraction of an administered dose of unchanged drug that reaches the systemic circulation, one of the principal pharmacokinetic properties of drugs. By definition, when a medication is administered intravenously, its bioavailability is 100%. However, when a medication is administered via other routes (such as orally), its bioavailability decreases (due to incomplete absorption and first-pass metabolism) or may vary from patient to patient (due to inter-individual variation). Bioavailability is one of the essential tools in Pharmacokinetics, as bioavailability must be considered when calculating dosages for non-intravenous routes of administration.

The effect of trituration on thermal degradation of sugar of milk can be studied by using a thermogravimetric analyser. A correlation between the rate of degradation with increased potency observed up to 600°C suggests that the vehicle plays an important role in the bioavailability of the drug. It can be compared between machine and hand triturated sugar of milk. For lower potencies (up to the 2x) machine triturated sugar of milk is found to degrade faster than hand triturated sugar of milk, whereas, at higher potencies, hand triturated sugar of milk showed faster degradation as compared to machine triturated sugar of milk.

Mechanism of Drug Action

Unlike allopathic medicines, there is no proven mechanism by which homoeopathy works. Allopathic drugs work by the interaction of the drug with systems in the body, but that cannot be the case in homoeopathy. Many of the homoeopathic medicines are so diluted that according to the known laws of physics and chemistry, they couldn't possibly have any effect. Once you get beyond a certain point—24x or 12c—there is probably not even one single molecule of the original active substance remaining. This fact is often pointed to by critics of homoeopathy as they dismiss the effect of homoeopathy as merely due to placebo effect.

And yet, according to homoeopathic principle and experience, the more diluted the solution, the more potent it is. Homoeopaths contend that the medicines work—and they see no reason to stop using them simply because we do not understand how they work. They often argue that pharmacologists cannot explain exactly how most conventional drugs work. For example, even aspirin is not fully understood in terms of how it works, but physicians have no difficulty in recommending its use. Over the years several theories have been proposed to explain the action on homoeopathic potentisation.

We are now in a position to provide a rational and scientific explanation to the molecular dynamics of homoeopathic cure. It has been known that low potency and high potency medicines contain different classes of active principles, and, hence, their mode of actions are also entirely different.

A drug means a sample of substance containing chemical molecules, that can interact with biological molecules, effecting deviations in biological processes.

Normally, when a drug substance is introduced into an organism, the constituent drug molecules exhibit their action as:

1. Acting on various structural membranes, deranging their permeability.
2. Engaging in chemical reactions with various molecular substrates and metabolites inside the body.
3. Interacting with enzyme proteins, and other complex biomolecules, thereby inactivating or incapacitating them for biochemical processes.
4. Interaction with various structural proteins.
5. Interacting with carrier proteins.
6. Interaction with ion channels.
7. Binding to hormone receptors, and neurotransmitter receptors.

But the therapeutic properties of highly potentised homoeopathic medicines cannot be explained by any of these ways. Once we admit that there is not any chance of a single drug molecule being present in the higher homoeopathic potencies, we will have to seek some other models of drug action entirely different from those described above.

The Arndt-Schultz Law

Attempts to explain the properties of higher homoeopathic potencies basing on the phenomenon of 'hormesis' had been done by some people earlier. This phenomenon was proposed by Southam and Ehrlich and Stebbing. They proposed that a substance which acts as a toxin in high concentrations, acts as a stimilant in low concentrations. This phenomenon is known as 'hormesis'. There is a theory known as Arndt-Schultz rule or Schultz' law to explain this phenomenon. The

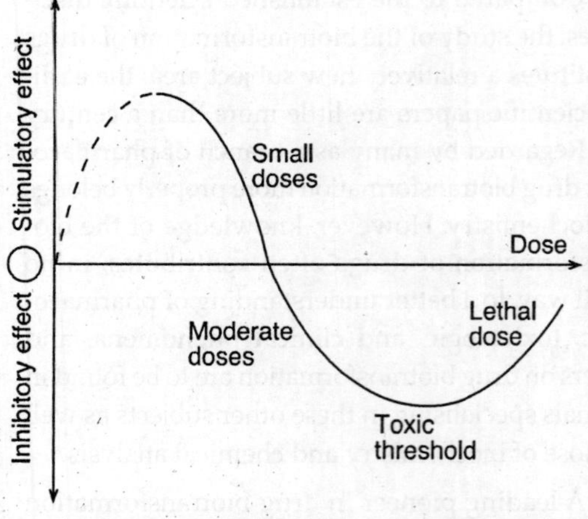

Fig. 27.1: Graphical representation of the Arndt-Schultz Law

Arndt-Schultz law is an early pharmacological law: 'for every substance, small doses stimulate, moderate doses inhibit, large doses kill' as shown in the diagram. The Arndt-Schultz Law states the homoeopathic principle of dilutions; homoeopathy operates in the area where stimulation occurs, whereas allopathy operates in the inhibitory area of dosages.

Over a century ago Schultz's experiments (1888) showed that many chemical agents had the effect of stimulating the growth and respiration of yeast. The phenomenon became known as the Arndt-Schultz Law and was widely referred to in the pharmacological literature for over 30 years and became one of the scientific principles.

Hueppe (1896) at about that time made similar observations on bacteria, apparently unaware of Schultz's experiments. His generalisation became known as Hueppe's Rule. Long before them both, the German alchemist and physician Theophrastus Bombastus von Hohenheim (1493-1541), who coined for himself the name Paracelsus, had recognised with respect to the medical use of small amounts of toxic chemicals that their efficacy depended principally on the dose. Such ideas are perhaps more easily accepted nowadays, when it is in the experience of most to use the stimulatory effects of alcohol, caffeine or nicotine, all of which are toxic at high concentrations.

Much later Southam and Ehrlich (1943) studied the effect of a natural antibiotic in cedar wood that inhibits the growth of wood-decaying fungi. They found that subinhibitory concentrations of the antibiotic had the reverse effect and stimulated fungal growth. The term "hormesis" was coined to describe it.

Toxins in their highly diluted form stimulates biological processes. In their concentrated forms the toxins inhibit or kills the biological processes. But even today it has not been made possible to explain this phenomenon scientifically.

The experiments conducted in Utrecht University, undertaken by a team under the leadership of scientists, Roeland van Wijk and Fred A. C. Wiegant tried to explain homoeopathy on the basis of 'hormesis'. Even though these experiments succeeded in proving the therapeutic properties of potentised drugs to a certain extent, they failed to explain the phenomenon on the basis of 'hormesis', and to uncover the molecular kinetics of 'hormesis.

Allopathic medicine, with its emphasis on moderate drug doses, works in the inhibitory part of the scale. The result is seen in the typically inhibitory medicines produced: antihistamines, antibiotics, antacids, cough suppressants, and so on, laying the basis for the so-called 'suppressant' effect of drugs. The allopathic recommendation of dosing lies at the point ED-50, at approximately 50% of the maximum dose—while homoeopathy uses the threshold dose at the beginning of the dosage scale.

Homoeopathic Medicine, on the other hand, begins at the stimulatory end of the curve, and moves to the left, into the smaller and smaller dose range. Its emphasis is on the stimulation of the body's natural balancing mechanisms, as seen in its philosophy of the natural regeneration of the body through rebuilding of vitality, a concept also in close agreement with naturopathic thought.

Homoeopathy—thanks to the work of Boyd in the early forties—works in accordance with the Arndt-Schultz law. Boyd found that while large doses of mercuric chloride inhibited the enzyme activity of malt distase homoeopathically prepared 61x solutions of mercuric chloride actually accelerated the activity of malt diastase—while the control of distilled water showed no inhibition or acceleration of enzymatic activity.

The D8 effect is a phenomenon that occurs in homoeopathically prepared solutions of differing potencies. Studies conducted have shown that 'the relation between amount of agent and effect is not

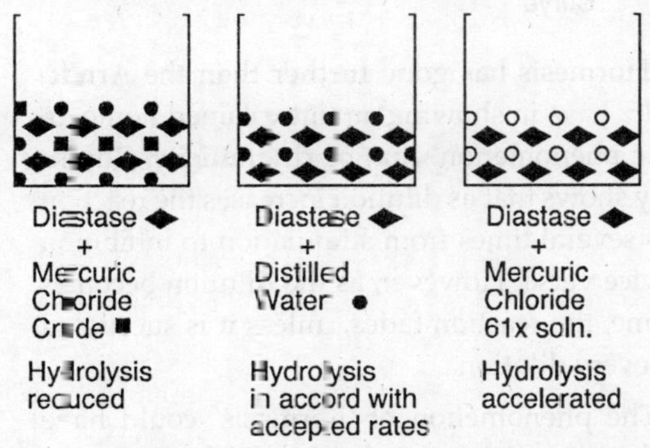

Fig. 27.2: The activity of malt diastase

linear'. The graph of effect against potency showed a maximum effect at the D8 potency; allopathy would predict that there would be the maximum effect at a much higher potency.

One of the results of the D8 effect and Arndt-Schultz Law—and also the high dilutions—is that homoeopathic remedies are not dangerous to healthy people or animals. Because of this, homoeopathic remedies can be given to animals in their drinking water, and if any other animals are to drink the treated water, they would not be affected, and the same is true for human homoeopathic remedies.

Hormesis is a relatively new subject—and many studies are incomplete—springing from the Arndt-Schultz Law, and studies began in the 1960s on the toxic effects of poisons at low dosages. Hormesis is, in fact, a phenomenon that demonstrates the now almost-forgotten Arndt-Schultz Law, that toxins have a stimulatory effect at low levels, and inhibitory effect at high doses.

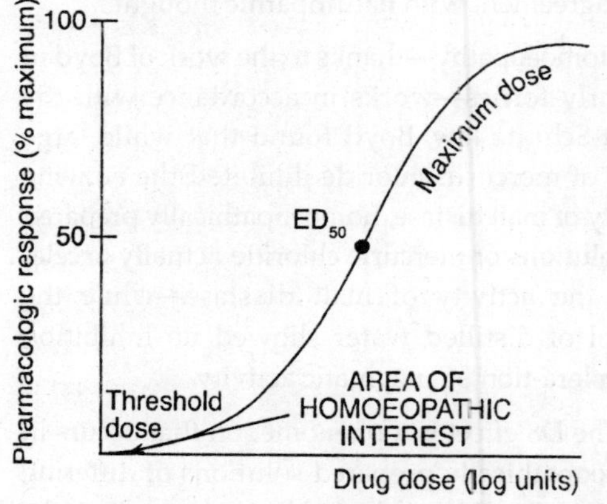

Fig. 27.3: A typical pharmacological dose—Response Curve

Hormesis has gone further than the Arndt-Schultz Law, in showing an unexplained homoeopathic phenomenon, that of rhythmicity. Rhythmicity shows that as dilution increases the reaction alters several times from stimulation to inhibition and vice versa. However, as the dilution becomes extreme, the reaction fades, unless it is succussed after every dilution.

The phenomenon of 'hormesis' could have been better explained on the basis of 'hydrosomes' or 'molecular imprints' of drug molecules, which are likely to be formed in the highly diluted solution of a toxic substance.

Obviously, molecular tracking protocols used in modern medical research are not applicable in the study of movements and targetting of potentised drugs inside the organism, since there is no drug molecules present. As for now, there is no scientific technology available for this purpose to track the molecular imprints inside the organism. Rational analysis and deductions based on available understandings alone are possible in this respect.

Some homoeopaths believe that potentised medicines can only act upon the brain and mind, being transported through nervous system as nerve impulses, and the mind, in turn, induces the cure of disease. The fact that we can prove the medicinal properties of potentised drugs in vitro, where nervous system is not present, clearly negates this theory. The theory that homoeopathic potencies directly act up on 'vital force' as a 'dynamic power', and cures diseases from that plane, is also disproved by the fact that these drugs can exhibit their effects in vitro experiments, as in clotting of blood, or antibody-antigen interactions. A more rational and scientifically viable model is required to explain the therapeutic effects of high potency homoeopathic preparations.

Potentised homoeopathic medicines, when introduced into the organism by any route, is carried in the body fluids, and transpoted to different parts of body. When they come in the vicinity of pathological foreign molecules, having similarity to the molecular imprints (complementary configuration) contained in them, these molecular imprints selectively bind to the pathological molecules. By this process, pathological foreign molecules are prevented from establishing contact with biological molecules, thereby relieving the biological molecules from pathological molecular blocks. This can be described as some sort of molecular scavenging or entrapping of pathological molecules, by hydrosomes or molecular imprints contained in the potentised medicines.

Energy Storage

Since Benveniste—who still stands by his theory of the memory of water—investigations have continued and one possible way that homoeopathic dilutions work is to be found in the field of biophysics.

Theoretical research has shown that the effect of homoeopathic remedies must come from the water that the solutions are made from, especially as there are no other molecules in the remedies except water molecules. All reactions, even biomolecular ones, require energy in order to occur, and that energy is contained within the reacting molecules. As a result, it is thought that homoeopathy works by the type of energy storage in the water molecules.

Water, along with all other molecules, stores energy in four quantised ways:

- In *translation*—the energy of moving the whole molecule from one place to another (also called kinetic energy).
- In *rotation*—the energy of spinning the whole molecule.
- In *vibration*—the energy of vibrating the molecular bonds.
- In *electronic excitation*—the energy associated with the electrons of the molecule.

Translational energy storage is the lowest energy required, and is the energy that triggers the majority of all chemical reaction, and is altered simply by collision between molecules, even if they are the same. For this reason it is thought to be too low to make homoeopathy work.

Electronic excitation, at the other end of the scale, is too high. In order to excite electrons, visible- or better still, ultraviolet-light is needed. Rotational energy is thought to be too low an energy. The frequency needed to rotate water molecules is 2.45×10^9 Hz, the frequency of a microwave —approximately 1.62×10^{-24} joules.

Vibrational energy, which lies between rotational and electronic energy, is an accepted means of storing energy in physics; it is also found in all three states of matter (gas, liquid and solid). It is now thought that succussion causes exchange of vibrational energy between the extract being diluted and the water. The water is left with a 'vibratory impact' that deepens with each further dilution as more and more succussion occurs.

The "image" of vibrational energy left on the water molecules differs with each extract used, as each extract has its own differing levels of vibrational energy; if a molecule absorbs energy it changes its shape according to the energy it has absorbed.

Homoeopathic remedies have been examined for structural changes (Callinan, P), which do appear. However, they only appear when the remedy has been prepared by succussion, and only when an extract has been used; a homoeopathic remedy cannot be made from water alone.

Ice crystal structures show the energy status of the water contained, and they effectively show the changes in structure in homoeopathic water, particularly where vibrational energy is concerned. As vibrational energy increases, the size of the ice crystals formed increases—and these largest crystals are to be found at the highest potencies of dilutions of homoeopathic remedies.

Benveniste—Champion or Charlatan

In one of the stranger episodes in the recorded history of scientific publishing, the prestigious British Research Journal **Nature**' recently published experimental results which, the editors say, they consider utterly impossible. The typically indigestible title of the paper is **"Human Basophil Degranulation Triggered by Very Dilute Antiserum Against IgE14"**, and the conclusions it proposes have been similarly indigestible to the medical community. The main players in the experiment were a special type of white blood cell known as a basophil and an antibody, IgE. When basophils are normally exposed to this antibody, their chemistry and internal structure change in a way that is easily checked by staining techniques. But what Benveniste and his colleagues found was that the changes occurred even when the antibody was used up to the 120x potency, a dilution at which it is virtually impossible for even one molecule of the antibody to remain. The results also showed the familiar rhythmic changes in basophil reactions as the potencies increased, a factor still unexplained, even by homoeopaths. The deputy editor of 'Nature' remarked that two centuries of observation and rational thinking about biology will have to be abandoned if the results stand, because they cannot be explained by existing physical laws.

The 13 member international research team headed by **Benveniste** conducted their experiments after being challenged by two eminent French homoeopaths to disprove homoeopathy once and for all, by conducting a sensitive, tightly controlled experiment in an accredited research centre. The centre chosen was at the University of South Paris, where Benveniste is a Research Director. "That was how it all started", he said. "They challenged us to prove them wrong, and we couldn't."

The furore surrounding this experiment has produced some unique reactions within the scientific community, and highlights an important question: how should the scientific establishment deal with anomalous findings which challenge the very roots of established thought? Nature journal had its own answer: it sent a fraud squad comprising one of its editors, a professional magician, and an investigator of scientific frauds from the USA to Benveniste's laboratories. Over a period of a week they criticised shortcomings in experimental design, studied the laboratory records, and interrogated the researchers. Finally, they failed to replicate the results in a double-blind trial, and declared the experiments "a delusion.". Benveniste, not unexpectedly, considered the investigation a witch hunt and an outrage. "I welcome any explanation for our findings" he said, "but not this kind of crap".

The homoeopaths of the world, together with interested onlookers, can be assured that the matter will not rest there. Further interesting reading on the bizarre reactions to homoeopathic experiments on the part of the scientific and medical establishments will surface. Benveniste will undoubtedly be back, with a more tightly controlled experiment which will probably decide, once and for all, the future of homoeopathy.

The Theory of High Dilutions

The Theory of High dilutions is a theory based on a new mathematical model and the quantum theory that has been put forward as an explanation to how homoeopathic remedies work. It was developed by a physician, Rolland Conte, a mathematician, Henri Berliocchi, and an allopathically trained doctor, Yves Lasne (who died in February 2001).

They observed changes in the infra-red spectrum of homoeopathic solutions—which should have the same infra-red spectrum as water—and when analysed with Nuclear Magnetic Resonance (NMR) data, the Cotonian frequency was developed. The Cotonian frequency is unique to each remedy, and produces quantifiable results. The Cotonian model is based on several quantum theories and involves more higher mathematics than is sensible to try and explain here. The mathematical theory uses Quantum Mathematics, as well as Berliocchi's Semiotic mathematics, which he deve-loped as part of his work on ethers.

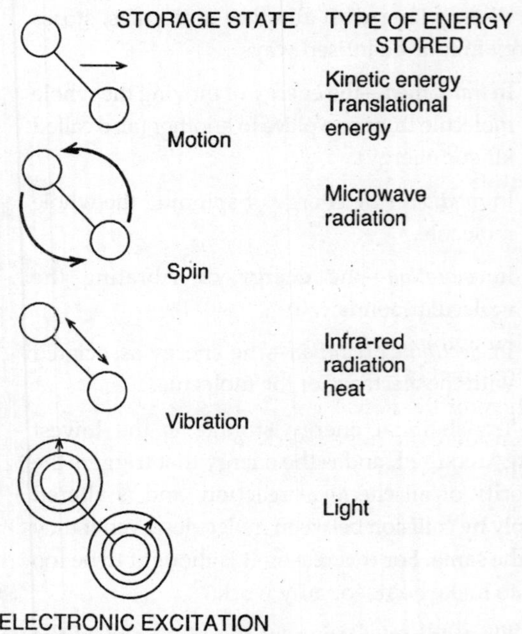

Fig. 27.4: Energy storage in molecules

The theory is that the disappearance of the extract molecules during dilution creates white holes in the solution; white holes are the opposite of black holes—the other side, as it were, of a spiral black hole through space-time—and are thought to be a small but nevertheless highly-energised area of space-time. These white holes are singularities that induce a remnant wave proportional to the amount of particles lost. With the regular appearance of singularities created by successive dilutions, a regular sequence of remnant waves is created, increasing the amplitude of the remnant wave. After a certain time, the wave energy is released as infrared radiation, and is easily measured.

The white hole and remnant waves trigger nuclear reactions that emit beta energy—which is associated with electrons—and also change the NMR data and the IR radiation. However, the nuclear reactions are known to have a low efficiency.

After the Avogadro limit is reached, at about 12°C, no more white holes can appear, as there are no molecules of the extract left to disappear. However, continued dilution and succussion stimulates hyperproton expansion. Hyperprotons are free protons with no mass or charge formed through the interaction of protons and white holes, which are thought to be able to pass in and out of space-time. Hyperprotons produce irradiation on matter surrounding them, and alter the structure of the water.

The Theory of Universal Wave Function was developed in order to explain the effect of high dilution on organisms. Toxic substances trigger disease indicated by vector and phase displacement, and treatment with a remedy containing the counteracting phase displacement restores health. Organisms have a continuous process of elimination within their cells—from metabolic reactions, presumably—that can create white holes, and therefore, remnant waves. Each organism can be considered to have its own remnant wave profile; illness disturbs this profile.

Conclusion

Homoeopathy is a discipline in medicine that is gaining status, perhaps not with some of the staunchest scientists, but certainly with doctors, vets and their patients. Some of homoeopathy's beliefs are a little incredible, hardly scientific explanations of what are undoubtedly scientific phenomena. However, it must be considered that, when some of those philosophies were formulated, the concept of a "vital force", even to a scientist, was entirely possible.

Homoeopathy is very different from allopathy—in both its belief system and its methods. However, there are a few similarities—both allopathic and homoeopathic drugs can be formed from plant or mineral extract, as the drugs used for heart failure show. Homoeopathic remedies, despite the obvious downsides that they take slightly longer to take effect, and that there is always the chance that, for that particular animal or person, they might not work (as is possible with allopathic medicines as well), have no side-effects. Homoeopathic remedies, because they use only a small amount of plant extract and water as their basic ingredients, are also inexpensive to produce, and often cheaper than allopathic drugs.

The theories as to how homoeopathy works are many and hugely different at times. They tend to use more and more biochemistry—and in the case of the High Dilution Theory—biophysics.

A lot of the problems that science has with accepting homoeopathy are that, by the rules of allopathic science, it should not work. However, placebo-controlled tests and isolated cell tests—with the exception of Benveniste's tests—show that homoeopathic remedies do work and there is pharmacological evidence to support it. There is no reason why homoeopathy should work along allopathic lines; as Mark Twain said: 'The reason why truth is so much stranger than fiction is that there is no requirement for it to be consistent.'

In *Theory of Energy Storage* to the *Theory of High Dilutions*—there seems to be more evidence for the former and you don't need a PhD in Quantum Mathematics to really understand it. Both theories work on the basis that homoeopathy works, and certainly in the Theory of High Dilutions, that white holes can be formed in a certain way can produce certain effects. If in the future one of those assumed actions is proved to be wrong, then those theories will no longer be important.

One thing has become apparent, and makes a link between homoeopathic philosophy and theoretical mechanisms: resonance. The concept expressed by Vithoulkas on resonance, is echoed in both the Energy Storage and High Dilutions theories. In the latter, the remnant wave profile of the body is disturbed by illness. In Energy Storage, the homoeopathic remedies have their own vibrational energy. This indicates that there might be a little truth in all of those theories and philosophies. We will just have to wait for the proof.

Adverse Drug Reaction (ADR)

An adverse drug reaction may be defined as "An appreciably harmful or unpleasant reaction, resulting from an intervention related to the use of a medicinal product, which predicts hazard from future administration and warrants prevention or specific treatment, or alteration of the dosage regimen, or withdrawal of the product." Such reactions are currently reported by use of WHO's Adverse Reaction Terminology, which will eventually become a subset of the International Classification of Diseases.

An adverse drug reaction is a term to describe the unwanted, negative consequences sometimes associated with the use of medications. It is more precise than, and usually preferred in the medical field, over the term "side-effect" as these purported side-effects may sometimes be therapeutically useful.

While ADR is probably the most precise term to describe the concept, it is not widely used in the community since it may be perceived as jargon and because of the negative-associations with the term "Drug". Alternative terms with equivalent meaning to ADR include: side-effect, adverse event, adverse effect, etc.

Adverse events to homoeopathic drugs exist and are distinguishable from homoeopathic aggravations, but are rare and not severe.

Generally there are no side-effects of Homoeopathic Medicine if prescribed in potencies of 3CH and above. However, some tinctures and triturates in very low potencies like 1x, 2x have some side-effects of minor nature. There are no life threatening side-effects but any homoeopathic medicine should only be taken under the guidance of a homoeopath.

Homoeopathic Medicines in high dilutions, prescribed by trained professionals, are probably safe and unlikely to provoke severe adverse reactions. It is difficult to draw definite conclusions due to the low methodological quality of reports claiming possible adverse effects of homoeopathic medicines.

Chapter 28

The Technique of Homoeopathic Drug Proving (Section 105-145)

Historical Perspective

Albrecht von Haller (1708-1777), (a well known physician, botanist, poet and novelist) was the first known person, besides Hahnemann, who felt the need of testing medicines for their pure and peculiar effects in deranging the health of man, in order to learn what morbid state each medicine is capable of curing (F.N. to Section 108).

Albrecht von Haller recommends the following in his '*Pharmacopoeia Helvetica*,' Basel; Im Hof 1771, p.12. Haller describes "Indeed, a medicine must first of all be assayed in a *healthy* body *without any foreign admixture*. When the odour and taste of the medicine have been examined, a small dose of it must be taken, and attention must be paid to every change that occurs, to the pulse, the temperature, respiration and excretions. Then, having examined the symptoms encountered in the healthy person, one may proceed to trials in the body of a sick person."

Hahnemann was competent in different languages (he knew 14 languages) and used to translate many works of considerable significance. In 1790, whilst translating **"A Treatise on Materia Medica"** (second volume) by **William Cullen** who was a professor of Medicine at London University, from English to German, Hahnemann came across the statement made by Cullen in the book regarding the action of Cinchona bark in the cure of Malaria, i.e., by virtue of bitterness and the tonic effect on the stomach, the drug cured malaria. Cullen remarked: *"I have endeavored to explain in my first outlines of practical medical science, that the bark in this instance acts through its tonic effect on the stomach, and I have found nothing in any writings which could make me doubt the truth of my statements."*

But this statement did not satisfy Hahnemann as there were plenty of bitter drugs but not possessing the malaria curative power. He attacked this statement vigorously in his notes: *"By combining the strongest bitters and the strongest astringents we can obtain a compound which, in small doses, possesses much more of both these properties than the bark, and yet in all eternity no fever specific can be made from such a compound. The author should have accounted for this. The undiscovered principle of the effect of the bark is probably not easy to find."*

Then he thought of testing the positive action of Cinchona bark on his own body. Hahnemann therefore resolved to ascertain, by the natural method of experience, wherein lay the power of cinchona bark to allay intermittent fever. He says—

"I took for several days, as an experiment, four drachms of good Cinchona twice daily. My feet and finger tips, etc. at first became cold; I became languid and drowsy; then my heart began to palpate, my pulse became hard and quick; an intolerable anxiety and trembling (but without a rigor), prostration in all the limbs, then pulsation in the head, redness of the cheeks, thirst; briefly, all the symptoms usually associated with intermittent fever appeared in succession, yet without the actual rigour. To sum up: all those symptoms which to me are typical of intermittent fever, as the stupefaction of the senses, a kind of rigidity of all joints, but, above all, the numb, disagreeable sensation which seems to have its seat in the periosteum over all the bones of the body—all made their appearance. This paroxysm lasted from two to three hours every time, and recurred when I repeated the dose, not otherwise. I discontinued the medicine and I was once more in good health." i.e., Hahnemann experienced symptoms similar to malaria after taking this drug. He had discovered a great principle—The drugs cure diseases that they can produce on a healthy person. This event led to the development of a new therapeutic system—Homoeopathy.

Drug after drug, specific after specific, was tested by Hahnemann on himself and on his family and friends, all with one result—each remedy of recognised specific power excited a spurious disease resembling that for which it was considered specific. He verified his discoveries and observations by exploring volumes of recorded experiments on Materia Medica and history of poisonings.

Hahnemann made the induction that diseases which were cured by medicines are by the virtue of the power of the medicines to produce symptoms similar to those of diseases which it cured. After six years of careful study and observations he formulated the principle *"Similia similibus curantur"* (Let likes be treated by likes).

He published an article in 1796 in Hufeland's Journal (Vol II, parts 3 & 4, pages 391-439 and 436-561) under the title *"An Essay on a New Principle for Ascertaining the curative powers of Drugs"* in which he propounded the Homoeopathic therapeutic rule. In a few years more he was able to give an array of medicinal substances whose pure pathogenetic action he had ascertained by experiments on himself, his family, and few friends. The results of the laborious and painstaking experiments were published in 1805 in *"Fragmenta De Viribus Medica mentorum positivis sive Insano Corporo Humano observatis"*. It is the first published Materia Medica by Hahnemann. It was in Latin and published at Leipzig, Germany, and contains the pathogenesis of 27 drugs.

In 1805, he published his celebrated essay *"The Medicine of Experience"* and in this essay he details at length how experiments with medicinal substance are done in order to ascertain their pathogenetic effects.

After 6 years, in 1811 appeared the first volume of *"Materia Medica Pura"* containing 12 medicines, Volume II in 1816 with 8 medicines; Volume III in 1817 with 8 medicines; Volume IV in 1818 with 12 medicines, Volume V in 1819 with 11 medicines and Volume VI in 1821 with 10 medicines, of these medicines 22 were transferred from the Fragmenta.

Later, Die Chronischen Kranheiten (The Chronic Diseases, their peculiar nature and their Homoeopathic cure) (1828–1838) was published which contained 47 medicines.

Hahnemann conducted repeated experimental drug studies on himself and 64 volunteers whose names were listed in his Materia Medica Pura. In total he investigated 99 remedies over a period of about half a century, establishing the method which has came to be known as Proving (or testing) Medicines.

Developments in the field of Homoeopathic Drug-proving after Hahnemann

1. **Germany:** After Hahnemann, in the field of homoeopathic drug-proving, firstly appeared **Johann Christian Gottfried Jorg,** a professor of the University of Leipzig, Germany. He published at Leipzig in 1825 a first volume of the results obtained.

After that, two distinguished members of the homoeopathic school, Hartlaub and Trinks, took up the work of instituting and publishing drug-proving. Their work was published at Leipzig in 3 volumes, dated 1828, 1829, and 1831, respectively.

The next name on our list is that of **Johann Ernst Stapf** (1788-1860). This physician, one of

Hahnemann's oldest and most valued disciples, began in 1822 to publish a Journal generally known simply as the Archive, or very often 'Archive'. The whole work makes a very valuable volume and, it has been rendered into English by **Charles Julius Hempel** (1811-1879).

2. **Austria:** In Austria, from 1842 onwards, the Homoeopathic Society of Vienna undertook numerous reproving, as well as establishing new pathogenesis. Most of them have been translated into English with more or less completeness. All Austrians were forbidden by a strict law to send anything outside of Austria to be printed; hence not only Nenning, but all other Austrians appeared in our literature with only initials. Nenning's symptoms were obtained in the true way, viz., by proving on the healthy body.

3. **France:** In France, some indigenous proving were done by David Roth, Jahr, Antoine Petroz (1781–1859) of Paris, Ozanam, Teste, Molin, and Imbert Gourbeyre and published in the French homoeopathic journals.

4. **England:** In England, some medicines were proved by homoeopathic physicians.

John Henry Clarke (1853-1931) proved many important nosodes. He has the credit of introducing the following remedies in the Homoeopathic Materia Medica:

Pertussin, Morbillinum, Carcinosinum, Parotidinum, Epihysterinum, Scarletinum, Bacillinum testinum, Scirrhinum.

The proving of *Kali bichromicum* done by **Drysdale**, *Naja* by **Russell**, *Cedron* by **Casanova**, *Cotyledon umbilicus* by **Douglas Craig** (1901-1995), and the *Uranium nitricum* by **Edward Blake**.

5. **Spain: Jose Nunez,** (1805–1879) was a Spanish orthodox physician who converted to homoeopathy and received an Honorary Doctorate in 1867 from the Homoeopathic Medical College of Pennsylvania, to become one of the first Spanish homoeopaths, was the founder of the Hahnemann Society of Madrid, of the Homo-eopathic Institute and the San Jose Hospital, Honor President of Liga Medicorum Homoeopathica Internationalis. In 1864, Jose Nunez conducted a proving of *Tarantula hispanic.*

6. **Italy:** In Italy, Rocco Rubini (1805-1886) introduced the drug *Cactus grandiflorus.* The Cactus grandiflorus published by him in 1864 has been translated into all the languages, and at present forms a valuable part of every treatise of pure Materia Medica and of therapeutics.

7. **Brazil:** In Brazil, proving of plants and animal venoms (e.g., *Elaps, Crot-c, Hura,* and *Manc*) indigenous to that country was instituted by **Benoit Jules Mure** (1809–1858), author of *Provings of The Principal Animal and Vegetable Poisons of The Brazilian Empire,* published in English, 1854.

8. **America:** In America, some homoeopathic physicians contributed for the homoeopathic drug-proving. Honoured names among the American contributors to our Materia Medica, Constantine Hering (1800–1880), Timothy Field Allen (1837–1902), Edwin Moses Hale (1829–1899), James Tyler Kent (1849–1916), Charles S. Neidhard (1809-1895), Jacob B. Jeanes (1800–1877), Walter Williamson (1811–1870), Joslin, Carroll Dunham (1828–1877), Conrad Wesselhoeft (1884–1962). The chief investigation and collection of the drug-proving of the United States has proceeded from the American Institute of Homoeopathy (AIH).

(a) **Constantine Hering (1800–1880):** He proved 72 drugs, out of which the followings are most important ones: *Lachesis, Cantharis, Colchicum, Iodum, Mezereum, Sabadilla, Sabina, Psorinum, Nux moschata, Crotalus, Apis mel, Hydrophobinum, Phytolacca, Platina, Glonoine, Gelsemium, Kalmia, Ferrum met, Fluoric acid, Phosphoric acid* etc. Hering describes the **five steps** involved in drug-proving protocol in the preface of Vol. 1 of his ***'Guiding Symptoms of Homoeopathic Materia Medica'*** (1892). They are:

(i) **Probability:** When a symptom occurs in a proving, there is first a certain probability that it belongs to the remedy picture.

(ii) **Confirmation:** When several volunteers have the same symptom during their proving.

(iii) **Corroboration:** Which means to look for physiological or pathological effects of the drug, when taken as a raw substance, i.e., by accidental poisoning or otherwise.

(iv) **Verificaiton:** When a clinical verification is made by seeing if the remedy cures when given according to symptom similarity to seek patients having the same symptoms.

(v) **Characteristics:** When the symptom is consistently verified by clinical cures, then it becomes characteristic of that remedy.

(b) **Timothy Field Allen (1837-1902):** Of New York in the USA, contributes Encyclopedia of Pure Materia Medica in 10 volumes with the active cooperation of Richard Hughes.

(c) **Edwin Moses Hale (1829-1899):** A new fountain of Materia Medica was opened in 1865 by E.M. Hale, of Chicago. The result was the volume entitled *'New Remedies in Homoeopathic practice'*.

(d) **Richard Hughes (1836-1902) and Jabez Philander Dake (1827-1894):** They compiled and edited a Homoeopathic Materia Medica called *'A Cyclopedia of Drug Pathogenesy'* (1888), included 412 medicines but Richard Hughes in his *'A Manual of Pharmacodynamics'* (1868) included only 300 medicines.

(e) **James Tyler Kent (1849-1910):** Of New York in the USA, proved many new medicines, which he has described in his books *New Remedies, Clinical cases, Lesser Writings, Aphorisms and Percepts.*

Kent's view of Drug-proving:

(i) A master prover is decided upon, who will prepare for the proving a substance unknown to the class and to all the provers, known only to himself.

(ii) Potentise it to the 30th potency, putting a portion of that potency into a separate vial for each member.

(iii) The provers do not know what they are taking, and they are requested not to make known to each other their symptoms.

(f) **Prof. Howard Perry Bellows (1852-?):** In the United States, the proving technique was perfected by the use of placebos as control during proving and reproving. In two reproving of *Belladonna* carried out in Boston in 1906, one by the American Homoeopathic Ophthamological and Otorhinolarygological Society and second conducted under the direction of **Howard P. Bellows** (three reproving of *Belladonna* conducted by him), the general instruction for the conduct of proving specify without any ambiguity, the use of placebos, double blind technique and cross-over studies.

(g) **Francois Lamasson (1907-1975):** The former President of the International Homoeopathic Medical League, has discussed the experimental conditions which should apply in modern proving. In the *Annales Homoeopathiques Francaises* of 1965, he insists on the necessity of single or double blind technique, on varied subjects, using a range of dilutions, and at different times of the year.

(h) **William Gutman (1903-1991):** The **International Institute for Homoeopathic Research** chaired by the late **William Gutman** of New York put forward certain recommendation s for the conduct of proving.

History of Homoeopathic Drug-proving in India

The idea of proving indigenous drugs of India first originated in the mind of S. C. Ghose in1886 as he found that it is very unfortunate that the homoeopaths of India have done nothing to add to the dignity and usefulness of homoeopathy. So he proved *Ficus religiosa* in 1887, without any assistance or friendly advice of the homoeopathic fraternity of India, except the help of L. Salzer, of the university of Vienna, came to Kolkata and voluntarily encouraged and appreciated him. He was fortunate enough to win the sympathy and active cooperation of several eminent foreign homoeopaths, notably Cowperthwaite, Hughes, H. C. Allen, Nash, Halbert, Dudgeon, E. H. Porter, Clarke, Shedd and others.

S. C. Ghose proved several new indigenous drugs of India and and gave them to his patients in low potency with great results. These proving were incorporated by J. H Clarke in his *'Dictionary of Practical Materia Medica'*.

S. C. Ghose compiled a book named *'Drugs of Hindustan'* in which proving of 51 Indian drug are included. Unfortunately, nobody noticed this book until 1970-1971, when the "Central Council for Research in Indian Medicine and Homoeopathy" (CCRIM & H) unearthed the book and a number of drugs were proved.

Pratap Chandra Majumdar (-1922) edited *'Indian Homoeopathic Review'* second oldest homoeopathic Journal in India. He along with D. N. Roy established Calcutta Homoeopathic Medical College in 1881 and came into the field of drug-proving and proved three or four indigenous drugs of India.

Pramada Prasanna Biswas of Pabna, Kali Kumar Bhattacharya of Coochbehar, have proved several indigenous drugs.

P. Sankaran conducted drug-proving on *Aqua marina, Hirudo officinalis, and Pituitaria glandula.*

Drug-proving now termed as Homoeopathic Pathogenetic Trials (HPT) are conducted now by Central Council for Research in Homoeopathy, (C.C.R.H) since the emergence of Homoeopathy the process and and methodology of HPTs have improved greatly.

Proving conducted by

S. C. Ghose: Ficus religiosa, Nyctanthes arbortristis, Justicia adhatoda, Terminalia arjuna.

D. N. Roy: Abroma augusta, Saraca indica or Jonosia asoka.

Pramada Prasanna Biswas: Andersonia or Amoora rohitaka, Andrographis paniculata, Aegle folia, Oldenlandia herbacea, Trichosanthes dioica.

Pratap Chandra Majumdar: Azadirachta indica.

Kali Kumar Bhattacharya: Caesalpinia bonducella, Atista indica, Gentiana or Swertia chirata.

Definition of Drug-proving

'Drug-proving' is the process of acquiring a knowledge of instruments intended for the cure of the natural diseases (§105).

It is the systematic and orderly way of investigating the pathogenetic power of a medicine on a healthy person. By 'drug-proving' we mean the positive effects of drugs upon living organism, i.e., to know the pathogenetic effects of the drug. Drug-provings are experiments with drug substances on healthy human beings to note the disease-producing powers known as 'curative powers' of the particular drugs.

Pre-requisition (essentials) of Drug-proving (Ref. H. A. Roberts)

1. *Drug:* The quality of the drug must be pure, it must be free from all mixture with other drugs, and it must possess all its active properties.
2. *Prover:* The prover must possess the proper balance in functions and be in a normal, healthy state, so that we can estimate and weigh the amount of the disturbance caused when we deliberately upset the balance of health.
3. *Environment:* The circumstances surrounding the prover must be those of his normal surroundings.

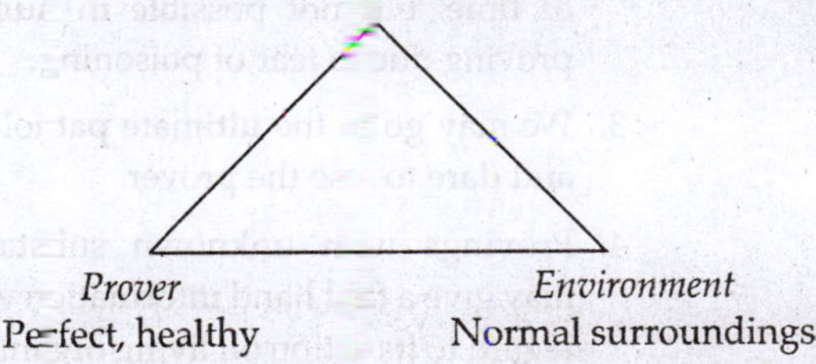

Objects of Drug-proving

1. To know the pathogenetic effect, i.e., disease-producing effect upon healthy human beings.
2. To observe and record the alterations of the normal sensations by the production of subjective symptoms.
3. To observe and note deviations in the appearance of the surface, changes in the tissues, organs, changes in the physiological functions etc.
4. To produce the characterisitcs of the drug as they manifest in the disease states.
5. To assay the physiological action of drugs.

Selection of Prover

A. Animal proving

(a) **Disadvantages:** Proving on lower animals should not be done due to defects as:

1. Subjective and mental symptoms cannot be studied as they cannot express themselves by speaking.
2. Modalities and finer sensations are lacking to make a symptom complete.
3. The effect of same drug on animals and on humans are different.
4. Proper individualisation of the knowledge of drugs is never possible on animal provings.
5. The question of susceptibility and idiosyncrasy is difficult to judge from animal provings.

(b) **Advantages**

1. The drug may be proved in any quantity, but not possible in human proving due to the toxicological effects of drugs.
2. The drug may be proved for any length of time, but not possible in human proving due to fear of poisoning.
3. We may go to the ultimate pathology and dare to lose the prover.
4. Provings with unknown substance may give a first hand information with regard to its action on living organism.

B. Human proving

(a) **Proving on sick persons (§107) should not be done because:**

1. The true effects of medicine can seldom be distinctly observed as the symptoms of the natural disease and the peculiar alterations of medicine are mixed up, even though they be administered singly and alone.
2. In diseased state the person may be hypersensitive or hyposensitive and so the intensity of the symptoms may be increased or decreased accordingly.
3. If accidentally the symptoms of the medicine are similar to his disease, he will be cured or partially relieved. Neither the symptoms of the disease nor of the drug shall be visible externally.
4. If the drug used is of opposite nature to his disease, it shall bring temporary relief.
5. If the drug is dissimilar to the disease, either there will be no effect or will form a complex disease.

(b) **Proving on healthy human being (§108):**

The best possible way of ascertaining the pure and peculiar effects of medicines is to make a proving by administering several medicines experimentally, on healthy human beings, in moderate doses.

Advantages: Except the negligible amount of disadvantage, human proving serves all our purposes. They are:

1. Subjective and mental with their modalities and concomitants may only be recorded in the human proving.
2. From such proving we get pure and accurate pathogenetic effect of medicine, which help to cure the natural disease on the basis of symptom similarity.
3. Administration of medicine on healthy human being gives response properly according to the full capability of the vital force.

4. **Peculiar characteristic of the drug**—the rare unusual symptoms that distinguish it from all others is only possible during human proving specially from this susceptible one.

(c) **Qualities of human prover:**

1. ***Ideal prover:*** The qualities of an ideal prover are:
   (i) *Healthy:* The prover must possess sound health, free from disease, and individual can determine the effects of medicine very distinctly.
   (ii) *Intelligent.*
   (iii) *Delicate, irritable and sensitive* (§121).
   (iv) Lover of truth, temperate in all respects of delicate feelings, who can direct the most minute attention to his sensations (§137). He must avoid all over-exertion of mind and body, disturbing passions and distractions.
2. ***Best prover (§141):*** The healthy, unprejudiced and sensitive physician himself is the best prover.
3. ***Idiosyncratic prover:*** The idiosyncratic person is a best possible prover of the substance to which he is idiosyncratic.

(d) **Choice of prover:**

The medicines must be tested on both sexes—males and females, in different ages, and many individuals with various constitutions:

1. **Both males and females (§127):** Drug-proving must be done on both sexes, because of the following causes:
   (i) In order to reveal the alterations of the health they produce in the sexual sphere (§127).
   (ii) Males and females are different in anatomical, physiological and psychological sphere. So to treat the diseases of both sexes, we must know the pathogenetic power of medicines in the sexual sphere.
   (iii) Moreover, there are certain diseases which are specific for male and some for female. So, for the treatment of specific diseases, we must know the effects of drugs through drug-proving, on both sexes.
2. **Different ages:** Drugs should be proved in persons of different ages because of the following reasons:
   (i) Physical appearance, anatomical development and functions vary according to the age. We have to treat the persons of different age-groups. So we must be certain of the curative powers of medicines in different age-groups.
   (ii) There are diseases which are more common in certain age groups e.g., measles, whooping cough, rheumatic fever are common in children, whereas enlarged prostate and cataract are common in aged individuals.
   (iii) Susceptibilities and physical irritability varies with age.
3. **Many individuals (§136):** Drug-proving must be done on many individuals. All the symptoms peculiar to a medicine do not appear in one person, nor all at once, nor in the same experiment, but some occur in one person chiefly at one time, others again during a second or third trial (§134). So, in order to get the whole pathogenetic power of a medicine, proving should be done on many different individuals, varying in their corporeal and mental constitution (§136).

Method of preparation of drugs for proving (§123)

1. **Indigenous (native) plants:** They should be administered in the form of freshly expressed juice, mixed with a little alcohol to prevent its spoiling.
2. **Exotic (foreign) vegetables:** Exotic substances are prepared in the form of powder or tincture, with alcohol, when they were in the fresh state, and afterwards, mixed with a certain proportion of water.
3. **Salts and gums:** Salts and gums, however, should be dissolved in water just before being taken.

4. **Dry and weak medicinal substances:** Dry plants (esp. herbs) available only in dry state, are cut into small pieces and an infusion is made by pouring boiling water on it and are swallowed while still warm. Alcohol is not added because all expressed vegetable juices, and all aqueous infusion of herbs, rapidly passes into fermentation and decomposition, if preserved.

Dose and mode of administration

1. **Strong medicines:** Strong, heroic medicines are liable even in small doses to produce changes in the health even of robust persons (§121).
2. **Milder medicines:** Medicines having milder power must be given in more considerable quantities (§121).
3. **Weakest medicines:** Weakest medicines should be proved on healthy, delicate, irritable, sensitive persons, those are free from disease and are given in much larger quantities (§121).
4. **Mode of administration:** Potentised medicines should be given to the prover, on an empty stomach, daily from 4-6 globules of the 30th potency, moistened with a little water for several days (§128).

Only potentised (i.e., dynamic) medicine should be employed for proving purposes because:

(i) Most recent and advanced observation shows that the crude drug substance—when administered for proving—does not give idea about full amount of signs and symptoms. Many of the properties of a drug remains in the dormant or hidden form, but, by potentisation, the latent curative power of drugs are developed and roused into activity to an incredible extent.

(ii) Potentisation brings medicines to dynamic plane so that it can act on dynamic vital force.

(iii) Only potentised medicine when applied upon healthy organism produce generic (i.e., common dynamic) symptoms, which serve to distinguish from one class to another.

5. **More medicine if indistinct:** If the effects of dose are slight, a few more globules may be taken daily, until they become more distinct (§129) stronger and the alterations of the health become more conspicuous.

Recording of symptoms

(a) **Symptoms to be recorded during proving:**

(i) *Except narcotics:* Symptoms produced by primary action of all medicines are recorded, except narcotics (§114).

(ii) *Narcotic substances:* In case of narcotic substances, symptoms of secondary action are to be recorded (§113).

(iii) *Alternating actions:* Which are produced by some medicines are also to be noted (§115).

(iv) *Modalities (§133):* In order to determine the exact character of symptom the modalities are recorded. Which means slight intensification or decrease of symptoms in relation to time, position, weather etc. by various factors.

(v) *Any alternations from normal health:* Should be recorded (§138).

(vi) *Proving on sick persons (§142, F.N.-2):* Symptoms which, during the course of disease, might have been observed or never before, consequently new ones, belonging to the medicines.

(b) **How to note the above symptoms:**

(i) *Literate prover (§139):* he must note down distinctly the sensation, sufferings, accidents and changes of health he experiences at the time after the ingestion of the drug. The physician looks over the report in the presence of the experimenter immediately after the experiment is concluded or, if the trial lasts several days, he does this every day, so that everything is still fresh in his memory to question him about the nature of everyone of these circumstances.

(ii) *Illiterate prover (§140):* If the prover cannot write, the physician should enquire everyday concerning the nature of symptoms and the manner of their appearance. The physician must note down his sensations chiefly from voluntary narration without asking any leading questions.

(iii) *Physician is prover (§141):* When physician himself is prover, recording will be more accurate.

Physician is the best prover because of the following advantages:

(i) The physician knows with the greatest certainty the things he has experienced in his own person (§141). When the physician proves a medicine upon himself, then any uncertainty in respect of exact changes in health are entirely removed.

(ii) The medicinal qualities of all drugs lie in the changes of health he has himself undergone from the medicine he has proved, and the morbid states he has himself experienced from them becomes for him an incontrovertible fact (§141, F.N. 1).

(iii) By such noteworthy self-observation, the physician will himself be trained to be— what every physician ought to be— a good observer.

(iv) These experiments on himself promise to give him a reliable knowledge of the true value and significance of the instruments of cure that are still to a great degree unknown to our art (§141, F.N. 1).

(v) Well-conducted drug-proving never produces any injurious effect on health of the prover. On the contrary, experience shows that the body of prover becomes more resistant to disease by removing the external morbific influences. His health becomes more unalterable. He becomes more robust. Moreover, immune power are greatly increased against all kinds of infections (§141, F.N. 1).

Precautions to be taken during proving

A. Regarding the medicine

1. Medicines to be proven must be well-known and its purity, genuineness and energy are to be thoroughly assured (§122).

2. It must be taken in a perfectly simple, unadulterated form (§123).

3. Every medicinal substance must be taken quite alone and perfectly pure (§124).

   Only one drug should be proved at a time because the individual properties of the particular drug will be known, there will be no mixture of the symptomatology of the different drugs with suspicion of the sequential order of their appearance.

4. The medicines must not be given for several successive days in over-increasing doses, as too frequent repetition confuses the symptoms (§1[illegible]).

5. Administration of large doses of medicines should be avoided as they bring out secondary reaction but hurried appearance of primary symptoms unsuitable for study (§137).

B. Regarding the prover

1. **Medicinal restrictions (§124):** Those substances which have any medicinal property should not be taken on the same day, nor yet on the subsequent days, nor during all the time, we wish to observe the effects of the medicine.

2. **Dietetic restriction (§125):** During the whole period of experiment the diet of the prover must be strictly regulated:

   a) Nature of diet: Diet during proving should be purely nutritious and simple.

   b) Vegetables:

   (i) Allowed: young green peas, green French beans, carrots.

   (ii) Avoided: green vegetables, roots, all salads, herb soups and spices.

(c) Beverages: Tea, coffee, alcohol must be avoided by the prover during proving experiment.

3. **Mental restrictions (§126):**

(a) He must avoid all over-exertion of mind and body, all sorts of dissipation and disturbing passion.

(b) He should have no urgent business to distract his attention.

(c) He must devote himself to careful self-observation and not to be disturbed whilst so engaged.

(d) He must possess sufficient amount of intelligence to be able to express and describe his sensation in accurate terms.

When can a medicine be considered to have been thoroughly proved?

A medicine can be considered to have been thoroughly proved in the following conditions (§135):

1. It must be proved on suitable persons of both sexes and of various constitutions.
2. Subsequent experiments can notice little of a novel character from its action.
3. Almost always the same symptoms as had already been observed by others are exhibited during re-proving.
4. The symptoms most carefully recorded are complete with regard to their specific sensations, locations, modalities and concomitant factors—so that a complete individual picture of the drug has been established.
5. Clinically verified and has not exhibited any clinical symptoms even after repeating.

Relative demerits and merits of employing large and moderate doses (§137)

A. **Demerits of employing excessively large doses:**

1. The toxic and poisonous effects of the drug may develop.
2. The primary action of medicine will appear in such hurried confusion and with such violence that nothing can be accurately observed.
3. The symptoms of primary action will get mixed up with secondary action.
4. Drugs produce different types of symptoms in different doses (Ref: Carroll Dunham).

(i) In large doses, the medicines produce their own chemical action.

(ii) In small doses, the medicines produce generic action which give symptoms common to all members of a certain class of drugs.

(iii) In very small doses those produce 'specific action' which manifests the characteristic symptoms of the medicines.

B. **Merits of employing moderate doses:**

1. The symptoms of primary action are more distinctly observed.
2. The symptoms of primary action occur without any admixture of symptoms of secondary action or reactions of the vital force.

Other sources, besides drug-proving, to know the curative properties of drugs.

Drug-proving is the only reliable source to know the curative properties of drugs, but, however, we can acquire knowledge about the drugs to some extent through:

(a) Histories of poisonings, narcotics or any toxic substances (toxicology);

(b) Empirical sources;

(c) Chemistry;

(d) Biochemistry.

Explanation:

1. *Poisonings:* The symptoms collected from the cases of poisoning has been of immense value. Those have great curative properties. Those are occupied in materia medica as 'clinical symptoms'. These give information about the sphere of action, chemical action and common symptoms of a drug. Even poisonous substances, when used in minute quantity, produce finer

symptoms. The knowledge of toxic effect of a substance helps in the identification of power of a drug but not in obtaining complete knowledge of curative properties of it. Many dreadful poisons like Lachesis, Crotatus and other snake poisons, Arsenic, Stramonium, Croton tig etc. are found to be very useful homoeopathic medicines when they are given on their toxicological symptoms in minimum doses.

2. *Empirical:* Empirical knowledge gave only superficial view and did not help in acquiring the complete and rational knowledge about the curative powers of drug.
3. *Chemistry:* From the chemistry we got the general information about the authenticity, standardisation and active principles of drugs. Chemical action of a drug is different from its dynamic action. Chemical action produces only the common symptoms of the medicine. But it does not give a knowledge about dynamic properties of a drug.
4. *Biochemistry:* It gives information about the biochemical actions of drugs, which deals with the sphere of action of drugs on one or two systems or organs. As a result, this knowledge is suitable only for palliative treatment. In homoeopathy, only few drugs have been included because of their biochemical action.

Research on Drug-proving

1. **Proving of new-drugs:** proving of antibiotics, steroids and other modern drugs should be done over healthy human beings, in potentised form, to get many valuable data. These drugs may be effective in curing many obstinate and complicated chronic diseases. When well-selected medicines fail to produce any favourable effect, in continued fever, chloromycetin (i.e., chloramphenicol) cured the patient. In vertigo, potentised streptomycin are very useful. Equally good results are obtained from Aspirin in acute migrainous headache. So, we should get the full proving picture of these Isode group of drugs. If we get full picture of these drugs (i.e., steroids, antibiotics) we can easily combat the iatrogenic diseases coming from allopathic system.
2. **Proving and reproving of nosodes and sarcodes:** The nosodes and sarcodes which are not proved at all or partially proved and are empirically used, require thorough reproving or new proving. The nosodes and sarcodes have great role in curing chronic complicated and incurable diseases. Even in acute diseases, complete cure is unnecessarily delayed unless a dose of the indicated nosode is administered. The drugs like Thyroidinum, Insulin, Carcinosin, Lyssin, Scirrhinum, X-ray and bowel nosodes require proper proving or reproving.
3. **Proving on lower animals:** Homoeopathic drug-proving is not continued up to the stage of organic changes on healthy human being. Because, it may be hazardous on the life of a prover to continue proving till the end of organic changes. But to get a complete picture

Table 28.1: Differences between Fully-proved and Partially-proved Drug

Points	Fully proved	Partially proved
1. Method	Hahnemann's method of drug-proving of medicines	Toxicological, empirical, clinical observations
2. Symptoms	Wide range	Short range
3. Pathogenesis	Specific, dynamise (belonging to causes and idiosyncrasis both)	Specific only (belonging to diseases only)
4. Composition of symptoms	Generals, keynote, particular, and causes	Guiding symptoms and causes
5. Action	(i) Deep and all round (ii) Primary, alternating and secondary action	(i) Superficial (ii) Primary, local, focal and general actions
6. Relationship	With other remedies	No relationship with other remedies

Table 28.2: Sources of Drug Knowledge

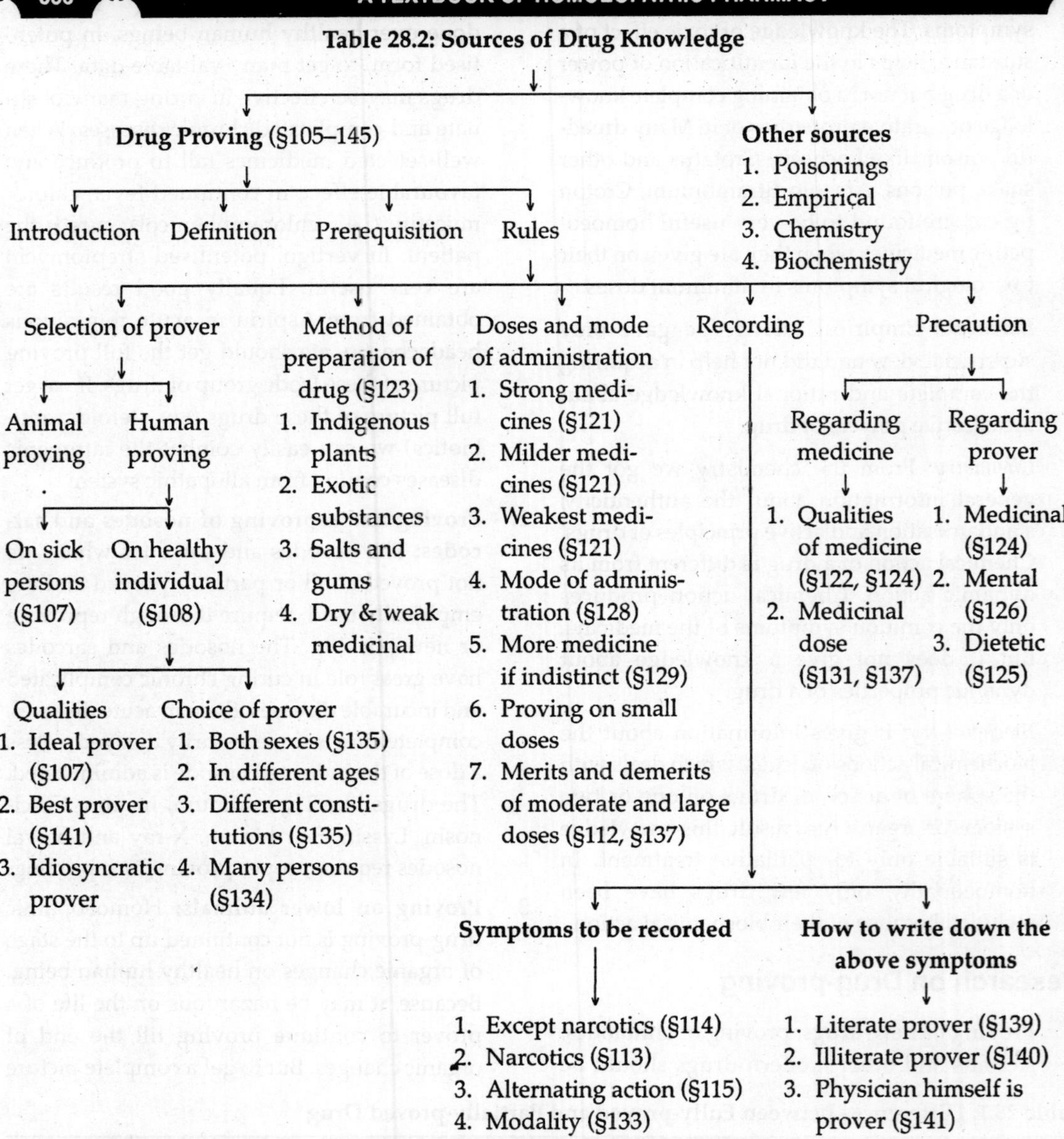

of a drug pathogenesis, we should know the various structural changes in different organs. So, there is no other alternative than to prove the medicines on lower animals. Only well-proved and fully proved drugs should be used for proving on lower animals to find out the organic changes (organic pathology), where the picture of dynamic pathololgy is known to us.

Methodological Flaws in Hahnemannian Drug-provings

1. **The absence of a control group as standard:** A control group is a very useful and widely used method of reducing bias. There are several features which introduce bias into trials that do not use control groups. These include temporal effects, which simply refer to the fact

that people change over time regardless of any intervention. In relation to HPTs, those who are healthy at the beginning of a trial may very well develop a whole range of symptoms during that trial that would have happened anyway and are not linked to the remedy being tested.

A number of studies have shown that many symptoms occur spontaneously in daily life even in the most apparently healthy groups of individuals, with up to a third of individuals reporting six or more symptoms in a 3 day period.

Observer expectancy effects are well-known in social science. People tend to see what they want to see or expect to see. Assessors and participants in HPTs are usually homeopaths and are likely to be predisposed to expect new symptoms to occur during such trials.

Symptoms recorded as new or different during the course of HPTs may be partly or entirely due to temporal effects, factors relating to selection and recruitment of participants, observer expectancy effects and other potential sources of bias. One useful way to determine whether effects are really caused by the remedy is to see whether they are qualitatively and quantitatively different in a group receiving the remedy in comparison to a control group not receiving the remedy. Alternatively researchers have also developed methodologies in which the participant forms his or her own control at different points of the trial.

2. **The absence of random allocation:** If it is accepted that control groups are essential for detecting real differences attributable to an intervention, then it is important to ensure that the control and the intervention groups are as similar as possible. It is widely accepted in the health sciences that random allocation is the only way to ensure this. Indeed some argue that random allocation is the essence of the RCT. Randomisation is by far the best way of controlling temporal changes, regression to the mean, and selection bias (selecting people who are different on some measures at the start and who are, therefore, likely to show different outcomes). There is good evidence that non-randomised trials yield consistently larger estimates of treatment effects than the randomised ones, although other studies have cast some doubts on this, and there remains uncertainty about the magnitude of any differences.

3. **The absence of blinding:** Trials that do not use blinding tend to show larger treatment effects than those that do. This is not surprising, unless both participants and investigators are blinded as to who is receiving the active intervention, people will react in ways which are biased towards a particular favoured outcome. The use of control groups and blinding are central features of modern pharmacological trials. Whilst these were not requirements in Hahnemann's times, those were introduced by later homeopathic researchers, and indeed, it can be claimed that those were significant innovations in these areas.

4. **The inclusion of trivial and pre-existing symptoms:** To know the pathogenetic effects produced by a remedy in HPTs close observation is certainly necessary. Such effects may be rare, subtle, and short lived, and will only be recorded if the volunteer applies careful attention and has good supervision. However, the daily and detailed recording which takes place in HPTs is highly likely to lead to the inclusion of many naturally occurring and pre-existing symptoms that a person becomes aware of. Because of the unusually close monitoring of the body and self required for the trial. Hawthorne effects refer to the tendency for people to change their behaviour when receiving the kind of special interest and attention which occurs when they are part of a trial. Hawthorne effects are known to be a significant non-specific effect of participation in trials, and the kind of close scrutiny which takes place in HPTs is only likely to increase this phenomenon. Again, the use of a control group receiving an identical placebo intervention will help to control Hawthorne effects by ensuring that they are spread equally between the two groups.

5. **Lack of definition of the healthy state:** Hahnemann grappled with this idea and admitted that health is relative, for instance, when he stated in Organon §126 that the

participant must be "in what is for him a good state of health". Whilst it has become a platitude that only healthy volunteers should be enlisted in HPTs, remarkably very few authors have defined what is meant by "healthy", or actually measured it in some way. From extensive health-related research it is known that even the healthiest among people experience day-to-day fluctuations in symptoms, and over the course of a trial these may give rise to significant background noise. Therefore, without careful checks and definitions of health, it is likely that some pre-existing symptoms of illness will be recorded as proving symptoms.

6. **The use of well-known acquaintances as volunteers:** There are good arguments for having volunteers in HPTs who have an understanding of homeopathy. They may be more likely to record the type of symptoms that are useful in homeopathic terms. It is perhaps for this reason that Hahnemann suggested in Section 141 of the Organon that experiments "which the sensitive physician experiences on himself" are the best of all. However, it is also the case that placebo effects are heightened in trials in which participants have strong expectations and, for example, believe strongly in the intervention on trial.

7. **The sudden prohibition of all medicinal drugs and foodstuffs:** We know that Hahnemann was very specific in this matter. However, we should be aware that an unintended consequence might be that volunteers who suddenly abstain at the start of a trial from what may be frequently consumed substances, may experience withdrawal symptoms and abstinence effects, and that such symptoms may be wrongly attributed to pathogenetic effects of the remedy.

Homoeopathic Pathogenetic Trial (HPT) versus Phase I Clinical Trials

1. **Similarities:** HPT is similar in conception to the Phase I clinical trials according to the FDA regulations developed in the 1960s.
   (i) Both trials comprise healthy provers (volunteers).
   (ii) Subjective and objective changes are observed in both trials.
   (iii) Both trials have multiple or more specific end-points.
   (iv) Controlled trial or placebo groups are applied in both trials to avoid any bias or influences in experimenter and provers.
   (v) Small number of subjects (20-100).

2. **Differences:**

HPT	Phase I Clinical Trial
1. **Dose:** Ultramolecular dose.	Pharmacological dose.
2. **Symptoms:**	
(i) Expecting more subjective and objective symptoms.	Close monitoring of objective changes (Lab tests).
(ii) The more reliable symptoms, the better.	The fewer symptoms, the better.
(iii) High level of detail for every reported symptom.	Raw symptoms.
3. **Reaction:** Tendency to produce type B reactions, but without serious effects.	Apt to produce type A reactions.

RECENT ADVANCES IN DRUG-PROVING

Drug-proving now termed, as Homoeopathic Pathogenetic Trials (HPT) is a process in which drug substances are put into trial over healthy volunteers and their pathogenetic effects are observed and noted for therapeutic purposes. Therefore, it is the only and unique method, which is based on the nature's law of cure, i.e. *Similia Similibus Curantur* which states that likes are cured by likes, i.e. a drugs capacity for eradicating a disease, lies in its capacity to produce the same.

Hahnemann preferred proving drug substance on himself and his trusted fellowmen. All these proving were either open or single blind, i.e. Hahnemann knew the medicine he was proving on himself and others. With passage of time, however things changed. In order to eliminate false signs/

symptoms and subjective bias, Dr. J. J. Drysdale proposed the double blind method for the proving of drugs in healthy volunteers where neither the proving master nor the prover knew the name of drug conducted for the proving.

In 1996, Dr. Flavio Dantas, University of Uberlandia, coined the new term for Drug-proving—'Homoeopathic Pathogenetic Trial' (HPT).

HPT is the first systematic experimental approach to detecting changes in the healthy volunteers after exposure to a drug. HPT is a clinical trial to investigate the effects of potentially toxic or pathogenetic substances diluted and attenuated according to the homoeopathic Pharmacopoeias, in non-patient volunteers in relatively stable health conditions.

Current Proving Protocol

The three basic components of HPT are:

1. The Test Substance
2. The Proving Team—Personnel
3. The Methodology.

1. The Test Substance

The Drug-proving is conducted on healthy human beings to note the disease producing power i.e. disease curing power of a particular drug. The drug is tested singly and alone as because in homoeopathic system medicines are prescribed on the basis of Law of Similia, i.e. simple single substance are prescribed at one time.

The test drug should be obtained from a reliable pharmaceutical company and detailed record should be kept of that company for future reference.

(a) **The Test Dose:**

(i) *Source:* The test drug should be proved singly and in a pure, unadulterated form. The test drug should be natural, authentic. Detail records regarding source, collection, preservation of the drug substance should be maintained.

(ii) *Nomenclature:* The Latin name of the drug substance should be used wherever possible. The name should be unique to the substance proved, so that it can be accurately identified. Proving from similar sources should be differentiated by a unique name specifying subspecies, or some individual characteristics.

(iii) *Preparation:* Detailed description about the preparation of tested drug (maceration or percolation; mode of succussion or trituration) should be mentioned. Details of the vehicle and the scale of preparation should be mentioned. The type of succussion (manual or automatic) applied should be mentioned.

(iv) *Potency:* The proving is conducted with different range of potencies in centesimal, decimal and fifty millesimal scale including mother tinctures to get all aspects of tested drug.

(v) *Toxicology:* Before starting any proving, the physiological and toxicological action of the drug should be studied in crude or material doses in lower animals.

(vi) *Placebo:* To avoid any bias or influences on the part of volunteer and the master prover, the placebo is employed, which should be of the same colour and texture as that of the test drug and should be administered in the same way as that of the experimental group. Use of placebo serves as a means to increase provers attention, it increases reliability and enables clearer deduction of symptoms when set against those arising spontaneously in the general population.

(b) **Determination of Dosage (as per H. A. Roberts):** In Drug-proving, the drug may be used in crude form, in low potency or high potency depending upon the nature of drug.

(i) **Any drug which in its natural state affects the vital energy but little will develop a proving only in a high potency.** e.g., *Carbo vegetabilis, Graphites, Lycopodium.*

Substances that are inert in the natural state will not develop a proving and it needs to be tested only after potentisation.

(ii) **Any drug which in its natural state disturbs the vital energy to functional manifestations only may be proven in a crude form**, e.g. *Cicuta, Ipecacuanha, Lobelia, Tabacum*. Such substances may and should be tested also in the mother tincture. Such substances act as remedies in the tincture form. At the same time, these should also be proved in different range of potencies.

(iii) **Any drug which in its natural state disturbs the vital energy to destructive manifestations should be proven only in a potentised form**. e.g., heavy metals, poisons, venom. These substances are fatal in the natural state. Hence, the pharmacopoeia gives cautionary details for dispensing of potencies of these remedies. These instructions are listed in a different part of this literature. Potentisation reduces the toxicity of these drugs and also makes them more potent.

2. The Proving Team—Personnel

The proving team comprises (a) Master Prover (or Project Director), (b) Advisor/Expert, (c) Proving Supervisors, and (d) Provers.

The Drug-proving is a cooperative venture and teamwork of the different personnel, working towards the common goal for the study of pathogenetic effect of drugs. Each member of the proving team has great role during the process of Drug-proving.

(a) **Master Prover (or Project Director):** The Master Prover is the chief person responsible for the entire proving project from start to end.

The Master Prover must have a qualified education in homoeopathy, well-acquainted with homoeopathic principles and methodology of proving and should have sufficient practical experience in the process of proving. It is preferable for the Master Prover to have actively participated in completed proving as a prover, to have enough experience in supervision of provings and also participated in post-proving compilation, analysis, collation, extraction and publication of proving.

He plans the entire proving, right from the pre-proving protocol to post-proving task of analysing the proving. He has to ensure that the methods followed conform to the highest standards.

The Master Prover decides on the protocol to be followed, decides upon the drug, its potency.

He coordinates with the different group of people involved in the proving.

He is responsible for the safety of provers, the quality of work of supervisors, the extraction, collation and editing of the symptoms.

He should be closely familiar with all the details as well as have an overview of the entire project.

In order to ensure freedom from prejudice, the Master Prover should be blinded to the remedy that is being proved and to the provers.

(b) **Advisor (or Expert):** The Advisor assists the Project Director and provides him information regarding the details of the drug to be proved, its toxicity—both in toxic and hypotoxic doses.

He may be a qualified Botanist, Zoologist, Chemist or Microbiologist providing the characteristics of the drug to be proved. He also provides information about the pharmacological action of the drug as well as the biological study of the drug on laboratory animals. The advisor may also be a qualified physician who certifies the health of the prover and conducts necessary examination and investigation into the provers health before, during or after the proving.

(c) **Proving Supervisors (or Panel of Investigators):** The Proving Supervisors or the Investigators are the crucial and vital link between the Prover and the Project Director. They monitor the responses and the records of the Prover, inquiring in detail into each symptom recorded in the provers daybook.

Good attentive supervision is one of the key factors in ensuring successful and fruitful proving.

Supervisors also should be qualified and experienced homoeopaths.The Proving Supervisors, preferably, should have the experience of participating as provers in previous proving.

They take the prover's case before the proving and need to keep a close contact with the prover from the moment of the first dose and has to be available for eliciting symptoms thereafter. They need to pay the utmost attention and receptive to any change in the state of the prover and make sure that it is recorded in the provers notebook as well as in their own elaboration book.

Supervisors have a duty to notify the coordinator of any changes in the state of the prover that might potentially affect the safety of the provers.

The Supervisors need to maintain the same fidelity in eliciting the right, true and complete picture of the deviations as noticed by the prover, as is required in tracing the portrait of the disease. This demands freedom from prejudice, sound senses and attention in observing from the Proving Supervisors.

They also need to be blinded from the medicine that is proved and also from the provers that receive the test dose, so as to obtain a pure and unbiased proving record.

(d) **Provers:** The best possible way of ascertaining the pure and peculiar effects of drugs is by proving drugs on healthy human beings. These healthy subjects on whom the drug is tested to obtain the portrait of the medicine are called 'provers'.

3. The Methodology

Proving is not only the intake of the test drug and recording the changes in health, but requires a meticulous planning and study before and after the proving. Hence the proving experiment is best studied under three different protocols:

A. The Pre-proving Protocol

B. The Proving Protocol

C. Post Proving Protocol

A. THE PRE-PROVING PROTOCOL

(a) **Study of Test Drug:** The Proving master undertakes the study of the drug, covering areas of pharmacognosy, standardisation, pharmacology and toxicology. An antidote to the test drug, if any, is confirmed. The Proving Master decides on the test drug and is responsible for its procurement from a reliable source. The Proving master undertakes the project of proving of either a new drug or a reproving of existing drugs from the Materia Medica. Homoeopathic Drug-proving tend to be exploratory in nature, especially when the properties are not known, whereas, in reproving, it is confirmatory as well as exploratory.

(b) **Selection of Supervisors:** The Proving Master selects the panel of investigators or supervisors and instructs them about the ethics and conduct of proving. Supervisors also should be qualified and experienced homoeopaths. The Proving Supervisors, preferably, should have the experience of participating as provers in previous proving.

The Supervisors prepare the Initial Medical Report Proforma.

(c) **Selection of Provers:** Apparently healthy individuals are selected as provers from different regions of the country in order to ascertain whether ecological, socio-economic, climatic, regional factors and food habits, variation in physical constitution of the volunteers affects the drug pathogenesis in any form.

A consent form having name, age, sex, address and an undertaking is used to take the consent of the prover.

Persons selected must be between the age group of 18-45 yrs, as

(i) they are intelligent enough to understand the seriousness of the experiment and able to record the subjective symptoms properly.

(ii) the natural bodily degenerative changes which come with age will not be present.

The drug must be proved on both males and females to get the changes produced in the sexual sphere.

Ethical Considerations

(i) The subject or prover should be in such a mental, physical and legal state as to be able to exercise fully his or her power of choice.

(ii) Consent should be, as a rule, obtained in writing from the subject. However, the responsibility always remains with the investigator, or investigating team. It never falls on the prover even after the consent has been obtained.

(iii) The nature and purpose of the Drug-proving must be explained to the subject or prover.

(iv) Proving should never be done in toxic doses. For toxic symptoms we must rely solely on the reports of accidental provings recorded in toxicological literature.

(v) The investigator or investigating team should discontinue the provings if in his, her, or their judgment, the proving, if continued, would be harmful to the subject.

Inclusion Criteria

The person should be reasonably healthy and well-balanced in body, soul and spirit.

The prover must be well-acquainted with Homoeopathic Methodology and must have good knowledge of symptomatology found in Materia Medica so that the particular deviations which may manifest during the experiment are fully appreciated.

The subject must be able to lead a life which is as normal as possible during the course of the proving so as to allow a definite time for sleep, for working, for eating etc.

The subject must be intelligent enough to properly appreciate and record the subjective symptoms as deviations from his normal condition of life. These subjective symptoms are of utmost value.

Honesty is a prerequisite of a good prover, for he must be very careful to record all phenomena from the very beginning of the trial.

Exclusion Criteria

(i) The persons who are hysterical or displaying anxieties and emotionally disturbed stated should not be included in the proving trials, as such individuals display a high incidence of "Placebo effect".

(ii) Persons suffering from allergic manifestations, particularly pertaining to respiratory system and skin, should not be included.

(iii) Those who note down a lot of emotional symptoms. Too many symptoms in these realms confuse the final results.

(iv) Those who obviously omitted to recall symptoms or who exhibited superficiality in reporting.

Instructions to Provers

Before starting the proving, the following instructions are given to the prover so as to get a clear picture of the proving:

(i) Not to make any major change in their daily routine and lifestyle, specifically food habits, sleep, exercise etc.

(ii) Those who are habitual for tobacco chewing, smoking, tea, coffee, alcohol etc. are advised to minimise the use of such stimulants. These can, however, be withdrawn if the prover does not suffer from any ill-effects from the withdrawal of these habits or stimulants and beverages.

(iii) To restrict any other medication during the course of the proving.

(iv) To avoid use of other drugs and medicaments—especially of camphor—during the proving and also the use of table condiments and highly spiced and seasoned food.

(v) To avoid over-exertion—both mentally and physically.

(vi) To report everyday to the proving master or write down all the details by themselves.

(vii) To mention in the provers report about any probable precipitating factor which could have produced the symptoms such as over-exertion, night watching, any excitement, excess intake of coffee/tea, over-eating, indiscretion in diet etc.

(viii) To avoid any extraneous influence as this may distort the result.

(d) **Primary Coding of Remedy:** The Proving master is responsible for the primary coding of the remedy. The test drug as well as the control (placebo of a similar vehicle) is coded. The different doses that are received by a single prover are also numbered. The provers are also assigned code numbers. The coding should necessarily be done by a committee that shall not be involved in the direct supervision of the records of the provers. Blinding also signifies Blind Assignment of the codes. A detailed record of the coding should be maintained that is unlocked after the initial blind assessment at the termination of the actual testing of the drug.

B. THE PROVING PROTOCOL

Hahnemann recommended the preparation of the test drug by the actual provers, so that they can rely on them. The provers were, hence, fully aware of the nature of the substance that they were proving. Modern proving have deviated and modified from this concept and the entire process is more scientific in outlook, though complex. It is to be remembered at the same time that the rich Materia Medica of today was derived from the proving of the old:

(a) **Multicentric Trials:** Keeping the variations in lifestyles, food habits, climate, constitutional and temperamental factors in view, multicentric trials are undertaken for the proving of a drug. The studies should be conducted at least at three different centres under the same protocol before releasing the data for professional use. Ideally, the proving should be conducted at three different locations, in the mountains, on the low plains and the seashore.

(b) **Orientation Meeting:** Orientation meetings are arranged at the commencement of the proving. The aim of the orientation meeting is to explain the importance and conduct of the proving process in detail to the provers and supervisors and to stress to all participants the depths of observation needed. Each prover and each supervisor should be given a thorough written briefing in the form of an "instruction letter" They should study it carefully and familiarise themselves with the details. Any queries regarding the nature, process, outcome, complications, etc should be cleared at the onset, so that the participants are without any preconceived bias or prejudice. The day-books are also provided to the provers for the recording of the proving.

(c) **Nature of Trials:** Since 1948, **Randomised Control Trial (RCT)** has become the standard design for drawing valid conclusions on the efficacy of the medicine.

The requests of an RCT are:

(i) *Randomised Trials.* Randomised trials are those in which the subjects of an experiment are randomly placed either in treatment groups or in placebo groups. The researchers attempt to place people with similar characteristics in equal numbers in treatment and placebo groups. This process is helpful for reducing the bias.

(ii) *Double-blind Trials:* Double-blind trials refer to experiments in which neither the experimenter nor the subjects know, whether a specific treatment was prescribed or a placebo (a fake medicine that looks and tastes like real homeopathic medicines). The double-blind modification in proving trials was suggested by Drysdale, wherein neither the Proving Masters nor the provers (volunteers) knows the name of the drug and its potencies of the drug or the control received by each of the provers.

In India the authority has adopted Hahnemann's concept of proving of drugs on healthy human volunteers with modifications based on Drysdale's Double-Blind Technique. The cross-over design is followed during the entire course of the proving.

The test drug as well as the control (placebo of a similar vehicle) is coded. The different doses that are received by a single prover are also numbered. The provers are also assigned code numbers.

The **coding** should necessarily be done by a committee that shall not be involved in the direct supervision of the records of the provers. Blinding also signifies Blind Assignment of the codes. A detailed record of the coding should be maintained that is unlocked after the initial blind assessment at the termination of the actual testing of the drug.

(iii) *Crossover Studies (Double Control Studies):* Crossover studies refer to experiments in which half of the subjects of a study are given a placebo during one phase of a study and then given the active treatment during the second phase, while the other half begin with the active treatment and then receive the placebo during the second phase. Crossover studies sometimes do not test a placebo and instead compare one type of treatment with another type of treatment.

(iv) *Controlled Trial-Placebo:* The use of placebo is aimed at giving a picture of the remedy response, separate from the physiological and emotional aspects of the doctor-patient relationship, to exclude the charisma of the physician and such factors as expectation, motivation and suggestion. A trial can be described as controlled only if it includes a method of elimination. The control medicine must be a similar preparation that is identical in all other respects except there is no other original and specific substance to be mixed and potentised with the vehicle. It would be ideal to triturate or succuss the placebo dose to remove bias following the potentisation of the vehicle.

(d) **The Committee:** It is recommended to have a committee of homoeopaths and experts for a proving to assist the Proving Project Director. The committee's tasks should be:

(i) To select remedy, the different potencies, communicate with the pharmacy and prepare the test doses.

(ii) To do the primary coding of the test doses in a randomised fashion. this is known as blind assignment.

(iii) The provers are also coded. This is blinding of the prover and is also done in a randomised fashion.

(iv) To keep the records of remedy codes and which prover got which remedy.

(v) To distribute the remedies and the day-books.

(vi) To ensure the double-blind principle all along the proving. Hence, at a given time, the Prover master shall be unaware of the identity of a given test dose—drug or placebo—and he shall also be unaware of the nature of dose received by the prover. The Supervisors, while assessing the patient, shall also not be prejudiced by the nature of the dose that the prover has. The prover is also unaware of the nature of the dose that is being tested and will hence result in a pure proving of the test dose along with the effects of the placebo. This is **exploratory trial**, where each member of the entire team is unaware of the outcome.

(vii) To organise the typing and the publication of the proving.

(viii) To keep a clear account of the proving protocol.

(e) **The Protocol:**

(i) The process of proving commences with the orientation meeting.

(ii) Instructions regarding the proving are detailed to the prover and the day books are distributed.

(iii) Drugs are provided to the provers in coded phials and provers are divided into two groups, one receives 'placebo' and other 'actual drug' to distinguish between the false and true symptoms.

(iv) The drug is administered, in doses of 4-6 globules, four times a day for 14 days. Mother tincture is given 10-20 drops (1 drop per kg body wt), 4 times daily for a period of 14 days unless the symptoms arise earlier. The drugs are proved in ascending or descending order of potencies. As stated by Dunham, it is better to start first with higher potencies so that susceptible prover may be known right from the beginning as they will give us finer and more detailed symptoms. If there is no response, then lower potency or mother tincture may be employed.

(v) Once a prover develops any signs/symptoms, administration of drug is stopped immediately and is not re-administered till the sign(s) and symptom(s) persist. Disappearance of sign(s) and symptom(s) is followed by a washout (drug free) period of 7 days and, in case of no recurrence of sign(s) and symptom(s), the drug is readministered, till the completion of one quota. Next quota is administered after a washout period of seven days.

(f) **Recording of Proving:** The recording of the proving is the most important aspect of the entire proving exercise; for it is on the experiences of the provers that the pure Homoeopathic Materia Medica is derived. Hence it is important that the observations of the prover have to be recorded in meticulous detail and in a systematic way, so as to ease the post-proving analysis of the records.

(g) **Proforma Lay Out:**

(i) *Initial Medical Report Proforma (IMRP):* As it is nearly impossible nowadays to find perfectly healthy provers, a format is designed to minimise recording of any pre-existing pathological symptoms. This is known as pre-medical examination proforma. With the help of pre-trial medical examination the details of physical and clinical examination along with constitutional, both mental/emotional and physical traits are recorded in this form. The pre-trial medical examination is conducted by Honorary Consultants in the field of Medicine, Psychiatry, Ophthalmology, Otorhino-laryngology, Dermatology, Pathology and Gynaecology (in case of female provers). Pathological, Biochemical and serological tests are required to be performed to facilitate correlation between the subjective and objective changes as far as possible.

(ii) *Prover's Day-book/Log-book:* The prover's day-book or the log-book is a properly designed format wherein the prover makes data entries in chronological order as per instructions. Each prover is provided with sufficient number of predesigned ***'Prover's Day Book Proforma'*** to record all the signs and symptoms, subjective and objective, they might observe during the course of the proving. The provers are directed to report to the proving master everyday, and hand over the recorded symptomatic data.

Guidelines for the recording of symptoms

- Adherence to the protocol, honesty and sincerity are prerequisites both on the part of investigators and the subject.
- The provers must make day-book entries at least 3 times a day—to prevent even minor memory lapse.
- Each entry should record even the slightest deviation from the subject's normal life.
- Intensity and duration of the symptoms should be carefully recorded.
- Possible exciting causes should be recorded meticulously.
- A detailed record of the order of appearance of all the symptoms should be made.
- Duration and the modifying characters of the symptoms, together with concomitants, should be properly recorded.
- Recording should be done without biased ideas about the outcome of the proving.

Way of minimising errors

- The subject is assured that the information will be treated as confidential.
- There should be frequent meetings between investigators and subjects, to record the elaboration and clarification of each symptom.

(iii) *Response Monitoring Proforma (RMP):* The proving master should take care to ascertain and record environmental changes, alteration in daily routine and lifestyle of the provers, if any, to ensure a true and realistic evolution of drug pathogenesis.During the course of the proving, the proving master should interrogates the provers with regard to their symptomatic presentation and records them with his own observation in respect of location, sensation, modalities, concomitants, extensions (if any) and duration of each reported symptom in the 'Symptoms Elaboration Proforma'. During the period of the trial the clinical, laboratory and radiological investigations are also to be recorded.

(iv) *Post-trial medical examination:* After the completion of the experiment, the provers are required again a thorough physical and clinical examination. Along with this, similar lab investigations as carried out at the time of the pre-medical examination are also done. This is known as 'post-trial medical examination proforma'. Any variation in pre- and post-trial findings is also to be recorded.

C. POST-PROVING PROTOCOL

The primary objective of a proving is to discover the nature of a remedy so it can be used to restore the sick to health, to cure. In order to do this it is necessary to process the information and put it into a form that will easily reveal the nature of a drug and the characteristic features that make it different from other drugs.

1. **Completion of Proving:** No time scale can be fixed for the proving of drugs as drugs vary in their intrinsic nature and in the development of their properties. A proving can actually never said to be complete, as there is always a scope for further reproving.

Any group discussions about the proving should only be conducted after notebooks have been handed to the coordinator.

The proving records are thoroughly screened and analysed.

The symptoms collected from all the provers is to be sifted in such a manner that all the relevant data collected is not lost, but shall have a proper flow of thought, so that the mental, physical and functional state of the drug is understood.

Adequate data indexing is done as per the pattern of *Kent's repertory* so that the data is rendered clinically useful.

2. **Analysis of Proving Records:** Extracting, collating, analysing, theming into Materia Medica and repertorising are the most laborious, painstaking and time-consuming stages of carrying out a proving. An appreciation of the work involved in this part of the work should be carefully considered before embarking on a proving. A well-balanced group for this task should be a mixture of experienced homeopaths, who are well-acquainted with the different repertories and repertory language and the Master Prover who has an overview of the whole process from start to end. A good working knowledge of the native language of the provers is also required:

(i) ***Extraction:*** This process involves the conversion of written diaries or day-books into the format of the Materia Medica and the valid symptoms are extracted. The observations and experiences of all the provers are thoroughly screened, analyzed and compared with their Initial Medical Report Proforma (IMRP), and lastly, compared with the test, control (i.e., placebo) and crossover groups.

(ii) ***Collation:*** After the completion of analysis and conversion of prover symptoms into the language of the Materia Medica, the aim of the collation stage is to synthesise the proving from all the separate accounts of each prover as if it belonged to and evolved in a single person. All the provers separate sheets are put together. Symptoms with a common denominator are grouped together under each section.

(iii) ***Repertorisation:*** The aim of the repertorising stage is to accurately and truthfully interpret the proving information into repertorial language. Each symptom is accurately analysed and translated into a rubric. Certain symptoms may require creating new rubrics. The remedy is then considered for addition into the rubrics.

(iv) *Theming the Symptoms:* These symptoms are studied for its peculiar pattern that emerges out of the proving. The physical generalities, the constitutional affinity, the peculiar characteristic state of mind and disposition is then studied. This theming of the proving is the practical outcome of the painstaking effort of the entire project and is understood and implemented.

3. **Publication:** The publication of the proving should contain all the data of the logbooks, the medical records and a summary of the proving, with discussion and conclusions. Data indexing should be as per the schema followed in Kent's repertory. The final publication, in book form or in a journal or electronic form, should include the Materia Medica, the repertorisation, information about the substance and its toxicology. This introduction should explain why they chose that substance and give their view of the remedy picture.

Minimum standard for Homoeopathic Drug-provings Protocols given by European Committee of Homoeopathy (Subcommitee on Drug-provings)

To meet today's standards of methodology, the ECH Subcommittee on Drug-proving (European Committee for Homoeopathy, 1994) have formulated a Minimum Standard for Homoeopathic Drug-proving Protocols which is given as:

1. **Qualification of the Proving master: For** Homoeopathic Drug-proving the following qualifications are considered to be adequate: All investigators, who are in direct contact with volunteers, must have a qualified education in homeopathy, must have a **minimum 5 years of experience in homoeopathic practice** (treating patients) and **must have proven at least 3 homoeopathic remedies personally as a volunteer**. The principal investigator of the proving must additionally have at least 2 years of experience in HDPs.

2. **Case taking (before pre observation phase), case taking is obligatory:**

(i) For the safety of the volunteer, to make sure that they are healthy enough to take part in a proving.

(ii) To give baseline of the actual state of health and symptoms.

(iii) To make sure that the volunteer has properly understood the purpose and procedure of the proving, is reliable (Section 126) and is able to express their symptoms precisely enough.

3. **Inclusion Criteria:**

(i) The volunteer must be healthy in the sense that they do not show severe psychic or physical symptoms and do not consider themselves to be in need of medical treatment. The proving doctor should not see any necessity for treatment. A medical history and physical examination should confirm this.

(ii) The person must be trustworthy, able and ready to express and describe his experiences during the Proving (Section 126,139).

(iii) There should be no plans for important life changes like moving, change of job, marriage etc The usual habits and conduct of life should be continued.

(iv) The person should not plan to begin medical treatments like dentistry, surgery or psychotherapy during the drug-proving.

(v) Age: Over 18 years.

4. **Exclusion Criteria:**

(i) Current medical treatments or Homoeopathic drugs in the preliminary observation period or during the Proving.

(ii) Prescription of drugs (including Homoeopathic) in the past four weeks.

(iii) Contraceptive pills in the past three months. (IUP's mark in the accounts)

(iv) Surgical treatment within past 2 months.

(v) Pregnancy, breast feeding.

(vi) Under the age of 18.

5. **Preliminary observation period:** During this phase, lasting for one week, the volunteers are required to fill out the diaries the way they have been shown. The Proving doctor will contact each person every two or three days to test her or his compliance. Failure in keeping the diary properly may lead to exclusion from the Homeopathic Drug-proving.

6. **Drug administration:**

   (a) *Definition of the remedy:* Origin and identification, way of manufacturing (e.g., Fresh plants, trituration or mother tincture, way of potentisation, solvent etc.).

   (b) *Dosage and potency:* Normally 12c or 30c, 3 globules every 2 hours (if another application form or dosage is given, please explain), as long as no symptoms occur, maximum 6 times, during one day, stop drug intake immediately if symptoms occur.

7. **Documentation of symptoms:**

   (a) *Duration of observation of symptoms:* Minimum 4 weeks.

   (b) *Supervision:* Intense contact between proving master and volunteer has to be secured i.e., daily phone calls, schedule of meetings.

   (ç) *Symptoms should include:* location, sensation, modalities in regated to time also), concomitants and chronological records (illustrating how long after the commencement of the proving each symptom arose) and should be presented following the head to foot scheme, in distinct categories:

   (i) New symptom (NS).

   (ii) Return of old symptom (OS).

   (iii) Altered symptom (AS) i.e., a symptom that has changed its character, modality or concomitant.

   (iv) Cured symptom (CS) i.e., one which has disappeared.

Complete original notes should be kept from each volunteer and proving doctor excluded.

8. **The legal requirements of a country must be considered:** At the time of Hahnemann, laboratory investigations and modern techniques to assess the effects of the drugs on prover were not available. This has resulted in difficulties to evaluate the physiological, anatomical, biochemical and pathological changes of the system on which the proving took place.

   So, to make the Materia Medica more pure and scientific, all the possible investigations will be taken up during the proving of the drug.

Reproving of Homoeopathic Medicines

There is necessity for reproving of homoeopathic medicines, in our country keeping in view the varying ecological, environmental, psychological, nutritional factors etc. If the true pathogenetic power of the drugs can be ascertained through appropriate methodology, under scientific scrutiny, then the new findings can be valuable additions to the Materia Medica. CCRH has already reproved I10 medicines on a standard protocol, data of which have been published in the form of books and articles in Council's journal.

Proving of New Drugs in Homoeopathy—Countrywise

A. United Kingdom (UK):

1. ***Clayton Collyer and Jackie Davis:*** Lavendula angustifolia.

2. ***Jacqueline Houghton and Elizabeth Halahan:*** Lac humanum (Human breast milk).

3. ***Misha Norland (1943-.........), School of Homoeopathy:*** Agathis australis (Kauri tree) (1993-95), Aids nosode (1994-95), Carbo fullerenum (Carbon 60), Cladonia rangiferina (Reindeer or Caribou moss) (2000), Falcon peregrinus disciplinatus (Wing feather, blood spot) (1997), Knopper Oak Galls (Gall on Quercus penduncilata) (1998), Latex vulcani (Vulcanised rubber prepared from a Condom) (2001), Lava Arizona (Basaltic lava from Arizona) (1994), LSD (D-lysergic acid diethylamide) (1999), North Wales slate (Slate) (1996), Passer domesticus (House sparrow), Positronium (Antimatter) (1998).

4. ***Penny Stirling, in Bristol:*** Cygnus columbianus bewickii (Bewick's swan) (2002), Salix fragilis (Crack willow) (1998).

5. ***Bocock Richard:*** Aspartame (N-(L-α-Aspartyl)-L-phenylalanine, 1-methyl ester, $C_{14}H_{18}N_2O_5$) (2002), Chlamydia trachomatis (Sexually transmitted bacteria) (2000)
6. ***Stirling Penelope:*** Cygnus bewickii (Bewick swan) (2002)
7. ***Lidia Hogan/Anya Kropacz:*** Pilus equinus (Horse hair) (1994)
8. ***Biggs / Gwillim:*** Placenta humana (Placenta) (2000)
9. ***Alastair Gray (1966-……):*** Chironex fleckeri (Box jellyfish), Culex musca (Culex pervigilans), Ficus macrophylla (Moreton bay fig), Lampona cylindrata (White tailed spider)
10. ***Misha Norland and Peter Fraser:*** Galium aparine (Mutton chops)
11. ***Peter Fraser:*** Pavo cristatus (Peacock feather)
12. ***Steve Smith:*** Mobile phone radiation (Radiation from mobile phone)
13. ***Mary English:*** Naufragium helvetia (Shipwreck) (2003), Stanton Drew Stone (2004), Tempesta (Thunderstorm) (1999).

B. United State of America (USA):

1. ***David Riley, MD. (1952-……):*** AMP (Adenosinum monophosphoricum acidum) (1996), Anthraquinone (9, 10-dioxoanthracene), ATP (Adenosinum triphosphoricum acidum) (1996), Baryta oxalsuccinata, Cartilago suis (Cartilage of pig) (1994), Chorda umbilicalis (Umbilical cord) (1994), Coenzyme A (1996), Colibacillinum (coli.) (1995), Embryo suis (Embryo of pig) (1994), Fumaricum acidum, Funiculus umbilicalis, Geranium robertianum, L. cysteinum, Manganum phosphoricum, Medulla ossis suis (pigs bone marrow) (1995), Mucosa nasalis (Mucous membrane of human nose) (1993), Natrum pyruvicum, Oxalis acetosella, Pancreas suis (Pigs pancreas) (1995), Placenta suis (pigs placenta) (1994), Riboflavinum, Sinusitisinum (1994), Staphylococcinum (1995), Streptococcinum (1995), Veronica officinalis.
2. ***Greg Bedayn:*** Corvus corax (Northern Raven,Common Raven, corv-cor.)(1995), Tungsten.
3. ***Nancy Herrick:*** Lac delphinum (Bottlenose dophin milk) (1993), Lac equinum (Milk of the horse) (1998), Lac leoninum (Milk of the lion) (1996), Lac loxodonta africana (Milk of the elephant) (1995), Lac lupinum (Milk of the wolf) (1999), Limenitis bredowii californica (California sister butterfly) (1995-1998), Maiasaura lapidea (The fossilised bone of the dinosaur) (1998), Sanguis soricis (Blood of the Norway Rat) (1998), Sanguis ursus arctos horribilis (Blood of the grizzly bear) (2000).
4. ***Todd Rowe MD(H), CCH, DHt:*** Alligator mississippiensis (The American alligator) (2001), Argemone pleiacantha (Crested prickle poppy), Carnegia gigantea (Saguaro cactus), Cathartes aura (Turkey vulture) (1999), Geococcyx californianus (Greater roadrunner)(2004), Heloderma suspectum (Gila monster), Larrea tridentata (creosote-bush), Turquoise (Hydrated Copper Aluminum Phosphate), Urolophus halleri (Roundtail stingray (1998).
5. ***Steven Olsen:*** Abies canadensis, Acer circinatum, Alnus rubra, Angelicae sinensis, Arbutus menziessi, Borrago officinalis, Pinus contorta (Shore pine), Spirostachys africanus sond(Tambootie tree), Taxus buccata, Taxus brevifolia(Western pacific yew), Tsuga menziessii.
6. ***Teresa Beernard:*** Sambucus nigra.
7. ***Jeremy Yaakov Sherr (1955-……), The Dynamis School:*** Adamas, Androctonus amoreuxii hebraeus (Scorpion, Israel), Brassica napus (Rape seed), Calopteryx splendens (Damsel fly) (2002), Chocolatum (Chocolate), Cygnus cygnus (Whooper Swan) (2001), Dama dama (Fallow deer) (2003) Germanium metallicum, Haliaeetus leucocephalus (Bald Eagle) (1995), Hydrogen, Iridium metallicum, Neon, Plutonium nitricum.
8. ***Shore Jonathan:*** Atrax robustus (Veno-

mous spider, Sydney funnel web spider, a spinner mygale from Australia) (1995).

9. *Susan Sonz/Kushner/Robert Stewart:* Musca domestica (Housefly) (1999).

10. *Karen Allen:* Sus scrofa (Wild boar) (2000).

11. *Donald Brown, Andrew Lange:* Candida parapsilosis (Candida arkrusei, Monilia parapsilosis, Thrush fungus, cand.)(1989).

C. Canada:

Lous Klein, RSHom (1951-……): Carboneum diodum (Carbon dioxide), Coriandrum sativum (Coriander), Helodrilus caliginosus (Earthworm), Loxosceles reclusa (Brown recluse spider).

Shepard Cynthia: Calypte anna (Anna's humming bird) (2003)

D. France:

Phou Souk-Aloun: Brucella melintensis (Brucel), Calamus aromaticus, Cyclosporinum (Cyclosporine cyclsporin A, cyclosp.), Diazepam, GABA, Interferon, Propanololum.

E. Ireland:

Nuala Eising: Granitum, Ignis alcoholis (Fire), Limestone, Succinum(Amber), Vacuum, White marble.

F. New Zealand:

Sue Balance: Pinus contorta, Salix alba.

G. Denmark:

Friedrich Ritzer: Placenta.

H. Australia:

Robins Philipp: Aqua marina (Sea water), Aristolochia clematitis (Birthroot), Dioxinum (Chlorinated dioxins and furans, halogenated organic compounds, most common being polychlorinated dibenzofurans and polychlorinated dibenzodioxins) (2000), DNA(Deoxyribo nucleic acid), Meditatio, Phascolarctos cinereus (Australian Koala secretion), Sol (Sunlight), Vibhuti Sai Baba.

Alastair Gray, DSH, PCH, RSHom: Chironex fleckeri (Box jelly fish), Ficus macrophylla, Melaleuca alternifolia (Tea tree).

I. India:

Pichiah Sankaran, LIM, FCEH, DFHom (London), DHT (USA), FHMS (Maha.) (1922-1979), India: Atrax robustus (venomous spider, Sydney funnel web spider, a spinner mygale from Australia) (1969), Pituitaria glandula (Pituitrinum, Entire gland Hypophysis) (1965 and 1967)

Rajan Sankaran MD (1960-……), Mumbai, India: Bacillinum burnett (bac.) (1993), Coca cola, Crotalus cascavella (Crotalus durissus terrificus, Neotropical rattlesnake) (1995), Dendroaspis polylepis (Black mamba) (1998), Lac caprinum (goat's milk) (1994), Lac humanum (human breast milk of one woman) (1995), Lac leoninum (Milk of the lion) (1996), Lac vaccinum defloratum (Skimmed milk) (1995), Tinea unknown species (Ringworm Nosode) (1993)

F. J. Master MD. (1957-……), in Mumbai, India: Ancistrodon piscivorus, Toxicophis pugnax (Agkistrodon piscivorus, Water moccasin snake) (1998), Bitis Arietans arietans (Clotho arietans, Common African puff adder) (2003), Bungarus fasciatus (Banded krait)(2002)

Shukla Chetna: Agamemnon graphium (tailed jay), Carassius auratus (red cap veil tail gold fish) (2003), Pavo cristatus (Peacock) (2001),

Thakar Munjal, in Mumbai: Blatta orientalis (Indian cockroach)(1995)

Jayesh Shah: Rattus rattus (Rat) (1995)

Burch Melissa: Stychodactyla gigantea (Indo Pacific sea anemone, Giant carpet anemone) (2004)

Mahendra Singh: He is doing clinical proving of Phyllanthus niruri (Bhui amla), Cyperus rotundus (Mutha), Leucas aspera (Goma), Mimosa pudica (Lajjabati) and from the toxin of Plotosus anguillaris (Kan majur)

J. Austria:

Hildebrandt Jörg: Acanthaster planci (crown-of-thorns starfish) (1998)

Santos Uta: Boa constrictor (Red tailed boa) (1996), Cerastes cerastes (Desert horn viper)

Flick Reinhard: Conchiolinum (Mother-of-pearl) (1992)

W. Gluck: Botulinum (Botulism Nosode, botul.) (1993), Veintiquattro Paraponera calvata od. Diponera grd (3 cm large poisonous ant from Venezuela) (1996)

Krassnig: Ambra grisea (Whale ambergris

from the intestine of the Sperm Whale found on beaches or floating in the sea) (1985)

H. Lesigang: Latrodectus mactans (Black widow spider) (1989).

K. Germany:

K-J. Müller: Acipenser sturio ex ovis (Caviar, acip-st-ov.) (1996), Apeira syringaria (a butterfly), Dens elephantum (Ivory) (1998), Dermatophagoides farinae (House Dust Mite), Dermatophagoides pteronyssinus (House Dust Mite), Lamprohiza splendidula (Glowworm, firefly) (2004), Serinus canaria (Canary bird) (1997), Morbillinum (Nosode of Measles, morb.) (1997), Parotidinum (Nosode of Mumps) (1998)

Becker Jürgen: Bombus sylvestris (Bumblebee), Vespula germanica (Wasp, vespul-germ.) (1993)

Schulz Elisabeth: Buteo jamaicensis (Common Red Tailed Hawk) (1995), Cygnus olor (Swan feathers) (1997)

Anne Schadde: Cypraea eglantina (Cowries-nail) (1996), Lapis lazuli, Ozone.

Eberle Hans/Ritzer Friedrich: Excrementum caninum (Dog excrements, canis-exc.) (1996), Haliaeetus leucocephalus (Bald eagle) (1997), Lac pan troglodytes (Chimpanzee's milk) (1994), Urina equina (Horse's urine) (1997)

Holling Andreas/Shah Jayesh: Folliculinum (Corpus luteum, luteum, foll.) (1999)

Neuhöfer/Zeising: Lac suinum (House pig's milk, lac-sui.) (1997)

Fink Wilfried: Larus argentatus (Sea Gull) (1996)

Klotzsch Brigitte: Portia fimbriata (Jumping spider) (2005), Python regius (Royal python) (2001)

Heck Günter: Tegenaria atrica (Hauswinkel-spinne, Central European Spider) (2000)

Wichmann Jörg: Tyto alba (Barn owl wing) (2004)

Geisler Michael: Candida albicans (Monilia albicans, moni., Thrush Fungus) (2001).

The Current Status of Drug-proving

The Central Council of Homoeopathy, through its research wing—Central Council for Research in Homoeopathy (CCRH) at its Clinical Verification Unit situated in different parts in India. At present, drug-proving is carried out at the following centres in India.

1. Drug-proving Research Unit, Ghaziabad, Uttar Pradesh.
2. Drug-proving Research Unit, Kolkata, West Bengal.
3. Drug-proving Research Unit, Midnapore, West Bengal.
4. Homoeopathic Drug Research Institute, Lucknow, Uttar Pradesh.
5. Regional Research Institute, New Delhi.

List of Drugs proved so far by CCRH

1. Abroma augusta folia Q. B. Vol. 19 (3-4), 1997
2. Acalypha indica Q. B. Vol. 18 (1-2), 1996; (Homoeopathic Drug provings) (2005)
3. Acid butyricum Q. B. Vol. 24 (3-4), 2002 (Drug-proving Special-IV)
4. Acorus calamus
5. Aegle folia Q. B. Vol.9 (3-4), 1987 (Drug-proving Special I)
6. Aegle marmelos Q. B. Vol. 27 (3), 2005
7. Agave americana (Homoeopathic Drug-provings, Vol.2) (2007)
8. Alfalfa (Homoeopathic Drug-provings) (2005)
9. Andrographis paniculata
10. Aranea diadema (Homoeopathic Drug-provings) (2005)
11. Aranea scinencia Q. B. Vol. 12 (1-2), 1990 (Drug-proving Special II)
12. Argemone mexicana (Homoeopathic Drug-provings, volume 2)
13. Arsenicum bromicum (Q. B. Vol. 24 (3-4), 2002) (Drug-proving Special-IV)
14. Atista indica Q. B. Vol. 12 (1-2), 1990 (Drug-proving Special II)
15. Azadirachta indica (Homoeopathic Drug-provings) (2005)
16. Bacopa monniere
17. Baryta iodata Q. B. Vol. 2 (3), 1980
18. Bellis perennis Q. B. Vol. 26 (3), 2004

19. Boerhaavia diffusa (Homoeopathic Drug-provings) (2005)
20. Calotropis gigantea (Homoeopathic Drug-provings) (2005)
21. Carica papaya (Homoeopathic Drug-provings) (2005)
22. Cassia fistula(New Drugs-proved by CCRH) (2008)
23. Cassia sophera (New Drugs-proved by CCRH) (2008)
24. Cephalandra indica (Homoeopathic Drug-provings, volume 2) (2007)
25. Chelone
26. Chromium kali sulphuratum Q. B. Vol. 24 (3-4), 2002
27. Clerodendron infortunatum
28. Coleus aromaticus
29. Cornus circinata
30. Cup. oxydatum nigrum (Homoeopathic Drug-provings) (2005)
31. Curcuma longa (New Drugs-proved by CCRH) (2008)
32. Cuscuta reflexa (New Drugs-proved by CCRH) (2008)
33. Cynodon dactylon Q. B. Vol. 2 (4), 1980
34. Embelia ribes (Homoeopathic Drug-provings) (2005)
35. Euphorbia lathyris (Homoeopathic Drug-provings) (2005)
36. Ficus religiosa (Homoeopathic Drug-provings, Vol.2) (2007)
37. Formicum acidum (Homoeopathic Drug-provings) (2005)
38. Glycyrrhiza glabra (New Drugs-proved by CCRH) (2008)
39. Holarrhena antidysenterica (Homoeopathic Drug-provings) (2005)
40. Hydrocotyle asiatica (Homoeopathic Drug-provings) (2005)
41. Ichthyolum (Homoeopathic Drug-provings) (2005)
42. Juglans regia
43. Kalium muriaticum Q. B. Vol. 3 (1), 1981
44. Lapis alba (Homoeopathic Drug-provings) (2005)
45. Leucas aspera
46. Liatris spicata
47. Magnesia sulphuricum Q. B. Vol. 19 (1-2), 1997 (Drug-proving Special-III)
48. Malaria officinalis
49. Mangifera indica (Homoeopathic Drug-provings) (2005)
50. Mimosa humilis (Homoeopathic Drug-provings, Vol.2) (2007)
51. Mygale (Homoeopathic Drug-provings) (2005)
52. Nyctanthes arbortristis (Homoeopathic Drug-provings) (2005)
53. Ocimum canum (Homoeopathic Drug-provings) (2005)
54. Ocimum sanctum
55. Oxytropis lamberti (Homoeopathic Drug-provings) (2005)
56. Paraffinum (Homoeopathic Drug-provings, Vol.2) (2007)
57. Phyllanthus niruri (New Drugs-proved by CCRH) (2008)
58. Pothos foetidus (Homoeopathic Drug-provings, Vol.2) (2007)
59. Pyrus americana (Homoeopathic Drug-provings) (2005)
60. Rauwolfia serpentina (Homoeopathic Drug-provings) (2005)
61. Ricinus communis (Homoeopathic Drug-provings) (2005)
62. Saraca indica(Homoeopathic Drug-provings, Vol.2) (2007)
63. Senega
64. Skookum chuck (Homoeopathic Drug-provings, Vol.2) (2007)
65. Staphylococcinum Q. B. Vol. 24 (3-4), 2002 (Drug-proving Special-IV)
66. Tarentula cubensis (Homoeopathic Drug-provings) (2005)

67. Tarentula hispanica Q. B. Vol. 9 (3-4), 1987 (Drug-proving Special I)
68. Tela aranea Q. B. Vol. 12 (1-2), 1990 (Drug-proving Special II)
69. Terminalia arjuna (Homoeopathic Drug-provings) (2005)
70. Terminalia chebula (Homoeopathic Drug-provings) (2005)
71. Thea chinensis (Homoeopathic Drug-provings) (2005)
72. Theridion (Homoeopathic Drug-provings) (2005)
73. Thymolum (Homoeopathic Drug-provings) (2005)
74. Thyroidinum
75. Tinospora cordifolia
76. Tribulus terrestris (Homoeopathic Drug-provings) (2005)
77. Tylophora indica (Homoeopathic Drug-provings) (2005).

Chapter 29

Posology and Homoeopathic Posology

Etymology

The term 'Posology' originates from the Greek and POSOS meaning how much and LOGOS meaning study or discourse.

Definition of Posology

Posology means knowledge of doctrine of doses of medicine. The terminology of "dose" is derived from the Greek word *"dosis"* which means 'a giving' the quantity of a drug or other therapeutic agent to be taken or applied all at a time or in fractional amounts within a stated period. (Ref. Stedman's Medical Dictionary).

Definition of Homoeopathic Posology

A homoeopathic "dose" means the particular preparation of medicine used, the quantity and form of that preparation as well as the number of administration of the medicine. In short, homoeopathic "dose" includes potency, quantity, form and number of administration of the medicine.

The study of the doctrine of these doses is known as "Posology".

Difference between Homoeopathic and Allopathic concept of Doses

Allopathic concept of dose: In allopathy "dose" means so many drops by measure or so many grains by weight—enough to produce the direct positive or physiological effect and not enough to endanger the patient. Allopaths relate the word "dose" to the material quantity of the medicine used.

Example: In constipation, recommended dose is 1 to 3 grains.

Homoeopathic concept of dose: In common speech a homoeopathic "dose" of anything means an infinitesimal dose:

1. In the first place, the "dose" related to the particular preparation of medicine used, e.g., in constipation, Opium mother tincture or the 6th, 12th or 30th potency.
2. In the second place, the "dose" related to the quantity of that preparation and the form of that preparation, e.g., Opium 30 was given. It may have been given as one drop liquid under the tongue, one or two globules, one drop liquid is dispensed with purified water or sugar of milk.
3. In third place, the "dose" related to the number of administration of the medicine—repetition, e.g., Opium 30, it may be a single dose or may be repeated every 4 hours or every

week—according to the condition of the patient.

Selection of Potency

Introduction

Selection of proper potency is another great difficult task, after proper selection of medicine for a homoeopathic physician.

It has been shown experimentally that in spite of the correctly selected medicine on the basis of totality of symptoms, it will not act curatively unless it is given in proper potency.

The medicine may fail to produce any favourable effect in lower potencies in a case but may show unexpected good results in higher potencies. It does not indicate, that lower potencies do not act at all in such cases. They do act, but their favourable effects are not perceived properly.

Discussion

There are different opinions in this regard as to which potency one should prescribe, though there is consensus over the broad divisions of potency, namely:

(i) Low: potencies below 30

(ii) Medium: potencies between 30 to 1M

(iii) High: potencies above 1M

Voisin has clearly stated that low potencies are organotropic, medium potencies influence function, and higher potencies are for the psyche.

There is no hard and fast rule for the selection of potency. Susceptibility is the only guide for the selection of potency. To assess the susceptibility of a patient, the physician must be qualified through the knowledge of allied subjects and must possess unbiased experience, freedom from prejudice, attention in observing, as well as clear conception of fundamental principles of homoeopathy and second prescription. There is no such parameter to judge the susceptibility of a patient. The axiom which is used for this purpose is *"More the susceptibility—higher the potency, less the susceptibility—lower the potency"*. But the modern life with its complexities, sophistications and over-drugging very often comes in front of the physician, as an obstacle to determine the susceptibility of a patient.

Various factors contribute to assume the susceptibility of a patient. They are: age, sex, habit and environment, constitution and temperament, nature and depth of the disease, structural changes, various suppressions, vitality, mental and physical reactions to environmental stimuli etc.

1. **Age:** Child and young adults require higher potencies as there is no wear and tear of organs and tissues.

   But in old age, susceptibility becomes gradually low due to wear and tear as well as different degenerative changes. So, they generally require low or medium potencies.

2. **Sex:** Females in villages of our country are usually less exposed to mental stress and strain, worries and anxieties, their nervous system are generally quiet in nature having a moderate degree of susceptibility. They require medium potencies.

   Males of irritable, sensitive nature, having a higher susceptibility, require higher potencies.

3. **Habit and environment** (Ref. Stuart Close)

   Higher potencies are best adapted to:

   (i) Persons engaged in highly intellectual and mental work (e.g., doctors, lawyers, ministers etc.)

   (ii) Sedentary occupations.

   (iii) Excitement of the imagination and emotions.

   (iv) Long sleep.

   (v) An effeminate life.

   Lower potencies are best adapted to:

   (i) Persons engaged in physical labour without much mental exertion.

   (ii) who sleep little.

   (iii) whose food is coarse.

   (iv) Persons exposed to the continual influence of drugs such as tobacco-workers and dealers.

   (v) Distillers and brewers and all connected with the liquor and tobacco trade.

   (vi) Druggists, perfumers, chemical workers etc.

   (vii) Idiots, imbeciles, and the deaf and dumb.

But where their illness is directly caused by some particular drug influence, a higher potency of the same or similar drug may prove to be the best antidote.

4. **Constitution and temperament**

Higher potencies are best adapted to (Ref. Stuart Close):

(i) Sensitive persons of a nervous, sanguine or choleric temperament.

(ii) Intellectual persons, quick to act and react.

(iii) Zealous and impulsive persons.

Lower potencies and frequent doses are suited to (Ref. Stuart Close):

(i) Torpid and phlegmatic individuals, dull of comprehension and slow to act.

(ii) Coarse fibred, sluggish individuals of gross habits.

(iii) Those who possess great muscular power but who require a powerful stimulus to excite them.

Lower potencies but repeated at long intervals

(i) *Oversensitive patients:* Sensitive patients will prove every remedy given in high potency and will fail to have their sickness cured. Such patient must be given the indicated drug, very low, 3rd to 30th potency or in drop doses of tincture, a single dose at a time with long intervals elapsing between doses in order to bring about curative action (Ref. A. H. Grimmer).

(ii) *Idiosyncratic patients:* They possess the higher susceptibility but must not be given in high potency. It is sufficient to inhale few globules of 30th potency only for few seconds. The dose may be repeated after 2 to 3 or even after 6 months if needed. Otherwise, these patients have no chance of cure.

5. **Nature and depth of the disease**

(a) *Acute diseases:* No structural change is usually effected in such a case. Naturally, susceptibility of the patient remains higher. Moreover, sudden onset, rapid progress and more or less fixed duration of disease indicate higher susceptibility. So an acute disease (e.g. chicken pox, measles, influenza, whooping cough, meningitis, common cold) requires high potency. Here, repeated doses of higher potencies are effective to arrest the progress of the disease.

(b) *Acute diseases with lowered vitality:* In severe dehydration (e.g. diarrhoea, vomiting), shock, collapse, extreme prostration, severe bleeding, typhoid state etc. the patient requires low potencies in repeated doses to overcome the inhibitory state of the vital dynamics. Here, preferable potencies are 3, 6, 12 or maximum 30th potency.

(c) *Acute manifestations of chronic diseases:*

(i) With gross organic changes—require low or medium potencies.

(ii) At the beginning of organic change or in functional plane—require high potencies.

(d) *Chronic diseases:*

(i) Without gross organic changes—higher potencies act curative if given in single or repeated doses, e.g., migraine, neuralgia, neurosis, most of the paralyses.

(ii) With gross organic changes—as the susceptibility becomes gradually low because of long continued suffering and organic changes, low or medium potencies are required. Too low potencies in repeated doses even in organic chronic disease may lead to Kent's 10th observation (New symptoms appear after the remedy) while too high potencies in comparison to patients susceptibility leads to Kent's 3rd observation (The aggravation is quick, short and strong with rapid improvement of the patient) and the patient may have to pass through grievous suffering before cure takes place.

(iii) Mental diseases—the susceptibility is generally very high, but high potencies are contraindicated in such cases to start with because of the possibility of too violent an aggravation.

(e) *Difficult and incurable diseases:* The patients with difficult and incurable diseases, will avoid severe aggravation and get palliation of their symptoms and a prolonging of their life if the physician prescribes remedies of a more superficial nature and in potencies not above 30th or 200th. But 50 millesimal potency is best for this purpose. Even the incurable case may turn into curable stage after the use of successive potencies in this scale.

(f) *Seat of the disease:* Where an important viscus, i.e., an internal organ, has been considerably deteriorated, material doses of the medicine are necessary to check it. This naturally belongs to chronic cases, e.g., in ischaemic heart disease: *Cactus* Q or *Spongia tosta* Q, 10-15 drops doses may be used.

(g) *The previous treatment of the disease:* Patients who have taken many crude drugs homoeopathic or allopathic—often require higher potency for their use.

(h) *Stage of the disease:* The disease process manifested in two stage—dynamic pathology and organic pathology. Dynamic pathology denotes the stage from the very beginning of the disease till structural changes start. During this period only functional disturbances are reflected, so the susceptibility of the patient is greatly higher. So, this kind of chronic disease must be treated with higher potency, in single dose. By frequent repetition in these cases, the patient will turn from "dynamic pathology" to "organic pathology".

On the other hand, "Organic Pathology" denotes the stage from the beginning of structural changes up to the end of the disease process. During this period, the susceptibility to disease is gradually decreased. As a result, the potency should be lower.

Different miasmatic states:

(i) Primary manifestations of psora, sycosis and syphilis require high potencies in repeated and large doses for an early and permanent cure.

(ii) Secondary manifestations of different miasmatic states require medium or low potencies to start with.

6. **Nature of medicine**

(a) *Nosodes:* The nosode group of medicines should be administered in higher potencies for its true effect.

(b) Some medicines work best in low potency or tincture such as *Crategus* in valvular heart disease, *Sabal serrulata* in benign hyperplasia of prostate (B.H.P.), *Arsenicum iodatum* in some cases of influenza, *Calc iodatum* in goitre and enlarged nodes, *Polygonum* sag in urinary stone.

(c) With some remedies their effect is reputed to vary with the potency used. Hepar sulph is said to abort infections if used high early in the process. It has resolve abscessed teeth and osteomyelitis of the jaw when used in low potency.

(d) Great care must be taken in selection of potency of deep acting remedies in serious chronic diseases.

Examples:

(i) *Lachesis* 200 had a most unpleasant effect, later antidoted by a dose of Sepia (—*M.L. Tyler*).

(ii) In some drugs 200 is a wicked potency, particularly of *Lycopodium*, a physician dreaded to use it (—*M.L. Tyler*).

(iii) Be careful of using *Lycopodium* in potencies much higher than **12C** in a case of severe pain (duodenal ulcer) or may precipitate a perforation (—*H.W. Boyd*).

(iv) It is dangerous to give *Phosphorus* in high potencies to patients with advanced phthisis as it may start a hoemorrhage that may prove fatal (—*M. L. Tyler*).

(v) *Phosphorus, Silicea* and *Lachesis* are three very dangerous remedies if there is pre-tubercular tendency. The wrong potency or too frequent repetition may drive the patient into an active tuberculosis (*—E. W. Hubbard*).

Various kinds of Doses

Maximum dose

It is the maximum or largest possible quantity of medicine, not harmful to human life which can be taken at a time by an individual.

In homoeopathy, maximum or large dose should not be administered for treatment purpose except in cases of primary manifestations of psora, sycosis and syphilis. Here, large doses, as well as repeated doses, of the indicated medicine are to be administered; otherwise the disease will not be cured, rather go on increasing along its course.

Lethal or fatal dose: It is also known as toxicological or narcotic dose. It is such amount of dose which can cause death of a living being. The fatal dose of different substances may be different, which depend upon their toxicity. A fatal dose of a milder narcotic or poison will obviously be more than that of a stronger narcotic or poison.

"Minimal lethal dose" is the smallest dose that has been recorded as fatal to a healthy person.

Booster dose: A subsequent dose given to enhance the action of the initial dose.

Fractional or refractive or divided dose: It is the fraction of a full dose, which is taken at short intervals.

Physiological dose: Physiological doses are those which stimulate the normal physiology or functions of the different organs or systems of our body and, hence, the symptoms thus appearing are known as physiological symptoms.

W. M. Boericke, in his *"A Compend of the principles of Homoeopathy"* states: "It is the physiological dose—that is, a dose large enough to produce symptoms. Opium constipates the bowels, produces insensibility. For these purposes a recognised, fixed quantity is necessary, not less than one-half to one grain. This constitutes its physiological dose".

Physiological dose is sufficient quantity and strength of a drug to produce a definite, predetermined effect or group of symptoms.

It bears these characters:

(i) It is injurious to the patient.

(ii) Its action is toxic in nature.

(iii) Its action is the exact opposite of curative action.

(iv) It is never employed in homoeopathic practice for curative purpose.

Infinitesimal dose: Dictionary meaning of "infinitesimal" is, "infinitesimal small quantity" and by extension "very small". The homoeopaths are divided into two groups. For one, that which is immeasurable is infinitesimal, though they remain below the Avogadro's number. For the other, the infinitesimal is beyond the Avogadro's number, i.e., the spiritual dilution.

Average dose: It is the prescriber's adjusted dose according to requirement of the patient. H.P.U.S. gives this kind of dose.

Single dose: It means that only one dose should be given in a day.

Daily dose: It is the total amount that can be given in a day—either as a single dose or the total amount divided into three or four doses.

Total dose: It means the total amount to be given in a day which should not be exceeded.

Minimum dose

Definition

It is that dose which is sufficient to overpower and annihilate the disease and capable of producing slight homoeopathic aggravation scarcely observable after the ingestion (Section 280).

It is that amount of medicine which, though smallest in quantity, produces the least possible excitation of the vital force, and yet sufficient to effect the necessary changes in it (Section 246).

It bears these characteristics:

(i) It is beneficial to the patient.

(ii) It is curative in action.

(iii) It is not toxic in nature.

(iv) Its action has been proved.

Nash has defined minimum dose as: "It is a dose crude or potentised, capable of affecting the patient curatively, without unnecessary aggravation when given according to Law of Similars".

Stuart Close says: "Minimum dose is a dose so small that it is not capable of producing symptoms, when used therapeutically. Homoeopathy requires that the therapeutic dose must be capable of producing a slight temporary aggravation or intensification of existing symptoms and never of producing symptoms".

Evolution of concept of minimum dose

Hahnemann at the beginning used large doses of medicine like allopathic system:

1786: He used large and repeated doses of *mercury* for Lues venerea.

1796: He prescribed *Verat alb* for bronchial asthma, 3 grains, every morning, for 4 weeks and *Arnica mont* several grains for dysentery.

1797: He prescribed 4 grains *Verat alb*, once daily, for colic. He also prescribed 5 grains of *Ipecac*, 4 grains of *Nux vom* and 1.5 drachum of *Cinchona* in different cases.

1801: Here we get the first indication of "infinitesimal doses".

1813: He stated that smallest dose is sufficient to cure disease and there might have been severe aggravation following large doses of medicine.

To avoid excessive aggravation, he decided to diminish the dose—which results after ingestion of medicinal dose.

In this way, Hahnemann reaches to the concept of minimum dose.

Reasons behind the application of minimum dose

In homoeopathy, use of minute dose has certain advantages. On the other hand, application of large dose has some disadvantages. Due to these reasons homoeopathy advocates minimum dose of medicine in practice.

A. **Disadvantages of using large dose**

(a) ***Too large a dose of homoeopathic medicine is injurious***

Too strong a dose of medicine, though quite homoeopathic, in spite of its remedial nature, will produce an injurious effect by its magnitude. Its qualities, as well as its homoeopathic similitude, will produce an unnecessary, too strong impression upon the vital force, which, in its turn, acts upon the most sensitive parts of the organism, already most seriously affected by the natural disease (Section 275).

For this reason, a medicine even homoeopathically suited to the case of disease does harm in every dose that is too large. It does more harm, the greater the homoeopathicity is and higher the potency selected. It does much more injury than an equally large doses of allopathic medicine that is un-homoeopathic and in no respect adapted to the morbid state (Section 276).

In that case, the so-called homoeopathic aggravation (i.e., the artificial and similar drug disease, called forth in the diseased parts of the body by the excessively large dose, and the reacting vital force (Aphor. 157-160) will rise to an injurious height. But the same similar drug disease, if of appropriate intensity, would have gently effected a cure (Aphor. 276).

(b) ***Produces violent medicinal disease***

Too large doses of an accurately chosen Homoeopathic Medicine, and especially when frequently repeated, bring about much trouble as a rule. They often put the patient in danger of life or make the disease almost incurable.

They do indeed extinguish the natural disease as far as the sensation of the life principle is concerned. The patient will no longer suffer from the original disease which had been homoeopathically cured, yet he will have to suffer from the excessively violent medicinal disease which is most difficult to destroy. (Aphor. 276, 6th edition).

B. **Advantages of minimum dose**

(a) In order to act really in conformity with nature, the true physician will prescribe his well-selected medicine in minute dose which is exactly as small as will just be sufficient to overcome and extinguish the disease.

But as human skill and caution sometimes fail in the selection of the remedy, the injury arising from small dose of wrongly selected appropriate medicine will be insignificant.

Moreover, harm done by the smallest possible dose is so slight that it may be immediately extinguished, or repaired by the natural vital powers, as well as by the speedy administration of an equally small dose of a more suitably selected similar remedy (Aphor. 283).

(b) A medicine whose selection has been accurately homoeopathic must be all the more salutary; the more the dose is reduced to the degree of minuteness appropriate for a gentle remedial effect (Aphor. 277).

(c) By applying minimum dose **unwanted aggravation** can be avoided.

(d) The specific dynamic action which produces uncommon, characteristic, distinguishing symptoms of the drug is produced by the minimum quantity of the drug.

(e) The smallness of the dose does not allow the drug to do any organic damage nor is there any risk of drug-addiction and drug-effects.

(f) To take the full advantage of finer and finest **curative property** of the remedies, they should be administered in minimum dose.

(g) In order to maintain the similarity of the sequence of the disease and the drug, minimum dose is suitable.

(h) The concept of minimum dose is verified by Arndt-Schultz Law—"Small doses stimulate, medium doses paralyse and large doses kill".

Repetition of Doses

(Pharmacopollaxy or Medicamental Repetition)

Introduction

To achieve rapid cure, three conditions are to be fulfilled (Section 246, 5th edition):

(i) *Similimum:* The medicine selected with utmost care should be perfectly homoeopathic.

(ii) *Minimum dose:* The medicine should be given in minimum dose, so as to produce the least possible excitation of the vital force, and yet sufficient to effect the necessary changes in it.

(iii) *Repetition:* The minutest yet powerful dose of the best selected medicine should be repeated at suitable intervals.

In homoeopathy, the selection of proper medicine is probably the most essential thing that matters but after the remedy has been selected and administered in proper potency, the physician should be able to watch out for, understand and interpret the remedy reaction and should know the proper "period for repeating the dose". This is considered so important that Kent warned us that a case may be completely spoiled by improper repetition of the dose.

Factors responsible for repetition of doses

In repetition of dose,—the following factors should be considered:

1. Condition and progress of the patient.
2. Nature of the disease.
3. Nature of the remedy.

1. Condition and progress of the patient

(a) *Perceptible and continued progress of improvement contraindicates repetition (Section 245, 5th edition).*

Perceptible and continued progress of improvement in an acute or chronic disease contraindicates the repetition of any medicine, because the beneficial effect the medicine continues to exert is rapidly approaching its perfection. Under these circumstances—every new dose of medicine even of the last one that proved beneficial would disturb the process of amelioration.

(b) *Repeat the dose only when improvement ceases.*

To allow a dose or remedy to act as long as the improvement produced by it is sustained is a good practice. But to attempt to fix arbitrary limits to the action of medicine, as some have done, is contrary to experience.

(c) *Repetition may be continued till either recovery ensues or different groups of symptoms arise and, thus, demands different remedy (Section 248, 5th edition).*

The dose of the same medicine may be repeated several times if necessary, until recovery ensures, or until the same medicine ceases to do good. At that period, the rest of the disease presenting a different group of symptoms demands another homoeopathic remedy.

2. **Nature of the disease**

A. ***Acute disease***

(a) *As per 5th edition* (in Centesimal scale): In acute diseases, the medicine may be repeated every twenty-four hours, twelve, eight or four hours. In most acute cases, every hour, up to as often as every five minutes.

(b) *As per 6th edition* (in 50-Millesimal scale): In acute diseases, every 2, 3, 4 or 6 hours interval may be repeated (e.g. Diarrhoea, Dysentery, Malaria, Typhoid etc.) In very urgent cases, medicine may be repeated every hour and oftener (e.g., Chicken-pox, Tetanus, Cholera etc.)

B. ***Chronic disease***

(a) *As per 5th edition* (in centesimal scale): The medicine may be repeated at intervals of fourteen, twelve, ten, eight, or seven days. Repetiton of higher potency—a single dose of higher potency is administered and then a wait follows till its action is over.

Repetition of lower potency: Frequent repetition of lower potency in chronic diseases acceptable.

(b) *As per 6th edition* (in 50-millesimal scale):

(i) Recent chronic diseases (F.N.I., Section 282): In chronic diseases where primary manifestations of psora, syphilis and sycosis (their first cutaneous manifestions) are present without any history of suppression, in that case Hahnemann advised to use the indicated medicine in large doses and repeated doses. This is the only exception from the administration of minimum dose. If we administer minimum dose in primary psora, syphilis and sycosis the disease will not be cured—rather progressed.

As for example—for **Psora**: recently developed eruption with vesicle, burning and itching.

As for example—for **Syphilis**: untreated primary chancre.

" " " for **Sycosis**: Condylomata.

These localised diseases (and not local) do not only tolerate, but demand immediate administration of **large doses** (large table-spoonful or even mouthfuls) repeated daily or even several times a day of their specific remedies in *ascending repetition*. This procedure does not involve any danger of causing medicinal aggravation, and since the physician has the advantage of observing the progress of the treatment day by day until the disappearance of these (local) lesions, they convince him of a perfect cure.

(ii) Old chronic diseases: In chronic diseases, every correctly selected homoeopathic medicine—even those whose action is of long duration—may be repeated daily for months with ever-increasing success.

If the solution is used up (in 7-15 days) it is necessary to add to the next solution of the same medicine if still indicated—one or several globules of a higher potency. Thus, higher and higher potencies of the medicine may be continued so long as the patient experiences continued improvement without encountering one or another complaint that he never had before in his life.

If new symptoms appear, then another homoeopathically related medicine must be chosen in place of the last and administered in the same repeated doses, modifying the solution of every dose with thorough vigorous succussions, thus changing its degree of potency and increasing somewhat.

"Homoeopathic aggravation" may occur towards the end of the treatment of chronic disease. In that case, the doses must be reduced still further and repeated in longer intervals and possibly stopped several days, in order to observe if the convalescent need no further medicinal aid. The apparent symptoms (not real symptoms) caused by the excess of the homoeopathic medicine will soon disappear and leave undisturbed health in its wake.

3. **Nature of remedy**

The repetition of the remedy depends also on the nature of remedy:

(a) *Potency:*

(i) Medicine in lower potency: Frequent repetition

(ii) Medicine in higher potency: Not frequently repeated.

(b) *Duration of action:*

(i) Deep-acting remedy: Medicines obtained from elements, compounds (inorganic and organic), minerals, and nosodes have longer duration of action and, hence, repeated less frequently.

(ii) Short-acting remedy: Medicines obtained from vegetable and animal sources have shorter duration of action and, hence, their repetitions had been more frequent.

(c) *Medicines having alternating action* (Section 251, 5th edition):

There are some medicines, which produce two opposite states alternating with each other in human health. These alternating opposite states are produced by the primary action of the medicine. This action of producing two opposite states in the primary action of medicine is termed as Alternating Action of Medicines; e.g., *Ignatia, Bryonia, Rhus tox,* sometimes *Belladonna.* If after prescribing properly selected medicine, on strict homoeopathic principles, no improvement follows, another small dose of the same medicine is prescribed. In most of the cases, the improvement ensues after the second dose of the same medicine. The second dose may even be administered within a few hours after the administration of the first dose in acute diseases.

Kent's Instructions of Repetition of Doses:

J. T. Kent has given clear instructions about the rules of repetition in the second prescription:

The first medicine should be repeated:

1. When improvement remains standstill.
2. When the original symptoms return after a temporary disappearance having the same general and particulars as formerly (Kent's 11th observation).

Single Medicine

[Monopharmacy (Simplex) or Polypharmacy]

Hahnemann was against mixing of two or more remedies at a time as only the most similar or the similimum is needed in Homoeopathy.

Hahnemann clearly states about the application of single medicine at a time, in Organon, Sections 272, 273 and 274.

Section 272: In no case is it requisite to administer more than one single, simple medicinal substance at one time.

Section 273: It was more consistent with nature and more rational to prescribe single simple medicine at one time in a disease.

Section 274: As the true physician is enabled to cure natural diseases safely and permanently by the simple medicine, administered singly and uncombined, so it is wise to follow the maxim "It is wrong to attempt to employ complex means when simple means suffice".

Section 272. F.N.I.: Some physicians have tried the plan of administering two medicines at a time, or nearly so, in cases where one of the remedies seemed to be homoeopathic to one portion of the symptoms of the diseases, and where a second remedy appeared adapted to the other portion. Hahnemann warned seriously against such an attempt, which will never be necessary even if it should proper.

Reasons for applying only single simple medicinal substance at a time

1. The homoeopathic medicines were proved singly and the Materia Medica was built up on the observed effect of drugs given singly, either in planned proving or in accidental proving.
2. The action of single medicine is certain, but in mixture form it is uncertain.
3. The homoeopathic medicine is administered singly so that its action is complete and unmodified by other drugs.
4. If more than one medicine are used, then it is difficult for the physician to assess which of the symptoms are removed by what medicine.
5. It is quite impossible for the physician to select a medicine of "Second prescription", when

more than one medicine is prescribed at one time.

6. Application of "**Polypharmacy**" for prolonged period in a patient ultimately will develop Iatrogenic disease (or artificial chronic disease or drug disease).
7. In homoeopathy, cure takes place by secondary curative action, due to reaction of vital force. But if the physician gives more than one medicine at a time the vital force cannot react in three or four different ways. So, cure is not possible in such a case.
8. Well-selected homoeopathic medicine is capable of effecting cure. But administration of few more or less similar medicines will only palliate some of the symptoms, never cure the patient as a whole. Prolonged palliation in such cases usually develop suppression of the symptoms.
9. The comparison of symptoms of single medicine is easily done and observed. Each medicine has its symptomatic individuality.
10. Administration of several medicines at a time may contraindicate each other or antidote the action of the other medicines. Moreover, the physician is unable to know which element was curative and one source of future guidance is thereby obscured.
11. In polypharmacy prescription, one out of many medicines may help to remove certain similar symptoms in a patient but others may do harm to other parts of the body.
12. In monopharmacy, when the medicine does not work or harms, we can change or antidote the medicine but in polypharmacy we are not able to know which is acting and which medicine is to be given for antidote of mixture if any harmful effect is being experienced.
13. In homoeopathy, single medicine is administered in minimum dose for effective cure, but in poly-prescription large doses are usually given, which may develop harmful effects.
14. The single medicine is quite enough to remove a disease, either simple or complicated. But it is not possible while several medicines are administered at a time, because the mixture of medicines have not been proved on healthy human beings and, as such, the symptoms that they can produce in the system is quite unknown to us.
15. The scientific data on drug action or estimation of curative drug action can be determined only when the medicine is administered singly.
16. Alternation or rotation of remedies is reprehensible since it leads away from accurate and definite knowledge of drug-effects and, sooner or later, to polypharmacy which is the most slovenly of all practices.
17. Since we have no proving of combination of drugs, it will be impossible to prescribe them with scientific accuracy.

Chapter 30

Weights and Measures (Metrology)

Introduction

One of the most essential functions of a pharmacist is the ability to perform *accurate pharmaceutical measurements, calculations and conversions.* Without this ability, a pharmacist is not able to apply their knowledge of pharmacology in a practical manner during their everyday work functions. This is important as one incorrect calculation, conversion or measurements will affect a dosage, and can potentially harm a patient. Therefore pharmacist should have a thorough knowledge about weights and measures, which are used in the calculations.

Note: The term 'Metrology' is derived from the Greek word 'Metron' meaning *'measure'*. Metrology is a science that deals with the measurements of weights and volumes.

Weights

1. It is the measure of the respective gravitational force acting on a body.
2. It is directly proportional to the body's mass. The latter, being a constant based on inertia, never varies.
3. It varies slightly with latitude, altitude, temperature, and pressure. The effect of these factors usually is not considered unless very precise weighing and large quantities are involved.

Measures

1. It is the determination of the volume or extent of a body.
2. Temperature and pressure have a pronounced effect, especially on gases or liquids. These factors, therefore, are considered when making precise measurements.

All standard weights and measures in the US are derived from or based on the United States National Prototype Standards of the Metre and the Kilogram. The standards are made of platinum-iridium, and are in the custody of the *National Institute of Standards and Technology* (NIST) in Washington, DC.

Different Measurement Systems

There are two systems for the "weights and measures" of drug substances.

A. Metric System (Decimal System)

B. Imperial System

A. Metric System (Decimal System)

1. **Definition**: The international System of

Units (SI), formerly called the metric system, is the internationally recognised decimal system of weights and measures with all multiples and divisions based on a factor of 10. It was implemented in India from 1st April, 1964 in pharmacy profession.

2. **Advantages**: The units are divided into tenth, the unit of volume and length are related and unit of volume is comparable to the unit of weight. It allows for quick and easy conversions between different systems of measurements.

3. **Fundamental units**: The Metric System made up by three basic units:

(a) Unit of Length – Metre

(b) Unit of Capacity – Litre

(c) Unit of Weight – Gram

(a) Unit of Length – Metre (m)

(i) Definition: It is defined as the distance at 0°C *between the axes of the two median lines engraved on a Platinum (90 part) and Iridium (10 part) bar*, known as, "International Prototype Metre" which is deposited at the International Bureau of weights and measures in Paris.

The metre is defined as 165063.73 wave lengths of the orange radiation in vacuum of the krypton 86 isotype-1960.

(ii) Uses: It is used for measuring the **lengths.** It has limited application in pharmacy practice.

(b) Unit of Capacity – Litre (l)

(i) Definition: The standard of capacity is the litre, which is the volume of one kg of purified water at its maximum density (approx 4°C). Microlitres (L) are used to measure volumes of solutions used in chromatographic procedures for the separation and quantitative determination of some official drugs.

(ii) Uses: It is used for measuring **liquids.**

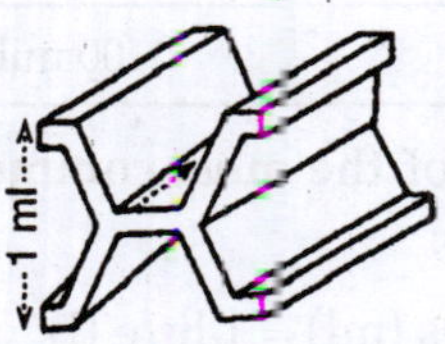

International Prototype Metre

(c) Unit of Weight – Gram (g)

(i) Definition: Originally defined as 'the absolute weight of a volume of pure water equal to the cube of the hundredth part of a metre, and at the temperature of melting ice' (later at 4°C, the temperature of maximum density of water).

The modern definition of a "gram" is a one-thousandth of the International Prototype kilogram.

(ii) Uses: It is used for measuring **mass/solid substances.**

Tables for Metric System Measurement

1. Measures of Weights (Mass)

The table of Metric Weight:

Weights	
1 kg	1000 g
1 g	1000 mg
1 mg	1000 μg, mcg.

Equivalencies of the most common weight denominations:

- 1000 micrograms (g/mcg) = 1 milligram (mg)
- 1000 milligrams (mg) = 1 gram (g)
- 1000 grams (g) = 1 kilogram (kg)

Metric System

Length (L) | Mass (M) | Weight (W) | Volume (V) | Density (D) | Temperature (T)

2. **Measures of Capacity (Volumes)**

The table of Metric Volume:

Volume	
1 litre (l)	1000 millilitres
1 millilitre	1000 μl
1 decilitre	100 millilitre

Equivalencies of the most common volume denominations:

- 1000 millilitres (ml) = 1 litre (l)

3. **Measures of Linear (Lengths)**

The table of Metric Length:

Length	
1 kilometre	1000 metres
1 metre	100 centimetres
1 centimetre	100 millimetres
1 millimetre	1000 microns (μ)
1 micron	1000 mμ, nm
1 mμ, nm	10 angstrom Å

Equivalencies of the most common volume denominations:

- 1000 millimetres (mm) = 100 centimetres (cm)
- 100 centimetres (cm) = 1 metre (m).

B. Imperial System

It is an old system of weights and measures. Weight is a measure of the gravitational force acting on a body and is directly proportional to its mass. The imperial system is divided into two parts for the purpose of measurements of weight. These are:

(a) Avoirdupois System (UK),

(b) Apothecary System (USA).

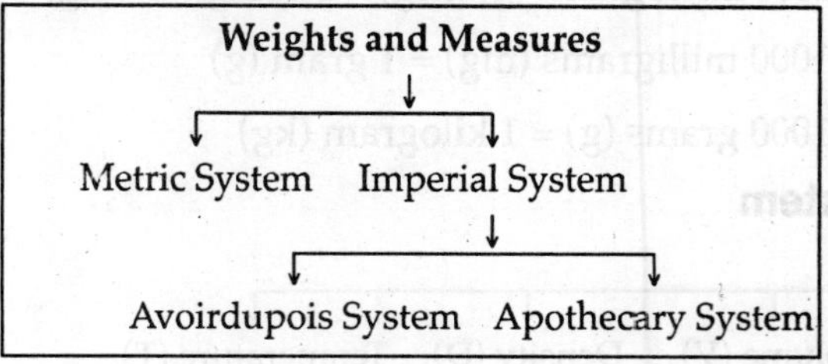

(a) Avoirdupois System (UK)

(i) Introduction: This system is Roman in origin, has a French name, and mostly used in United Kingdom as a standard for weights in commerce. It is formerly recognised by the British Pharmacopoeia (BP).

(ii) Fundamental units: In this system pound (lb) is taken as the standard of weight (mass).

Tables for Avoirdupois System Measurement

Weight		
Measurement Unit	**Unit Equivalent within System**	**Metric Equivalent**
1 grain (gr)		0.06 g
1 ounce oz	437.5 gr	30.00 g
1 pound (lb)	16 oz or 7000 gr	454.00 g 2.20 kg

(b) Apothecary System (USA)

(i) Introduction: The Imperial System includes a set of special weight termed as Apothecaries. It is also known as Troy system, developed by Romans. Apothecary System usually used by the practitioners during their prescription writing as well as by the pharmacists while dispensing medicines even in retail trade. Apothecary system was widely used until the beginning of the 20th century.

(ii) Fundamental units: The grain is the standard unit in this system and all other weights are derived from it.

Tables for Apothecary System Measurement

1. **Measures of Weight (Mass)**

Weight	
1 drachm	34 g
1 ounce	℥ 30 g
1 grain (gr)	0.06 g
1 scruple (Ə)	20 gr = 1.2 g
1 pound (lb)	373.2 g

2. Measures of Capacity (Volume)

Volume	
1 fluid drachm	Fʒ 4 ml
1 fluid ounce	F℥ 30 ml
1 minim (min)	0.06 ml
1pint (pt)	480 ml
1 quart (qt)	960 ml
1 gallon (gal)	3840 ml

3. Measures of Linear (Length)

Length	
1 inch	2.5 cm

Measurement Conversion Tables

Approximate Measures: Liquids

1 fl oz	=	30 ml
1 cup (8 fl oz)	=	240 ml
1 pint (16 fl oz)	=	480 ml
1 quart (32 fl oz)	=	960 ml
1 gallon (128 fl oz)	=	3800 ml
1 teaspoon	=	5 ml
1 tablespoon	=	15 ml

Approximate Measures: Weights

1 oz	=	30 g
1 lb (16 oz)	=	480 g

15 grains	=	1 g
1 grain	=	60 mg

Apothecary Equivalents: Weight

1 scruple	=	20 grains (gr)
60 grains	=	1 dram
8 drams	=	1 ounce
1 ounce	=	480 grains
16 ounces	=	1 pound (lb)

Apothecary Equivalents: Volume

60 minims	=	1 fluid dram
8 fluid drams	=	1 fluid ounce
1 fluid ounce	=	480 minims
16 fluid ounces	=	1 pint (pt)

Exact Equivalents

1 g	=	15.43 grains
1 grain	=	64.8 mg
1 ml	=	16.23 minims
1 Minim	=	0.06 ml
1 oz	=	28.35 g
1 lb	=	453.6 g (0.4536 kg)
1 kg	=	2.2 lb
1 fluid oz (fl oz)	=	29.57 ml
1 pint (pt)	=	473.2 ml
1 quart (qt)	=	946.4 ml
0.1 mg	=	$\frac{1}{600}$ grain (gr)
0.12 mg	=	$\frac{1}{500}$ gr

Conversion Table for Domestic Measures

Domestic Measure	Imperial system	Metric System
1 drop	= 1 minim	= 0.06 ml
1 teaspoonful	= 1 fl. Drachm	= 4.00 ml (5 ml for all practical purposes)
1 desert spoonful	= 2 fl. Drachm	= 8.00 ml (10 ml for all practical purposes)
1 tablespoonful	= 4 fl. Drachm	= 16.00 ml (15 ml for all practical purposes)
2 tablespoonful	= 8 fl. Drachm	= 32.00 ml (30 ml for all practical purposes)
1 wine glassful	= 2 fl. Ounce	= 60.00 ml
1 teacupful	= 4 fl. Ounce	= 120.00 ml
1 tumblerful	= 8 fl. Ounce	= 240.00 ml

Note: one drop is often considered to be one minim, but this is incorrect, as drops are variable.

0.15 mg	=	$\frac{1}{400}$ gr	0.6 mg	=	$\frac{1}{100}$ gr
0.2 mg	=	$\frac{1}{300}$ gr	0.8 mg	=	$\frac{1}{80}$ gr
0.3 mg	=	$\frac{1}{200}$ gr	1 mg	=	$\frac{1}{65}$ gr
0.4 mg	=	$\frac{1}{150}$ gr	1 kg	=	1000 g
0.5 mg	=	$\frac{1}{120}$ gr	1 g	=	1000 mg
			1 mg	=	1000 mcg

Chapter 31

Prescription Writing

ABBREVIATIONS COMMONLY USED

Abbreviations are most useful in prescription writing. It saves the valuable time of the prescriber and gives the clear direction to the pharmacist in very short space. Following is the mode of writing abbreviations/notations in prescription writing. Abbreviations are given below with Latin or Greek words and their **English meaning:**

Abbreviation	*Latin or Greek words*	*English meaning*
AA, Aa, aa	*Ana*	Of each
A.C., a.c.	*Ante cibum*	Before food, Before meal
Ad	*Ad*	To, Up to
Add	*Adde*	Add, Let them be added
Ad lib	*Ad Libitum*	To the desired amount
Ad us exter	*Ad usum externum*	For external use
Aeq	*Aequales*	Equal
Agit	*Agita*	Shake or stir
Agit a us	*Agita ante usum*	Shake before using
Alb	*Albus*	White
Alt. hor.	*Alternis horis*	Every other hour
Alt. noct.	*Alternis nocta*	Every other night
Ante	*Ante*	Before
Aq	*Aqua*	Water
Aq. bull.	*Aqua bulliens*	Boiling water
Aq. comm.	*Aqua communis*	Common water
Aq. dest.	*Aqua distillata*	Distilled water

Abbreviation	*Latin or Greek words*	*English meaning*
Aq. ferv.	*Aqua fervens*	Hot water
Aq. pur.	*Aqua pura*	Pure water
Aur.	*Auris*	The ear or ears
Aut	*Aut*	Or
Bene	*Bene*	Well
Bib.	*Bibe*	Drink
Bis.	*Bis*	Twice
B.D., Bis in d	*Bis in dies*	Twice daily
B.I.D.	*Bis in dies*	Twice in a day
Bid	*Bidare*	Drink
Bol	*Bolus*	A large pill
B.P.	—	Boiling point
$\bar{C}$	*cum*	With
C	*Centum*	A hundred
C	*Congius*	A gallon
C.C.	—	Cubic centimetre
Cap.	*Capitat*	Let him take
Caps	*Capsula*	A capsule
Cera	*Cera*	Wax
Cerat	*Ceratum*	Cerate
Chart	*Charta*	A paper
Cib.	*Cibus*	Food or meal
Cito. disp.	*Cito dispensetur*	Let it be dispensed quickly
Cochl.	*Cochleare*	Spoonful
Cochl. ampl.	*Cochleare amplum*	A table spoonful
Cochl. mag.	*Cochleare magnum*	A large spoonful
Cochl. min.	*Cochleare minimum*	A small spoonful
Cochl. mod.	*Cochleare modicum*	A dessert spoonful
Cochl. parv.	*Cochleare parvum*	—
Co.	*Cola*	Strain
Coll. Collyr.	*Collyrium*	An eye wash
Collun	*Collunarium*	A nose wash
Collut	*Collutorium*	A mouth wash
Comp.	*Compositus*	Compound
Confricamen	*Confricamentum*	A liniment
Cong	*Congius*	A gallon
Cons.	*Conserva*	A conserve; keep
Contra	—	Against
Cort	*Cortex*	The bark
C.m	*Cras mane*	Tomorrow morning
C.n.	*Cras nocti*	Tomorrow night
C.v.	*Cras vespere*	Tomorrow evening
Cuj.	*Cujus*	Of which

Abbreviation	Latin or Greek words	English meaning
Cyath	*Cyathus*	A glass
C. vin.	*Cyathus vinarius*	A wine glass
D.	*Dosis*	A dose
d.	*Da*	Give
de	—	Of, from
dec	*Decanta*	pour off
Decem	*Decem*	Ten
de. d in d.	*De die in doe*	From day to day
det.	*Detur*	To be given, give
Dieb. alt	*Diebus alternis*	On alternate days
Dil.	*Dilutus*	Dilute, diluted
Dim.	*Dimidus*	One-half
Div.	*Divide*	Divide
D. inp aeq	*Dividatur in partes aequales*	Let it be divided into equal parts
d.t.d	*Dentur tales doses*	Give of such doses
e	*Ex*	From one of
Et.	*Et*	And
Ft.	*Fiat*	Let it be made
Ft. cerat	*Fiat ceratum*	Let a cerate be made
Ft. chart xii	*Fiat chartulae xii*	Let 12 powders be made
Ft. collyr.	*Fiat collyrium*	Let an eyewash be made
Ft. haust	*Fiat haustus*	Make a draught
Ft. linim	*Fiat linimentum*	Let a liniment be made
Ft. mist.	*Fiat mistura*	Let a mixture be made
Ft. pil.	*Fiat pilula*	Make a pill
Ft. pulv.	*Fiat pulvis*	Let a powder be made
Ft. solut.	*Fiat solutio*	Let a solution be made
Ft. ung.	*Fiat unguentum*	Let an ointment be made
Garg	*Gargarisma*	A gargle
Gm, g	*Gramme*	grams
Gr.	*Grana*	A grain
Gt.	*Gutta*	A drop
Haust	*haustus*	A draught
Habt.	*habeat*	Let him have
Hic, hoc	*Hic, hoc*	This
H.	*Hora*	An hour
H.D.	*Hora decubitus*	At bedtime
H.S.	*Hora somni*	At bedtime
Hor.	*Hors*	Hour
In, d.	*Indes, In die*	Daily, in a day
Lac.	—	Milk
Lat. Dol	*Lateri dolente*	To the painful side
Lin.	*Linimentum*	A liniment

Abbreviation	*Latin or Greek words*	*English meaning*
Lot.	*Lotio*	A lotion
M.	*Misce*	Mix
m.	*Minim*	A drop
Mag	*Magnus*	Large
Mane	—	Morning
M. et n	*Mane at nocte*	Morning and night
M.P.	—	Melting point
Mitt	*Mittes*	Send
Mitt tal	*Mitte tails*	Send such
Mist	*Mistura*	A mixture
Mod praescript	*Modo praescripto*	As prescribed
Mor. Dict	*Moro dicto*	To be used in the manner directed
M.D.U.	*Moro dicto utendum*	To be used as directed
N.O.	—	Natural order
No.	*Numero, numerus*	Number
Noct	*Nocte*	At night
Non	*Nox*	Not, do not
Non rep	*Non repetaur*	Do not repeat
Nox	*Nox*	Night
O	—	Mother substance
Oct, O	*Octaris*	A pint
Om	*Omnis*	All, every after
Omn. man	*Omni mane*	Every morning
Omn. noct	*Omni nocte*	Every night
Omn. hor	*Omni hora*	Every hour
Omn. bih	*Omni bihora*	Every two hours
O. d.	*Omni die*	Every day
O. P.	—	Over proof
P. ae	*Partes aequales*	Equal parts
Parvus	*Parvus*	Little
Phar	*Pharmaceutical*	Relating to pharmacy
Post	—	After
P.C.	*Post cibus*	After food
Pr. C.	*Pruis cibus*	Before food
P.R.N.	*Pro re nata*	When required
Prox.	*Proximo*	Next
Pt.	*Perstetur*	Continue
Puly	*Pulvus*	A powder
P. R., p.r.	*Per rectum*	By the rectum
P.v.	*Per vaginum*	By the vagina
Q	—	Mother tincture
Q.H., Q.U. hor.	*Quaque hora*	Each hour, every hour
Q.I.D., q.i.d	*Quarter in die*	Four times a day

Abbreviation	*Latin or Greek words*	*English meaning*
Q.L.	*Quantum libet*	As much as required
Q.P.	*Quantum placet*	As much as you please
Q.S.	*Quantum sufficiat*	A sufficient quantity
Q.v.	*Quantum vis*	As much as you wish
Rx	*Recipe*	To take
Rept.	*Repetatur*	Let it be repeated
S	*Signa*	Mark
SS	*Semis*	half
Ss	*Semi*	half
Semel	*Semel*	Once
Semel in d	*Semel in die*	Once a day
Semi h.	*Semi hora*	half an hour
Septimana	*Septimana*	A week
Sig.	*Signa*	Mark, label
Sine	—	Without
Sing.	*Singulorum*	Of each
Sol.	—	Solution
Solv.	*Solve*	To dissolve
S.L.	*Saccharum lactis*	Sugar of milk
S.O.S.	*Si opus sit*	If necessary
Sp. Gr., S.G.	—	Specific gravity
Stat.	*Statim*	Immediately
Sum	*Sume, Sumat*	Let him take
S.V.R.	*Spiritus vini rectificatus*	Alcohol
T.D. or TID	*Ter in die*	Thrice daily
Talis	*Talis*	Such, Like this
Ter	*Tere*	Rule
Tr.	*Tincture*	Tincture
Trit.	*Tritura*	Trituration
Una	—	Together
Uncia	*Uncia*	An ounce
Ung.	*Unguentum*	An ointment
Ut. dict	*Ut. dictum*	As directed
Vac ven	*Vacuo ventriculo*	In empty stomach
Vel	*Vel*	Or
Vol.	*Vol*	Volume
Wt.	—	Weight
ʒ I	—	One dram
ʒ ss	—	Half dram
℥ I	—	One ounce
℥ ss	—	half ounce
℥ iss	—	One and half ounce

Principles and Mode of Prescription Writing

Etymology: The word **"Prescription"** is derived from the Latin word *"Prescripto"* (para means "before" and scribo means "I write").

Definition: Prescription is a written direction given by a physician to his own compounder or any pharmacist for the preparation of medicine as well as instruction to the patient about mode of intake.

If the physician serves a prescription from his own medicinal stock, then there is no question of writing a prescription; in this case he just records in his diary or in a book exclusively kept for his future reference, along with the name, address and age of the patient and the prescribed remedy with potency and doses. But if the physician wants to serve a prescription by his own compounder or any other pharmacist, then he should write the prescription in such a way that a compounder faces no difficulty to dispense with his prescription.

It is a valuable document and must be properly written and must be preserved by the pharmacist, compounder or the patient, after it has been served. *Prescription is a legal evidence.*

Principles of writing an ideal prescription

1. *Norms (A rule; a pattern; a type):* Definite 'norms' is the most important in an ideal prescription. Prescription must be written in a definite pattern, i.e., Superscription, Inscription, Subscription and Signature. Inscription should never be written before Superscription. On the other hand supercription should never be written after subscription. Maintenance of proper arrangement as **Supercription, Inscription, Subscription** and **Signature** is essential for an ideal prescription.
2. *Forms (shapes; moulds; styles):* Prescription writing may be either in simple form or in Latin form. Simple form of prescription is generally used by most of the physicians nowadays.
3. *Legibility (i.e., easily read):* Prescription should be written in such a way that a compounder or pharmacist faces no difficulty with his prescription.
4. Accuracy and reliability of ingredients.
5. Administering the smallest dose that will cure (minimum dose).
6. Incompatibles (i.e., inimicals) are not to be used.

> *Note:* A prescription should not contain such ingredients which can counteract one another either physically, chemically, or physiologically, when mixed together. If they do so, they are known as incompatibles.

Different parts of a prescription

An ideal prescription consists of four parts: 1. The Superscription; 2. The Inscription; 3. The Subscription; 4. The Signature.

(a) ***The Superscription:*** It includes:

(i) *Name of the patient with address:* It should always be placed at the top of the prescription by the physican and should be transferred to the label by the compounder. The word "For" should be written before the name of the patient.

(ii) *Age and sex.*

(iii) Symbal R_x: It stands for the Latin word, *"Recipe"* which means, "to take". The oblique dash across the "R" is probably a relic of the symbol, that represented a prayer of Jupiter. The letter originally signifies the symbol of the planet of our Sun, "The Jupiter".

Values of each item in Superscription

(i) *Name of the patient:* For identification of the patient, the name is essential, while recording the case, for follow up of the case, as well as while investigating any tests that are written in prescription.

(ii) *Address:* Location, where the patient resides is most important. There may be prevalence of some diseases which attack persons in certain specific localities. By knowing the address, the physician may enquire about that. If the patient comes for his or her treatment from long distance, the physician usually faces great difficulty in treating the chronic disease. In this case, the physician must enquire how the patient will communicate with the doctor at proper time interval.

(iii) *Age:* From the age, the physician can assess the growth and development of the patient. There are certain diseases (e.g., adenoids) which especially attack children and others (e.g., enlarged prostate, cataract) in aged individuals. Moreover, during selection of potency the "Age" of the patient plays a very important role. As we know, susceptibility of children is more and, with the advancement of age, it gradually decreases. So, higher potencies are usually required in children and lower to medium potencies in aged individuals.

(iv) *Sex:* There are some specific diseases in relation to sexes (male/female). Nature of disease susceptible to each sex is different. So the physician must write the sex in prescription.

(v) *Symbol R_x:* Practically, it has less value for the treatment of the patient. The physician remembers the name of "God" before writing a prescription, just like the proverb, "I treat, He cures".

2. ***The Inscription*** (or the body of a prescription). It includes:

(i) Name of the remedy, its potency, its quantity.

(ii) Name and quantity of the vehicle.

Name of the remedy, potency and its quantity should be written at first, then the name and quantity of the vehicle is to be written.

The "inscription part" is most important than any other part of a prescription as this part contains the medicine as well as vehicle.

3. ***The Subscription:*** It includes the directions to the pharmacist as to how he is to dispense the remedy, e.g., "M. Ft. Mist", "M. Ft. Pulv." etc.

4. ***The Signature*** (from L. signature—let it be labelled): It includes:

(a) *Directions to the patient:* Make it a point to give directions in a definite manner. These should be brief, simple and to the point. That should be written in simple language and good hand-writing so that the patient can decipher the instructions:

(i) How to use the medicine. It is important to mention the hour of the day when medicines are to be administered.

(ii) When to report.

(iii) Some advices (if any): e.g.,

—Diet (to be allowed and to be avoided).

Specimen of a Model Prescription

[For
Miss Arpita Mondal
155/1 K. P. Roy Lane, Kolkata 78
Age: 9 years.] ...... Superscription

[R_x
Bryonia alba 30
Gtt. iv
Aqua dest ozi] ...... Inscription

[M. Ft. Mist
Make eight marks] ... Subscription

[To be taken twice daily morning
and night, in an empty stomach,
Stop when improvement starts.
Adv... Blood for T.C., D.C., E.S.R., Hb%
... Chest X-ray (P.A. view)

Sd/-
B. Mondal
25.2.2003
Regn. No. 13936] Signature

Note

Some authors divide a model prescription into six parts:

1. Superscription (or the heading).
2. Name of the patient.
3. Inscription (or name and quantity of ingredients).
4. Subscription (or direction to the pharmacist).
5. The sigma (or direction to the patient).
6. The signature of the physician, date and registration no., of Medical Council.

—Yoga and physiotherapy.

—Investigations (such as pathological, radiological, U.S.G., endoscopy etc.)

(b) *Signature of the physician* with date and registration number obtained from Homoeopathic Council.

Precautions to be taken while writing prescription

In writing prescription the following precautions should be taken:

1. Each line must always begin with a capital letter.
2. The name of the medicine and its potency must be written first, then the name of the "vehicle" and quantity.
3. The name of the medicine should be written in Latin (or generic name). Even Latin names should be used for the directions to the compounder or dispenser.
4. Directions to the patient should be written in simple language and good handwriting. But the dispenser must write the directions on the label either in English or in vernacular of the locality.
5. When in doubt, always write in English. It is important that the dispenser should understand the meaning of expression(s) used.
6. Never handover the prescription without reading it over again.

Justify: *Prescription writing is compulsory of a physician; Or, Prescription writing is MUST for a physician; Or, Enumerate the values of a prescription; Or, Mention the utility of serving the prescription.*

Every homoeopathic physician must write a prescription and that should be handed over to the patient.

Prescription writing has great advantages

A. **Advantages for the patient**

(i) The patient can take the prescribed medicine in proper time and proper form (i.e., by dissolving in water or taking directly over the tongue), (ii) The patient can follow the advices regarding the diet (which food items are to be taken or to be avoided) and other auxiliary measures, written in the prescription, (iii) Different investigations that should be done are written in prescription. So the patient can take help of this prescription for doing so, (iv) Moreover, the patient can communicate easily with the physician, in urgent cases, over phone or directly to the physician's chamber or residence, as phone no. and address are written in the prescription. (v) Medico-legal importance: In case of fatal or serious condition of the patient following wrong treatment—the patient can put a case against the physician. (vi) It is helpful for the patient to know the academic qualification of the physician written on the prescription.

B. **Advantages for the physician**

(a) *For the patient under treatment*—(i) The physician can easily look on the previous case record of the patient on the basis of date, name of the patient and reference no., if any; (ii) It is easy for the physician to select a medicine for "second prescription" in respect of previous prescribed medicine, written in prescription; (iii) The physician can follow up the case properly—whether the patient improved or deteriorated, in respect of previous prescription.

(b) *For the patient coming from other physician*—(i) If the patient can supply the name of the homoeopathic medicine lastly taken from the prescription, then it is easy for the physician to select a medicine thereafter. (ii) If the patient still continues the medicine of the prescription and its action still persists, then physician usually supplies some unmedicated substances for some time and after that indicated medicine is given. (iii) If the patient comes from allopathic physician, developing some adverse effect, then the medicine lastly taken by the patient should be known from the prescription and "Tautopathic medicine" may be administered to antidote the case. (iv) Previous prescription or prescriptions helps the physician to know—about the way of treatment—single medicine therapy or poly-prescription.

Some homoeopathic physicians treat their patient by noting the medicines in their record book, without serving any prescription to the patient. In that case, if the patient goes to another physician for the treatment of some disease, then it will be very difficult for the physician to treat the patient homoeopathically.

So every homoeopathic physician must serve prescription to his patient, which **bears a legal evidence.**

Vehicle used in homoeopathic prescriptions: Following vehicles are used in homoeopathic prescriptions:

1. Sugar of milk. 2. Globules. 3. Tablets. 4. Cones. 5. Purified water. 6. Glycerine. 7. Vaseline. 7. Olive oil.

Examples of prescription writing

A. Liquid medicine with purified water

(i) *Write a prescription for a lady suffering from acute follicular tonsillitis.*

(Internal only)

For

Mrs. Sarbani Saha

Age : 35 years

Rx

Phytolacca decandra 200

Gtt-ii

Aqua dest ozi

M. Ft. Mist

Put four marks

To be taken twice daily, morning and evening, in an empty stomach.

Stop when improvement starts.

Report thereafter.

Sd/-

Souri Ghosh

18.6.92

Regn. No. 5310

(ii) *Write a prescription for a person having a pus-forming abscess, few doses of a suitable drug to be taken four hourly in common form.*

For

Mr. Soumitra Saha

Age: 25 years

Rx

Hepar sulph. 6

Gtt-ii

Aqua dest ozii

M. Ft. Mist

Put six marks

To be taken every four hours interval.

Sd/-

Subhasis Chakraborty

12.3.92

Regn. No. 8957

B. Liquid medicine with sugar of milk

(i) *Write a prescription for a baby suffering from diarrhoea.*

For

Baby Sonali

Rx

Nux vomica 30

Gt-ii

Sac. lac, Grs.vi

M. Ft. Pulv.

Make four packets (powders)

1 such to be taken tric. hor.

Sd/-

Tapas Koley

10.6.92

Regn. No. 9939

(ii) *Write a prescription for a lady requiring Pulsatilla 30—6 drops in 18 grains of sugar of milk to be divided into six doses—one to be taken twice daily.*

For

Miss Debarati Banerjee

Rx

Pulsatilla 30

Gt-vi

Sac. lac, Grs. xviii

M. Ft, Pulv

Make six packets

To be taken twice daily.

Medicine must be stopped when improvement starts.

Report thereafter.

Sd/-

Mita Dhar

12.4.92

Regn. No. 7321

C. Liquid medicine with globules

As a medical man, how will you write a prescription for a girl who is suffering from acute tonsillitis? (The medicine to be served in globules).

For

Miss Malati Mandal

Age: 14 years

℞

Belladonna 30

Gtt-viii

Globule No. 20, in dr i phial.

Add and mix well

Four globules to be taken at a time, in an empty stomach, thrice daily, for four days.

Report thereafter.

Sd/-

Debasish Mandal

12.3.92

Regn. No. 8032

D. Globules with purified water

(i) *Write a prescription for a baby suffering from acute fever with coryza.*

For

Baby Rinku

℞

Acon nap 6

8 globules No. 20

Aqua dest oz i

M. Ft. Mist

Put 12 marks

To be taken every two hours' interval. Stop when improvement starts.

Report thereafter.

Sd/-

Shampa Dey

18.3.92

Regn. No. 1207

(ii) *Write a prescription for a lady suffering from menstrual disorders. The medicines are to be supplied in liquid form.*

For,

Swati Roychoudhury

℞

Pulsatilla 30

10 Globules No. 20

Aqua dest oz i

M. Ft. Mist

Put six marks

To be taken every morning on an empty stomach for six days.

Stop the medicine when improvement starts.

Report thereafter.

Sd/-

Sanat Pandit

17.9.91

Regn. No. 6554

E. Globules with sugar of milk

(i) *Write a prescription for a child suffering from worm troubles and vomiting.*

For

Master Santu

Age: 6 years

℞

Cina 30

8 Globules no. 20

Sac. lac. grs xvi

M. Ft. Pulv

Make four packets.

To be taken twice daily—morning and night, on empty stomach.

Sd/-

Ranjan Dey

8.4.92

Regn. No. 7589

(ii) *Write a prescription for a lady suffering from digestive trouble.*

For

Seema Kapila

℞

Nux vomica 200

4 Globules No. 20

Sac. lac., grs vi

M. Ft. Pulv. one

To be taken c.m.

Followed by:

℞

Sac. lac., grs xx
M. Ft. Pulv.
Make five packets.
One packet is to be taken omn. noct.

Sd/-
Partha Mandal
27.6.92
Regn. No. 13920

F. Prescriptions with three vehicles

(i) *As a medical man, how will you write a prescription for a baby suffering from diarrhoea and requiring two doses of medicines at two hourly intervals followed by a dose of Sac. lac?*

For

Baby Rintu

(a) ℞

Nux vomica 30
2 Globules No. 20
Aqua dest oz ii
Mix, put two marks
Each mark is to be taken every 2 hour interval.
Followed by

(b) Sac. lac. 30
Grs. ii
One dose

Sd/-
Rebati Sarkar
2.6.92
Regn. No. 8324

(ii) *Write a prescription for a lady who is suffering from severe headache.*

For

Putul Nandi

℞

Nat mur 200
8 Globules No. 20
Aqua dest oz i
With the addition of 2 minims of R.S.
M. Ft. Mist.
Put 4 marks
To be taken twice daily.

Sd/-
Nirmal Paul
12.08.92
Regn. no. 12336

G. Prescription for both internal and external use

(i) *Write a prescription for a lady for internal and external use, who is suffering from erosion of cervix of the uterus.*

Internal

For

Ruma Kundu

℞

Argentum nitricum 200
Gtt-II
Aqua dest oz i
M. Ft. Mist
Put two marks
Twice daily

External

℞

Hydrastis can Q
3 ml. Q in 27 ml. of glycerine.
Mix it thoroughly by shaking.
Apply on the affected part by a cotton swab.
B. D. × 10 days.

Sd/-
Jayasree Sarkar
10.6.92
Regn. No. 11334

(ii) *Write a prescription for a gentleman who is suffering from septic tonsillitis (both internal and external).*

Internal

For

Himangshu Koley

℞

Phytolacca decandra 30
4 globules No. 20
Aqua dest oz ii
M. Ft. Mist
Put eight marks
One mark, three times a day
Stop when improvement starts
Report thereafter.

External

℞

Phytolacca decandra Q
3 ml Q in 27 ml of Glycerine

Mix it thoroughly by shaking

Apply on the effected tonsil by a cotton swab.

Twice daily × 10 days.

Sd/-

Samir Dey

14.6.92

Regn. no. 3006

H. Prescription in Latin form

(i) *Write a prescription for a person who is suffering from fever.*

For

Bijoy Mondal

R_x

Kali mur 3x trit.

Grs. VII

Ft. 7D.

Cito. disp

Cap. omn. hor.

Sd/-

Nirmal Dutta

5.5.92

Regn. No. 9937

(ii) *Write a prescription for a lady who is suffering from hyperemesis gravidarum.*

For

Sujata Pillai

R_x

Ipecac 30

6 Globules No. 20

Aqua dest oz ii

M. Ft. Mist

Mark 6D

T.D. vac. ven.

Sd/-

Rita Dhar

13.4.92

Regn. No. 13605

(iii) *Write a prescription for a baby suffering from parotiditis requiring one dose of Merc proto iod. 200 followed by 8 doses of placebo powders.*

Use the following abbreviations.

O.M.; Pulv.; Vac. ven.; Gtt.; M.Ft.; Grs.; XX; Cap.; Aqua dest; 200; R_x; Sac. lac; Idosis; ℨ ii

For

Baby Soumen

(a) R_x

Merc proto iod. 200

Gtt. ii

Aqua dest ℨ ii

M. Ft. I dosis

Cap. vac. ven.

followed by,

(b) Sac. lac.

Grs. XX

M. Ft. pulv.

Make 8 packets.

Cap. o.m.

Sd/-

Ramesh Hari

18.6.92

Regn. No. 9998

I. Prescription in 50-Millesimal scale of potency

For

Mr. Kalyan Mukherjee

48 M.G. Road

Kolkata 9

Age: 29 years

R_x

Sulphur 0/3

I Globule No. 10

Sac. lac. grs-11

Aqua dest ℨ ii

Rectified spirit Gtt xii

M. Ft. Mist

Mark 8D

Give ten equal and uniform downward strokes.

Before taking each dose, ten stroke, are to be given. Each dose is to be taken in a glass of pure water. Then one teaspoonful is to be taken orally, remaining portion is to be thrown away. Each dose is to be taken every morning in an empty stomach.

Remaining doses should be used in similar way.

Sd/-

B. Mandal

15.6.92

Regn. No. 13936

Chapter 32

Dispensing of Medicines

Introduction

The homoeopathic medicines are routinely dispensed in the form of tinctures and solid or liquid potencies with the help of a suitable vehicle (i.e., menstrua or solvents). These are called as **dosage forms.**

Homoeopathic medicines are usually dispensed in the form of mother tinctures, liquid potencies or in the form of powder triturates for oral use.

1. **Mother tinctures (Q)** are dispensed diluted in **purified water** or mixing with a sweet vehicle **simple syrup** which gives the flavour. Mother tinctures may be transformed into tincture trituration (TT) and dispensed.
2. **Liquid potencies**, which are the most frequently used by the physician, are rarely dispensed in their original form as drops. This is because these are prepared in alcohol, which creats a burning taste.

   Liquid potencies are dispensed

   (a) by medicating globules.

   (b) by adding medicated globules to sugar of milk.

   (c) by adding medicated globules and sugar of milk to purified water.

   (d) by medicating sugar of milk

   (e) by medicating purified water
3. **Powder triturates** are potencies, usually upto 6X or 3CH, which are insoluble in a liquid vehicle. These are not dispensed in the solid form above 6X or 3CH as these are conveniently converted into a liquid potency. But, this is not the case in the Biochemic system of medicines where potencies in the decimal scale are dispensed as tablets above 6X potency also. Powder triturates of the desired potency are dispensed in their original form in measured doses as medicated powders.

Forms of Vehicles for Dispensing

Dosage forms are preparations that provide the physician with the appropriate form in which the medication is to be dispensed to the patient.

Dosage forms in homoeopathy may be solid or liquid:

1. Vehicles for solid dosage forms are globules, cones, sugar of milk and tablets.
2. Vehicles for liquid dosage form are distilled water and syrup simplex.

Sometimes, homoeopathic medicines may be dispensed in their original form (e.g., homoeopathic lower triturations upto 6X or 3CH) without adding any vehicle for dispensing.

Pharmaceutical Dosage Forms

1. Solid dosage forms

In orthodox medicine, tablets and capsules are made in different forms to control the speed at which the active ingredient is delivered. This is not necessary in homoeopathy, so the choice of 'vehicle' is governed by convenience rather than therapeutic efficiency. Solid dosage forms are the more popular category of dispensing agents. Vehicles usually preferred are globules or pillules, sugar of milk, cones, and tablets.

Advantages: These show a greater stability than liquid dosage forms. These are more convenient to carry as compared to liquids.

2. Liquid dosage forms

The oral use of liquids is advantageous on the basis of ease of administration to those individuals who have difficulty in swallowing solid dosage forms. A drug administered in solution is immediately available for absorption. It is more rapidly and more efficiently absorbed than the same drug and dose in a solid dosage form.

Methods of Dispensing

1. Mother tinctures dispensed with purified water

Mother tinctures are usually dispensed in sufficient amount of purified water. It should not be taken directly, which will cause burning sensation on the tongue.

Examples: Avena sativa Q, is prescribed for nerve weakness. The patient should take the required quantity of medicine after mixing with 15 to 30 ml of purified water 2 to 3 times daily, as directed by the physician.

2. Mother tinctures dispensed with sugar of milk

Tincture Triturations

These are preparations of sugar of milk saturated with the mother tincture of the desired drug. They are used for dispensing **lower potencies of vegetable drugs.**

In making 1X potency of Tincture Trituration (T.T.), 10ml of the desired mother tincture and 10 gm of sugar of milk are taken.

After having the sugar of milk and the mortar moderately heated, the tincture is mixed with the sugar of milk and triturated for one hour. It will be found that the menstrum is completely volatilized and a stable and perfectly dry substance is obtained.

It is labeled 1X with the name of the drug as (T.T.) tincture trituration.

The 2X and all succeeding tincture-triturations are to be prepared by adding 1 part of the preceding tincture-triturate to 9 parts of sugar of milk and triturating for one hour to dryness.

Examples: Azadirachta indica 1X, *Bacopa monnieri* 1X, *Echinacea angustifolia* 1X, *Ginkgo biloba* 1X, *Ginseng* 1X, *Glycyrrhiza glabra* 1X, *Hypericum perforatum* 1X, *Syzygium jambolanum* 1X, *Baptisia tinctoria* IX, *Crataegus oxyacantha* IX, *Daphne indica* IX, *Quercus robur* IX, *Rauwolfia serpentina* IX.

3. Liquid potencies dispensed with globules

(i) A perfectly dry, clean, round phial and a new non-porous velvet cork is taken.

(ii) Name of medicine and potency (here, e.g., Bell. 30, is written over the top of the cork.

(iii) Then fresh non-medicated globules are poured in the phial filling up to ¾th part of it.

(iv) Then requisite quantity of liquid medicine (here, Bell. 30) is poured upon the globules, to moisten them uniformly. Then the phial is closed by the cork and kept standing on the cork for 8 hours.

(v) After this period, excess liquid medicine (if any) is drained out by losing the cork a little.

(vi) Then the cork is again closed. A label is pasted over the body of the phial, writing the name and potency of the medicine.

(vii) These medicated globules are kept for 24 hours and then it becomes ready for use.

Utility

(i) The globules retain their virtue from 18 to 20 years, if they are protected from heat and sunlight and the bottle is only opened in places odourless and free from dust.

(ii) These serve a convenient dosage form when a large number of doses are to be dispensed for frequent or repeated use.

Precaution

In medicating cane sugar globules, care should be exercised not to use a dilution having an alcoholic strength of much less than 88 percent or that of dispensing alcohol.

Globules have to be discarded, in any of the following conditions:

(i) When there is a change in the colour of the globules, i.e. they become 'yellow'.

(ii) When the globules stick to each other or to the walls of the container. This occurs when the globules absorb moisture or the water content in the medication is high. Globules do not stand medication in these cases.

(iii) When there is a change in the taste or the odour of the globules.

(iv) Presence of impurities.

4. Liquid potencies dispensed with sugar of milk

The number of drops (or minims) of the prescribed medicine are poured on measured quantity of sugar of milk in the proportion of 1 grain, 2 grains or 4 grains as desired and packed in paper envelope.

5. Liquid potencies dispensed by adding medicated globules and sugar of milk to purified water

Liquid potencies can be dispensed in purified water in different ways:

(i) Homoeopathic liquid potency can be given, dissolved in 30 to 60 ml of water without any addition, e.g., 1 drop of Rhus tox 30CH is put in a phial of 30 ml purified water and then taken by the patient.

(ii) The doses, prepared either in globules or sugar of milk can be dissolved in purified water and dispensed in aqueous medium, taking care that the dose is in every case modified a little in its degree of dynamisation.

(iii) Medicines prepared according to fifty millesimal scale are dispensed only in aqueous medium.

Disadvantages

1. The dispensing of aqueous vehicles has this disadvantage—they are less stable than solid dosage forms, since deleterious changes take place more readily in solution.

Medicines to be dispensed in distilled water must be recently prepared, for immediate use, because deterioration is likely if they are stored longer. The patient is to be warned against long storage by a label instructing that any unused part must be discarded after a specified date. There is no official recommendation as to the shelf life of such a preparation.

2. They are bulky to carry around.
3. A spoon is needed to administer the dose.
4. Accidental breakage of the glass container results in complete and messy loss of the contents.
5. Unpleasant flavour of tinctures is difficult to mask, if dispensed in water.

The preparation should be stable. It should maintain a status quo with reference to its curative properties. Preservation is necessary to prevent changes and microbial growth.

Since water commences to deteriorate after a few days, whereby the power of the small quantity of medicine contained is destroyed, the addition of a little alcohol is necessary, or, where this is not practicable, or if the patient cannot bear it, add a few small pieces of hard charcoal to the watery solution.

> *Note:* (i) Such a globule, placed dry upon the tongue, is one of the smallest doses for a moderate recent case of illness. Here but few nerves are touched by the medicine. A similar globule, crushed with some sugar of milk and dissolved in a good deal of water and stirred well before every administration, will produce a far more powerful medicine for the use of several days. Every dose, no matter how minute, touches, on the contrary, many nerves. (Sec. 272)
>
> (ii) There are numerous patients of so excitable a nature that they may be sufficiently affected by the dose of a small pellet laid dry upon the tongue, in slight acute ailments. It is most useful to give to the patient the powerful homoeopathic pellet or pellets only in solution, and this solution in divided doses.

6. Powdered triturates dispensed singly

Triturations are generally dispensed without mixing with any other vehicle.Taking several pieces of perfectly new white paper, packets of triturations of the drug of one grain, two grains, or three grains each, according to the prescription of of physician, are to be prepared and served.

Advantages

(i) Powders show a greater stability than liquid dosage forms.

(ii) The smaller particle size of powders give a greater and more rapid diffusion than that obtained from other solid forms like globules and tablets.

(iii) In this form, each dose can be separately enclosed as unit dose.

7. Powdered triturates dispensed in the form of tablets

Tablet triturates (Molded tablets)

The desired drug is to be triturated with sugar of milk in a given proportion for at least two hours until thorough comminution is obtained. Tablet triturates are then made by making a stiff paste of the medicinal powder with 60% alcohol. The apparatus used for their preparation consists of a stainless steel upper plate with perforations that correspond in size, position and number to the range of pegs fixed in a lower stainless steel plate. The plates are made in a range of sizes: ½ to 4 grains and about 50 to 250 tablet triturates are prepared at a time. Plates may be designed to produce tablets in various shapes. The stiff paste prepared is pressed into the perforations of upper plate. A spatula is used to ensure that each cavity is filled and to smooth off the excess. The filled paste is then pressed down on the lower plate, thus leaving the paste in the form of tablets, resting on each peg. The tablets are then left to dry for 1 to 2 hours. The alcohol evaporates and the partially dissolved sugar of milk rapidly recrystallises and is ready for administration.

These act as effective, cohesive and protective excipient of the drug. Tablet triturates are powders that are molded in the form of a tablet. The tablet triturates retain their shape under normal conditions and may be swallowed whole or crushed into a powder. The tablet triturates are allowed to dissolve on the tongue or in a teaspoonful of water.

Quality Assurance while Dispensing Homoeopathic Medicine

Dispensing of homoeopathic medicines **needs to be standardised and quality assurance.** At present, homoeopathic medicines are mostly being dispensed in substandard way by practioner themselves. They use the cheap quality plastic container, mostly re-cycled. We need to use **food grade containers, glass bottles** need to be made of neutral glass. The traditionalists still favour neutral glass containers, suggesting that there is a possibility of chemicals leaching into the plastic. Little work has been done to investigate whether the fears of those eschewing plastic have a firm foundation. There have also been suggestions that the glass may play some part in 'holding' the potency.

Blister pack is especially used by so called top doctors with their name printed, the one sealed by aluminium foil needs to be discouraged as aluminium reacts—even if placebo packed would have trace of Aluminium metal.

Globules, Diskets are safe provided they are manufactured with pharmaceutical grade sugar.

Liquids are packed in glass dropper bottles. The major suppliers use amber screw cap bottles with a plug in the neck, with a channel that facilitates the delivery of one measured drop (0.05 ml). Silicon rubber teat droppers are rarely used as, again, there is some concern over leaching.

> *Note:* A food grade container is one that will not transfer non-food chemicals into the food and contains no chemicals which would be hazardous to human health.

Chapter 33

Drug Administration

As homoeopathy bears a speciality and originality in the field of medicine, its route and mode of administration also bear a speciality.

Routes or Channels for Administration (Sec. 284–285)

The subject dealing with the route or channel of administration of drugs and medicines is termed **"Pharmaconomy"**.

The following are the various routes or channels through which homoeopathic medicines can be introduced into the system for their action after absorption:

1. *By oral route (ingestion through mouth).*
2. *By olfaction (inhalation through nose or mouth).*
3. By application to the skin:
   (a) Rubbing or Friction (Innuction or Epidermic)
   (b) Enepidermic.
4. *Others:* (a) Eye; (b) Ear etc.

By oral route

The homoeopathic medicines are usually administered singly and orally. The medicines given orally seem to act effectively and promptly. Homoeopathic potentised medicines seem to require no digestion but are absorbed directly from the mouth and then act through the cerebro-spinal or ganglionic nervous system. Sub-lingual administration of medicines is sometimes adopted in case of coated tongue which interferes with the absorption and action of medicines. For local action, we use gargle, e.g., Phytolacca gargle in acute tonsillitis.

> *N.B.:* Gargles (Gargarisma)—These are solutions of drugs for local action in mouth or throat.

By olfaction

Olfaction' means 'Act of smelling'.

It is a method of administering medicine to a patient through the nose and mouth by the act of smelling. Hahnemann administered medicines by oral route for many years. But in his last years he favoured the olfactory route.

In Aphorism 288/1 F.N. Hahnemann states that homoeopathic remedies act most surely and most powerfully when the medicinal aura that is always emanating from the medicine is inhaled for a short time.

Method of olfaction: For this, globules (or a single globule) are moistened with the medicinal fluid and placed dry in a small phial. The homoeopathic physician allows the patient to hold the open mouth of phial first in one nostril, and, in the act of inspiration, draw the air out of it into himself. Then, if it is wished to give a stronger dose, the patient is asked to inhale the same vapour with the other nostril, more or less strongly, according to the strength intended.

If both the nostrils are stopped up by coryza or polypus, the patient should inhale by the mouth holding the orifice of the phial between the lips. In little children it may be applied close to their nostrils while they are asleep with the certainty of producing an effect. The medicinal aura thus inhaled comes in contact with the nerves in the walls of the spacious cavities and, thus, produces a salutary influence on the vital force—in the mildest yet most powerful manner.

The interval of repeating the olfaction should be same as that of oral route.

Indication: This method is applicable in the following conditions:

(a) In Idiosyncratic patients;

(b) When it is not possible to give medicine through mouth — (i) during fit of epilepsy or hysteria, (ii) in locked-jaw or Tetanus.

By application to the skin

(a) *Rubbing or friction (Innuction or Epidermic)*— Friction through the whole cutaneous surface of the body, wherever the epidermis is sound, as epigastrium, inner parts of thighs, lower part of abdomen, back, arms, legs, testicles, labia majora etc.

Aphorism. 292 F.N. 1: "Rubbing-in appears to favour the action of medicine only in this way—friction makes the skin more sensitive and the living fibres thereby more capable of feeling, as it were, the medicinal power and of communicating to the whole organism this health-affecting sensation".

Examples: Application of lotions, ointments liniments over the unbroken skin.

(b) *Enepidermic:* In this method, drugs are simply kept in contact with the unbroken skin without friction or rubbing.

Examples: plasters, poultices, ointments, etc. are thus applied.

Others

(a) Eye: as eye-drop, e.g., Cineraria maritima succus.

(b) Ear: as ear-drop, e.g., Mullein oil.

(c) Nose: as nasal drop, e.g., Sanguinaria.

Principles of Drug Administration

1. Routes

Oral and olfaction method is satisfactory for drug administration.

2. Forms

(a) *Liquid form:* Medicine may be administered after being dissolved in greater quantity of liquid vehicle, thus it comes in contact with much larger surface of sensitive nerves (Aphor. 286).

(b) *Solid form:* Medicine may also be administered in form of medicated globules, sugar of milk or tablets.

3. Doses

(a) 'In no case is it requisite to administer more than one single, simple medicinal substance at a time.' (Aphor. 272)

(b) "It is wrong to attempt to employ complex means when simple means suffice." (Aphor. 274)

(c) The smaller the dose of the homoeopathic remedy is, so much the slighter and shorter is this apparent increase of the disease.

It is better to give a small poppy seed like globule soaked with the medicinal substance and then to serve it either by dissolving it in a small quantity of purified water or sugar of milk.

4. Repetition of doses

(a) Perceptible and continued progress of improvement contraindicates repetition (Aphor. 245).

(b) Repeat the dose only when the improvement ceases.

(c) Repetition may be continued till either recovery ensues or different groups of symptoms arise and thus demands different remedy (Aphor. 248).

(d) In chronic diseases, medicine may be repeated at intervals of fourteen, twelve, ten, eight or seven days.

In chronic diseases resembling cases of acute disease—should be repeated at still shorter intervals.

In acute diseases—at very much shorter period—every twenty four, twelve, eight, four hours.

In acutest—every hour, even at every five minutes.

5. Proper time of administration of medicines

(a) *In intermittent fever*—most appropriate time is immediately after the end of the paroxysm (Aphor. 236).

(b) *In menstrual disturbances*—the best time is the post-menstrual period (Aphor. 236).

> *Note:* Medicine should not be given during their aggravation time (day or night).

6. Diets and regimens

Everything which can have any medicinal action should be removed from the diet and regimen of the patient during administration of medicine, so that the small dose may not be overwhelmed and extinguished or disturbed by any foreign medicinal irritant (Aphor. 259).

(a) Nothing should be taken at least ½ hour before or after taking the medicine.

(b) No new habits or addictions should be indulged in during the taking of medicine.

(c) All emotional stress and strains and excitements should be avoided.

Chapter 34

Drug–Medicine–Remedy

DRUG

(Apho. 19-23 and 105-116)

Definition

The word "Drug" is derived from the French word *drogue* meaning a dry herb.

Drug is a therapeutic agent, prepared pharmaceutically from standerdised drug-substances according to the rules and regulations of pharmacopoeia, which is sufficiently capable of affecting the sensations and functions, even the structural change and may be even cause of death, if continued for a sufficient time and dose.

1. The **Scientific Group of WHO** has defined drug as 'Any substance or product that is used or intended to be used to modify or explore the physiological system or pathological states for the benefit of the recepients'.
2. As per **H. A. Roberts:** 'A drug is any material agent, in however attenuated form, the ingestion of which is capable of so disturbing this balance of the vital forces that the functioning of one or more organs of the body is no longer carried out to the best of the whole; and any material substance capable of so acting on the living organism is a drug'.
3. **Hahnemann** said (Sec. 19, Organon of Medicine): 'Now, as diseases are nothing more than alterations in the state of health of the healthy individual, they express themselves by morbid signs, and cure is also only possible by a change to a healthy condition of the state of health of the diseased individual, it is very evident that medicines could never cure diseases if they did not possess the power of altering man's state of health which depends on sensations and functions, indeed, that their curative power owes solely to this power they posseses of altering man's state of health'.
4. **Richard Huges** says that, 'Drugs are substances which have the power of affecting the animal body in health and disease'.

Types

1. **Mother tincture:** It is the drug pharmaceutically prepared from the drug substance of vegetable and animal kingdom, using strong alcohol as a vehicle (solvent) by the process of immersion, maceration and percolation.
2. **Mother solution:** It is the drug pharmaceutically prepared from the drug substance of mineral and chemical source as the strongest alcoholic, or aqueous solvent by the process

dissolving in alcohol or purified water or exposing as the case may be.

3. **Mother substance:** It is the drug pharmaceutically prepared from the drug substance of any source insoluble in liquid vehicle as the strongest solid solvent by the process of trituration with sugar of milk.

Character of Drugs

The science of identifying crude drugs is very important to a homoeopathic pharmacist and, hence, an acquantance with the chief physical and chemical properties of the drugs is of much value.

Knowledge of physical characters of each drug is acquired by comparision of the description of the particular drug with its actual specimen, when particular care should be taken about the character, taste, smell, shape, colour, weight etc., of the drug.

Impurities of Drugs

Impurities in drugs may arise from various causes, the following are the common ones:

1. **Imperfect selection:** This is due to the ignorance of collectors of crude vegetable drugs, those are imperfectly acquinted with their botanical characters and, therfore, fail to distinguish those from allied species; hence the substitution of an inferior or allied article for the genuine one.
2. **Imperfect preservation:** This is one of the causes of deterioration of many drugs. Several drugs are materially affected by light and air, others by the lapse of time.
3. **Imperfect preparation:** Impurities are of two kinds—(i) Those which exist in the crude drug, (ii) Those which arise as byproducts during the process of preparation.

   These can be avoided only by scrupulous care on the part of the manufacturing pharmacists.
4. **Adulteration:** It is the intentional and fraudulent admixture of foreign substances with drug. All highly priced drugs are liable to adulteration.

The Homoeopathic Pharmacopoeia of India (HPI 1) maintains the limits of permissible impurities in crude drugs. A knowledge of this is of utmost importance to the pharmacist for the supply of drugs conforming with the pharmacopoeial standards of purity and activity.

Crude Drugs

By 'Crude drugs' are meant the commercial forms of drugs taken from the vegetable, animal and mineral kingdoms as are brought to the market and utilised for the purpose of preparing medicines.

Difference between Crude Drugs and Low Potencies

Difference between crude drugs and low potencies (triturations) should be specially noticed. Even though both contains same drug molecules, their therapeutic properties are found to be different. In crude form, drug molecules are packed tightly, often their bonds saturated due to interactions with various other molecules. Hence, they are not free to exhibit all their potentials. Whereas in triturations and low potencies, the drug molecules are free or ionised, and they can exhibit all their properties. Hence, pathologic and therapeutic potentials of triturations and low potencies are much higher to crude forms. We know that various drugs which are seemingly inert in crude forms become very potent in triturated forms. Difference between crude Silicea and *Silicea* 3x, crude Lycopodium and *Lycopodium* 3x etc. are examples.

Crude Vegetable Drugs

The word 'Herb' should be taken to mean 'all of those parts' of the plant kingdom that we utilise for medicinal purposes. All such substances, when in the natural or dried state, are referred to as 'crude' drugs, i.e. drugs that have not been converted to a form that ensures maximum absorbency and effect.

Crude Drugs

Barks	Fungi	Rhizomes	Seaweeds
Flowers	Leaves	Roots	Tubers
Fruits	Lichen	Seeds	Woods

All of the above plant parts are classified as 'organised' drugs, in that they have a well-defined cellular structure. Another class of crude drugs is the exudations.

Natural Exudations

Balsams	Fixed oils	Oleo resins
Essential oils	Gums	Resins
Fats	Oleo gum resins	Waxes

Those substances are said to be 'unorganised', meaning that they do not have a cellular structure.

Classification and Naming of Drugs

In this universe each and every drug has one official name for ultimate convenience and safety. The drug may be placed in any of the classes as:

1. **Non-proprietary Name (Generic, Approved):** These are homoeopathic medicines (consonant with the homoeopathic scope of practice) which are formulated and/or prepared by a registered homoeopathic medicine manufacturer which is not available in the market/trade. The official name of medicines are derived from the official homoeopathic pharmacopoeias (e.g., HPI, HPUS, GHP/HAB, BHP).
2. **A Proprietary Name:** These are registered medicines (consonant with the homoeopathic scope of practice) that are available in the open market or trade, or which are bought in bulk from manufacturers or wholesalers and dispensed to patients in smaller volumes without any compounding or manipulation. Viburcol, a proprietary homoeopathic medicine often used in Europe, can be very effective for acute colic. It contains Chamomilla, Belladonna, Dulcamara, Plantago major, Pulsatilla, and Calcium carbonicum.

   Single ingredient shall not bear **proprietary** name on its label.
3. **Pharmacopoeial Name:** The drugs which are named as specified in different homoeopathic pharmacopoeias (e.g.HPI, HPUS, GHP/HAB, BHP).
4. **The full Botanical Name:** It is applicable for those medicines which are derived from vegetable source. The botanical name is used world-wide to indicate the various names given to a particular plant in different regions or place and by different languages.
5. **The full Zoological Name:** It is applicable for those medicines which are derived from animal source. The zoological name is used world-wide to indicate the various names given to a particular animal in different regions or places and by different languages.

> *Note:* (The Drugs and Cosmetics Act, 1940 (India), Chapter 1—Introductory) **"Patent or Proprietary Medicine"** means—(i) in relation to Ayurvedic, Siddha or Unani Tibb systems of medicine all formulations containing only such ingredients mentioned in the formulae described in the authoritative books of Ayurveda, Siddha or Unani Tibb systems of medicine specified in the First Schedule, but does not include a medicine which is administered by parenterate route and also a formulation included in the authoritative books as specified in clause (a).
> (ii) in relation to any other systems of medicine, a drug which is a remedy or prescription presented in a form ready for internal or external administration of human beings or animals and which is not included in the edition of the Indian Pharmacopoeia for the time being or any other Pharmacopoeia authorised in this behalf by the Central Government after consultation with the Drugs Technical Advisory Board constituted under Section 5.

Abbreviations of Drugs

In homoeopathic system the scientific name of a drug is used in Latin form. English name is used only where no accepted Latin name. Abbreviation of a drug is necessary for easy handling during the process of manufacturing, marketing and clinical application.

The abbreviation of a drug has two parts: (a) Root; (b) Extension.

(a) **Root:** It is used to indicate where the drug contain only one part, e.g. Bor. for Borax, Caust. for Causticum, Op. for Opium.

(b) **Extension:** It is used to indicate the second part of the drug, e.g., carb. for carbonica, ind. for indica, alb. for alba.

MEDICINE

Definition

When a drug has been potentised homoeopathically and proved on healthy human beings in both sexes (male and female), all ages and in different constitutions—producing abnormal signs and symptoms (both subjective and objective), is called medicine, e.g., Nux vomica 30.

Homoeopathic medicines include any substance which is recorded in standard books of materia medica from Hahnemann down to the present-day authorities with symptoms gathered from proving on healthy human beings or symptoms, not found during provings but observed to have been actually cured by the substances during their administration to sick persons, or symptoms observed either accidentally or by controlled experiment; or observed as toxicological effects on human beings or animals and which are being prepared as per homoeopathic pharmacy and administered to the sick according to symptom similarity.

Genuine Medicine

The medicine which has been prepared pharmaceutically, under the guidance of qualified and honest pharmacist, by obeying the rules and regulations of homoeopathic pharmacopoeia is supposed to possess all the active properties of the drug substance from which it has been prepared and, as such, when potentised, is quite capable of curing dynamic disease This genuineness of the medicine may be tested by administering the same to some healthy human beings—as done by drug-proving, to know whether it can produce the signs and symptoms which have been previously recorded by the physicians on previous occasions. If the signs and symptoms totally correspond to the previous records it will be said as the genuine medicine.

In disease, having the same set of signs and symptoms, if we administer this medicine on the basis of symptom similarity it will definitely be able to cure the disease. Therefore, it is justly said, "Genuine medicines are only the weapons in the hand of the physicians"

The true physician must be provided with genuine medicine of unimpaired strength, so that he may be able to rely upon their therapeutic powers. He himself must be able to judge their genuineness (Aphorism 264).

Drug	Medicine
1. Drug is a therapeutic agent, prepared pharmaceutically from standardised drug substance according to the rules and regulations of pharmacopoeia, which is sufficiently capable of affecting the vitality of living organism by altering the sensations and functions, even the structural change and may be cause of death, if continued for a sufficient time and dose.	1. When a drug has been potentised homoeopathically and proved on healthy human beings—in both sexes (male and female), all ages and in different constitutions—producing abnormal signs and symptoms (both subjective and objective) it is called medicine.
2. They are in crude form and cannot cure dynamic diseases but can suppress temporarily.	2. They are in potentised form and can cure dynamic diseases but cannot suppress temporarily.
3. As they are crude, they are very often poisonous and, as such, produce very dangerous effects when administered in large doses.	3. The large doses of homoeopathic potentised medicines cannot do so.
4. Due to the crudeness of their action, it is not possible to bring out the physical and mental symptoms which they can produce in their potentised state—when administered to a healthy human being.	4. Due to fineness of their action, they can bring out the very fine physical and mental symptoms in healthy man who is very susceptible to a particular medicine.
5. Drug has an affinity to effect at the periphery.	5. Medicine has an affinity to affect at the centre.
6. Physico-chemical property remains.	6. Physico-chemical property more or less absent but dynamic power is in full form.

Hahnemann advises the physician, 'to be thoroughly convinced in every case that the patient always takes the right medicine'. Therfore, he must give the patient the correctly chosen medicine prepared, moreover, by himself (Aphorism 265).

The homoeopathic physician uses so little medicine that it behaves him to have that which he does use absolutely pure and perfect in every sense of the word, and that he cannot tell without some knowledge of pharmacy.

REMEDY

Definition

When a particular medicine is prescribed for a particular diseased condition, according to symptom similarity and when the diseased condition is cured totally, the medicine is called a remedy of that particular case.

A "drug" becomes a "remedy" when it satisfies the law of similars, though loosely they are used in the same sense.

Aphorism 3

'Choice of the remedy, the medicine indicated', so a remedy is an indicated medicine.

Examples: A patient suffering from tonsillitis having following symptoms:

(a) Rosy-redness of the part; < by hot application.

(b) Puffy swelling.

(c) Thirstlessness.

(d) Great sensitiveness to touch.

According to symptom similarity Apis mel 30 is applied and cure takes place.

So *Apis mel* 30 becomes a remedy.

Short-acting remedy

A remedy whose action lasts for a comparatively short period:

e.g., Acon nap.; Aethusa cynapium; Allium cepa; Avena sativa; Belladonna; Chamomilla; Colocynth; Ipecacuanha.

Deep-acting remedy or Long-acting remedy

A remedy whose action lasts for a comparatively long period.

e.g., Anthracinum; Bacillinum; Calcarea carb; Calcarea fluor; Carcinosin; Kali carb; Lachesis; Lycopodium; Malandrinum; Nat. mur; Pertussin.

Polychrest remedy

A remedy which has produced a wide range of symptoms in the provings and can, therefore, treat a wide range of problems:

e.g. Ars. alb; Ac. hydrocyanic; Ac. mur; Ac. nit; Acid phos; Acid sulph; Aesc hip; Aethusa cya; Agar; Agnus cast; Aloe soc; Ammon carb; Anac; Ant. tart; Apis mel; Arg nit; Arn mon; Bapt; Bell; Bryo; Calc. carb; Calc. phos; Cimicifuga; China; Caust; Chamo; Caulo; Con; Colch; Digit; Dros; Dulc; Eup per; Gels; Hamam; Hyos; Ign; Iod; Ipecac; Kali bi; Kali carb; Kreos; Lach; Led; Lyco; Medo; Mez; Merc sol; Nat s; Nux m; Nux v; Op; Petro; Phyto; Plantago; Podo; Psor; Puls; Pyro; Rheum; Rhodo; Rhus tox; Sabad; Sab; Samb nig; Sec cor; Sep; Sil; Spong; Staph; Stram; Sulph.

Simillimum

Word meaning

The word, 'simillimum', has originated from the Latin *'similis'* meaning 'like'. *Simile means an explicit likening of one thing to another*.

Hahnemann uses this word in Sec. 56 F.N. of Organon of Medicine.

Definition

The word 'simillimum' denotes the most similar remedy. The simillimum or the most similar medicine will be that which is similar in all respects to the disease condition for which it is given. For this reason the medicine has to be similar in six ways to the disease.

The six factors are:

(i) Seat of action (selective affinity)

(ii) Kind of action (disease process)

(iii) Causative modifications (modifying conditions)

(iv) Character of sensation (nature of sensation aroused)

(v) Concomitant

(vi) Sequence of symptoms (chronological appearance)

Some authors have suggested that simillimum is not only the most similar remedy but *'the most similar remedy in most appropriate potency and dose which cures a patient.'*

Remedy Relationship (Pharmacokinship)

By the term relationship of remedies—it relates to 'the chief allies of each remedies'.

Dewey suggest the following type of relations which the drug do bear to each other:

A. Complementary
B. Antidotal
C. Inimical
D. Concordant
E. Family.

A. Complementary relationship

The word complementary comes from *complementation*. The complement means that one drug which completes the cure that has been began by the former but the former drug was unable to terminate in cure, which the latter drug performs. Thus these two drugs are said to be complementery:

1. **Clarke** says, "When a remedy has done all that it can in a case, then another remedy is likely to follow up and complete its action, both being related to the case."

2. **Boenninghausen** says that some remedies are in harmony with others. The most similar one as a rule becomes complementary, that antidotes each other's bad effects, follow each other well and often make up for the deficiencies of the other. Other with a lesser degree of similarity may be used at a greater interval of time and finish up the works started by the former.

3. **Hahnemann:** Though he does not use the term complementary, we can consider his second prescription after a partial simillimum as 'complementary', as it often helps to complete the action of the first. "Hahnemann was guided in the selection of an antidote by the symptoms of the medicine actually present, in others he did not follow this rule, but was led by something else, probably experiment and observation,to give substances as antidotes, the Homoeopathicity of which to the symptoms sought to be removed could not be proved." (Lectures on the theory and practice of Homoeopathy—R. E. Dudgeon—Page 536.)

4. **J. T. Kent:** He says complementary medicine completes the action of the first, when the first one is no longer acting. He continues that the selection is purely symptomatic. "When *Pulsatilla* has been of great service in a given case and finally cure no more,while the symptoms now point to *Silicea,* the latter will be given with confidence as its complementary relation has long been established." (Page 425)

5. **E. A. Farrington:** The drug which completes a cure which the other begins, but is unable to effect. Such a relation exists between *Belladonna* and *Calcarea.*

6. **H. A. Roberts:** The most similar ones, as a rule are complementary; those antidote each other's bad effects, follow each other well and often make up for the deficiencies of the others.

7. **H. L. Chitkara:** These are remedies which completes the action of the first prescription. Acute and Chronic remedies also come under this.

8. **C. L. Olds:** Very often in the treatment of a patient, no matter whether the disease be acute or chronic, we find that after a longer or shorter period of time, the remedy indicated in the beginning of the treatment no longer benefits the patient. We say that the remedy has run out and that another remedy must be selected. If, after the administration of this remedy, the patient progresses toward health, the second remedy, because it completes the work of the first in a greater or lesser degree, is called a complement of that remedy. (C. L. Olds, The Homeopathic Recorder, April 1928)

9. **Garth Boericke:** Work done by one remedy is completed by another. This relationship is especially useful in organic diseases where the person is under medication for a long time.

Inimical relation—lack of harmony between drugs though they have similar disease producing power.

Acute compliments of Chronic remedies and Chronic compliments of Acute remedies

1. **Kent:** Kent has given more specialised class of complementary remedies and that is the acute complements of chronic remedies. He says that a chronic patient may be suffering from an acute disease and the physician on being called may think that it is necessary to take the totality of the symptoms but if he should not do that in an acute disease, mixing both chronic and acute symptoms together. The two things must be separated here. The group of symptoms that constitutes the image and appearance of the acute miasm must now be prescribed for.
2. **Elizabeth Wright:** Remedies which carry on or complete most successfully the action of other given remedies. (A Brief Study Course in Homoeopathy, Page 59.)

   Examples:

   Acon nap: Sulph.; Bac: Calc. phos.; Ars. alb: Thuja.; Hepar: Sil.; Coloc: Staph.; Bell: Calc. carb; Puls: Sil.; Nux. v: Sep.; Bry: Alum or Nat. m (Page 61)

Remedies in Series

Kent: Another type of complementary remedies described by Kent is one on which the least work has been done. Most of the data are being sprinkled around in Kent's Materia Medica and it is remedies in series. For instance, Calc.-Lyc.-Sulph, Ign.-Nat. mur.-Sepia, Puls.-Sil.-Fluor. ac., Ars.-Thuja-Tarant., All. cep.-Phos.-Sulp., It will be noted that all three of these are chronic remedies. They must be used in this order and not the opposite one.

Examples:

Acon – Spong – Hep (Wright)
Sulph – Calc – Lyc (Wright)
Sulph – Sars – Sep (Wright)
Ign – Nat-m – Sep (Wright)
Puls – Sil – Fl-ac (Wright)
Ars – Thuj – Tarent (Wright)
All-c – Phos – Sulph (Wright)
Merc – Hep – Sil (Kent)
Sulph – Ars – Sulph (Kent)
Arn – Rhus.t – Calc (Kent)
Puls – Sil – Kali.s (Kent)

B. Antidotal relationship

Stadesman Medical Dictionary suggests that 'anti' means 'against' and 'dotas' means 'what is given', i.e. an agent which neutralises a poison or counteracts its effects.

A substance/thing that counteracts something unpleasant or a substance that opposes the effects of a remedy is called as antidote.

1. **Dewey** classically explains that antidote is a substance which modifies or opposes the effect of a remedy.
2. **Clarke** reports that it is necessary to know the antidotal relation of remedies in order to be able to control of overaction of any remedy that has been administered previously.
3. **Hahnemann:** In Aphorism 249, he suggests "If the aggravation be considerable (after a medicine), be first partially neutralised as soon as possible by an antidote before giving the next remedy chosen more accurately according to similarity of action." His words tells us indirectly that antidote is not selected on the basis of symptom similarity.

Hahnemann says, when writing about drug-proving, that "The subsequent dose often removes, curatively, some one or other of the symptoms caused by the previous dose." (Aphorism 131). Here he suggests the second dose to be an 'Increasing dose'. From this we may make a conclusion that higher potency of the same medicine act as an antidote.

4. **R. E. Dudgeon:** Dudgeon quotes Trinks. "The antidotarial influence of medicines on one another depends solely upon the homoeopathic principle." (Page 535) He says, "The necessity for the administration of an antidote in consequence of the too violent effects of an infinitesimal dose is, I apprehend, very rare." (Page 537). According to him, "A fresh dose of the same medicine is the best antidote" (Page 537). He explains the modus operandi of antidotes with no symptom relation as this. "Thereby a stronger but transient and different

effect is produced upon the nerves, whereby the feebler impression of the medicine previously given is effaced and the new action being evanescent, the nervous system is speedily restored to its normal equilibrium." (Page 537)

5. **E. A. Farrington:** The medicines which modify the effects of a wrongly selected potency or an apt potency—but in an 'idiosyncracy' patient. The symptoms are opposite, not so much in the phraseology in which those are expressed, for those may read almost exactly alike, but those are results acting in opposite directions. Those act by modifying the effects and not by suppressing the symptom, e.g., Belladonna and Hyoscyamus in skin symptoms. Nux vomica and Coffea.

6. **J. T. Kent:** It is employed when there appears new symptoms. The selection is,"The new symptoms combining with the old ones must be again studied and the second remedy must correspond more particularly to the new than to the old." (Lectures on Homoeopathic Philosophy, Page 238)

7. **Stuart Close:** These are commonly divided into three classes, according to their mode of action: (a) Physiological or Dynamical (b) Chemical and (c) Mechanical.

Physiological or dynamical antidoting requires that the antidotal substance shall be pathogenically similar to the poison, but opposite in the direction of its action.

He quotes Boenninghausen "Medicines producing similar symptoms are related to each other and are mutually antidotal in proportion to the degree of their symptom similarity." (The genius of Homoeopathy, Page 107)

He cites the incidences where the higher potency of the same drug becoming the antidote. i.e., in a case, chronic disease of the liver or some other organ from suppression of malaria with massive doses of quinine or arsenic (Page 120).

8. **Garth Boericke:** Homoeopathic remedies work as a antidote and destroy the existing action of a remedy in the body.

9. **H. L. Chitkara:** Antidotes of poisons. Antidotes for the bad effects of indiscriminate use of homoeopathic remedies. Antidote for the violent homoeopathic aggravation of the simillimum.

C. Inimical relationship

There are drugs which are in relation of enemity amongst them. They may be resembling each other apparently, but will not follow one another with any satisfaction. They seem to be mixed up the case. It can also be said that they do harmful effects if they follow or spoils the action of the former. Such drugs are said to be inimical between them.

1. **Boger:** The common experience that the continued thoughtless and injudicious use of the same medicine often does more harm than good, and that two very similar remedies do not follow each other well, has its origin in this fact (Boger's Repertory. Page viii)

2. **J. T Kent.** He says 'they do not like to work after each other.'

3. **H. L. Chitkara:** Which do not follow each other well. He says,in practice it was found that their use immediately after the other produced complications in the smooth management of the case.

Examples

Acon & Acet.ac.; Am.c & Lach.; Apis & Rhus; Aur.m.n & Coffea; Bell & Dulc.; Cham & Nux or Zinc.; China & Psor.; Cocc & Coffea.; Ign & Nux; Ign & Tab.; Lach & Dulc, Psor.; Led & Chin.; Merc & Sil.; Phos & Caust.; Psor & Sep.; Sep & Lach.

D. Concordant relationship

The drugs whose actions are similar but are of dissimilar origin to another are said to be concordant and they follow each other well.

E. A. Farrington: The drugs which have present marked similarities in action though dissimilar in origin. These are said to be "concordant". Drugs which hold a concordant relation may follow each other well.

Examples of concordant remedies are China and Calcarea, Pulsatilla and Sepia, Nitric acid and Thuja, Belladonna and Mercurius, Ignatia and Zinc.

E. Family relationship

The relation existing between drugs whose origin is similar.

1. **E. A. Farrington** says: family relation, derived from their similarity in origin. When drugs belong to the same family they must of necessity have a similar action. (Clinical Materia Medica, Pages 23, 24)
2. **Garth Boericke:** He has explained Remedy relationship as of practical importance in the application of Materia Medica. Different relationships given by him are similarity of origin or family relations which indicate a group of drugs belongs to the same botanical family or chemical group.

Examples: An example of a family of remedies is halogens like Bromine, Chlorine and Iodine; snake remedies like Lachesis and Crotalus; nut remedies like Ignatia and Nux vomica of the Ranunculaceae family.

Explanation: The snake remedies Lach. and Crot. hor. in many of their characters have resemblance, but they may not follow each other well.

Nut remedies Nux vomica and Ignatia belong to the same family but they do not follow each other well.

Conclusion

We could find out the symptom relation of the complementary, antidote and inimical remedies by studying some examples.

Complimentary: Acon & Coffea in fever (Key Note).

Acon: Internal heat with external chill., in the evening after lying down (HCMM).

Coffea: External heat with internal chill., in the evening after lying down (HCMM), i.e., in most instances, the complementary remedy will be having similar symptomatology but opposite modalities or conditions. This is not true in all the cases. They are related some times by their occurrence in nature. (Ars: Phos) (Nat.m: Sep) and sometimes by constituents. (Badiaga: Iodum.) (Puls: Kali.sul.) (Bell: Calc.) (Carb.v: Kali.c) these examples are not given by Dudgeon.

Inimical: Most of the authors relate it to the symptomatology, e.g., Apis and Rhus tox have similar symptomatology in eruptive diseases. Phos and Caust have much similarity in paralytic affections. "Inimical to Lachesis (Am.c) similar in action." (Materia Medica. Boericke, page 42). Contents of the medicine also suggests the inimical, e.g., Lyco contains Sulph.

Antidotes: Medicines with similar symptoms but acting in opposite directions make the antidotes to many authors. But, the suggestions of Dudgeon are the most valuable in this subject. He says that Hahnemann recommends Camphor as an antidote to an immense number of medicines, to all of which it can assuredly not be said to have a homoeopathic relationship.

FOOD

Introduction

Food (la. *cibus*) is any substance or material eaten or drunk to provide nutritional support for the body and/or for pleasure. It usually consists of plant or animal origin, that contains essential nutrients, such as carbohydrates, fats, proteins, vitamins, or minerals, and is ingested and assimilated by an organism to produce energy, stimulate growth, and maintain life.

Functions of Food

1. **Growth:** Food is essential for growth. Without food a living organism will stop growing. The living cells in our body multiply after getting nourishment from the food we eat. Insufficient or a wrong type of food does not help healthy growth.
2. **Repair:** Living organisms sometimes damage their parts by accident. Constant work also causes wear and tear of the body parts. If we get a wound or cut, it heals up after some time. If we damage our skin due to some burn etc., it regains its shape in due course. The body needs food for all these functions.
3. **Energy:** We spend our energy when we do work. That is why after doing considerable work, we get tired. We then need food and rest to regain the lost energy. If we do not get food, we would become weak.
4. **Protection from Diseases:** We need to protect our body from diseases and keep it healthy. For this, we need vitamins and mineral salts in our food. Vitamins neither provide energy nor

do they repair or replace the worn-out parts. But they are essential for our proper health.

Comparison between Drug and Food

1. Drug is prepared from various substances in the pharmaceutical laboratory as per rules and regulations of different pharmacopoeias. Foods are not essentially prepared in the laboratory, rather, they are collected from nature in the usual form. Only synthetic foods are prepared in the laboratory.
2. Drug has both preventive and curative value in relation to the disease. Food has only preventive value in relation to the disease.
3. Drug has no nutritive value for the maintenance of the health. Food has nutritive value for the maintenance of the health.
4. Action of drugs on the body may cause morbid changes. Food causes only indisposition if overeaten.
5. Action of drugs on the body may be long lasting. The effects of foods on the body will be transient.
6. Drug has no direct role in the synthesis of proximal principle of body. Food has direct role in the synthesis of proximal principle of body by its constituents carbohydrate, protein and fat.

COSMETICS

The word Cosmetics derives from the Ancient Greek '*kosmetike*', meaning 'the art of dress and ornament', from '*kosmetikos*', meaning 'skilled in ordering or arranging' and that from '*kosmos*', meaning amongst others 'order' and 'ornament'.

Cosmetic means any article intended to be rubbed, powered, sprinkled or sprayed on, or introduced into, or otherwise applied to, the human body or any part thereof for cleansing, beautifying, promoting attractiveness, or altering the appearance, and includes any article intended for use as a component of cosmetic. [The Drugs and Cosmetics Act, 1940 (India), Chapter 1—Introductory].

Homoeopathic cosmetics are available in the form of Homoeopathic soaps, Homoeopathic shampoo, Homoeopathic oil, Homoeopathic creams, Homoeopathic skin treatment creams, Homoeopathic paste etc. Homoeopathic cosmetics catalyse the speed of recovery in cosmetological disorders.

Homoeopathic cosmetics are useful for hair falling(alopecia), dandruff, gray hairs, acne, pimples, black heads, blemishes, pigmentation, eczema, psoriasis, scar marks, warts, molluscum, moles, keloids, skin tags, beautifying hair, skin, and nails.

For all above complaints, conventional medicine does give relief but many times patients face reccurrence. For this homoeopathy has a tremendous scope as it not only considers the disease from the diagnosis point of view but will go the root of disease finding the underlying cause and treat man as a whole.

So, to conclude for the treatment of cosmetic problems external application has an immense role to play but along with it we have to administer internal medicine—the constitutional medicine which will correct the economy from within and balance the system.

POISONS

Introduction

Poison is a substance that can cause disturbances due to chemical reactions—usually on a molecular scale, when a sufficient quantity is absorbed by an organism. Poison is a general term for substances that are harmful or may be lethal in small amounts that may be from chemical or biological source to any type of living organisms. In medicine, a poison is often distinguished from a toxin and a venom.

A **toxin**, strictly speaking, is a poison that is produced naturally by living cells or organisms that is active at very low concentrations. Toxins can be small molecules, peptides, or proteins and are capable of causing disease on contact or absorption with body tissues by interacting with biological macromolecules such as enzymes or cellular receptors. Toxins vary greatly in their severity, ranging from usually minor and acute (as in a bee sting) to almost immediately deadly (as in botulinum toxin).

Venoms are usually defined as biological toxins that are injected by a bite or sting to cause their effect, while other poisons are generally defined as substances which are absorbed through epithelial linings such as the skin or gut.

Paracelsus, the Father of Toxicology, once wrote: "All things are poison and nothing is without poison, only the dose permits something not to be poisonous" or, more commonly, "The dose makes the poison."

Venom vs Poison

The terms venom and poison are often used interchangeably. Although both venomous and poisonous animals have potentially dangerous toxins in their bodies, the way that toxin is delivered differs.

Venom is injected. Venomous animals have an active delivery system and may use their toxin for protection or to help them catch food. There are venomous lizards, venomous snakes, venomous mammals, venomous insects, jellyfish. Unlike poisonous animals, venomous animals store their toxin in venom glands. They inject their toxin into their predator or prey using fangs, pinchers, spines, or any other sharp body part that is hollow, grooved or breaks the skin to introduce venom. In other words, venom is used to get food, poison is used to not be food.

Poison is eaten or absorbed. Poisonous animals have a passive delivery system and use their toxin for protection only. They store their toxin in their meat or skin. If someone or something eats the animal, the predator may get sick or even die. When this happens, you can be sure the predator won't make that mistake again! An example of a poisonous animal is a poison dart frog.

Poison and Homoeopathy

It is a singular distinction of homoeopathy to have used poisons for positive and curative effects on human and animal health. Homoeopathic Materia Medica includes a large number of medicines prepared from most of the known poisons, including organic, inorganic, synthetic, herbal and snake poisons—but that does not mean that homoeopathic remedies are poisonous and harmful to take. The secret lies in the way they are prepared, potentised and used. The special pharmaceutical process of raising the potency of the medicine called "potentisation" is done in such a way that every next higher potency prepared from the previous potency has a reduced content of the source substance. After a certain stage, the physical content of the drug disappears leaving the medicine totally non-toxic. Thus any homoeopathic medicine made from a poison, when taken in a higher potency, is non-toxic and safe—there is nothing to worry about.

Chapter 35

Scope of Homoeopathic Pharmacy in Relation to Materia Medica, National Economy and Organon of Medicine

Scope of Homoeopathic Pharmacy in relation to Materia Medica

From the study of pharmacy we get knowledge of:

A. Sources of drugs.
B. Mode of collection of various drug-substances and their method of preservation.
C. Knowledge of preparations, scales and preservation.
D. Potentisation.
E. Knowledge of prescriptions and serving them.
F. The posology or the Doctrine of doses.
G. Drug-proving.

Explanations

A. Sources of drugs

(a) Drugs prepared from vegetable kingdom (with some exceptions) are short-acting in nature. In acute disea ses, short-acting remedies work well.

(b) Drugs prepared from nosodes, mineral kingdoms and many drugs of animal kingdoms are deep-acting in nature.
In chronic diseases, deep-acting or long-acting medicines work very well.

(c) In diseased condition, due to deranged vital force, certain fundamental functions of the human body should continue to be discharged to help eliminate poisons accumulated and it is the duty of the attending physician to see that they are so done before prescribing medicines from any of the three (vegetable, animal and mineral) groups.

Thus, it is important to see that excretory functions are in working order before prescribing medicines from the vegetable group, that heart and kidney functions are not impaired and the state of vitality is not too low while prescribing medicines from the animal group and that if the condition of a local lesion is grave, no medicine from the mineral group is prescribed.

(d) Drugs belonging to the same family (vegetable, animal or mineral) must of necessity have a similar action e.g.

Vegetable Kingdom

(i) *Arum triphyllum and caladium* belong to the same family Araceae but are inimical to each other.

[ATBOHP 29]

(ii) *Nux vomica* and *Ignatia* belong to the same family Loganiaceae but are inimical to each other.

(iii) *Belladonna* and *Dulcamara* belong to the same family Solanaceae but are inimical to each other.

(iv) *Ranunculus bulbosus* and *Staphysagria* belong to the same family Ranunculaceae but are inimical to each other.

(v) *Aloe soc., Allium cepa, Allium sativum* and *Scilla maritima* belong to the same family Liliaceae, but do not follow each other.

Animal Kingdom

All snake-venoms of the same family of Ophiotoxin possess some similarity in many of their actions, but they do not follow each other well, e.g., *Lachesis; Crotalus horridus; Naja; Elaps.*

Mineral Kingdom

The halogens, Chlorine, Iodine, Bromine and Fluorine have many similitudes, because they belong to one family.

(e) Some medicines (e.g. nosodes) are very much harmful in their low potencies but they act better in high and highest potencies.

(f) If the treatment started with a medicine obtained from vegetable kingdom and metals are used in the later part of the course of treatment then better results are obtained.

B. Modes of collection of various drug-substances and their methods of preservation

The drug substances do not possess equal amount of medicinal properties throughout the whole year. During a particular time or season their medicinal properties are highest. So, effects of medicine varies if the drug substances are collected in different times of the year.

Example

Rhus tox plants are to be collected in the damp weather, rainy season, and in the evening time because at that time Rhus tox plant possess more medicinal property.

The preservation of drug substance is most important in the preparation of drugs. The methods of preservation of plant substances and animal substances are different. The animal substances should be used immediately after collection.

The proper study of pharmacy gives the above information regarding collection and preservation of drug substances which supplement the knowledge of Materia Medica.

C. Knowledge of preparation, scale and preservation

To be a true practitioner, the physician must know the exact mode of preparations of medicine. The true physician must be provided with genuine medicine of unimpaired strength so that he may be able to rely upon their therapeutic powers.

Medicines are prepared from crude drug substances under certain definite scale (centesimal, decimal, 50-millisimal) and definite fixed pharmaceutical formula and procedures (drug power and potentisation).

The mother preparation and potentised medicine should be properly preserved according to the pharmaceutical directions, otherwise they will lose their efficacy on storing. Pharmacy provides all these information.

D. Potentisation

A man may be sick in three planes—physical, mental and casual. A medicine selected on the law of Similia cannot always cure a sick patient. Here, proper selection of potency is required so that it may have the capability to reach the plane in which the person has been affected. If the potency selection is improper, then there will be no cure. Here the knowledge of Materia Medica will be of no value to the physician if he has no knowledge of potency of the medicine and different methods of potentisation. It may help the physician in other way. There are many medicinal substances which are highly toxic in their crude state—their curative power can only be developed after proper potentisation.

E. Knowledge of prescriptions and serving them

The physician should know the ideals of an ideal prescription. He must have proper idea about the 'norms' and 'forms' of a prescription.

He must also know about dispensing of medicines. All medicines cannot be dispensed in every vehicle. The doses of triturations cannot be prepared in purified water, cannot be dispensed in globules. The medicine can be served in either liquid form (e.g. purified water, dispensing alcohol) or solid form (e.g. sugar of milk, globules etc.). Pharmacy gives us the above knowledge.

F. The 'Posology' or the Doctrine of doses

Highest ideal of cure not only depends upon the proper selection of remedy but also on the proper doses of medicine. A homoeopathic physician must know about the doses of selected medicine because a very large dose may cause violent aggravation. Without proper knowledge of poso-logy a well-selected remedy never brings on ideal cure and unwanted aggravation can never be avoided. The knowledge of dose helps the 'Simillimum' to act properly. So the knowledge of pharmacy supplements the knowledge of Materia Medica.

G. Drug-proving

Drug proving is an integral part of homoeopathic pharmacy. Efficacy of homoeopathy can only be proclaimed if the latent curative power of drugs is well understood. Different observations obtained from drug-proving on healthy human being increase the correct knowledge of materia medica—that means the latent curative power of the drug and the effects of the drug on healthy, irritable, intelligent, susceptible and idiosyncratic persons. This improved the knowledge of Materia Medica.

Scope of Homoeopathic Pharmacy in relation to National Economy

National economy is especially related to two factors: (i) National wealth, and (ii) Per Capita Income of people.

The current population of India as in 2011 is 1, 210, 193, 422 (1.21 billion), and is the second most populous country in the world, while China is on the top with over 1, 350, 044, 605 (1.35 billion). The figure shows that India represents almost 17.31% of the world's population, which means one out of six people on this planet live in India. So, India (a developing country) suffers from population problem. The population of India is greater than the capability of maintaining them at a reasonable standard of living. Due to economic development, the living condition improves and also medical help becomes more obtainable resulting in decreased death rate (in July, 2011 est., 7.48 deaths/1000 population) and at the same time there is increased birth-rate (in July, 2011 est., 20.97 births/1000 population), thereby increase of population.

There has been no uniform measure of poverty in India. The Planning Commission of India has accepted the Tendulkar Committee report which says that 37% of people (in rural area: 41.8% and in urban area: 25.7%) in India live below poverty line (BPL) Due to this poverty, there is lack of capital which prevents the expansion of our national income.

Our national economy is unstable since independence because of the conflicts created by different catastrophies like—

(i) The last great war (World War II—1939-1945).

(ii) Influx of refugees from eastern and western neighbouring zones of the country.

(iii) Lack of integrated attempt to explore the natural wealth adequately.

Besides this, international crisis is persisting. All these factors not only have shaken our economy but also the people. Due to insufficient wealth our foreign exchange resources are utilised to meet different emergencies—resulting in inflation which become a prominent one in our economy.

To combat the shortfall, India will have to depend on: (i) manpower, including technical personnel, and (ii) national resources.

The primary and essential duty of all governments is to provide the minimum health coverage to the people by arranging to prevent diseases and to supply all requirements to cure diseases.

The Government of developed countries spends around 9-10% of GNP (Gross National Product) on health care, whereas India (a developing country) spends only 5% of GNP on health care.

India spends around 85% of its total health budget on Allopathic system, 12% on Homoeopathic system and remaining 3% on other system of medicine.

In this context, homoeopathy can play an important role. For this, two essential factors are: (i) trained technical medical personnel, and (ii) requisite medicines.

The source of requisite medicines in the pharmaceutical manufacturing concern may be either public or private sector. In homoeopathy, with the least expenditure, requisite medicines can be served to the patient. Not only the cheapness but its efficacy has also been established clinically. Preparation of medicine is also very easy and simple.

Besides this, most of the homoeopathic drugs have the capability to grow or to collect—in different meteorological conditions for which the government exchange has to spend a minimum amount.

Almost 85% of the sources of necessary drugs can be procured and may be manufactured at comparatively much less cost and without drainage of precious foreign exchange.

If these indigenous sources and materials and unexplored talents be properly utilised, homoeopathy shall never be a burden to our economy. Moreover, it can add to the national wealth providing at least a minimum health coverage to our people.

Now, homoeopathy has gradually proved its efficacy in different parts of the world. If properly nourished, this system of medicine will be expanded as there is ample scope. Under these circumstances homoeopathy may even be helpful in earning foreign money for India.

Scope of Homoeopathic Pharmacy in relation to Organon of Medicine (§264-§272)

§264: Physician's responsibility—genuine unimpaired medicine

The physician has to be fully satisfied that his patient is getting genuine medicine that he prescribes. It becomes a part of his personal responsibility. The physician must be provided with genuine medicines so that he may be able to rely upon their therapeutic power.

§265: Employment of correct medicine

Hahnemann advises the physician to be thoroughly convinced in every case that the patient always takes the right medicine. Therefore, he must give the patient the correctly chosen medicine prepared by himself.

§266: Medicines—vegetable and animal kingdom—are more potent in crude state

Medicinal substances belonging to vegetable and animal kingdom possess their medicinal properties during their raw state.

§267-§268: Preparation of medicines from vegetable substances

1. ***Medicines from indigenous (native) plants (§267)***

Collection of fresh plant
↓
Mixed with equal parts of alcohol
↓
Kept in close-stoppered bottle for 24 hours
↓
Deposition of fibrinous and albuminous matters
↓
Supernatant fluid is decanted off
↓
Fermentation is prevented by alcohol
↓
Kept in close-stoppered bottle and protected from sunlight, heat and strong-smelling substance.

2. ***Medicines prepared from exotic (foreign) substances (§268)***
   - (i) It is difficult to secure exotic plants, barks, seeds and roots in fresh form, they are to be collected dry.
   - (ii) In order to ensure their identity the material is to be collected whole rather than in the form of powder.
   - (iii) Those will then be pulverised and dehydrated by exposing to heat. A flat tin saucer with raised edges is taken. The powder of the plant is then spread on the saucer, which is placed to float in a vessel of boiling water and thoroughly stirred to get the entire moisture evaporated.
   - (iv) The powder is then placed in well-stoppered bottle in closed chest—

protected from daylight. In this way, the powder retains its medicinal properties for long.

3. *Medicines prepared from plants containing thick mucus or albumin (§267 F.N.)*

When plants contain much of thick mucus (e.g., *Symphytum officinale, Viola tricolor* etc.) or an excess of albumin (e.g., *Aethusa cynapium, Solanum nigrum* etc.), their freshly expressed juice one part is to be mixed with two parts of alcohol.

4. *Medicines prepared from plants that are deficient in juice, i.e., dry (§267 F.N.)*

(i) Plants that are deficient in juice (e.g., *Oleander, Ledum, Sabina* etc.) should be pounded up into a moist, fine mass. Then it is stirred up with double quantity of alcohol so that the juice may mix with the alcohol and then pressed out by extraction.

(ii) They can also be dried and triturated with sugar of milk. Then they may be further diluted and potentized.

§269: Dynamisation of drugs—development of medicinal power

The homoeopathic system of medicine develops spirit-like medicinal powers of crude drug substances to a unparalleled degree by a process which has never been attempted before, and which causes medicines to penetrate the body, and thus to become more efficacious and remedial; it is applicable even to those substances which, in their crude state, give no evidence of the slightest medicinal power on the human body.

§270-§271: Method of dynamisation in centesimal scale

(i) 2 drops of fresh vegetable juice is mixed with equal part of alcohol and diluted with 98 drops of alcohol and potentised by 2 succussions—this is the 1st development of power (potency) (§270).

(ii) The same process is repeated with 29 successive vials, each vial to contain 99 drops of alcohol, filling 3/4th of the vial; this 2nd vial is then to be shaken twice, and so on the 30th development of power (potency) (§270).

(iii) This is the potentised decillionth dilution (X), and Hahnemann advises to use in all cases of chronic diseases (§270).

(iv) Pure metals, their oxides and sulphurates and other minerals e.g., *Petroleum, Phosphorus* etc (excepting *Sulphur*) are first to be potentised to the millionfold dry or powder dilution, by triturating them for 3 hours; then 1 grain of trituration to be dissolved and diluted in 27 successive vials, up to the 30th potency (§271).

§272: Administration of single remedy.

In no case it is required to administer more than one single, simple medicinal substance at one time.

Chapter 36

Doctrine of Signature (DOS) – The Sign of Nature

Introduction

According to Oxford Dictionary, 'Doctrine' is "what is taught; a body of instructions"; "a set of principles". 'Signature' means "identification, indication".

Doctrine of signature or Organoleptic sense is the relation between the external physical characters of drug substances and the signs and symptoms of the medicines produced during pathogenetic trial on healthy human beings. According to DOS, physical characteristics of plants (including shape, color, texture, and smell) reveal their therapeutic value.

The doctrine of signature, is an age old concept in history of medicine, plays an important role in folk medicine from the middle ages until the early modern era.

The doctrine of signature, in its true sense and originality was not formulated for the medical profession. It is based on a spiritual philosophy and simple concept that Almighty had marked everything he had created with a sign.

Historical Background

1. **Paracelsus**: Paracelsus (1493 – 1541), a Swiss physician developed the concept Doctrine of Signatures writing that *"Nature marks each growth ...... according to its curative benefit"*. Doctrine of Signature also has a more specific meaning. It is believed that the Creator gave physical clues about the value he imbued to plants. According to Paracelsus *"We see that the internal character of a man is often expressed in his exterior appearance, even in the manner of his walking, and in the sound of his voice. Likewise the hidden character of things is to a certain extent expressed in their outward forms"*. His law of signature is an application of medicine on the basis of similarity of anatomical structures, colors and smell between the plants and the human body. Paracelsus also proposed the concepts such as similar cures the similar, scorpion cures scorpion, mercury cures mercury, etc.
2. **Oswaldus Crollius**: Oswaldus Crollius (1560 – 1608), in his *"Treatise of Signatures of Internal Things"*, writes, the occult properties of plants; first, those endowed with life, and second, those destitute of life; are indicated by resemblances; for all exhibit to man by their signatures and characteristics, both their powers by which they can heal and in the diseases in which they are useful. Not only by their shapes, form and colours, but also by their actions and

qualities, such as their retaining, or shedding their leaves. They indicate what kind of service they can render to man, and what are the particular members of his body, to which they are especially appropriate.

3. **Jakob Bohme**: Jakob Bohme (1575 – 1624) suggested that God marked objects with a sign, or "signature", for their purpose. Plants bearing parts that resembled human body-parts, animals, or other objects were thought to have useful relevance to those parts, animals or objects. This doctrine became popularised after the publication of a book named, "*Signature Rerum*" (The Signature of All Things) in 1621. This doctrine also adopted by various schools of medicine, which states "*by observation, one can determine from the colour of the flowers or roots, the shapes of leaves, the places of growing, or other signatures that can be determined by the observation of the plant's purpose in God's plan*".

4. **William Coles**: William Coles (1626 – 1662), an English botanist considered in his books "*The Art of Simpling*" and "*Adam in Eden*" that walnut was good for treating brain diseases because it looks like a brain. Similarly, the little holes in the leaves of Hypericum resembles the skin, which is a hint for its use in all sorts injuries affecting the skin.

5. **R. H. True**, a plant physiologist and historian, succinctly explained the doctrine: "*... every plant having useful medicinal properties bears somewhere about it the likeness of the organ or of the part of the body upon which it exerts a healing action*".

Views of Homoeopathic Stalwarts

Many stalwarts like Dr. John H. Clarke, Dr. H. A. Roberts, Dr. C. M. Boger, Dr. Constantine Hering, Dr. William Boericke, Dr. James C. Burnett and Dr. Von Grauvogl had supporting attitude towards this doctrine.

1. **John H. Clarke**: Clarke stated in his '*A Dictionary of Practical Materia Medica*' under the heading 'Characteristics' of 'Magnesia phosphorica' that, "*it is only right to say that Schuessler arrived at them by a way of his own, which shows that there are other means besides proving of finding the keynote symptoms of remedies*".

   The second reference supporting the doctrine of signature in the Clarke's '*A Dictionary of Practical Materia Medica*' under the heading 'Characteristics' of 'Magnesia carbonica' where he wrote that "*it is often found that the physical characteristics of the substances correspond with their dynamic influences*".

2. **Herbert A. Roberts**: According to H. A. Roberts in his '*The principles and Art of Cure by Homoeopathy*' under the chapter of 'Drug Proving' stated that "*The preparation and administration of medicines was kept as a mystery for centuries, and the medicine man was held as superior and revered as a little more than mortal for his powers. Various doctrines of healing sprang up through the years; perhaps the most interesting of these was the doctrine of signature, founded on the belief that each member of the vegetable kingdom carried within itself the likeness of some organ or part of the human economy, as a sign that this particular plant was applicable to disturbances of that organ. That was probably the most consistent method among all the very ancient systems of applying drugs*".

3. **Cyrus M. Boger**: Dr. Boger (1861 – 1935) in his '*Lesser Writings*' under the chapter 'Reason and Facts', stated that "*The doctrine of signatures has been derided and said to rest upon pure fancy; but I know of no accidents in nature and everything has an adequate cause, hence we should not be too ready to attribute such things to mere coincidence. Such correspondences are too numerous as well as much too striking to be lightly passed over. It seems rather a case of not knowing just what they mean or what the real connection is*".

4. **Constantine Hering**: Hering stated that "If our school ever gives up the strict inductive method of Hahnemann we are lost and deserve to be mentioned only as a caricature in the history of medicine". He says, the remedy *Chelidonium* from Middle ages, was administered in serious complaints in hepatic derangements according to 'law of signature'. Arnica this wonderful remedy was used in domestic practice.

5. **William Boericke**: Boericke says that "The lungs of a fox must be specific against asthma – because this animal has a very vigorous respiration. *Hypericum*, having red juice, ought, therefore, to be use in hæmorrhage. *Euphorbia*, having a milky juice, must be good for increasing the flow of milk. *Sticta*, having some likeness to the lungs, was called pulmonaria (Lung wort) – and esteemed as a remedy for pulmonary complaints".

6. **Von Grauvogl**: As per Von Grauvogl "Digitalis must be used in blood dyscrasia – because its flowers are adorned with blood-coloured dots. *Euphrasia* (Eyebright) was famous, from ancient times, as a medicine for the eyes – because it had a black spot in its corolla – which looked like a pupil".

7. **J. C. Burnett**: Dr. J. C. Burnett (1840 – 1901) had a supporting attitude towards this doctrine. He writes in his work on 'The Diseases of the Liver', "The interaction of the human organism with its environment has generally been recognized in every age according to the views current at the time, the relations of the microcosm to the macrocosm used to be a big chapter in medical doctrine".

   He also says "The old doctrine of signatures is laughed at by almost all physicians, inclusive of the homoeopaths, and yet it is not without considerable foundation in fact; and, indeed, facts in great numbers may be drawn from homoeopathic literature in support of its real practical value. It has often helped me and I have long since ceased to ridicule it. Of course, it can easily be turned upside down and made to look silly, but still there it is and in the long run will most certainly be justified by science".

   Though pioneers like **John H. Clarke, Herbert A. Roberts, Cyrus M. Boger, James C. Burnett, Constantine Hering, William Boericke, Von Grauvogl** supported this Doctrine of Signature but our master **Dr. Hahnemann** was against this concept.

8. **Hahnemann**: Hahnemann was against the speculation and proposed the rational medicines based on pure experimentation exact observation and correct interpretation. He gave cardinal principles of homoeopathy and prove that permanent annihilation of disease is possible only by prescribing medicine on the similarity of symptoms which are already proved by drug proving on healthy human being.

   (i) **In Sec. 108** of Organon he writes, "There is, therefore, no other possible way in which the peculiar effects of medicines on the health of individuals can be accurately ascertained - there is no sure, no more natural way of accomplishing this object, than to administer the several medicines experimentally, in moderate doses, to healthy persons".

   (ii) **In F. N. of Sec. 108** of Organon he says, "not one single physician, as far as I know during the previous two thousand five hundred years, thought of this so natural, so absolutely necessary and only genuine mode of testing medicines for their pure and peculiar effect in deranging the health of the man, in order to learn what morbid state each medicine is capable of curing, except the great and immortal Albrecht Von Haller".

   (iii) **In Sec 110.** of Organon he said it is wrong to treat patients based on the idea of doctrine of signature and mixture prescription. As per Hahnemann the medicinal powers of drug can be ascertained only by drug proving and not by speculation, smell, colour, taste or appearance of the drugs, nor by chemical analysis.

   (iv) **In Sec. 144** of Organon he writes, "All conjecture, everything merely asserted or entirely fabricated, must be completely excluded from such a materia medica; everything must be the pure language of nature carefully and honestly interrogated".

   (v) And in his 1830 preface to the **"Materia Medica Pura Vol I"** he writes, "In my Organon of the healing art, 1 teach the principle that diseases can only be cured by remedies which produce analogous symptoms upon the healthy organism, and I moreover assert and prove, that every system of therapeutics in order to become a safe guide in the treatment of disease, ought to exclude all empty assertions and conjectures, as regards the supposed virtues of medicines, and ought to furnish a correct description of the symptoms by which remedial agents manifest their action upon the healthy organism. Anyone who admits the truth of these positions, will gladly seize the means which I here offer him, of relieving the affections of mankind in a speedy, durable, and much more certain manner".

Doctrine of Signature

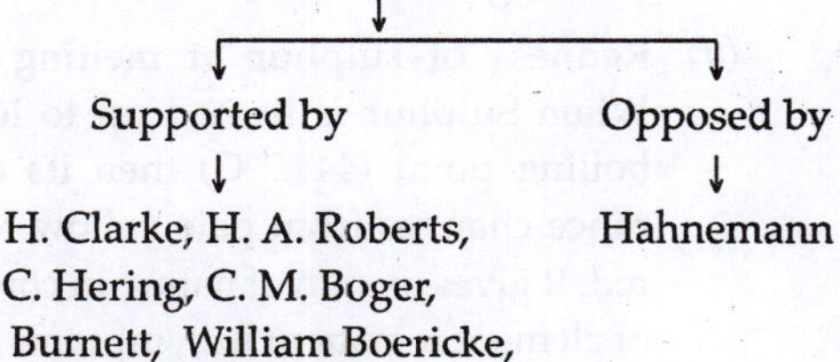

Examples:

The doctrine of signature can be observed from the general therapeutic study of a drug. Some examples of doctrine of signatures among Homoeopathic drugs:

Actaea racemosa: Herb is very soft and it is perennial plant 1 to 2.5 met., root is knotted and root of it appears as a Ganglia of Nerve. This medicine is used for nerve and muscle diseases.

Agaricus Muscarius: Sliced mushrooms resemble human ear, so are ancestors believed these were the perfect vegetable to cure earache.

Belladonna: The plant grows in the lime ($CaCO_3$) rich soil; from this we get the relation that Belladonna is the acute and complementary to Calcarea carb.

Blatta orientalis: Lives in cracks, crevices, damp places. Useful for asthma of people living in damp basements and cellars.

Bryonia: Bryonia is prepared from the root, which is fleshy, yellowish white in colour, rough with acidic and bitter taste, its odour is nauseating. Bryonia patient is also to some extent fleshy, with yellowish-white coated tongue with rough irritating temperament and has bitter taste in mouth.

Calcarea carbonica: It has hard shell to protect the soft body. The patient of Calcarea carb, also needs protection.

Carbo vegetabilis: The colour of wood charcoal is black; hence the patient looks bluish-black due to cyanosis.

Chelidonium majus: The yellow colour of it resembles bile; hence it is well known medicine for Jaundice and Hepatic diseases.

Corralium rubrum: The colour of this coral is red; hence it helps to cure red chancres or coral red eruptions.

Digitalis: It is useful in diseases of blood vessels, because its flowers are adorned to blood coloured dots.

Drosera: Drosera can be best remembered with its doctrine of signature. It is a carnivorous plant, a plant behaving almost like an animal. Hence it is prescribed in violent insanity. The plant preys on insects, it deceives the insect by keeping calm and when it comes near, and the plant traps it, chokes the insect and kills it. Similarly, we find the symptoms of being persecuted, deceived, trapped, choked and killed.

Euphorbia officinalis: Euphorbia, having a milky juice, must be good for increasing the flow of milk.

Euphrasia officinalis: It was famous as a medicine for the eye diseases, because it had a black spot in its corolla, which looked like a pupil.

Ficus religiosa: The leaves of Ficus religiosa resemble to the shape of the heart and uterus, so it treats the diseases of the circulatory system and uterus. On cutting the bark of a tree, it produces bright-red discharge which can treat diseases of the circulatory system.

Gelsemium sempervirens: It is prepared from yellow jasmine and the colour of its flower is yellow, hence it is used in conditions where the skin turns yellow, i.e. Jaundice.

Hamamelis virginica: The plant having red juice ought, hence use in bleeding which is dark and clotted.

Hypericum: It has red juices, hence used in haemorrhages.

Lachesis: The snake always protrudes its tongue unsteadily, similarly the patient always trembles the tongue when it protrudes.

Lycopodium: It is prepared from the spores of stick moss. The spores are externally very hard but once broken, they are very soft internally. Similarly, the patient does not fully cooperate with the doctor at the beginning, but becomes cooperative as soon as he begins to trust the doctor.

Phosphorus:

(i) Phosphorus is transparent in its pure form. Phosphorus constitution is also transparent, i.e. open.

(ii) It is an active element; reaction is very fast, cannot remain in atmosphere without any bond with other element. Active personality making friends very easily. Cannot remain anywhere without friendship.

(iii) At room temperature it burns like fire hence should be kept carefully under water in a cool and dark place protected from light. Burning is the keynote. General amelioration in the dark, cold food and cold water.

Pulmo vulpis: This is prepared from the fresh lungs of wolf hence used in lung diseases, i.e. Bronchial asthma.

Rhus tox: Rhus tox plants are collected in damp weather, rainy season, in the evening, because at that time Rhus tox plant possess more medicinal properties. These are also its modalities.

Sanguinaria canadensis: When the roots of the plant are cut, a red coloured juice comes out and appears like blood. Similarly, this medicine is useful in disorders relating to blood.

Sulphur:

(i) Chemically reactive substance: Due to high reactivity of substance we get a clear image of patient in relation to defective reactivity against stimuli.

(ii) Occurrence of sulphur: Sulphur is product of the volcanic eruptions and we know that volcanoes have tendency to erupt anytime. According to signature from here we get image that person also has a tendency to erupt either symptoms are in mental and physical form.

(iii) Pale yellow colour: The colour of the element is pale yellow, so according to doctrine of signature all the discharges of the sulphur are yellowish and offensive in nature.

(iv) Burning in the air with a blue flame: Sulphur burst out with blue flames and gives burning sensation to our body when come in contact, from here we get a guideline symptom relation of medicine to 'burning'.

(v) Redness of sulphur at melting point: When Sulphur is heated up to level of boiling point (444.7°C) then its appearance changes from pale yellow to dark red. It gives us sign of nature in corelation of element to patient in symptoms of redness of orifices of body like lips, ears, nose, eyelids, anus and vulva.

Tarentula hispanica: The Spanish spider comes out from the underground when a drum is beaten. From this we get that Tarentula patient has a characteristic symptom, i.e. hypersensitive to music.

Thuja occidentalis: This plant has pedunculated, wart like growths at the junction of the branch and the stem, or between two branches. Hence this medicine is very effective for pedunculated warts.

Zingiber officinale: Go through the structure of Ginger root, it looks like the stomach. And Ginger is a good medicine for stomach cramp or irritation of stomach.

Conclusions

In an ancient world where destiny of human beings are determined by the stars and planet; there is no modern facilities for treatment of suffering humanity – Doctrine of Signature plays a significant role in folk medicine to filled up this vacuum. This concept is found throughout the world though modern botanists dismiss it as a "primitive" or "pre-scientific" idea.

Though Doctrine of signature helps us to understand the basic nature of the plants and their relation for treatment but Hahnemann warned us against this concept in his Organon of Medicine under Sec. 108, F.N. to Sec. 108, Sec. 110, Sec. 144 even in Materia Medica Pura that we should go through Drug proving on healthy human beings to get the proper sign and symptoms which will be helpful for our Materia Medica.

In Homoeopathic system of medicine it is still gets an importance because it helps to study our Materia Medica in an easy and interesting manner by compare and remember some symptoms.

Chapter 37

General Knowledge of Legislation in Relation to Homoeopathic Pharmacy

Introduction

Homoeopathic system of medicine is about two hundred years old. In India, first time it was introduces and patronised by Raja Ranjit Singh in 19th century. In 1969 first time homoeopathic got a legal status and it was introduced in Drug and Cosmetics Act, 1940. The Drug and Cosmetics Act regulate the import, manufacture, distribution and sale of drugs. The Homoeopathic Acts and Rules are formed by sub-committee of Drugs Technical Advisory Board (DTAB) for Homoeopathy. The Government analysts, drug inspectors and import of homoeopathic medicines are governed by the same rule as applicable for modern medicine.

Legal Definition of Homoeopathic Medicines

Homoeopathic medicines include any drug which is recorded in homoeopathic provings or the therapeutic efficacy of which has been established through long clinical experience as recorded in authoritative homoeopathic literature of India or abroad, and which is prepared according to techniques of homoeopathic pharmacy but does not include a medicine which is administered by parenteral route.

Quality of Drugs

Quality of drugs for import and for manufacture is given in Chapters III & IV, respectively.

As per Drugs and Cosmetics Act, quality of drugs are given as:

Standards of Quality:

Standard of quality means:

(a) In relation to drugs that the drug complies with the standard set out in the (Second Schedule) and

(b) In relation to a cosmetic that the cosmetic complies with such standard as may be prescribed.

Misbranded Drugs

A drug shall be deemed to be misbranded:

(a) If it is so coloured, coated, powdered or polished that damage is concealed or if it is made to appear of better of greater therapeutic value than it really is; or

(b) If it is not labelled in the prescribed manner; or

(c) If its label or container or anything accompanying the drug bears any statement, design or device which makes any false claim for the drug or which is false or misleading in any particular.

Adulterated Drugs

A drug shall be deemed to be adulterated:

(a) If it consists in whole or in part, of any filthy, putrid or decomposed substance; or

(b) If it has been prepared, packed or stored under insanitary conditions whereby it may have been contaminated with filth or whereby it may have been rendered injurious to health; or

(c) If its container is composed, in whole or in part, of any poisonous or deleterious substance which may render the contents injurious to health; or

(d) If it bears or contains, for the purposes of colouring only, a colour other than one which is prescribed; or

(e) If it contains any harmful or toxic substance which may render it injurious to health; or if any substance has been mixed therewith so as to reduce its quality or strength.

Spurious Drugs

A drug shall be deemed to be spurious:

(a) If it is manufactured under a name which belongs to another drug;

(b) If it is an imitation of, or is a substitute for, another drug or resembles another drug in a manner likely to deceive or bears upon its label or container the name of another drug unless it is plainly and conspicuously marked so as to reveal its true character and its lack of identity with such other drugs; or

(c) If the label or container bears the name of an individual or company purporting to be the manufacture of the drug, which individual or company is fictitious or does not exists; or

(d) If it has been substituted wholly or in part by another drug or substance; or

(e) If it purports to be the product of a manufacturer of whom it is not truly a product.

Standard to be followed

Second Schedule covers the standards to be complied with by imported drugs manufactured for sale, sold, stocked or exhibited for sale or distributed.

Homoeopathic Medicines are also covered under Second Schedule 4(A) which is given below*

The Drugs and Cosmetics Act and Rules

The Drugs and Cosmetics Act, 1940, as amended by the Drugs (Amendment) Act, 1955, the Drugs (Amendment) Act, 1960, the Drugs

Table 37.1: Second Schedule 4(A)*

Class of Drugs	Standards to be complied with
(a) Drugs included in the HPI	Standards of identity purity and strength of drugs given in the HPI for the time being in force and such other standards as may be prescribed.
(b) Drugs not included in the HPI but which are included in the HPUS or the GHP	Standards of identity, purity and/strength prescribed for the drugs in the edition of such pharmacopoeia for the time being in which they are given and such other standards as may be prescribed.
(c) Drugs not included in the HPI or HPUS or GHP	The formula or list of ingredients displayed in the prescribed manner or the label of the container and such other standards as may be prescribed by the Central Government.

(Amendment) Act, 1962, the Drugs and Cosmetics (Amendments) Act, 1964, the Drugs and Cosmetics (Amendments) Act, 1972, the Drugs and Cosmetics (Amendments) Act, 1982, the Drugs and Cosmetics (Amendments) Act, 1986, and the Drugs and Cosmetics (Amendments) Act, 1995. and The Drugs and Cosmetics Rules, 1945, as corrected up to the 30th April, 2003.

Part VIA: Sale of Homoeopathic Medicines

67-A.(i) Appointment of licensing authority: The State Government shall appoint Licensing Authorities for the purpose of sale of homoeopathic medicine in specified areas.

(ii) **Application for the grant or renewal of a licence:** To sell, stock or exhibit for sale or distribution of homoeopathic medicines shall be made in Form 19-B, to the Licensing Authority with payment of rupees two hundred and fifty.

If the applicant applied for renewal of licence after its expiry but within six months of such expiry the fee payable of renewal of such licence shall be rupees two hundred and fifty plus an additional fee at the rate of rupees fifty per month or part thereof.

(iii) **Damage or loss of licence:** If the original licence is either defaced, damaged or lost, a duplicate copy thereof may be issued on payment of a fee of rupees fifty.

67-B. Power of Licencing Authority: A Licensing Authority may, with the approval of the State Government, by an order in writing, delegate the power to sign licences and such other powers, to any other person under his control.

67-C. Forms of licences to sell drugs: A licence to sell, stock or exhibit for sale or distribute homoeopathic medicines by retail or by wholesale shall be issued in Form 20-C or 20-D, as the case may be.

67-D. Sale at more than one place: A separate application shall be made and a separate licence shall be obtained in respect of each place—if drugs are sold or stocked for sale at more than one place.

67-E. Duration of licences: An original licence or a renewed licence shall be valid for a period or five years on and from the date on which it is granted or renewed.

The licence shall continue until orders are passed on the application—if the application for renewal of a licence is made before its expiry or if the applications is made within six months of its expiry, after payment of additional fee.

The licence shall be deemed to have expired if application for its renewal is not made within six months after its expiry.

67-EE. Certificate of renewal: The certificate of renewal of a sale licence in Forms 20-C and 20-D shall be issued in Form 20-E.

67-F. Conditions to be satisfied before a licence in Form 20-C or Form 20-D is granted

(i) The premises in respect of which the licence in form 20-C, the sale premises is in charge of a person who is or has been dealing in homoeopathic medicines and who is in the opinion of the Licensing Authority competent to deal in homoeopathic medicines.

(ii) Any person who is aggrieved by the order passed by the Licensing Authority under sub-rule (1) may within 30 days from the date of the receipt of such order, appeal to the State Government and the State Government may, after such enquiry into the matter as it considers necessary, and after giving the applicant an opportunity for representing his case, make such order in relation thereto as it thinks fit.

67-G. Conditions of licence: Licence in Form 20-C or 20-D shall be subject to the conditions stated therein and to the following further conditions, namely:

(i) The premises where the homoeopathic medicines are stocked for sale or sold are maintained in a clean condition.

(ii) The sale of homoeopathic medicines shall be conducted under the supervision of a person, competent to deal in homoeopathic medicines.

(iii) The licencee shall permit an Inspector to inspect the premises and furnish such information as he may require for ascertaining whether the provisions of the Act and the Rules made thereunder have been observed.

(iv) The licensee in Form 20-D shall maintain records of purchase and sale of homoeopathic medicines containing alcohol together with names and addresses of parties to whom sold.

(v) The licensee in Form 20-C shall maintain records of purchase and sale of homoeopathic medicines containing alcohol. No records of sale in respect of homoeopathic potentised medicines in containers of 30 ml or lower capacity and in respect of mother tinctures made up in quantities up to 60 ml need to be maintained.

(vi) The licensee shall maintain an Inspection Book in Form 35 to enable an Inspector to record his impressions and the defects noticed.

67-GG. Additional information to be furnished by an applicant for licence or a licensee to the Licensing Authority: The applicant for the grant of a licence or any person granted a licence under this part shall, on demand furnish to the Licensing Authority, before the grant of the licence or during the period the licence is in force, as the case may be, documentary evidence in respect of the ownership or occupation on rental or other basis of the premises specified in the application for licence or in the licence granted, *constitution* of the firm, or any other relevant matter, which may be required for the purpose or verifying the correctness of the statements made by the applicant or the licensee, while applying for or after obtaining the licence, as the case may be.

67-H. Cancellation and suspension of licences

(a) The Licensing Authority may, after giving the licensee an opportunity to show cause why such an order should not be passed, by an order in writing stating the reasons therefore cancel a licence issued under this Part or suspend it for such period as he thinks fit, if in his opinion, the licensee has failed to comply with any of the conditions of the licence or with any provisions of the Act or Rules made thereunder:

Provided that, where such failure or contravention is the consequence of an act or omission on the part of an agent or employees, the licence shall not be cancelled or suspended unless the Licensing Authority is satisfied:

(i) That the act or omission was not instigated or connived at by him or, if the licensee is a firm or company, by a partner of the firm or a director of the company, or

(ii) That the owner of the business or an agent or employee of the owner had not been guilty of any similar act or omission within twelve months before the date on which the act or omission in question took place, or where his agent or employee had been guilty of any such act or omission, the licensee had not or could not reasonably have had knowledge of that previous act or omission, or

(iii) If the act or omission was a continuing act or omission and the owner of business had not or could not reasonably have had knowledge of that previous act or omission, or

(iv) That the owner of the business had used due diligence to ensure that the conditions of the licence or the provisions of the Act or the Rules made thereunder were observed.

(b) A licensee whose licence has been suspended or cancelled may, within three months of the date of the order under sub-rule (1), prefer an appeal against that order to the State Government whose decision will be final.

Part VII-A: Manufacture for sale or for Distribution of Homoeopathic Medicine

85-A. Manufacture on more than one set of premises: If Homoeopathic Medicines are manufactured in more than one set of premises a separate application shall be made and a separate licence shall be obtained in respect of each such set of premises.

85-B. Application for licence to manufacture Homoeopathic Medicines

1. Application for grant or renewal of licences to manufacture for sale or for distribution of Homoeopathic medicine shall be made to the Licensing Authority appointed by the State Government for the purpose of this part and shall be made in Form 24-C.

2. The Application in Form 24-C shall be accompanied:

   (a) By a fee of (Rupees two hundred) for the manufacture of homoeopathic mother tinctures and potentised preparations and an inspection fee of (Rupees one hundred) for the first inspection of (Rupees fifty) in case of inspection for renewal of licence;

   (b) By a fee of (Rupees two hundred) for the manufacture of Homoeopathic potentised preparations only and an inspection fee of (Rupees one hundred) for the first inspection or (Rupees fifty) in case of inspection for renewal of licence;

   (c) By a fee of (Rupees two hundred) for the manufacture of potentised preparations from back potencies by pharmacies which are already licenced to sell Homoeopathic medicines by retail and an inspection fee of (Rupeed one hundred) for the first inspection or (Rupees fifty) in case of inspection for renewal of licence.

3. If a person applies for renewal of a licence after its expiry but within six months of such expiry, the fee payable for the renewal of such a licence shall be

   (a) (Rupees two hundred) plus an additional fee at the rate of (rupees one hundred) per month or part thereof and an inspection fee of (rupees fifty) for the manufacture of homoeopathic mother tinctures and potentised preparations;

   (b) (Rupees two hundred) plus an additional fee at the rate of (rupees one hundred) per month or part thereof and an inspection fee of (rupees fifty) for the manufacture of homoeopathic potentised preparations only;

   (c) (Rupees two hundred) plus an additional fee at the rate of (rupees one hundred) per month or part thereof and an inspection fee of (rupees fifty) for the manufacture of potentised preparations from back potencies by pharmacies who are already licensed to sell Homoeopathic Medicines by retail.

4. A fee of (rupees fifty) shall be paid for a duplicate copy of the licence for the manufacture of Homoeopathic Mother Tinctures and Potentised preparations issued under sub-rule (1) if the original is defaced, damaged or lost. While the fee to be paid for such a duplicate copy of the licence for the manufacture of Homoeopathic potentised preparations only shall be (rupees fifty).

5. Applications by licensee to manufacture additional items of Homoeopathic medicines shall be made to the Licensing Authority and such applications shall be accompanied by a fee of (rupees fifty) for each additional item.

85-C. Application to manufacture New Homoeopathic Medicine

Subject to the other provisions of these rules:

1. No 'New Homoeopathic Medicine' shall be manufactured unless it is previously approved by the Licensing Authority mentioned in Rule 21;

2. The manufacture of 'New Homoeopathic Medicine' when applying to the Licensing Authority, mentioned in sub-rule (1) shall produce such documentary and other evidence as may be required by the Licensing Authority for accessing the therapeutic efficacy of the medicine including the minimum proving carried out with it.

3. While applying for a licence to manufacture a 'New Homoeopathic Medicine' an applicant shall produce along with his application evidence that the 'New Homoeopathic Medicine' for the manufacture of which application is made has already been approved.

[*Explanation:* The term 'New Homoeopathic Medicine' in this rule shall have the same meaning as in Rule 30-AA.]

85-D. Form of Licence to manufacture Homoeopathic Medicines

Licence for manufacture of Homoeopathic medicines is a licence to manufacture potentised preparations from back potencies by Pharmacies who are already licensed to sell Homoeopathic medicines by retail shall be granted in Form 25-C.

85-E. Conditions for the grant of renewal of a licence in From 25-C

Before a licence in Form 25-C is granted or renewed, the following conditions shall be complied with by the applicant:

1. The manufacture of Homoeopathic medicines shall be conducted under the direction and supervision of competent technical staff consisting at-least of one person who is a whole time employee and who is

   (a) a graduate in Science with Chemistry as one of the subjects with three years' experience in manufacture of Homoeopathic Medicines; or

   (b) a graduate in Pharmacy with 18 months of experience in the manufacture of Homoeopathic medicines; or

   (c) holds qualification as defined under sub-clause (g) of clause (1) of Section 2 of Homoeopathy Central Council Act, 1973 (59 of 1973), with 18 months of experience in the manufacture of Homoeopathic medicines. Provided that the persons who are already in employment with five years' experience in the manufacture of Homoeopathic medicines and whose name was accordingly entered in any licence granted in Form 25-C for manufacture of different classes of Homoeopathic medicines included in them shall be deemed to be qualified for the purpose of this rule.

2. The factory premises shall comply with the requirements and conditions specified in Schedule M1: Provided that where the Licensing Authority considers it necessary or expedient so to do it may having regard to the nature and extent of manufacturing operations, relax or suitably alter the said requirements or conditions in any particular case for reasons to be recorded in writing.

3. The applicant for manufacture of Homoeopathic mother tinctures shall either (i) provide and maintain adequate staff, premises and laboratory equipment for identifying the raw materials and for testing the mother tinctures wherever possible, or (ii) make arrangements with such institution approved by the Licensing Authority (under part XV(A) of the rules) for some tests, wherever possible, to be regularly carried out on his behalf by that institution.

4. The premises where Homoeopathic medicines are manufactured shall be distinct and separate from the premises used for residential purposes.

5. Homoeopathic medicine shall not be manufactured simultaneously with drugs pertaining to other systems of medicine.

6. The applicant shall make arrangements for proper storage of Homoeopathic medicines manufactured by him.

Provided that in case potentised preparations are made in a Pharmacy holding licence in Form 20-C, the conditions (2) and (3) shall not apply. The licensee shall ensure to the satisfaction of the Licensing Authority that the products manufactured by it confirm to the claims made on the label.

85-EA. Inspection before grant or renewal of licence: Before a licence under this Part is granted or renewed in Form 25-C or Form 26-C the Licensing Authority shall cause the establishment, in which the manufacture is proposed, to be conducted or being conducted, to be inspected by one or more Inspectors appointed under the Act. The Inspector or Inspectors shall examine all portions of the premises, plant and appliances and also inspect the process of manufacture intended to be employed or being employed along with the means to be employed or being employed for standardising and testing the substances to be manufactured and inquire into the professional qualifications of the technical staff to be employed. He shall also examine and verify the statements made in the application in regards to their correctness, and the capability of the applicant to comply with the requirements of competent technical staff, manufacturing plants, testing equipments and the requirements of plant and equipment as laid down in Schedule M-I read with the requirements of maintenance of records as laid down in Schedule U.

85-EB. Report by Inspector: The Inspector or Inspectors shall forward a detailed descriptive report giving his or their findings on each aspect of inspection along with his or their recommendations after completion of his or their inspection to the Licensing Authority.

85-EC. Grant or refusal of licence

1. If the Licensing Authority after such further enquiry, if any, as he may consider necessary is satisfied that the requirements of the rules under the Act have been complied with and that conditions of the licence and the rules under the Act shall be observed, he shall grant or renew a licence in Form 25-C or Form 26-C.
2. If the Licensing Authority is not so satisfied, he shall reject the application and shall inform the applicant of the reasons for such rejection and of the conditions which must be satisfied before a licence can be granted or renewed and shall supply the applicant with a copy of inspection report.

85-ED. Further application after rejection: If with a period of six months from the rejection of an application for a licence, the applicant informs the Licensing Authority that the conditions laid down have been fulfilled and deposits an inspection fee of rupees two hundred and fifty, the Licensing Authority may, if, after causing further inspection to be made, he is satisfied that the conditions for the grant of licence have been complied with, issue a licence in Form 25-C or Form 26-C.

85-EE. Appeal to the State Government: Any person who is aggrieved by the order passed by the Licensing Authority refusing to grant or renew a licence under this Part may within ninety days from the date of receipt of such order, appeal to the State Government and the State Government may, after such enquiry into the matter as is considered necessary and after giving the said person an opportunity for representing the case, pass such order as it thinks fit.

85-F. Duration of Licence: An original licence or a renewed licence unless it is sooner suspended or cancelled shall be valid for a period of five years on and from the date on which it is granted or renewed. Provided that if the application for renewal of a licence in force is made before its expiry or if the application is made within six months of its expiry, after payment of additional fee, the licence shall continue to be in force until orders are passed on the application and the licence shall be deemed to have expired if application for its renewal is not made within six months of its expiry.

85-G. Certificate of renewal: The certificate of renewal of a licence in Form 25-C shall be issued in Form 26-C.

85-H. Conditions of licence: A licence in Form 25-C shall be subject to the conditions stated therein and to the following further conditions, namely:

(a) The licencee shall provide and maintain staff and premises as specified in Rule 85-E.

(b) The licencee shall allow an inspector appointed under the act to enter, with or without prior notice, any premises where the manufacture of a homoeopathic medicine in respect of which the licence is issued is carried on, to inspect the premises and to take samples of the manufactured homoeopathic medicines.

(c) The licencee shall allow an Inspector to inspect all registers and records maintained under these rules and shall supply to the Inspector such information as he may require for the purpose of ascertaining whether the provisions of the Act and the Rules made thereunder have been observed.

(d) The licencee shall maintain an Inspection Book in Form 35 to enable an Inspector to record his impressions and defects noticed;

(e) The licencee shall comply with the following conditions in respect of the mother tinctures manufactured by him:

(i) The crude drug used in the manufacture of the mother tincture shall be identified and records of such identification shall be kept for a period of five years;

(ii) The total solids in the mother tincture shall be determined and records of such tests shall be kept for a period of five years;

(iii) The alcohol content in the mother tincture shall be determined and records of the same shall be maintained for a period of five years;

(iv) The containers of mother tinctures shall preferably be of glass and shall be clean and free from any sort of impurities or adhering matter. The glass shall be netural as far as possible.

(v) In the process of manufacture of mother tinctures hygienic conditions shall be scrupulously observed by the licensee. Storage and handling conditions shall also be properly observed by the licensee according to Homoeopathic principles.

No colour shall be added to any Homoeopathic medicines: Provided that caramel may be added to combination of Homoeopathic preparations with syrup base,

(f) Records shall be maintained of Homoeopathic medicines containing alcohol and the quantities sold together with names and addresses of parties to whom sold.

85-HH. Additional information to be furnished by an applicant for the licence or a licensee to the Licensing Authority: The applicant for the grant of licence or any other person granted a licence under this Part shall, on demand, furnish to the Licensing Authority, before the grant of the licence or during the period the licence is in force, as the case may be, documentary evidence in respect of the ownership or occupation in rental or other basis of the premises, specified in the application for licence or in the licence granted, constitution of the firm or any other relevant matters which may be required for the purpose of verifying the correctness of the statements made by the applicant or the licensee, while applying for or after obtaining the licence, as the case may be.

85-I. Cancellation and suspension of licences

1. The Licensing Autority may, after giving the licensee an opportunity to show cause why such an order should not be passed, by an order in writing stating the reasons therefore, cancel a licence issued under this part or suspend it for such period as he thinks fit either wholly or in respect of some of the substances to which it relates if, in his opinion, the licensee has failed to comply with any of the conditions of the licence or with any provisions of the Act or Rules made thereunder.
2. A licensee whose licence has been suspended or cancelled may, within three months of the date of the order under sub-rule (1), appeal to the State Government, which shall decide the same.

Part IX-A: Labelling and packaging of Homoeopathic Medicines

Rule 106-A. No Homoeopathic Medicine shall be imported unless it is packed and labelled in conformity with Rules in Part IX-A (Rule 106 A).

Manner of Labeling of Homoeopathic Medicine

A. The following particulars shall be either printed or written in indelible ink and shall appear in a conspicuous manner on the label of the innermost container of any Homoeopathic Medicine and on every other covering in which the container is packed:

(a) The words 'Homoeopathic Medicine'.

(b) The name of the Medicine'—

(i) For drugs included in the HPI, HPUS BHP or GHP the name specified in that pharmacopoeia.

(ii) For other drugs, the name descriptive of the true nature of the drug.

(c) The Potency of Homoeopathic Medicine: For this purpose the potency shall be expressed either in decimal, centesimal or 50-millesimal systems.

(c-A) In case of a homoeopathic medicine containing two or more ingredients, the name of each ingredient together with its potency or proportion or both shall be stated on the label.

(d) Name and address of the manufacturer when sold in original containers of the manufacture. In case of a Homoeopathic Medicine is sold in a container other than that of the manufacturer the name and address of the seller should be on the packing.

(e) In case the Homoeopathic Medicine contains alcohol, the alcohol content in percentage by volume in terms of ethyl alcohol shall be stated on the label.

Provided that in case the total quantity of the Homoeopathic medicine in the container is 30 millilitres or less it will not be necessary to state the content of alcohol on the label.

B. In addition to the above particulars the label of homoeopathic mother tincture shall display the following particulars:

(i) A distinctive batch number, that is to say, the number by reference to which details of manufacture of the particular batch from which the substance in the container is taken are recorded and are available for inspection, the figures representing the batch number being preceded by the words "Batch No." or "Batch" or "Lot No." or "Lot" or any distinguishing prefix;

(ii) Manufacturing Licence Number, the number being preceded by the words "Manufacturing Licence Number;" or "Mfg. Lic. No." or "M.L.".

Explanation: This clause shall not apply to a Homoeopathic Mother Tincture manufactured outside India.

(iii) No Homoeopathic Medicine containing a single ingredient shall bear proprietary name on its label.

106-B. Prohibition of quantity and percentage: No Homoeopathic Medicine containing more than 12% alcohol v/v (Ethyl alcohol) shall be packed and sold in packing or bottles of more than 30 millilitres, except that it may be sold to hospital/dispensaries in packings or bottles of not more than 100 millilitres.

Ophthalmic Preparations in Homoeopathic Medicines

All Eye Ointment and other ophthalmic preparation should conform to the Schedule FF of Drugs and Cosmetics Rule.

SCHEDULE FF (See Rule 126-A): Standards for Ophthalmic Preparations

Part-A: Ophthalmic Solutions and Suspension

Ophthalmic Solutions and Suspensions shall

(a) be sterile when dispensed or sold in the unopened container of the manufacture, except in case of those ophthalmic solutions and suspensions which are not specifically required to comply with the test for 'Sterility' in the Pharmacopoeia.

(b) contain one or more of the following suitable substances to prevent the growth of micro-organisms:

(i) Benzalkonium Chloride, 0.01 per cent (This should not be used in solutions of nitrates or salicylates).

(ii) Phenyl mercuric nitrate: 0.001 per cent.

(iii) Chlorbutanol: 0.5 per cent.

(iv) Phenyl ethyl alcohol: 0.5 per cent.

Provided that solutions used in surgery shall not have any preservatives and be packed in single dose container.

Provided further that the licensing authority may in his discretion authorise the use of any preservatives or vary the concentration prescribed on being satisfied that its use affords equal guarantee for preventing the growth of microorganisms.

(c) be free from foreign matter;

(d) be contained in bottles made of either neutral glass or soda glass specially treated to reduce the amount of alkali released when in contact of aqueous, or in suitable plastic containers which would not in any way be incompatible with the solutions; The droppers to be supplied with the containers of ophthalmic solutions and suspension shall be made of neutral glass or of suitable plastic material and when supplied separately shall be packed in sterile cellophane, or other suitable packings.

(e) In addition to complying with the provisions of the labeling laid down in the rules the following particulars shall also be shown on the label of container:

(i) The statement 'Use the solution within one month after opening the container'.

(ii) Name and concentration of the preservatives, if used.

(iii) The words 'NOT FOR INJECTION'.

Of containers or Carton or Package leaflet:

(i) Special instructions regarding storage, wherever applicable.

(ii) A cautionary legend reading as

WARNING

(i) If irritation persists or increases, discontinue the use and consult physician.

(ii) Do not touch the dropper tip or other dispensing tip to any surface since this may contaminate solutions.

Part-B: Ophthalmic Ointments

Ophthalmic ointment shall

(a) be sterile when dispensed or when sold in the unopened container of the manufacture;

(b) be free from foreign matter.

(c) In addition to complying with the provisions for labeling laid down in the rules the following particulars shall be shown on the container or carton or package leaflet:

(i) Special instructions regarding storage wherever applicable.

(ii) A cautionary legend reading

WARNING

If irritation persists or increases discontinue the use and consult physician.

SCHEDULE K: Class of Drugs with Extent and Conditions of Exemptions

Class of Drugs

The homoeopathic medicines supplied by a registered homoeopathic medical practitioner to his own patient or any medicine specified in Schedule C supplied by a registered medical practitioner at the request of another such practitioner if it is specialy prepared with reference to the condition and for the use of an individual patient provided the registered medical practitioner is not

(a) keeping an open shop, or

(b) selling across the counter, or

(c) engaged in the importation, manufacture, distribution or sale of medicines in the provision of Chapter IV of the Act and the Rules thereunder.

Extent and Conditions of Exemption

All the provisions of Chapter IV of the Act and the Rules made thereunder, subject to the following conditions:

The homoeopathic medicines shall be purchased only from a dealer or a manufacturer licensed under 'The Drugs & Cosmetics Rules, 1945'.

Schedule K, item 31 provides permission for sale of some homoeopathic medicines through any registered dealer of medicines licensed under Rule 61.

Item 31 (Schedule K) includes some 32 single homoeopathic medicines in pills in 30C potency in original sealed packs, 12 biochemic tissue remedies, 4 ointments and Arnica hair oil. They are as follows:

(a) Arnica montana hair oil

(b) Homoeopathic ointments, each in 15 gm tube

1. Arnica montana
2. Cantharis
3. Calendula officinalis
4. Rhus toxicodendron

(c) Biochemic tissue remedies in tablet forms, in generic names only, each in 20 gm packing in 3x and 6x trituration:

1. Calcarea phosphorica
2. Calcarea sulphurica

3. Ferrum phosphoricum
4. Kali muriaticum
5. Kali phoshoricum
6. Kali sulphuricum
7. Magnesium phosphoricum
8. Megnesia sulphurica
9. Natrum muriaticum
10. Natrum phosphoricum
11. Natrum sulphuricum
12. Silicea

(d) Homoeopathic medicines, mentioned below, in pills, each in 30c potency, in sealed original packing of manufacturer of 8 gms:

1. Arnica montana
2. Aconitum napellus
3. Arsenicum album
4. Aloe socotrina
5. Apis mellifica
6. Allium cepa
7. Bryonia alba
8. Borax
9. Belladonna
10. Cantharis
11. Carbo vegetabilis
12. Cina
13. Colocynthis
14. Calendula offcinalis
15. Caulophyllum thalictroides
16. Cocculus indicus
17. Chamomilla
18. Drosera rotundifolia
19. Hepar sulphur
20. Ipecacuanha
21. Ledum palustre
22. Millefolium
23. Mercurius solubilis
24. Nux vomica
25. Pulsatilla nigricans
26. Podophyllum peltatum
27. Plantago major
28. Rhus toxicodendron
29. Ruta graveolens
30. Symphytum officinalis
31. Veratrum album

Ministry of Health and Family Welfare Notification

New Delhi, 2006

GSR 678(E): Whereas certain draft rules further to amend the Drugs and Cosmetics Rules, 1945 were published, as required by sections 12 and 33 of the Drugs and Cosmetics Act, 1940 (23 of 1940), in the Gazette of India, Extraordinary, part II, section 3, sub section (i), dated 2nd August, 2005, vide notification of the Government of India in the Ministry of Health and Family Welfare (Department of Health), number GSR 521 (E), dated the 2nd August, 2005, for inviting objections and suggestions from all persons likely to be affected thereby, till the expiry of a period of forty five days from the date on which copies of the Gazette containing the said notification were made available to the public; And whereas, copies of the said Gazette containing the said notification were made available to the public on And whereas, objections and suggestions received from the public on the said rules have been considered by the Central Government; Now, therefore, in exercise of the power conferred by sections 12 and 33 of the Drugs and Cosmetics Act, 1940 (23 of 1940) Act, the Central Government, after consultation with the Drugs Technical Advisory Board, hereby makes the following rules further to amend the Drugs and Cosmetics rules, 1945, namely:

1. (a) These rules may be called the Drugs and Cosmetics (Amendment) Rules, 2006.

   (b) They shall come into force on or after two years of their publication in the Official Gazette.

In the Drugs and Cosmetics Rules, 1945, for Schedule M-1, the following schedule shall be substituted, namely:

The Prevention of Illicit Traffic in Narcotic Drugs and Psychotropic Substances Act, 1988 (PIT NDPS Act)

The deterrent penal provisions of the Narcotic Drugs and Psychotropic Substances Act, 1985 and other legislative, administrative and preventive measures were found inadequate to control the illicit transit traffic in drugs. It was, therefore, felt that a preventive detention law should be enacted with a view to effectively immobilise persons engaged in any kind of illcit traffic in narcotic drugs and psychotropic substances. To achieve this objective the President promulgated the Prevention of Illicit Traffic in Narcotic Drugs and Psychotropic Substances Ordinance on 4 th July,1988. To replace this Ordinance the Narcotic Drugs and Psychotropic Substances Bill, 1988 was introduced in Parliament.

The Prevention of Illicit Traffic in Narcotic Drugs and Psychotropic Substance Bill, 1988 was passed by both the Houses of Parliament and was assented by the President on 6th September, 1988. It was deemed to have come in force on 4th July, 1988 as The Prevention of Illicit Traffic in Narcotic Drugs And Psychotropic Substances Act, 1988 (46 Of 1988).

The Act empowers Central Government and the State Governments have been empowered to make orders of detention with respect to any person (including a foreigner) if they are of opinion that it is necessary so to do with a view to preventing him from committing illcit traffic in narcotic drugs and psychotropic substances. The expression "illicit traffic" had been defined to include cultivation of any coca plant or gathering any portion of coca plants, cultivating the opium poppy or any cannabis plant, or engaging in the production, manufacture, possession, etc., of narcotic drugs or psychotropic substance.

The Drugs and Magic Remedies Act (Objectionable Advertisement) (21 of 1954) and The Rules (1955)

As it stands, the Drugs and Magic Remedies (Objectionable Advertisements) Act, 1954, basically prohibits four kinds of advertisements pertaining to drugs and magical cures.

Section 3 of the Act says that no person shall take any part in the publication of any advertisement promoting a drug or leading to the use of a drug for the procurement of miscarriage in women or prevention of conception in women; the maintenance or improvement of the capacity of human being for sexual pleasure; and correction of menstrual disorders in women.

Section 3 further prohibits any advertisement promoting drugs for the diagnosis, cure, mitigation, treatment or prevention of any disease, disorder or condition specified in the Schedule. The schedule lists a number of diseases, disorders or conditions such as appendicitis, atherosclerosis, blindness, blood poisoning, Bright's disease, cancer, cataract, deafness, diabetes, brain diseases or disorder, uterine diseases, disorder of menstrual flow disorders of nervous system, prostatic gland disorders, dropsy, epilepsy, female disease (in general), fever (in general), fits, forms and structure of the female breast, gallbladder stones, kidney stones, bladder stones, gangrene, glaucoma, goitre, heart diseases, high or low blood pressure, hydrocele, hysteria, infantile paralysis, insanity, leprosy, leucoderma, lock jaw, locomotor ataxia, lupus, nervous debility, obesity, paralysis, plague, pleurisy, pneumonia, rheumatism, ruptures, sexual impotence, small pox, stature of person, sterility of women, trachoma, TB, tumours, typhoid fever, ulcers of GI tract, veneral diseases including AIDS.

Section 4 of the Act prohibits those advertisements relating to a drug if they contain any matter which directly or indirectly gives a false impression regarding the true character of the drug or makes a false claim for the drug or is otherwise false or misleading.

Section 5 of the Act prohibits advertisements of magic remedies for treatment of certain diseases and disorders.

Violation of the law attracts imprisonment for six months or fine or both, for first conviction and for subsequent conviction, imprisonment for a year or fine or both.

The Medicinal and Toilet Preparation (Excise duties) Act, 1955 (No. 16 of 1955)

It provides for the levy and collection of duty of excise on medicinal and toilet preparations containing alcohol, opium, Indian hemp, or other narcotic drugs or narcotics. As the homoeopathic medicines comprise mainly of alcohol, a pharmacist must be conversant with the above legislations.

Dangerous Drugs Act, 1930 and Rules, 1957

This legislation relates to medicines containing opium, morphine, pethadine etc which are considered addiction—forming, dependence-producing drugs and regulates their manufacture, sales, possession etc.

Drug Prices (Display and Control) Order, 1966

This order has been made in order to make drugs available to the general public at fair prices. Any change in the wholesale and retail price of a drug can be effected only with the prior approval of the Central Government. Under a recent amendment to this order no such prior approval for a change in price is necessary in respect of a drug covered by the latest edition of the Homoeopathic Pharmacopoeias of U.K., U.S.A. and Germany and is without a specific brand name.

THE HOMOEOPATHY CENTRAL COUNCIL ACT, 1973

[NO. 59 OF 1973 (19TH DECEMBER, 1973)]

An Act to provide for the constitution of a Central Council of Homoeopathy and maintenance of a Central Register of Homoeopathy and for matters connected therewith.

Be it enacted by Parliament in the Twenty fourth year of the Republic of India as follows:

Chapter I (Preliminary)

Chapter II (The Central Council Act and Its Committees)

Chapter IIA

Chapter III (Recognition of Medical Qualifications)

Chapter IV (The Central Register of Homoeopathy)

Chapter V (Miscellaneous).

CHAPTER I (PRELIMINARY)

Short Title, Extent and Commencement

1. (i) This act may be called the Homoeopathy Central Council Act, 1973.

(ii) It extends to the whole of India.

(iii) It shall come into force in a State on such date as the Central Government may, be notification in the Official Gazette, appointing this behalf for such State and different dates may be appointed for different States and for different provisions of this Act.

Definition

2. 1. In this, Act, unless the context otherwise requires:

(a) "Board" means a Board, Council, Examining Body or Faculty of Homoeopathy (by whatever name called) constituted by the State Government under any law for the time being in force regulating the award of medical qualifications in, and registration of practitioners of Homoeopathy;

(b) "Central Council" means the Central Council of Homoeopathy constituted under Section 3;

(c) "Central Register of Homoeopathy" means the register maintained by the Central Council under this Act;

(d) "Medical Institution" means any institution within or without India which grants Degrees, Diplomas or licences in Homoeopathy;

(e) "Prescribed" means prescribed by regulations;

(f) "Recognised Medical Qualification" means any of the medical qualifications in Homoeopathy included in the Second or the Third Schedule;

(g) "Regulation" means a regulation made under Section 33;

(h) "State Register of Homoeopathy" means a register or registers maintained under any law for the time being in force in any State regulating the registration of practitioners of Homoeopathy;

(i) "University" means any University in India established by law and having a Faculty of Homoeopathy and includes a University in India established by law in which instruction, teaching, training or research in Homoeopathy is provided.

2. Any reference in this Act to a law which is not in force in the State of Jammu and Kashmir shall, in relation to that State, be constructed as a reference to the corresponding law, if any, in force in that State.

Amended vide Homoeopathy Central Council Amendment Act, 2002 (No. 51 of 2002) published in Gazette of India on 9th December, 2002.

CHAPTER II (THE CENTRAL COUNCIL ACT AND ITS COMMITTEES)

Constitution of Central Council

3. 1. The Central Government shall, by notification in the Official Gazette, constitute for the purposes of this Act, a Central Council consisting of the following members, namely:

(a) Such number of members not exceeding five as may be determined by the Central Government in accordance with the provisions of the First Schedule from each State in which a State Register of Homoeopathy is maintained, to be elected from amongst themselves by persons enrolled on that register as practitioners of Homoeopathy;

(b) One member from each University to be elected from amongst themselves by the members of the Faculty or Department (by whatever name called) of Homoeopathy of that University.

Provided that until any such Faculty or Department of Homoeopathy is started in at least seven Universities, the Central Government may nominate such number of members not exceeding seven as may be determined by the Central Government from amongst the teaching staff of medical institutions within India, so however, that the total number of members so nominated and elected under this clause shall in no case exceed seven;

(c) Such number of members, not exceeding forty percent of the total number of members elected under clause (a) and (b), as may be nominated by the Central Government from amongst persons having special knowledge or practical experience in respect of Homoeopathy or other related disciplines:

Provided that until members are elected under clause a) or clause b) in accordance with the provisions of this Act and the rules made thereunder, the Central Government shall nominate such number of members, being persons qualified to be chosen as such under the said clause (a) or clause (b), as the case may be, as that Government thinks fit; and references to be elected as including references to members so nominated.

2. The President and the Vice-President of the Central Council shall be elected by the members of the Central Council from amongst themselves in such manner as may be prescribed;

Provided that for two years from the first constitution of the Central Council, the President and the Vice-President shall be nominated by the Central Government from amongst the members of the Central Council and the President and the Vice-President so nominated shall, notwithstanding anything contained in sub-section (1) of section 7, hold office during the pleasure of the Central Government.

Mode of Election

4. 1. An election under clause (a) or clause (b) of sub-section (1) of section 3 shall be conducted by the Central Government in accordance with such rules as may be made by it in this behalf.

2. Where any dispute arises regarding any election to the Central Council, it shall be referred to the Central Government whose decision shall be final.

Restriction on Election and Membership

5. 1. No person shall be eligible for election to the Central Council unless he posses any of the medical qualifications included in the Second or the Third Schedule, is enrolled on any State Register of Homoeopathy and resides in the State concerned.

2. No person may at the same time serve as a member in more than one capacity.

Incorporation of Central Council

6. The Central Council shall be a body corporate by the name of the Central Council of Homoeopathy having perpetual succession and a common seal with power to acquire, hold and dispose of property, both movable and immovable, and to contract, and shall by the said name sue and be sued.

Term of Office of President, Vice-President and Members of Central Council

7. (a) The President, Vice-President or a member of the Central Council shall hold office for a term of five years from the date of his election or nomination, as the case may be, or until his successor shall have been duly elected or nominated, which-ever is longer.

(b) A person who hold or who has held office as President or Vice-President of the Central Council, shall be eligible for re-election to that office once, but only once.

(c) Members of the Central Council shall be eligible for re-election or re-nomination.

(d) An elected or nominated member shall be deemed to have vacated his seat if he is absent without excuse, sufficient in the opinion of the Central Council from three consecutive ordinary meetings of the Central Council or, in the case of a member elected under clause (a) of sub-section (1) of section 3, if he ceases to be enrolled on the concerned State Register of Homoeopathy, or in the case of a member elected under clause (b) of that sub-section, if he ceases to be a member of the Faculty or Department (by whatever name called) of Homoeopathy of the University concerned.

(e) A casual vacancy in the Central Council shall be filled by election or nomination, as the case may be, and the person elected or nominated to fill the vacancy shall hold office only for the remainder of the term for which the member whose place he takes was elected or nominated.

(f) Where the said term of five years is about to expire in respect of any member, a successor may be elected or nominated at any time within three months before the said term expires but he shall not assume office until the said term has expired.

Meetings of Central Council

8. (a) The Central Council shall meet at least once in each year at such time and place as may be appointed by the Central Council.

(b) Unless otherwise prescribed, one-third of the total number of members of the Central Council shall form a quorum, and all the acts of the Central Council shall be decided by a majority of the members presented and voting.

The Executive Committee and Other Committees

9. (a) The Central Council shall constitute from amongst its members an Executive Committee and such other committees for general or special purposes as the Council deems necessary to carry out the purposes of this Act.

(b) (i) The Executive Committee (hereinafter in this section referred to as the Committee) shall consist of the President and Vice-President who shall be members Ex-Officio, and not less than five and not more than seven members who shall be elected by the Central Council from amongst its members.

(ii) The President and the Vice-President shall be the President and Vice-President respectively of the Committee.

(iii) In addition to the powers and duties conferred and imposed upon it by this Act, the Committee shall exercise and discharge such powers and duties as the Central Council may confer or impose upon it by any regulations which may be made in this behalf.

Meetings of Committees

10. (a) The Committees constituted under section 9 shall meet at least twice in each year at such time and place as may be appointed by the Central Council.

(b) Unless otherwise prescribed, one-third of the total number of members of a committee shall be decided by a majority of the members present and voting.

Officers and Other Employees of Central Council

11. The Central Council shall

(a) appoint a Registrar who shall also act as Secretary;

(b) employ such other persons as it deems necessary to carry out the purpose of this Act;

(c) require and take from the Registrar or from any other employee, such security for the due performance of his duties as the Central Council deems necessary, and

(d) with the previous sanction of the Central Government, fix the remuneration and allowances to be paid to the President, Vice-President and members of the Central Council and to the members of the committees thereof and determine the conditions of service of the employees of the Central Council.

Vacancies in the Central Council and Committees thereof not to Invalidate acts, etc.

12. No act or proceeding of the Central Council or any committee thereof shall be called in question on the ground merely of the existence of any vacancy in, or any defect in the constitution of the Central Council or the committee, as the case may be.

CHAPTER IIA

Permission for Establishment of New Medical Institution, New Course of Study, etc.

12A. 1. Notwithstanding anything contained in this Act or any other law for the time being in force:

(a) no person shall establish a Homoeopathic Medical College, or

(b) no Homoeopathic Medical College shall

(i) open a new or higher course of study or training (including post-graduate course of study or training) which would enable students of each course or training to qualify himself for the award of any recognised medical qualification.

(ii) increase its admission capacity in any course of study or training (including the post-graduate course of study or training), except with previous permission of the Central Government obtained in accordance with the provisions of this section.

Explanation 1. For the purposes of this section, "person" includes any University or trust, but does not include the Central Government.

Explanation 2. For the purposes of this section, "admission capacity" in relation to any course of study or training (including post-graduate course of study or training) in a medical institution, means the maximum number of students as may be decided by the Central Council from time to time for being admitted to each course or training.

2.(a) Every person or medical institution shall, for the purpose of obtaining permission under sub-section (1) submit to the Central Government a scheme in accordance with the provisions of the clause (b) and the Central Government shall refer the scheme to the Central Council for its recommendations.

(b) the scheme referred to in clause (a) shall be in such form and contain such particulars and be preferred in such manner and be accompanied with such fee as may be prescribed.

3. On receipt of a scheme from the Central Government under sub-section (2), the Central Council may obtain such other particulars as may be considered necessary by it from the person or the medical institution concerned, and thereafter, it may:

(a) If the scheme is defective and does not contain any necessary particulars, give reasonable opportunity to the person or the medical institution concerned for making a written representation and it shall be open to such a person or medical institution to rectify the defects, if any, specified by the Central Council.

(b) Consider the scheme, having regard to the factors referred to in sub-section (7), and submit it to the Central Government together with its recommendations thereon within a period not exceeding six months from the date of receipt of the reference from the Central Government.

4. The Central Government may, after considering the scheme and the recommendations of the Central Council under sub-section (3) and after obtaining, where necessary, such other particulars as may be considered necessary by it from the person or medical institution concerned, and having regard to the factors referred to in sub-section (7), either approve (with such conditions, if any, as it may consider necessary) or disapprove the scheme and any such approval shall constitute as a permission under sub-section (1):

Provided that no scheme shall be disapproved by the Central Government except after giving the person or medical institution concerned a reasonable opportunity of being heard.

Provided further that nothing in this sub-section shall prevent any person or medical institution whose scheme has not been approved by the Central Government to submit a fresh scheme and the provisions of this section shall apply to such scheme, as if such scheme had been submitted for the first time under sub-section (2).

5. Where, within a period of one year from the date of submission of the scheme to the Central Government under the sub-section (2), no order is communicated by the Central Government to the person or the medical institution submitting the scheme, such scheme shall be deemed to have been approved by the Central Government in the form in which it was submitted, and, accordingly, the permission of the Central Government required under the sub-section (1) shall also be deemed to have been granted.

6. In computing the time-limit specified in sub-section (5), the time taken by the person or medical institution concerned in submitting the scheme, in furnishing any particulars called for by the Central Council, or by the Central Government shall be excluded.

7. The Central Council, while making its recommendations under clause (b) sub-section (3) and the Central Government, while passing an order, either approving or disapproving the scheme under sub-section (4), shall have due regard to the following factors, namely:

(a) whether the proposed medical institution or the seeking to open a new or higher course of study or training, would be in a position to offer the minimum standards of medical education as prescribed by the Central Council under Section 20;

(b) whether the person seeking to establish a medical institution or the existing medical institution seeking to open a new or higher course of study or training or to increase its admission capacity has adequate financial resources;

(c) whether necessary facilities in respect of staff, equipment, accommodation, training, hospital and other facilities to ensure proper functioning of the medical institution or conducting the new course of study or training or accomodating the increased admission capacity have been provided or would be provided within the time-limit specified in the scheme;

(d) whether adequate hospital facilities, having regard to the number of students likely to attend such medical institution or course of study or training or as a result of the increased admission capacity, have been provided or would be provided within the time-limit specified in the scheme;

(e) whether any arrangement has been made or programme drawn to impart proper training to students likely to attend such medical institution or the course of study or training by the persons having the recognised medical qualifications;

(f) the requirement of manpower in the field of practice of homoeopathic medicine in the medical institution; and

(g) any other factors as may be prescribed.

8. Where the Central Government passes an order either approving or disapproving a scheme under this section, a copy of the order shall be communicated to the person or medical institution concerned.

Non-recognition of Medical Qualifications in Certain Cases

12B.1. Where any medical institution is established without the previous permission of the Central Government in accordance with the provisions of Section 12A, medical qualification granted to any student of such medical institution shall not be deemed to be recognised medical qualification for the purposes of this Act.

2. Where any medical institution opens a new or higher course of study or training (including a post-graduate course of study or training) without the previous permission of the Central Government in accordance with the provisions of Section 12A, medical qualification granted to any student of such institution on the basis of such study or training shall not be deemed to be recognised medical qualification for the purposes of this Act.

3. Where any medical institution increases its admission capacity in any course of study or training without the previous permission of the Central Government in accordance with the provisions of Section 12A, medical qualification granted to any student of such medical institution on the basis of increase in its admission capacity shall not be deemed to be recognised medical qualification for the purposes of this Act.

CHAPTER III (RECOGNITION OF MEDICAL QUALIFICATIONS)

Recognition of Medical Qualifications granted by Certain Medical Institutions in India

13. 1. The medical qualifications granted by any University, Board or other medical institution in India which are included in the Second Schedule shall be recognised medical qualifications for the purposes of this Act.

2. Any University, Board or other medical institution in India which grants a medical qualification not included in the Second Schedule may apply to the Central Government to have any such qualification recognised, and the Central Government, after consulting the Central Council, may, by notification in the Official Gazette, amend the Second Schedule so as to include such qualification therein and any such notification may also direct that an entry shall be made in the last column of the Second Schedule against such medical qualification only when granted after a specified date.

Recognition of Medical Qualifications granted by Medical Institutions in States or Countries outside India

14. 1. The medical qualifications granted by medical institutions outside India which are included in the Third Schedule shall be recognised medical qualifications for the purposes of this Act.

2.(a) The Central Council may enter into negotiations with the authority in any Sate or country outside India, which by the law of such State or country is entrusted with the maintenance of a Register of practitioners of Homoeopathy for setting of a scheme of reciprocity for the recognition of medical qualifications in Homoeopathy and in pursuance of any such scheme, the Central Government may, by notification in the Official Gazette, amend the Third Schedule so as to include therein any medical qualification which the Central Council has decided should be recognised medical qualification only when granted after a specified date.

(b) Where the Council has refused to recommend any medical qualification which has been proposed for recognition by any authority referred to in clause (a) and that authority applies to the Central Government in this behalf, the Central Government, after considering such application and after obtaining from the Council a report, if any, as to the reasons for any such refusal, may, by notification in the Official Gazette declare that such qualification shall be a recognised medical qualification and the provisions of clause (a) shall apply accordingly.

Rights of Persons Possessing Qualifications included in Second or The Third Schedule to the Enrolled

15. 1. Subject to the other provisions contained in this Act, any medical qualification included in the Second or the Third Schedule shall be sufficient qualification for enrolment on any State Register of Homoeopathy.

2. No person, other than a practitioner of Homoeopathy who possess a recognised medical qualification and is enrolled on a State Register or the Central Register of Homoeopathy.

(a) shall hold office as Homoeopathic physician or any other office (by whatever designation called) in Government or in any institution maintained by a local or other authority;

(b) shall practise Homoeopathy in any State;

(c) shall be entitled to sign or authenticate a medial or fitness certificate or any other certificate required by an law to be signed or authenticated by a duly qualified medical practitioner.

3. Nothing contained in sub-section (2) shall affect:

(a) the right of a practitioner of Homoeopathy enrolled on a State Register of Homoeopathy to practise Homoeopathy in any State merely on the ground that, one the commencement of this Act, he does not possess a recognised medical qualification;

(b) the privileges (including the right to practise Homoeopathy) conferred by or under any law relating to registration of practitioners of Homoeopathy for the time being in force in any State, on a Practitioner of Homoeopathy enrolled on a State Register of Homoeopathy;

(c) the right of a person to practise Homoeopathy in a State in which, on the commencement of this Act, a State Register of Homoeopathy is not maintained if, on such commencement, he has been practising Homoeopathy for not less than five years.

(d) Nothing contained in sub-section (2) shall affect:

4. Any person who acts in contravention of any provision of sub-section (2) shall be punished with imprisonment for a term which may extend to one year, or with fine which may extend to one thousand rupees or with both.

Power to Require Information as to Courses to Study and Examination

16. Every University, Board of medical institution in India which grants a recognised medical qualification shall furnish such information as the Central Council may, from time to time, require as to the courses of study and examination to be undergone in order to obtain such qualifications, as to the ages at which such courses of study and examinations are required to be undergone and such qualification is conferred and generally as to the requisite for obtaining such qualification.

Inspectors at Examinations

17. 1. The Central Council shall appoint such number of medical inspectors as it may deem requisite to inspect any medical college, hospital or other institution where education in Homoeopathy is given, or to attend any examination held by any University, Board or medical institution for the purpose of recommending to the Central Government recognition of medical qualifications granted by that University, Board of medical institution.

2. The medical inspectors shall not interfere with the conduct of any training or examination but shall report to the President of the Central Council on the adequacy of the standards of education including staff, equipment, accommodation, training and other facilities prescribed for giving education in Homoeopathy, as the case may be, on the sufficiency of every examination which they attend.

3. The Central Council shall forward a copy of any such report to the University, Board or medical institution concerned, and shall also forward a copy with the remarks of the

University or medical institution thereon, to the Central Government.

Visitors at Examinations

18. 1. The Central Council may appoint such number of visitors as it may deem requisite to inspect any medical college, hospital or other institution where education in Homoeopathy is given or to attend any examination for the purpose of granting recognised medical qualification.

2. Any person, whether he is a member of the Central Council or not may be appointed as a visitor under this section but a person who is appointed as an inspector under Section 17 for any inspection or examination shall not be appointed as a visitor for the same inspection or examination.

3. The visitors shall not interfere with the conduct of any training or examination but shall report to the President of the Central Council on the adequacy of the standards of education including staff, equipment, accommodation, training and other facilities prescribed for giving education in Homoeopathy or on the sufficiency of every examination which they attend.

4. The report of a visitor shall be treated as confidential unless in any particular case the President of the Central Council otherwise directs:

Provided that if the Central Government requires a copy of the report of a visitor, the Central Council shall furnish the same.

Withdrawal or Recognition

19. 1. When upon report by the inspector or the visitor it appears to the Central Council

(a) that the courses of study and examination to be undergone in or the proficiency required from candidates at any examination held by any University, Board or medical institution, or

(b) that the staff, equipment, accommodation, training and other facilities for instruction and training provided in such University, Board of medical institution or in any college or other institution affiliated to the University

do not conform to the standard prescribed by the Central Council, the Central Council shall make a representation to that effect to the Central Government.

2. After considering such representation, the Central Government may send it to the Government of the State in which the University, Board or medical institution is situated and the State Government shall forward it alongwith such remarks as it may choose to make to the University, Board or medical institution with an intimation of the period within which the University, Board or medical institution may submit its explanation to the State Government.

3. On the receipt of the explanation or where no explanation is submitted within the period fixed, then on the expiry of that period the State Government shall make its recommendations to the Central Government.

4. The Central Government after making such further inquiry, if any, as it may think fit, may, by notification in the Official Gazette, direct that an entry shall be made in the Second Schedule against the said medical qualification declaring that it shall be a recognised medical qualification only when granted before a specified date or that the said medical qualification if granted to students of a specified college or institution affiliated to any University shall be recognised medical qualification only when granted before a specified date or, as the case may be, that the said medical qualification shall be recognised medical qualification in relation to a specified college or institution affiliated to any University only when granted after a specified date.

Minimum standard of Education in Homoeopathy

20. 1. The Central Council may prescribe the minimum standards of education in Homoeopathy required for granting recognised medical qualifications by Universities, Board or medical institutions in India.

2. Copies of the draft regulations and of all subsequent amendments thereof shall be furnished by the Central Council to all State

Governments and the Central Council shall, before submitting the regulations or any amendment thereof as the case may be, to the consideration the comments of any State Government received within three months from the furnishing of the copies as aforesaid.

CHAPTER IV (THE CENTRAL REGISTER OF HOMOEOPATHY)

The Central Register or Homoeopathy

21. 1. The Central Council shall cause to be maintained in the prescribed manner a register of practitioners of Homoeopathy to be known as the Central Register of Homoeopathy which shall contain.

(a) in Part I, the names of all persons who are for the time being enrolled on any State Register of Homoeopathy and possess any of the recognised medical qualifications.

(b) in Part II, the names of all persons, other than those included in part I, who are for the time being enrolled on any State Register of Homoeopathy.

2. It shall be the duty of the Registrar of the Central Council to keep and maintain the Central Register of Homoeopathy accordance with provisions of this Act and of any orders made by the Central Council and from time to time to revise the register and publish it in the Gazette of India and in such other manner as may be prescribed.

3. Such register shall be deemed to be a public document within the meaning of the Indian Evidence Act, 1872 and may be proved by a copy published in the Gazette of India.

Supply of Copies of State Register of Homoeopathy

22. Each Board shall supply to the Central Council three printed copies of the State Register of Homoeopathy as soon as may be after the commencement of this Act and subsequently after the first day of April of each year and each Board shall inform the Central Council without delay of all additions to, and other amendments in the State Register of Homoeopathy made from time to time.

Registration in the Central Registrar of Homoeopathy

23. The Registrar of the Central Council may on receipt of the report of registration of a person in a State Register of Homoeopathy or on application made in the prescribed manner by any person, enter his name in the Central Register of Homoeopathy provided that the Registrar is satisfied that the person concerned is eligible under this Act for such registration.

Professional Conduct

24. 1. The Central Council may prescribe standards of professional conduct and etiquette and a code of ethics for practitioners of Homoeopathy.

2. Regulation made by the Central Council under sub-section (1) may specify which violations thereof shall constitute infamous conduct in any professional respect, that is to say, professional misconduct and such provision shall have effect notwithstanding anything contained in any law for the time being in force.

Removal of Names from The Central Register of Homoeopathy

25. 1. If the name of any person enrolled on a State Register of Homoeopathy is removed therefrom in pursuance of any power conferred by or under any law relating to registration of practitioners of Homoeopathy for the time being in force in any State, the Central Council shall direct the removal of the name of such person from the Central Register of Homoeopathy.

2. Where the name of any person has been removed from State Register of Homoeopathy on any ground other than that he is not possessed of the requisite medical qualifications or where any application by the said person for restoration of his name to the State Register of Homoeopathy has been rejected, he may appeal in the prescribed manner and subject to such conditions, including conditions as to the payment of a fee, as may be prescribed to the Central Government whose decision, which shall be given be binding on the State Government and on the authorities concerned

with the preparation of the State Register of Homoeopathy.

Provisional Registration for Practice

25A. If the courses of study to be undergone for obtaining a recognised medical qualification in homoeopathy include a period has passed the qualifying examination and before such qualification is conferred on him, any such person shall, on application made by him in this behalf, be granted provisional registration in a State Register of Homoeopathy by the Board concerned in order to enable him to practice homoeopathy in an approved institution for the purpose of such training and for no other purpose for the period aforesaid.

Privileges of Persons who are Enrolled on The Central Register of Homoeopathy

26. 1. Subject to the conditions and restrictions laid down in this Act regarding practice of Homoeopathy by persons possessing certain recognised medical qualifications, every person whose name is for the time being borne on Part I of the Central Register of Homoeopathy shall be entitled according to his qualifications to practice Homoeopathy in any part of India and to recover in due course of law, charges in respect of such practice any expenses, charges in respect of medicaments of other appliances or any fees to which he may be entitled.

2. Subject to the provisions of sub-section (3) of Section 15, any person whose name is for the time being borne on Part II of the Central Register of Homoeopathy, may practise Homoeopathy in any State, other than the State where he is enrolled on the State Register of Homoeopathy with the previous approval of the Government of the State where he intendeds to practise.

Registration of Additional Qualifications

27. 1. If any person whose name is entered in the Central Register of Homoeopathy obtains any title, diploma or other qualification for proficiency in Homoeopathy, which is a recognised medical qualification, he shall, on application made in this behalf in the prescribed manner, be entitled to have an entry stating such other title, diploma or other qualification made against his name in the Central Register of Homoeopathy either in substitution for or in addition to any entry previously made.

2. The entries in respect of any such person in a State Register of Homoeopathy shall be altered in accordance with the alterations made in the Central Register of Homoeopathy.

Persons enrolled on Central Register of Homoeopathy to Notify change of Place of Residence on Practice

28. Every person registered in the Central Register of Homoeopathy shall notify any transfer of the place of his residence or practice to the Central Council and to the Board concerned within ninety days of such transfer, failing which his right to participate in the election of members to the Central Council or a Board shall be liable to be forfeited by order of the Central Government either permanently or for such period as may be specified therein.

CHAPTER V (MISCELLANEOUS)

Information to be furnished by Central Council and Publications Thereof

29. 1. The Central Council shall furnish such reports, copies of its minutes, abstracts of its accounts, and other information to the Central Government as that Government may require.

2. The Central Government may publish in such manner as it may think fit, any report, copy, abstract or other information furnished to it under this section or under Section 18.

Commission of Inquiry

30. 1. Whenever it is made to appear to the Central Government that the Central Council is not complying with any of the provisions of this Act, the Central Government may refer the particulars of the complaint to a commission shall proceed to inquire in a summary manner and to report to the Central Government as to the truth of the matter charged in the complaint and in case may charge of default or of improper action being found by the commission to have been established, the commission shall recommend the remedies if any, which are in the opinion necessary.

2. The Central Government may require the Central Council to adopt the remedies so recommended within such time as having regard to the report of the commission, it may think fit and if the Central Council fails to comply with any such requirement, the Central Government may amend the regulations of the Central Council or make such provision or order or take such other steps as may seem necessary to give effect to the recommendations of the commission.

3. A commission of inquiry shall have power to administer oath, to enforce the attendance of witnesses and the production of documents and shall have all such other necessary powers for the purpose of any inquiry conducted by it as are exercised by a civil court under the code of Civil Procedure, 1908 (5 of 1908).

Protection of Action taken in Good Faith

31. No suit, prosecution or other legal proceeding shall lie against the Government, the Central Council or a Board or any committee thereof or any officer or servant of the Government or the Central Council or the Board or the committee aforesaid for anything which is in good faith done or intended to be done under this Act.

Power to make Rules

32. 1. The Central Government may, by notification in the Official Gazette, make rules to carry out the purpose of this Act.

2. Every rule made under this section shall be laid, as soon as may be after it is made, before each House of Parliament, while it is in session for a total period of thirty days which may be comprised in one session or in two or more successive sessions, and if, before the expiry of the session immediately following the session or the successive sessions aforesaid, both Houses agree in making any modification in the rule or both Houses agree that the rule should not be made, the rule shall thereafter have effect only in such modified form or be of no effect, as the case may be; so however, that any such modification or annulment shall be without prejudice to the validity of anything previously done under that rule.

Power to make Regulations

33. 1. The Central Council may, with the previous sanction of the Central Government, make, by notification in the Official Gazette, regulations generally to carry out the purposes of this Act, and, without prejudice to the generality of this power, such regulations may provide for

(a) The manner of election of the President and the Vice-President of the Central Council;

(b) The management of the property of the Central Council and the maintenance and audit of its accounts;

(c) The resignation of members of the Central Council;

(d) The powers and duties of the President and Vice-President;

(e) The summoning and holding of meetings of the Central Council and the committees thereof, the times and places where such meetings are to be held, and the conduct of business thereat and the number of members necessary to constitute a quorum.

(f) The functions of the committees constituted under Section 9;

(g) The tenure of office, and the powers and duties of, the Registrar and other officers and servants of the Central Council;

(i) The form of the scheme, the particulars to be given in such scheme, the manner in which the scheme is to be preferred and the fee payable with the scheme under clause (b) of sub-section (2) of Section 12A;

(ii) Any other factor under clause (g) of sub-section (7) of Section 12A;

(h) The qualifications, appointment, powers and duties of, and procedure to be followed by, inspectors and visitors;

(i) The courses and period of study of practical training to be undertaken, the subjects of examination and the standards of proficiency therein to be obtained, in any University, Board or medical institution for grant of recognised medical qualification.

(j) The standards of staff, equipment, accommodation, training and other facilities for education in Homoeopathy.

(k) The conduct of professional examinations, qualifications of examinees and the conditions of admission to such examinations;

(l) The standards of professional conduct and etiquette and code of the ethics to be observed by practitioners of Homoeopathy;

(m) The particulars to be stated, and the proof of qualifications to be given in applications for registration under this Act;

(n) The manner in which and the conditions subject to which an appeal under Section 25 may be preferred;

(o) The fees to be paid on applications and appeals under this Act; and

(p) Any matter for which under this Act provision may be made by regulations.

2. The Central Government shall cause every regulation made under this Act to be laid, as soon as may be after it is made, before each House of Parliament, while it is made, before each House of Parliament, while it is in session for a total period of thirty days which may be comprised in one session, and if, before the expiry of the session immediately following the session or the successive sessions aforesaid, both Houses agree in making any modification in the regulation or both Houses agree that the regulation should not be made, the regulation shall thereafter have effect only in such modified form or be of no effect, as the case may be; so, however that any such modification or annulment shall be without prejudice to the validity of anything previously done under that regulation.

Chapter 38

Homoeopathic Practitioners' Professional Conduct, Etiquette and Code of Ethics

Regulations

In exercise of the powers conferred by clause (l) of section 33 read with section 24 of the Homoeopathy Central Council Act, 1973 (59 of 1973), the Central Council of Homoeopathy, with the previous sanction of the Central Government, hereby makes the following regulations, namely:

1. These regulations may be called the Homoeopathic Practitioners (Professional Conduct, Etiquette and Code of Ethics) Regulations, 1982:

I. Declaration and Oath
II. General Principles
III. Duties of Homoeopathic Practitioners to Their Patients
IV. Duties of Practitioners to The Profession
V. Duties of Practitioners In Consultation
VI. Duties of Practitioners to The Public
VII. Professional Misconduct

Declaration and Oath

2. (a) At the time of registration, each applicant shall submit the following declaration and oath read and signed by him to the Registrar concerned attested by the Registrar himself or by a registered practitioner of Homoeopathy:

(i) I solemnly pledge myself to consecrate my life to the service of humanity.

(ii) Even under threat, I will not use my medical knowledge contrary to the laws of humanity.

(iii) I will maintain the utmost respect for human life.

(iv) I will not permit considerations of religion, nationality, race, political beliefs or social standing to intervene between my duty and my patient.

(v) I will practise my profession with conscience and dignity in accordance with the principles of Homoeopathy and/or in accordance with the principles of biochemic system of medicine (tissue remedies).

(vi) The health of my patient shall be my first consideration.

(vii) I will respect the secrets which are confided to me.

(viii) I will give to my teachers the respect and gratitude which is their due.

(ix) I will maintain by all means in my power the honour and noble traditions of medical profession.

(x) My colleagues will be my brothers and sisters.

(xi) I make these promises solemnly, freely and upon my honour.

(b) Hahnemannian Oath: "On my honour I swear that I shall practise the teachings of Homoeopathy, perform my duty, render justice to my patients and help the sick whosoever comes to me for treatment. May the teachings of master Hahnemann inspire me and may I have the strength for fulfillment of my mission."

General Principles

3. **Character of Medical Practitioner:** The primary object of the medical profession is to render service to humanity with full respect for the dignity of man; financial reward is a subordinate consideration. Whosoever chooses this profession assumes the obligation to conduct himself in accordance with its ideals. A practitioner of Homoeopathy shall be an upright man, instructed in the art of healing. He shall keep himself pure in character and be diligent in caring for the sick. He shall be modest, sober, patient and prompt and do his duty without anxiety, and shall be pious and conduct himself with propriety in his profession and in all the actions of his life.

4. **Standards of Character and Morals:** The medical profession expects from its members the highest level of character and morals, and every practitioner of Homoeopathy owes to the profession and to the public alike a duty to attain such a level. It shall be incumbent on a practitioner of Homoeopathy to be temperate in all matters, for the practice of medicine requires unremitting exercise of a clear and vigorous mind.

5. **Practitioner's Responsibility:** A practitioner of Homoeopathy shall merit the confidence of patients entrusted to his care, rendering to each full measure of service and devotion. The honoured ideals of the medical profession imply that the responsibilities of a practitioner of Homoeopathy extend not only to individuals but also to the entire society.

6. **Advertising**

(a) Solicitation of patients directly or indirectly by a practitioner of Homoeopathy either personally or by advertisement in the news papers, by placards or by the distribution of circular cards or handbills is unethical. A practitioner of Homoeopathy shall not make use of, or permit others to make use of, him or his name as a subject of any form or manner of advertising or publicity through lay channels which shall be of such a character as to invite attention to him or to his professional position or skill or as would ordinarily result in his self-aggrandisement provided that a practitioner of Homoeopathy is permitted formal announcement in press about the following matters, namely:

(i) The starting of his practice;

(ii) Change of the type of practice;

(iii) Change of address;

(iv) Temporary absence from duty;

(v) Resumption of practice;

(vi) Succeeding to another's practice.

(b) He shall further not advertise himself directly or indirectly through price lists or publicity materials of manufacturing firms or traders with whom he may be connected in any capacity, nor shall he publish cases, operations or letters of thanks from patients in non-professional newspapers or journals provided it shall be permissible for him to publish his name in connection with a prospectus or a director's or a technical expert's report.

7. **Payment of Professional Service**

(a) A practitioner of Homoeopathy engaged in the practice of medicine shall limit the sources of his income to fees received from professional activities for services rendered to the patient. Remuneration received for such services shall be in the form and amount specifically announced to the patient at the time the service is rendered; in all other cases he shall deem it a point of honour to adhere to the compensation for professional services prevailing in the community in which he practices.

(b) Fees are reducible at the discretion of the practitioner of Homoeopathy and he shall always recognise poverty as presenting valid claims for gratuitous services.

(c) It shall be unethical to enter into a contract of "no cure no payment".

8. **Rebates and Commission:** A practitioner of Homoeopathy shall not give, solicit or receive, nor shall he offer to give, solicit or receive, any gift, gratuity, commission or bonus in consideration for the referring, recommending or procuring of any patient for medical, surgical or other treatment nor shall he receive any commission or other benefit from a professional colleague, trader of appliances, dentist or an occulist.

Duties of Homoeopathic Practitioners to their Patients

9. **Obligations to the Sick:** Though a practitioner of Homoeopathy is not bound to treat each and every one asking for his services except in emergencies, he shall, for the sake of humanity and the noble traditions of the profession, not only be ever ready to respond to the calls of the sick and the injured, but shall be mindful of the high character of his mission and the responsibility he incurs in the discharge of his professional duties.

10. **Practitioner's Responsibility**

(a) A practitioner of Homoeopathy is free to choose whom he will serve provided be shall respond to any request for his assistance in an emergency or whenever temperate public opinion expects the service.

(b) Once having undertaken a case, a practitioner of Homoeopathy shall not neglect the patient nor shall he withdraw from the case without giving notice to the patient, his relatives or his responsible friends sufficiently long in advance of his withdrawal to allow them time to secure another practitioner.

11. **Termination of Service**

(a) The following shall be valid reasons for his withdrawal:

(i) where he finds another practitioner in attendance;

(ii) where remedies other than those prescribed by him are being used;

(iii) where his remedies and instructions are refused;

(iv) where he is convinced that illness is an imposture and that he is being made a party to a false pretence;

(v) where the patient persists in the use of opium, alcohol, chloral or similar intoxicating drugs against medical advice;

(vi) where complete information concerning the facts and circumstances of the case are not supplied by the patient or his relatives.

(b) The discovery that the disease is incurable is no excuse to discontinue attendance so long as the patient desired his services.

12. **Acts of Negligence**

(a) No practitioner of Homoeopathy shall willfully commit an act of negligence that may deprive his patient of necessary medical care.

(b) A practitioner of Homoeopathy is expected to render that diligence and skill in services as would be expected of another practitioner of Homoeopathy with similar qualifications, experience and attainments.

(c) His acts of commission or omission shall not be judged by any non-homoeopathic standards of professional service expected of him but by those standards as are expected from a Homoeopath of his training, standing and experience.

(d) A practitioner of Homoeopathy shall use any drug prepared according to Homoeopathic principles and adopt other necessary measures as required.

13. Behaviour towards Patients: The demeanour of a practitioner of Homoeopathy towards his patients shall always be courteous, sympathetic, friendly and helpful. Every patient shall be treated with attention and consideration.

14. Visits: A practitioner of Homoeopathy shall endeavour to add to the comfort of the sick by making his visits at the hour indicated to the patients.

15. Prognosis

(a) The practitioner of Homoeopathy shall neither exaggerate nor minimise the gravity of a patient's condition. He shall ensure that the patient, his relatives or responsible friends have such knowledge of the patient's condition as will serve the best interest of the patient and his family.

(b) In cases of dangerous manifestations, he shall not fail to give timely notice to the family or friends of the patient and also to the patient when necessary.

16. Patience, Delicacy and Secrecy: Patience and delicacy shall characterise the attitude of a practitioner of Homoeopathy. Confidences concerning individual or domestic life entrusted by patients to a practitioner and defects in the disposition or character of patients observed during the medical attendance shall not be revealed by him to anyone unless their revelation is required by the laws of the State.

Duties of Practitioners to the Profession

17. Upholding honour of Profession: A practitioner of Homoeopathy shall, at all times, uphold the dignity and honour of this profession.

18. Membership of Medical Society: For the advancement of his profession a practitioner of Homoeopathy may affiliate himself with Medical Societies and contribute his time, energy and means to their progress so that they may better represent and promote the ideals of the profession.

19. Exposure of Unethical Conduct: A practitioner of Homoeopathy shall expose, without fear or favour, the incompetent, corrupt, dishonest or unethical conduct on the part of any member of the profession.

20. Association with Unregistered Persons: A practitioner of Homoeopathy shall not associate himself professionally with any body or society of unregistered practitioners of Homoeopathy.

21. Appointment of Substitutes: Whenever a practitioner of Homoeopathy requests another to attend to his patients during his temporary absence from practice, professional courtesy requires the acceptance of such appointment by the latter, if it is consistent with his other duties. The practitioner of Homoeopathy acting under such an appointment shall give the utmost consideration to the interests and reputation of the absent practitioner. He shall not charge either the patient or the absent practitioner of Homoeopathy for his services, except in the case of a special arrangement between them. All such patients shall be restored to the care of the absent practitioner of Homoeopathy upon his return.

22. Charges for service to Practitioners of Homoeopathy

(a) There is no rule that a practitioner of Homoeopathy shall not charge another practitioner of Homoeopathy for his services, but a practitioner of Homoeopathy shall consider it a pleasure and privilege to render gratuitous service to his professional brother and his dependents, if they are in his vicinity or to a medical student.

(b) There is no rule that a practitioner of Homoeopathy shall not charge another practitioner of Homoeopathy for his services, but a practitioner of Homoeopathy shall consider it a pleasure and privilege to render gratuitous service to his professional brother and his dependents, if they are in his vicinity or to a medical student.

23. (a) The practitioner of Homoeopathy called in an emergency to visit a patient under the care of another practitioner of Homoeopathy shall, when the emergency is over, retire in favour of the latter; but he shall be entitled to charge the patient for his services.

(b) When a practitioner of Homoeopathy is consulted at his own residence, it is not necessary for him to enquire of the patient if he is under the care of another practitioner of Homoeopathy.

(c) When a consulting practitioner of Homoeopathy sees a patient at the request of another practitioner of Homoeopathy, it shall be his duty to write a letter stating his opinion of the case with the mode of treatment he thinks is required to be adopted.

24. **Engagement for an Obstetrics Case**

(a) If a practitioner of Homoeopathy is engaged to attend to a woman during her confinement, he shall do so. Refusal to do so on an excuse of any other engagement shall not be considered ethical except when he is already engaged on a similar or other serious case.

(b) When a practitioner of Homoeopathy who has been engaged to attend on an obstetrics case is absent and another is sent for and delivery is accomplished, the acting practitioner of Homoeopathy shall be entitled to his professional fees; provided he shall secure the patient's consent to withdraw on the arrival of the practitioner of Homoeopathy already engaged.

25. When it becomes the duty of a practitioner of Homoeopathy occupying an official position to see and report upon an illness or injury, he shall communicate to the practitioner of Homoeopathy in attendance so as to give him an option of being present. The medical officer shall avoid remarks upon the diagnosis or the treatment that has been adopted.

Duties of Practitioners in Consultation

26. **Consultation shall be Encouraged:** In cases of serious illness, especially in doubtful or difficult conditions the practitioner of Homoeopathy shall request consultation. He shall also do so in perplexing illness, in therapeutic abortions, in the treatment of a woman who had procured criminal abortion, in suspected cases of poisoning, or when desired by the patient or his representative.

27. **Punctuality in Consultation:** Utmost punctuality shall be observed by a practitioner of Homoeopathy in meeting for consultation. If the consultant practitioner of Homoeopathy does not arrive within a reasonable time such as a quarter of an hour after the appointed time, the first practitioner of Homoeopathy shall be at liberty to see the patient alone provided he shall leave his conclusion in writing in a closed envelope.

28. **Patient referred to another Physician:** When a patient is referred to another practitioner of Homoeopathy by the attending practitioner of Homoeopathy, a statement of the case shall be given to the latter practitioner of Homoeopathy. The latter practitioner of Homoeopathy shall communicate his opinion in writing in a closed cover direct to the attending practitioner of Homoeopathy.

29. **Consultation for Patient's Benefit:** In every consultation, the benefit to the patient shall be of first importance. All practitioners of Homoeopathy interested in the case shall be candid with a member of the patient's family or responsible friends.

30. **Conduct in Consultation**

(a) In consultations, there shall be no place for insincerity, rivalry or envy. All due respect shall be shown to the practitioner of Homoeopathy in charge of case and no statement or remarks shall be made which would impair the confidence reposed in him by the patient. For this purpose, no discussion shall be carried on in the presence of the patient or his representatives.

(b) All statements of the case to the patient or his representatives shall take place in the presence of all the practitioners consulting, except as otherwise agreed; the announcement of the opinion to the patient or his relations or friends shall rest with the attending practitioner of Homoeopathy.

(c) Differences of opinion shall not be divulged unnecessarily; provided when there is an irreconcilable difference of opinion, the circumstances shall be frankly and impartially explained to the patient or his friends.

(d) It shall be open to them to seek further advice if they so desire.

31. **Cessation of Consultation:** Attendance of the consulting practitioner of Homoeopathy shall cease when the consultation is concluded, unless another appointment is arranged by the attending practitioner of Homoeopathy.

32. **Treatment after Consultation**

(a) No decision shall restrain the attending practitioner of Homoeopathy from making such subsequent variations in the treatment as any unexpected change may require; provided at the next consultation, reasons for variation are stated.

(b) The same privilege, with its obligations, belongs to the consultant when sent for in an emergency during the absence of the attending practitioner of Homoeopathy. The attending practitioner of Homoeopathy may prescribe at any time for the patient, but the consultant, only in case of emergency.

33. **Consultant not to take Charge of the Case**

(a) When a practitioner of Homoeopathy has been called as a Consultant then none but the rarest and most exceptional circumstances shall justify the consultant taking charge of the case.

(b) He must not do so merely on the solicitation of the patient or his friends.

34. **Bar against Consulting Non-registered Practitioner:** No practitioner of Homeopathy shall have consultation with any practitioner of Homoeopathy who is not registered.

Duties of Practitioners to The Public

35. **Practitioners as Citizens:** Practitioners of Homoeopathy, as good citizens, possessed of special training, shall advise concerning the health of the community wherein they dwell. They shall play their part in enforcing the laws of the community and in sustaining the institutions that advance the interest of humanity. They shall cooperate with the authorities in the observance and enforcement of sanitary laws and regulations and shall observe the provisions of all laws relating to Drugs, Poisons and Pharmacy made for the protection and promotion of public health.

36. **Public Health:** Practitioners of Homoeopathy engaged in public health work, shall enlighten the public concerning quarantine regulations and measures for the prevention of epidemic and communicable diseases. At all times the practitioners shall notify the constituted public health authorities of every case of communicable disease under their care, in accordance with the laws, rules and regulations of the health authorities. When an epidemic prevails, the practitioner of Homoeopathy shall conti-nue his labours without regard to the risk to his own health.

37. **Dispensing:** A practitioner of Homoeopathy has a right to prepare and dispense his own prescription.

Professional Misconduct

38. The following actions shall constitute professional misconduct:

(a) Committing adultery or improper conduct with a patient, or maintaining an improper association with a patient;

(b) Conviction by a Court of Law for offences involving moral turpitude;

(c) Signing of or giving by any practitioner of Homoeopathy under his name and authority any certificate, report or document of kindred character which is untrue, misleading or improper;

(d) Contravention of the provisions of laws relating to Drugs and regulations made thereunder;

(e) Selling a drug or poison regulated by law to the public or his patients save as provided by that law.

(f) Performing or enabling an unqualified person to perform an abortion or any illegal operation for which there is no medical, surgical or psychological indication;

(g) Issue of certificates in Homoeopathy to unqualified or non-medical persons provided that this shall not apply so as to restrict the proper training and instruction of legitimate employees of doctors, midwives, dispensers, surgical attendants or skilled mechanical and technical assistants under the personal supervision of practitioners of Homoeopathy.

(h) Affixing a signboard on a chemist's shop or in places where the practitioner of Homoeopathy does not reside or work;

(i) Disclosing the secrets of a patient that have been learnt in the exercise of profession, except in a Court of Law under orders of the presiding judge.

(j) Publishing photographs or case-reports of patients in any medical or other journal in a manner by which their identity could be made out without their permission, provided that if the identity of patients is not disclosed, their consent is not necessary;

(k) Public exhibition of the scale of fees provided that the same may be displayed in the physician's consulting or waiting room;

(l) Using of touts or agents for procuring patients;

(m) Claiming to be a specialist without having put on substantial number of years of study and experience in the subject concerned or without possessing a special qualification in the branch concerned.

Chapter 39

Recent Advances in Homoeopathic Pharmacy

1. New Addition of Drug Source

In homoeopathic pharmacy, two new source are included such as Allersodes and Isodes:

(a) **Allersodes:** Homoeopathic preparations of antigens, (substances which, under suitable conditions, can induce the formation of antibodies). Antigens include toxins, ferments, precipitinogens, agglutinogens, opsonogens, lysogens, venins, agglutinins, complements, opsonins, amboceptors, precipitins and most native proteins.

(b) **Isodes:** These are homoeopathic medicines prepared from plant, animal or chemical substances, including drugs, excipients or binders, which have been ingested or otherwise absorbed by the body and are believed to have produced a disease or disorder which interferes with homeostasis. Those may be called detoxodes. These also contains the preparations made from commonly used allopathic medicines. Those are prepared as per HPI. Those are prepared generally at physician/prescriber level. Generally isodes are not used below 6x potency. Awareness of side-effects of these drugs and their lower attenuations up to 3x is essential.

Examples: Acacia, Eucalyptus oil, Gelatin, Indigo carmine, Frusemide, Gentamycin, Ibuprofen, Isoniazid.

2. Advances in Pharmaceutics

Pharmaceutics is the subject that deals with the technology of preparation of medicines:

(a) **Pharmaceutical Dosage Forms:** There are certain changes in the preparation of tablets as well as in external applications such as ointments.

(i) **Tablets**—*Traditional uses:* Conventional compressed tablets. These are standard uncoated tablets made by either wet or dry granulation technique. Starch, talc, magnesium stearate etc. used as diluents and binders.

Current trends: Lozenges, tincture tablets. Fluid bed spray granulation techniques are used for their preparation. The purpose of spray granulation is to generate particles with a defined structure, shape, size and composition according to specification. Compared with other granulation process, spray granulation has major advantages to offer in terms of the quality of the final product. Typical final product characteristics are: (i) almost spherical shape, (ii) dust free, (iii) high bulk density, (iv) good flow characteristic, (v) narrow particle size distribution. Carboxy-methyl cellulose (CMC) are used as diluents and binders.

(ii) **Ointments**—*Traditional uses:* For the preparation of ointments previously hydrocarbon and absorption bases such as white petroleum jelly (Vaseline) and beeswax were used.

Current trends: Nowadays hydrophilic bases such as gels, creams are used.

(b) **Extra-neutral Alcohol (ENA):** E.N.A. is the alcohol produced by taking extraordinary precaution during the process of redistribution of rectified spirit after the addition of chemicals, and treatment by activated carbon. The spirit is made neutral. The concentrated rectified spirit from Pre-Rectifier column is fed to the Extractive Distillation column. Dilution water is fed on the top most of the column with a dilution ratio of 1 : 9. Extractive Distillation column serves to remove the impurities based on the principles of Hydro-Extraction. The water is fed to the column in such a way that it selects the higher alcohols and other impurities to move upwards and extracts ethanol down. The top vapours of the columns are condensed and fed to the recovery column.

The purified dilute ethanol is removed from the bottom of the column and fed to the rectification column, which concentrates ethanol to 96% v/v. Rectifier Column operates under pressure and condensing steam provides energy to this column through a vertical Thermosyphon reboiler. ENA draw is taken out from appropriate upper trays and fed to Simmering Column after cooling. Simmering Column is operated under high reflux for better separation of methanol and di-acetyls. Final ENA product draw is taken from the bottom of this column. The spent lees of the column are recycled as dilution water after a part of it is purged.

Lower side draw streams are taken from rectification column to avoid fusel oil build up in the column. These streams are sent to the Recovery Column where fusel oils are concentrated and then sent to decanter where these streams are diluted with water and fusel oil rich layer is separated. Washings are sent back to the column to recover alcohol. An impure spirit cut will be taken from top of this column.

Extra Neutral Alcohol are used in the preparation of Mother Tinctures, Dilutions and Specialities. This ensures the purity, pleasant taste and odour of an essential medium with which the higher energies of the dynamised medicines are carried over and as a whole, purity of all our finished products.

(c) **Manufacturing Techniques**

(i) ***Succussion—Manual:*** Handmade succussions were proposed by Hahnemann, probably inspired on alchemist technique. Hahnemann instructed that all these potencies be prepared by hand. He did not subscribe to the idea of using any mechanical contrivance. But this is reasonable as long as small quantities are to be prepared. Shaking large quantities of drugs in big bottles cannot be potentised.

(ii) ***Automatic Potentiser:*** Keeping abreast with the latest and high-precision technology, different manufacturing company has incorporated the use of 'Automatic Potentiser' to ensure-standardised potentisation of higher potencies. It is an easy to operate equipment that enables to raise 900 potencies per head in one-time operation. The calibrated potentiser operates as per the specifications of homoeopathic pharmacopoeia and can replace infinity manual working hours. The contact parts made of SS-316 make the operation hygienic. The operation stops automatically after a prefixed number of cycles and retains the data in memory, in case of power failure to restart the process from where it was shut off. Homoeopathic medicines are prepared all over the world by a serial process of dilution and shaking (*succussion*), named potentisation. The dilution is generally performed as decimal or centesimal (in volume) while *succussion* can be made by mechanical, handmade, vortex, among other procedures (Fontes, 2005; Martinez, 1990). The proposition of each one is based on cultural, technological, commercial or philosophical reasoning. Experimental results have demonstrated the efficacy of all these procedures, validating the different *succussion* techniques (Belon et al, 2004; Davenas et al, 1988; Bonamin et al, 2001; Varricchio et al, 2006).

(iii) ***Manual Triturators:*** The older method of mixing of constituents by hand in a mortar and pestle.

(iv) ***Mechanical Triturators:*** The newer method of mixing of constituents in a mechanical device or amalgamator.

(d) **Standardising safe lower limit for trituration:**

Lowest potencies—legal limits of prescription

Name of the drug	Legal position
Ars. sul. flv.	Not below 2x
Lachesis	Not below 6x
Calcarea ars.	Not below 3x
Bufo rana	Not below 3x
Baryta mur.	Not below 3x
Ars. iod.	Not below 3x
Ars. alb.	Not below 3x
Antim. ars.	Not below 3x
Baryta carb.	Not below 2x
Ars. sul. rub.	Not below 2x

All Arsenic, Baryta, Mercurius and Plumbum group of medicines : not below 3x.

All nosodes: not below 6x (3rd potency) for trading, not below 6th potency in practice.

All isodes: not below 6x.

All snake, viper, spider, toad and insect poisons: not below 3x (exceptions in **India–Blatta orientalis Q**).

Phytochemicals (HCN glyc.) etc.: not below 6x.

Special storage conditions (upto 3x)

Acid acetic, Acid nitric, Acid picric, Acid sulph, Apis mellifica, Bromium, Gels semp., Hydrast can, Iodium, Kreosotum, Physostigma, Rauwolfia serp, Secale cor, Zincum aceticum.

Stringent storage condition (upto 3x)

Ars. alb., Acid fluoric (hydrofluoric), Atropine sulph., Chininum ars., Glonoine, Lachesis, Naja, Merc. iod. flv., Merc. iod. rub., Phosphorus.

Level of testing in Homoeopathic Drugs

Biochemic drugs	—upto 6x; upto 12x by plasma
Triturations	—upto 6x; upto 12x by plasma
Mother tinctures	—upto 4x; upto 6x by HPLC
Mother tinctures	—upto 2x in combinations.
Combination drugs	—upto 2x
Dilutions	—upto 6x

Ointments, hair oils, eye-drops, etc.

3. Essential Pharmacognosy

A. Microscopical Examination of Plant Drugs

The microscopical study of an organised drug, either in entire or powered form, is one of the important aspects of its histological evaluation. The arrangement of tissues in transverse and longitudinal sections and types of cells and cell contents are revealed by suitable histological study of a crude drug with the aid of a microscope. Certain microscopical characteristics like stomata, trichomes, calcium oxalate crystals, starch grains, stone cells, fibres, vessels etc. are important anatomical characteristics of organised drugs. The microscopical evaluation of crude drug also involves linear measurements, study of surface preparation of leaves, quantitative microscopical aspects and chemo-microscopy.

1. ***Leaf constants or diagnostic characters of leaves:*** It includes stomatal number, stomatal index, palisade ratio, vein islet number and vein termination number.

(a) ***Stomatal number***

It is the average number of stomata present per square mm of the epidermis.

The actual number of stomata per square mm of leaf may vary for leaves of the same plant grown in different environmental conditions. Stomatal number is relatively a constant for particular species of same age and, hence, taken into consideration as a diagnostic character for identification of leaf drug.

No.	Species	Stomatal number
1	Datura stramonium	087- upper epidermis
2	Datura innoxia	141- upper epidermis
3	Hyoscyamus niger	125- upper epidermis

(b) *Stomatal index*

It is the percentage which the number of stomata form to the total number of epidermal cells, each stoma being counted as one cell. It can be calculated by a formula

I = (S/E + S) X 100 (1 sq mm/8-10 segments)

I = Stomatal index

S = Number of stomata per unit area

E = Epidermal cells in the same area

No.	Species	Stomatal index (range)
1.	Atropa belladonna	20.2 to 23
2.	Atropa acuminata	16.2 to 18.3
3.	Indian senna (Cassia angustifolia)	17 to 20
4.	Alexandrian senna (Cassia acutifolia)	10.8 to 12.6
5.	Digitalis purpurea	17.9 to 19.5
6.	Digitalis lanata	14.9 to 17.6

(c) *Palisade ratio*

It is the average number of palisade cells, beneath one epidermal cells, using four epidermal cells for the count.

The palisade ratio as defined above is constant for a particular species or genus.

No.	Name of plant	Range
1.	Atropa belladonna	05-70
2.	Azadhirachta indica	03-3.5
3.	Datura stramonium	4-7
4.	Digitalis purpurea	3.7- 4.2

(d) *Vein islet number*

Minute photosynthetic area encircled by conducting strands.

It is the number of vein islets per square mm of leaf surface.

It is a constant for a given species of the plant.

It doesn't alter with the age of the plant and is independent of the size of the leaf.

No.	Name of drug	Range
1.	Erythroxylon coca	8-12
2.	Erythroxylon truxillense	15-26
3.	Digitalis purpurea	2-5.5
4.	Digitalis thapsi	8.5-16
5.	Cassia angustifolia	19-23
6.	Cassia acutifolia	25-30

(e) *Vein termination number*

It is defined as the number of veinlet—termed vein termination per sq mm of the leaf surface midway between midrib and margin.

2. ***Stomata***

Types of stomata

On the basis of number and orientation of subsidiary cells, there are four types of stomata in dicotyledons:

Anomocytic (irregular celled) type—In this type, the stomata are surrounded by a limited number of epidermal cells which are indistinguishable from other epidermal cells.

Anisocytis (unequal celled) type—This type is characterised by the presence of three subsidiary cells of which one is distinctly smaller than the other two.

Paracytis (parallel celled) type—In this type, the stomata is accompanied on either side by one or more subsidiary cells which lie parallel to the long axis of the pore and the guard cells.

Diacytic (cross celled) type—In this type, the stomata is enclosed by a pair of subsidiary cells whose common wall is at right angle to the long axis of the guard cells.

3. ***Trichome (Hairs And Scales of Plants):*** Trichomes (from the Greek *trikhoma* meaning "growth of hair") are fine outgrowths or appendages on plants. These are specialised hair-like structures found on the plant epidermis. It can be present on stems, leaves, sepals, petals, stamens and ovarium. There are many kinds of trichomes, each kind with a different function.

Depending upon the structure and the number of cells present in trichomes, they are classified as given below:

(a) *Non-glandular trichomes (covering or clothing trichomes)*

(i) *Unicellular*

Examples: Lignified trichomes: *Nux vomica, Strophanthus.*

Short, sharply pointed, curved: *Cannabis indica.*

Large, conical, strongly shrunken: *Lobelia inflata.*

Short, conical, unicellular: *Thea cinensis.*

Strongly waved, thick walled: *Yerba santa.*

(ii) *Multicellular:* It may be unbranched and branched.

Branched type

Stellate: *Hamamelis.*

Peltate: *Humulus.*

Candelabra: *Verbascum thapsus.*

T shaped trichomes: *Artemisia maritima.*

Unbranched type

Uniseriate: 1. Bi-cellular, conical: *Datura*

2. Three celled-long: *Stramonium*

3. Three to four celled-long: *Digitalis purpurea*

4. Four to five celled-long: *Atropa belladonna*

Biseriate: *Calendula officinalis.*

Multiseriate: Male fern.

(b) *Glandular trichomes*

These are characterised by the presence of glandular (spherical) cell all the top of the trichome. They contain volatile oils and other secretions that are produced by the plants.

They are sub-classified as:

(i) Unicellular glandular trichome: The stalk is absent e.g., *Justicia adhatoda.*

(ii) Multicellular glandular trichome.

(c) *Special type of trichomes (hydathodes)*

These are organs of absorption or secretion of water developed in certain plants e.g., Piper betal, London pride etc.

4. *Quantitative microscopy:*

Lycopodium spore method—It is an important analytical technique for powdered drugs, especially when chemical or other methods of evaluation of crude drugs fail as accurate measures of quality. It is inexpensive technique with official status. Lycopodium spores are very characteristic in shape and appearance and exceptionally uniform in size (25 cubic micron). On an average, 94,000 spores per mg of powdered lycopodium are present.

A powdered drug is evaluated by this technique, if it contains (i) well-defined particles which may be counted, e.g., starch grains and pollen grains, (ii) single layered cells or tissues, the area of which may be traced under suitable magnification and actual area calculated or (iii) the objects of uniform thickness, the length of which can be measured under suitable magnification and actual area calculated. The percentage purity of an authentic powdered ginger is calculated by using the equation

$$\frac{N \times W \times 94{,}000 \times 100}{S \times M \times P} = \%\ \text{Purity of drug}$$

where

N = number of characteristic structures (e.g., starch grains) in 25 fields.

W = weight in mg of lycopodium taken.

S = number of lycopodium spore in the same 25 fields.

M = weight in mg of the sample, calculated on basis of sample dried at 105°C.

P = 2,86,000 in case of ginger starch grains powder.

Lycopodium spore method can be used for evaluation of powered clove, ginger, cardamom, nutmeg, umbelliferous fruits etc.

B. Preliminary Phytochemical Screening

The plant is a biosynthetic laboratory, not only for chemical compounds such as carbohydrates, protein and lipids that are utilised as food by man, but also for a multitude for compounds like glycosides, alkaloids, volatile oils, tannins etc. that exert a physiological and therapeutic effect.

(a) ***Successive Solvent Extraction (Quantitative):*** The air-dried powered plant material is extracted successively in petroleum ether, benzene, solvent ether, chloroform, acetone, ethanol and methanol. Finally the drug is macerated with chloroform water. Each time before extracting with the next solvent, the powered material is dried in hot air oven below 50°C. Each extract is concentrated by distilling off the solvent and then evaporating to dryness on water bath. The extract obtained with each solvent is weighed. Its percentage is calculated in terms of air-dried weight of plant material.The colour and consistency of the extract are noted. The extracts with different solvents can also be prepared by successively macerating (cold extraction) the powdered drug in order of increasing polarity.

(b) ***Qualitative Chemical Examination:*** Phytochemical screening is a process of tracing plant constituents. Phytochemical screening have attracted the attention of plant scientist due to development of new and sophisticated techniques. The phytochemical screening tests are helpful in finding chemical constituents in the plant material that may lead to their quantitative estimation and also in locating the source of pharmacologically active chemical compound.

There are simple but standard chemical tests to detect the presence of alkaloids, tannins, saponins, anthraquinones, cardenolides etc in a plant extract. Each time the operator is undertaking the plant phytochemical screening, there is always the need to carry out confirmatory tests because one can experience false-positive reactions in some non-alkaloidal extracts. Plants are subject to physiological changes before extraction, if the plants are not extracted on the day of collection and this could invariably affect the phytochemical screening results.

In testing for the presence of bioactive agents in a plant, an extract of the plant must first be prepared by macerating a known weight of the fresh plant with redistilled methylated spirit in a blender. Each extract will then be suction-filtered and the process is to be repeated until all soluble compounds had been extracted, as judged by loss of colour of filtrate. The total extract from each plant part is to be evaporated to dryness in vacuo at about 450°C and further dried to constant weight at the same temperature in a hot-air oven. The yield of residue is to be noted and a portion of it is to be used to test for the constituents of the medicinal plants.

(1) *Detection of Carbohydrates*

Molish's test: The test solution is combined with a small amount of Molisch's reagent (α-naphthol dissolved in ethanol) in a test tube. After mixing, a small amount of concentrated sulfuric acid is slowly added down the sides of the sloping test-tube, without mixing, to form a bottom layer. A positive reaction is indicated by appearance of a purple ring at the interface between the acid and test layers.

(2) *Detection of Reducing sugars*

Benedict's test: Aqueous glucose is mixed with Benedict's reagent, a solution of copper sulfate, sodium hydroxide, and tartaric acid. The mixture is heated. Carbohydrates which react with Benedict's reagent to reduce the blue copper (II) ion to form a brick red precipitate of copper (I) oxide are classified as reducing sugars.

(3) *Detection of Monosaccharides*

Barford's Test is a chemical test used for detecting the presence of monosaccharides. It is based on the reduction of copper (II) acetate to copper (I) oxide (Cu_2O), which forms a brick-red precipitate. The aldehyde group of the monosaccharide which normally forms acyclic hemiacetal is oxidised to the carboxylate. A number of other substances, including sodium chloride, may interfere.

(4) *Detection of Alkaloids*

1. Mayer's test: Mayer's reagent is a solution of potassium mercuric iodide in water. A positive result is indicated by a cream-coloured precipitate.

2. Hager's test: Hager's reagent is a salt solution of picric acid. A positive result is indicated by a yellow coloured precipitate.

3. Wagner's test: Wagner's reagent is a solution of iodine in potassium iodide. A positive result is indicated by a reddish-brown coloured precipitate.

4. Dragendorf's test: Dragendorf's reagent is a solution of potassium bismuth iodide. A

positive result is indicated by a orange or dark coloured precipitate.

(5) *Detection of Steroids*

There are two types of methods to test steroids:

1. Colorimetric method using tetrazolium blue salts: The Colorimetric method, is the routine method for testing steroids. In this test, the reaction depends upon the reduction of Tetrazolium Blue salts to give a highly coloured compound known as "Farmazan". Under controlled conditions the amount of "Farmazan" developed is proportional to the quality of steroids or any other Reducing sugars present in the material being tested. In fact for some years, tetrazolium salts have been used for determination of reducing sugars. So if the drug contains any lactose. it will impart a strong color with tetazolium blue salt which will give a false impression of the presence of a steroid. Secondly, if the alcohol used in this method is not completely free from aldehyde, it will interface with the characteristic color, which may again give a false positive reaction for a steroid. So this method is not advisable to determine the presence of steroids in the Homoeopathic medicines. In routine the dispensing materials used in homoeopathic medicines are: Lactose (Milk sugar), Pills (made of cane sugar). Both of these materials are reducing sugars, so they give a false test for steroids even when they are unmedicated. Another dispensing material used is Alcohol. If the alcohol used is not completely free from Aldehyde, it will interfere with the reaction and will impart some characteristic colour in the reaction that may again give a false positive impression of steroid. So this method is not at all advisable to determine the presence of steroids in homoeopathic medicines.

2. Liberman Buchard test (Thin layer chromatography method and UV absorption method): This is another method for the testing of steroids. All steroids show UV absorption between 235 to 240 nm in dehydrated alcohol or methanol in a clear solution. This is a reliable method for testing steroids in homoeopathic medicines.

(6) *Detection of Glycosides*

(a) Cardiac Glycosides

(i) Keller-Killani test: 0.5 of extract will be dissolved in 2ml of glacial acetic acid containing one drop of ferric chloride solution. This will then be underlayed with 1ml of concentrated sulphuric acid.

A brown ring obtained at the interface will indicate the presence of a deoxy sugar characteristic of cardenolides. A violet ring may appear below the brown ring while, in the acetic acid layer a greenish ring may form just above the brown ring and gradually spread throughout this layer (Evans, 2002).

(ii) Legal's test: The extract is to be dissolved in pryridine and a few drops of 2 per cent sodium nitorprusside together with a few drops of 20 per cent NaOH are to be added. A deep red colour which faded to a brownish yellow indicates the presence of cardenolodes.

(iii) Liebermann's test: 0.5g of the extract will be dissolved in 2ml of acetic anhydride and cooled well in ice sulphuric acid was then carefully added. A colour change from violet to blue to green will indicate the presence of a steroidal nucleus (i.e., aglycone portion of the cardiac glycoside) (Shoppee, 1964).

(b) Detection of Anthraquinone Glycosides

Borntrager's test Borntrager's test is used for the detection of anthraquinones. 5 g of each plant extract is to be shaken with 10 ml benzene, filtered and 5 ml of 10 per cent ammonia solution added to the filtrate. The mixture is to be shaken and the presence of a pink, red or violet colour in the ammoniacal (lower) phase indicates the presence of free hydroxyl-anthraquinones.

For bound anthraquionones, 5 g of each plant extract is to be boiled with 10 ml aqueous sulphuric acid and filtered while hot. The filtrate was shaken with 5 ml of benzene, the benzene layer separated and half its own volume of 10 percent ammonia solution added. A pink, or violet coloration in the ammonia phase (lower layer) indicates the presence of anthroquinones derivatives in the extract (Evans, 2002).

(c) Detection of Saponin Glycoside

Foam test: The ability of saponins to produce frothing in agueous solution and to haemolyse red blood cells is used as screening test for these compounds.

For the test, the method described by Wall et al. (1952 and 1954) can be used. About 0.5 g of each plant extract was shaken with water in a test tube. Frothing which persists on warming was taken as preliminary evidence for the presence of saponins. In order to remove "False-positive" results, the blood haemolysis test needs to be performed on those extracts that frothed in water.

About 0.5g of each extract is to be boiled briefly with 50ml phosphate butter, PH 7.4, and then allowed to cool and filtered, 5ml of the filtrate is to be passed for 3 hrs. through an asbestos disc (1.5mm thick about 7mm in diameter), which has been previously soaked with two or three drops of 1 per cent cholesterol in ether and dried.

After filtration, the disc should be washed with 0.5ml of distilled water, dried and boiled in 20ml of oxylol for 2hrs to decompose the complex formed between cholesterol and any saponins in the extract. The disc should then be washed in ether, dried and placed on 7 percent blood nutrient ager. Complete heamolysis of red blood-cells around the disc after 6hrs. is taken as further evidence of presence of saponins.

(7) *Detection of Flavonoids*

1. Shindo's test
2. Test with Lead acetate solution
3. Alkaline reagent test.

(8) *Detection of Tannins*

Test with $FeCl_3$ solution: About 5 g of each portion of plant extract will be stirred with 10ml distilled water, filtered, and ferric chloride reagent will then be added to the filtrate. A blue-black, green or blue-green precipitate is taken as evidence for the presence of tannins (Evans, 2002).

4. Pharmaceutical Analysis

Chromatography

The chromatography is useful in qualitative and quantitative analysis of drugs especially mother tinctures and lower potencies. Thin Layer Chromatography (TLC) and Paper Chromatography (PC) are usually employed in the H.P.I. assays and tests.

Thin layer chromatography (TLC) is a simple, quick, and inexpensive procedure that gives a quick answer as to how many components are in a mixture. TLC is also used to support the identity of a compound in a mixture when the Rf of a compound is compared with the Rf of a known compound (preferably both run on the same TLC plate). Rf is the retention factor, or how far up a plate the compound travels.

HPTLC (High Performance Thin Layer Chromatography) is a sophisticated and automated form of TLC. The procedure simultaneously processes the sample and standard that results in better analytical precision and accuracy at a faster pace. It allows several analysis to be done at the same time.

HPTLC is a highly sophisticated equipment used for the qualitative (finger printing) as well as quantitative analysis of drug ingredients i.e. glycosides, alkaloids etc. that are present in tinctures and extracts. It is also used for developing in-house standardisation of mother tinctures, and developing analytical methods for testing mother tinctures.

HPTLC method is very simple, powerful, rapid, reliable and cost effective with respect to the accuracy of the result based on both qualitative and quantitative analysis.

For homoeopathic formulations, development of standard procedure through HPTLC is a new approach which may lead to proper standardisation of different homoeopathic tinctures based on fingerprinting characteristics. This investigation shows that these particular characteristics may be used as standardisation tool for homoeopathic tinctures more effectively and most accurately and is utmost essential which could enable the society in general to have quality homoeopathic formulations in one hand and to gain a momentum in homoeopathic medicine in the other.

Spectrometric/Spectroscopic Analysis

Spectroscopy is a technique that uses the interaction of energy with a sample to perform an analysis. The data that is obtained from spectroscopy is called a spectrum. A spectrum is a plot of the intensity of energy detected versus the wavelength (or mass or momentum or frequency, etc.) of the energy. A spectrum can be used to obtain information about atomic and molecular energy levels, molecular geometries, chemical bonds, interactions of molecules, and related processes. Often, spectra are used to identify the components of a sample (qualitative analysis). Spectra may also be used to measure the amount of material in a sample (quantitative analysis). There are several instruments that are used to perform a spectroscopic analysis. In simplest terms, spectroscopy requires an energy source (commonly a laser, but this could be an ion source or radiation source) and a device for measuring the change in the energy source after it has interacted with the sample (often a spectrophotometer or interferometer).

COMMON TYPES

(i) **Ultraviolet-Visible Spectroscopy or Ultraviolet-Visible Spectrophotometry (UV-Vis or UV/Vis):** It refers to absorption spectroscopy in the ultraviolet-visible spectral region. This means it uses light in the visible and adjacent (near-UV and near-infrared (NIR)) ranges. The absorption in the visible range directly affects the perceived colour of the chemicals involved. In this region of the electromagnetic spectrum, molecules undergo electronic transitions.

It is used to perform quality control assays on drug substances obtained from different sources in order to compare their spectra with that of standard spectrum for the same drug substance.

(ii) **IR Spectroscopy:** It offers the possibility to measure different types of inter atomic bond vibrations at different frequencies. It is applicable in structure determination and identity of organic and inorganic compounds-quantitative analysis.

(iii) **Raman Spectroscopy:** Raman scattering of light by molecules may be used to provide information on a sample's chemical composition and molecular structure.

(iv) **Nuclear Magnetic Resonance (NMR) Spectroscopy:** Nuclear Magnetic Resonance is an analytical technique where a sample is immersed in a magnetic field and irradiated with radio waves. Using this technique to study a molecule enables the recording of differences in the magnetic properties of the various nuclei, protons, electrons and neutrons present as well as what positions these hold within the molecule. This is directly influenced by the environment of, for example, a proton, and thus enables predictions concerning the structure of the liquid.

A variety of different tools have been used to investigate homoeopathic remedies, such as infrared spectra, electronic spectra and NMR spectroscopy (Sukul et al, 2001), diffraction, Raman spectroscopy (Berezin, 1994).

NMR spectroscopy has been shown to be a valuable tool in the assessment of the differences of the physico-chemical properties of homoeopathic substances. Although it is not yet known how the difference in chemical shift and mean integration values of the recorded NMR spectra of various homoeopathic remedies can be translated into an absolute indicator of specific structural differences, it does indicate that there is a structural difference (Demangeat et al, 2001).

Ives (2000) has stated that she believes the most promising line of research has come with the use of NMR spectroscopy. This is due to the fact that NMR spectroscopy can record energy transitions of protons, which are reliant on their precession rates and electronic environments.

NMR spectroscopy is a powerful tool used to determine the structure of molecules. The chemical environment of specific nuclei is deduced from information obtained about the nuclei. NMR takes advantage of the fact that the nuclei of these molecules have an intrinsic spin. The process of NMR entails placing the sample in a simple magnetic field and irradiating it with radio waves. NMR spectra then arise from the so-called spin property. The spin is a quantum effect where spin is quantised, i.e. having two directions, up or down.

Earlier research was conducted by **Smith and Boericke (1966)** on Sulphur potencies to evaluate homoeopathic drug structure. Distinct changes were noted in the hydroxyl part of the spectrum. They concluded that the solvent structure is changed in unsuccussed serial dilutions as compared to undiluted solvent. They established further differences in succussed serial dilutions, and the changes became more extreme as the potencies passed Avogadro's limit. This led them to believe that there is a physical rearrangement in the solvent, most likely in the form of self-replicating polymers. A further study by **Smith and Boericke (1968)** with higher potency levels up to 60X level with bracykinin-triacetate, only compounded the evidence that the act of succussion increased the area of the hydroxyl spectrum as opposed to identical unsuccussed dilutions.

The employment of NMR spectroscopy as an experimental technique on homoeopathic potencies, has proven very useful (Schulte, 1999), however problems have been reported by various investigators assessing this tool [Bol (1997), Demangeat and Poitevin (2001)].

Sukul et al (2001) conducted an experiment comparing the effects of Nux vomica 30c successed and unsuccussed on adult toads as well as the NMR spectra of the above mentioned compared to a range of variations. In the preparation of their samples they used 10 succussions except with the samples that were unsuccussed. They concluded that the ethanol-water mixture has the capability to imbibe some specific properties of drug molecules or particles during the dynamisation process, but that succussion is not an essential factor in producing an effective homoeopathic potency. The possibility remains that there is a threshold in the number of succussions that need to be used before its effect on the remedy will be evident.

The employment of NMR Spectroscopy as a method for the analysis of structure within homoeopathic potencies and as a method for the analysis of the differences between the respective homoeopathic potencies and a lactose-based control and differences between parallel potencies and a control has been well substantiated (Ross, 1997).

(v) **Atomic Absorption Spectroscopy (AAS):** It is a spectro-analytical procedure for the qualitative and quantitative determination of chemical elements employing the absorption of optical radiation (light) by free atoms in the gaseous state. In analytical chemistry the technique is used for determining the concentration of a particular element (the analyte) in a sample to be analysed. AAS can be used to determine over 70 different elements in solution or directly in solid samples.

(vi) **X-ray Spectroscopy:** This technique involves excitation of inner electrons of atoms, which may be seen as X-ray absorption. An X-ray fluorescence emission spectrum may be produced when an electron falls from a higher energy state into the vacancy created by the absorbed energy.

Discussion

(i) UV–VIS, IR, FTIR, and Raman Spectroscopy are used for the bulk "liquid" which in most cases is either water or a mixture of water and ethanol (95% ethanol). UV–VIS spectroscopy and Raman spectroscopy proved to be useful tools to investigate the subtle but significant changes in the structural parameters in both water and alcohol based remedies.

(ii) It should also be noted that different homoeopathic remedies and different dilutions of the same remedy have been distinguished from each other using Raman and infrared spectroscopy, even though all should theoretically contain nothing but water. Such findings may relate to complex processes such as the formation, during succussion, of colloidal nanobubbles that could contain the remedy source material.

(iii) In physical researches the most striking results indicating water memory were obtained from NMR, UV and X-ray spectroscopy of ultra-highly diluted water (ultra high dilution means a dilution of a substance in which there is high probability that not even one molecule is left; it is practically pure water).

(iv) Using Raman and Ultraviolet–Visible (UV–VIS) spectroscopy Roy et al distinguished two different homeopathic medicines (Nux vom and Nat mur) and differentiated their 6c, 12c, and 30c potencies.

(v) Potentisation may alter permanently the physical-chemical properties of the solvent water. It changes the structure of water molecule. Standard physico-chemical techniques, thermo-luminescence, Raman and UV–VIS spectroscopy and other methods have shown that water displays large changes in its physico-chemical properties.

(vi) **Heinz** studied the physical action of dilutions using the **infra-red spectroscopy (IR)** and stressed on the specific value of succussion. He found ihe rhythmicity indicating some favourable points in the curve of dilution.

Conclusion

(i) Homoeopathic remedies are spectroscopically distinct from the original solvent (water/ethanol).

(ii) Different potencies can be distinctly distinguished by the UV-VIS and the Raman spectroscopy.

(iii) Nat mur and Nux vomica are distinctly different while the same potencies with different succussion also show a clear evidence of difference in the structure of the individual samples.

(iv) No studies/claims whatsoever on the clinical effects of the remedies are made.

Electro-chemical Techniques

(i) **Potentiometry:** Potentiometry is the field of electroanalytical chemistry in which potential (or voltage) is measured under the conditions of no current flow. The measured potential may then be used to determine the analytical quantity of interest, generally the concentration of some component of the analyte solution. The potential that develops in the electrochemical cell is the result of the free energy change that would occur if the chemical phenomena were to proceed until the equilibrium condition has been satisfied.

(ii) **Conductometry:** Conductometry means measuring the conductivity—a conductometer measures the electrical conductivity of ionic solutions. This is done by applying an electric field between two electrodes. The ions wander in this field. The anions migrate to the anode and the cations to the cathode. In order to avoid substance conversions and the formation of diffusion layers at the electrodes (polarisation), work is carried out with alternating voltage. The rule of thumb is that the frequency of the alternating voltage must be increased as the ion concentration increases. Modern conductometers automatically adapt the measuring frequency to the particular measuring conditions.

(iii) **Polarography:** It is also called **polarographic analysis**, or **voltammetry**, in analytic che-mistry, an electrochemical method of analysing solutions of reducible or oxidisable substances. It was invented by a Czech chemist, **Jaroslav Heyrovský**, in 1922. In general, polarography is a technique in which the electric potential (or voltage) is varied in a regular manner between two sets of electrodes (indicator and reference) while the current is monitored. The shape of a polarogram depends on the method of analysis selected, the type of indicator electrode used, and the potential ramp that is applied.

The majority of the chemical elements can be identified by polarographic analysis, and the method is applicable to the analysis of alloys and to various inorganic compounds. Polarography is also used to identify numerous types of organic compounds and to study chemical equilibria and rates of reactions in solutions.

(iv) **Titrimetry:** Chemical analysis by titration, the determination of a given component in solution by addition of a liquid reagent of known strength until a given end point (e.g., a change in colour) is reached.

Moisture content in drug substance can be determined by this chemical method named as Karl Fischer Titration. This is particularly applicable for drugs containing small quantities of moisture. The reagents and solutions used in this method are sensitive to water and precautions must be taken to prevent exposure to atmospheric moisture. The Karl Fischer reagent used for this purpose consists of a solution of iodine, sulphur dioxide and pyridine in dry methanol. This is titrated against a sample containing water, which causes a loss of the dark brown colour. At the end-point, when no water is available, the colour of the reagent persists.

5. Experimental Pharmacology

Introduction

Samuel Hahnemann was the founder of homoeopathy. He established the fundamental principles of the science and art of homoeopathy.

He is called the Father of Experimental Pharmacology because he was the first physician to prepare medicines in a specialised way; proving them on healthy human beings, to determine how the medicines acted to cure diseases. Before Hahnemann, medicines were given on speculative indications, mainly on the basis of authority without experimental verification.

The term pharmacology is often confused with the term pharmacy, but they are not synonymous. Pharmacy is the profession dealing with the effective use of medication while pharmacology is more closely linked to chemistry—a study, not a practice.

Pharmacology is the study of drugs and their effects. Experimental pharmacology is study through experimental use in controlled situations. Human and animal drug testing falls into the category of experimental pharmacology. Scientists design drugs as well as they can without experimental evidence and then test them on humans or on animals in an experimental setting to gather more information and to perfect their drugs.

Research involving experimental pharmacology is generally conducted long before pharmacists or consumers have access to the drugs being tested.

The basis of homoeopathic medicine is experimental pharmacology (drug proving or homoeopathic pathogenetic trial-HPT, as known in homoeopathy). This essentially calls for that the raw material should be one used in the proving.

AIMS

The main aims of experimental pharmacology in homoeopathy are:

(i) To study the mechanism of action of potentised homoeopathic drugs in animal models.

(ii) To study the site of action of homoeopathic drugs.

(iii) To study the toxicity of crude drugs.

(iv) To find out a therapeutic agent suitable for human use.

6. Recent Advances in Drug-Proving (Human Pathogenetic Trial—HPT)

Drug-Proving now termed, as Homoeopathic Pathogenetic Trials (HPT) is a process in which drug substances are put into trial over healthy volunteers and their pathogenetic effects are observed and noted for therapeutic purposes. Therefore, it is the only and unique method, which is based on the nature's law of cure i.e., Similia Similibus Curantur which states that likes are cured by likes i.e. a drug's capacity for eradicating a disease, lies in its capacity to produce the same.

In 1996, Flavio Dantas coined the new term for drug proving-'Homoeopathic Pathogenetic Trial' (HPT).

HPT is the first systematic experimental approach to detecting changes in the healthy volunteers after exposure to a drug. HPT is a clinical trial to investigate the effects of potentially toxic or pathogenetic substances diluted and attenuated according to the homoeopathic Pharmacopoeias, in non-patient volunteers in relatively stable health conditions.

In India the authority has adopted the methodology of proving is based on **Drysdale's Double Blind Technique** where neither the Proving Master nor the Prover (volunteer) knows the name of the drug and its potencies being proved on them.

7. Good Manufacturing Practices (GMP)

There have been amendments to Drug Rules in October 2006 affecting homoeopathic medicines —Good Manufacturing Practices (GMP).

Government now differentiates single medicines and formulations.

It now differentiates indirectly low potencies and high potencies.

It now requires that the containers should be neutral glass.

In the manufacturing area no spitting, smoking, chewing, littering, etc. are permitted.

A standard operating practices (SOPs) is required for all processes, drugs and material movements.

The manufacturer shall use back-potencies procured from licensed manufacturers and the firm shall maintain proper records of purchase or shall prepare own back-potencies with records.

Different droppers shall be used for different medicines and different potencies.

Potentisation shall be done using Hahnemannian method (change of bottle at each stage of potentisation).

In case of formulation the following has been added:

1. Compound formulations shall preferably be in liquid and solid forms and the potency of the ingredients shall be in detectable quantity preferably be in 3x except in case of highly poisonous material and toxins which should not be below 6x.
2. The ingredient shall be compatible to each other.

3. Complete pharmacopoeial name of each ingredient shall be printed on the label along with composition.

In case of Laboratory Controls the following has been added:

1. Tests as per the pharmacopoeia and requirements shall be carried out on products and materials.
2. The stability of the products shall be established by proper methods.
3. Sterility tests, wherever applicable, shall be carried out.
4. Control samples shall be preserved for not less than three years after the last sales.

For the first time expiry date for homoeopathic medicines has been prescribed.

8. Fundamental Research in this Field

Basophilic Degranulation Test

One of the famous experiments carried out was by **Jacques Benveniste**, who published the results in his paper *'Human basophilic degranulation triggered by very dilute antiserum against IgE'*. In this experiment he treated basophils having IgE attached to it with anti IgE. Basophils were found to undergo degranulation. The antiserum containing anti IgE was then diluted up to 10"2 to 10"120 times, until no molecules of the original anti IgE existed. This diluted antiserum was then treated with IgE attached to it. Surprisingly, basophilic degranulation still occurred. So even in the absence of original IgE molecules, the reaction or cure can take place.

Water-Memory Theory

French biologist Jacques Benveniste formulated the idea that water retains a "memory" of what has been dissolved in it and that it is this memory that results in the homoeopathic effect.

In 1988 Dr. Benveniste published a study in the journal *'Nature'* in support of his water-memory theory. He claimed his experiments showed that an ultra-dilute solution exerted a biological effect.

The 'memory of water' is a popular phrase that is mostly associated with homoeopathy and Jacques Benveniste following his and others' allergy research work. The main evidence against water having a memory is that of the very short lifetime of hydrogen bonds between the water molecules.

In the absence of other materials or surfaces, the specific hydrogen bonding pattern surrounding a solute does not persist when the solute is removed any more than would a cluster around any specified water molecule, or else water would not know which of its myriad past solutes took preference.

A recent **NMR spectroscopic study** shows no stable (>1 ms, >5 μM) water clusters are found in homoeopathic preparations. It should, however, be noted that the lifetime of hydrogen bonds does not control the lifetime of clusters in the same way that a sea wave may cross an ocean, remaining as a wave and with dependence on its history, but with its molecular content continuously changing. Also, the equilibrium concentration of any clusters is governed by thermodynamics not kinetics. As applied to homoeopathy, the 'memory of water' concept should also be extended to the memory of aqueous ethanol preparations. Addition of ethanol to water adds an important further area of complexity. Ethanol forms solutions in water that are far from ideal and very slow to equilibrate.

Theory of IE Crystals (ICE Electrical Field Crystals)

This theory is contributed by **Dr. Shui-Yin-Lo,** a research scientist.

Even though this concept was not put forward to explain the action of homoeopathic medicine, homoeopaths think that there is a possible link between IE Crystal theory and the action of homoeopathic medicine. According to this theory water can exist as minute ice crystals in a solution. The shape of these crystals is influenced when a substance is placed in distilled water and vigorously shaken and diluted. And these crystals, even though minute in size are extremely stable in a wide variety of environments. Applying this to homoeopathy we can possibly state that potentised medicines contain IE crystals having specific shapes depending on the original drug molecule. Dr. Lo claims that these crystals are capable of interacting with immune system.

Theory of High Dilutions (New Methods of Drug Dissociation)

This theory is developed by a physician, **Rolland Conte and a group of scientists.** They observed, some changes in the infra-red (IR) spectrum of homoeopathic high dilutions that should have same infra-red spectrum of water. After the analysis of same with nuclear magnetic resonance (NMR) data, they developed the Contonian frequency. The Contonian frequency is unique to each remedy and can be measurable.

Nuclear Magnetic Resonance (NMR) Spectroscopic Study

NMR study showed that twenty-three different homoeopathic remedies and potencies tested had distinctive readings of submolecular activity, while the placebos did not. This demonstrates Homoeopathy's energetic function overriding chemical one. As chiropractors, one observes dramatic clearing of sensory nerve interference and pathological reflex activity causing chronic recurring subluxation activity and disease. [Adam Sacks—"Nuclear magnetic resonance spectroscopy of homoeopathic remedies," Journal of holistic medicine, 5 (fall-winter 1983): 172-175: RB. Smith and G. W. Boericke—"Changes caused by succussion on N.M.R, patterns and bioassay of bradykinin triacetate (BKTA) succussions and dilution," Journal of the American institute of homoeopathy, 61 (November-December 1968): 197-212.]

Positronium Complex Formation

It is known today that wherever there is an electro-magnetic field, there is spontaneous creation of electron-positron pair of positronium.

Positronium is a system consisting of an electron and its anti-particle, positron bound together into an "exotic atom".

The orbit of the two particle and the set of energy level is similar to that of the hydrogen atom.

Two types of positronium are seen:

1. Para positronium (having a mean lifetime of 125 pico seconds and decays preferentially into two gamma rays)
2. Ortho positronium (decay into three gamma rays)

But observation became difficult due to

- Low concentration of positronium available.
- Relatively high velocities of atoms of such small mass at thermal energies.

Positronium units are said to be moderately more stable when clumped together, competent to take part in chemical and biochemical reactions.

It has been possible to postulate scientifically that in the process of homoeopathic potentisation, a strong electromagnetic field is created through production of frictional electricity due to succussion/trituration.

Simultaneously, the electron-positron pairs or positronium units and complexes are also created around drug molecules, i.e. highly specific, imitating the electronic configuration of the drug molecules.

The specific positronium complexes thus formed, due to their very light or micro-isotope like character, retain the properties of the original drug molecules, even in their absence. These light isotopic molecules also act as auto-catalysts giving rise to the next generation of positronium complexes resembling drug molecules. Thus potencies become more and more powerful with higher dyna-misation.

Laboratory Evidence

The "infinitesimal" nature or the dilution principle of homeopathy has been the main criticism of the scientific community. Homoeopaths do agree that once a remedy is diluted beyond 24x or 12c potencies, it is diluted beyond Avogadro's number (6.23×10^{-23}) which theoretically indicates that no molecules are present in the original substance. However, both laboratory and clinical results over the last 200 years have demonstrated definite effectiveness with homeopathic remedies beyond this dilution.

Hydroxyl Ion Theory

The molecules of lactose, water and ethanol have only –OH group in common. The oxygen atom in the –OH group, due to sp3 hybridisation, has four equivalent valency orbitals. Two of these have bond pair electrons and the other two unshared lone pair electrons. The latter—having no definite higher energy levels—can be raised, in small steps, to any desired energy level and, hence, play the basic role here. The organic solvent DMSO (Dimethyl-Sulphoxide) has lone pair electrons but no –OH group and does not serve as a diluent medium, emphasising the role of the lone pair electrons of the –OH groups [Davenas, E. et al, Nature 333 (30 June 1988) 816-818].

Resonant Promotion Theory

During forceful triturations and impacted succussions the outermost electron shell of the solute drug molecules comes repeatedly in close proximity with those of the diluent molecules. This induces resonant promotion of the lone pair electrons of the diluent -OH groups, in small steps, to energy levels of the chemically active electrons of drug molecules. The diluent molecules thus acquire the chemically exchangeable energy and, hence, the chemical specificity of the drug molecule to get "potentised" with the drug. During serial dilutions of potency preparation the original drug molecules get eliminated and the diluent molecules resonantly promoted by them take over the resonant promotion of the unpromoted diluent molecules. These considerations have experimental support [Smith RB Jr & Boericke GW. Modern instrumentation for the evaluation of homoeopathic drug structure. Hahnemannian Gleanings 41 (1974) 99-119. Boiron J & Vinh CLD. Contribution to the study of the physical homoeopathic dilution by Raman laser effect. Hahnemannian Gleanings 43 (1976) 455-467].

Light Isotopic Model

Light isotopic model is proposed by **Dr. A. C. Dutta** to explain the action of potentised medicine. According to him, in the process of homoeopathic potentisation, increasingly strong electrical fields are produced, which help in the formation of electron-positron pairs otherwise called positronium units. In the vicinity of drug molecules, these positronium complexes imitate the electronic arrangement of drug molecules. These positronium complexes behave like drug substances and have therapeutic properties even in their absence. These light isotopic molecules also act as auto-catalysts giving rise to the next generation of positronium complexes resembling drug molecules. Thus potencies become more and more powerful with higher dynamisation.

Biological Specificity and Resonant Promotion of Lone Pair Electrons

The concept of 'biological specificity and resonant promotion of lone pair electrons' is put forward by **Dr. Rati Ram Sharma**. The open International University of Complementary Medicine, Colombo, even nominated his studies for the prestigious Nobel Prize. According to this concept, the lone pair of electrons in the vehicle molecules (alcohol, water and lactose) gets resonantly promoted during dynamisation. During this process, the vehicle molecules achieve the same number of active electrons and same exchangeable energies as the drug molecules. Thus the vehicle molecules exhibit the properties of drug molecules. He also introduces a new concept of Xenobiotics, which he equates to drug molecules, foreign bodies or any disease–causing organisms and explains all biological phenomenon on the basis of it.

Forward and Reverse Reaction of Biomolecules/Biotemplates on Water

This concept is introduced by **Dr. Mahata**. According to him water molecules are capable of taking the imprint of foreign molecules in their vicinity. Therefore, highly potentised medicine will contain water molecules having the imprint of original drug molecules.

Mahata says that disease occurs by forward reaction, of Jajoternplatei/biomolecules upon water, i.e. diseased biomolecules of body give a specific imprint to the water content of the cells. Thus the imprint of the disease is stamped on the water content of the cells. The reversed reaction of water upon biomolecules/biotemplates is brought about by potentised medicine. Here the water molecules having the imprint of drugs exert a corrective influence upon biomolecules thus changing them into healthy form.

Bioinformatics

Bioinformatics is built upon the concept of genome. Human Genome Project states that there are 30,000 genes in a human being. Understanding how the gene works provides a clue to how diseases are caused and how a cure can be effected. Human genome points out the need of individual medicine for each person's peculiar genetic make up. Modern Medicine is finally thinking of the concept of individualisation, which homoeopathy was insisting on for the past 200 years.

P. N. Varma, the renowned homoeopathic scientist and the founder of Homoeopathic Pharmacopoeia Laboratory (HPL) and of Central Council of Research in Homoeopahty (CCRH) uses bioinformatics to give an explanation for homoeopathy. He took inspiration from the works of scientists of Kalyani University, who suggested gene expression as possible model of action in 'radiation protection' (protection from the hazardous effects of radiation) by homoeopathic medicine Ginseng 200c on biological models. P. N. Varma says that the idea of individualistic medicine suggested by genomics is similar to 'constitutional medicine' which homoeopathy has upheld for long. He uses immunology to explain that the self-regulatory mechanisms of body, which is, in turn, controlled by genes, could be influenced by homoeopathic medicines. He replaces the word 'vital force' with a new terminology 'biological responses'.

He says this concept requires more scientific work so that gene expression can be linked to homoeopathy. This scientific model based on bioinfomatics explains the concept of health, cure, vital force (biological responses) and the action of medicines to effect a cure. Many such concepts are now proposed,so also many new discoveries are adopted by homoeopaths to suggest a possible scientific explanation for the system of Homoeopathy.

Stimulating Homeostatic Mechanism

If all biochemical reactions in human body are balanced and dependent on each other, this balance is called homeostasis. The disturbance in above balance is due to mal-synthesis, introduction of protein in human such as vaccination, insect bite, bacterial toxin, toxins from killed bacteria after antibiotics, etc. Disturbed homoeostasis impairs immunity and causes physical and mental symptoms. Homoeopathic medicines stimulate the body's homeostatic mechanism so that body heals itself by dealing with the sources of symptoms. This stimulus assists the body system in clearing itself of any expressions of imbalance.

Molecular Clusters

An alternative mechanism is suggested by the results of research on molecular clustering in water solutions, which has shown that as a solution is made more and more dilute, very stable and larger 'clumps' of material develop in dilute solutions rather than in more concentrated solutions. This means that residual molecular clusters of the original substance might be present in homeopathic dilutions. There are many variable-size clusters of water molecules found in potentised remedies. Ethanol acts more than just preservative. Ethanol forms its own cluster. Interestingly, ethanol forms clusters with water also (Wisniewski, 2001).

Transient Localised Regions

Succussion might also be responsible for crea-ting very tiny bubbles (nano-bubbles) that could contain gaseous inclusions of oxygen, nitrogen, carbon dioxide and possibly the homoeopathic source material. This means the succussion process gene-rates nano-bubbles and transient localised regions of high pressure topping 10,000 atmospheres that have been hypothesised to alter the water in a significant and persistent way.

Matching Wavelength

Homoeopathic medicine's main action is through taste buds, oesophageal canal, stomach and intestine (part of immune system). Action begins as the homoeopathy medicine touches the moist surface of tongue from where it is absorbed by mucous membranes and goes into circulation of a huge network of nerves which is spread like electric wires in miles in the body and from the tongue or olfactory nerves it reaches to a very specific point of weakness in immune system and starts correcting or boosting or strengthening it.

Likewise, one can imagine how accurate the potency and wavelength of the homoeopathic remedy—each of which carries a very specific wavelength and identity—can enter the weak points of a diseased individual in matter of microseconds when the drug and the disease is matched accurately! So remedy which is not similimum does not bring about any cure, and is mere waste of effort.

And in response to antigenic attack on body very specific antibodies are released which destroys the antigenicity of the organisms and there is no drug resistance as such, because body's own defense systems comes into action each time there is an attack of organisms.

Study of Thyroxin in Tadpoles

The study of Thyroxin 30x in **tadpoles**, has showed the inhibition of growth of tadpoles. Also, when a glass bottle containing homoeopathic dilution of Thyroxin hormone (30x) is suspended in the tank of tadpoles, without any contact with the water, the growth of tadpoles was inhibited. The research was replicated at several laboratories with consistency in results. The implications of this study are significant, in showing that homoeopathic medicines have some type of radiational effect through glass. This radiational effect may be tested with various homoeopathic medicines and the results recorded for further studies.

Histamine Dilutions and Basophil Activation

Many such studies have been carried out on stimulating the basophil by highly diluted histamine. Histamine is known to elicit a negative feedback effect on anti-IgE and allergen-induced basophil activation. A series of experiments performed between 1981 and 1995 using a manual method showed biological activity of highly diluted histamine. J. Benveniste's work on this is significant. Most of the experiments used histamine in the range 10–30 (15C)–10–36 M (18C). These results were confirmed by automated flow cytometry. This method is based on the selection of basophils by anti-IgE and analysis of basophil activation by anti-CD 63.

Antiviral Studies

A double-blinded study has shown that out of ten, eight homoeopathic remedies inhibited viruses in **chicken embryos** from 50 to 100 percent depending on the potencies used. [L. M. Singh and G. Gupta, "Antiviral efficacy of homoeopathic drugs against animal viruses," British Homoeopathic Journal, 74 (July 1985): 168-174.]

Allergy Studies

Studies have shown that homoeopathic **Apis mel and Histaminum hydrochloride** have a significant effect on reducing the release of certain allergy causing chemicals from basophils, which demonstrates one reason for homoeopathy's positive effects on allergies. [Jean Boiron. Jacky Abecassis and Philippe Belon- "The effects of Hahnemannian potencies of 7c Histaminum and 7c Apis mellifica upon basophil degranulation in allergic patients." aspects of research in Homoeopathy (Lyon: Boiron, 1983), pp. 61-66].

Rheumatoid Arthritis Studies

A double-blind homoeopathy experiment on patients with rheumatoid arthritis has shown that 82 per cent of the patients treated with homoeopathic medicine experienced some relief of symptoms, while only 21 per cent of those given a placebo experienced any similar degree of improvement. [R. G. Gibson, s. L.M. Gibson, Ad. Macneil. et al, "Homoeopathic therapy in rheumatoid arthritis: evaluation double-blind controlled trial," British Journal of Clinical Pharmacology, 9 (1980): 453-459].

Dental Neuralgia Studies

A double-blind homoeopathy trial was conducted on patients with dental neuralgic pain following tooth extraction. 76% of those given the homoeopathic medicine **Arnica and Hypericum** experienced relief of pain. [Henry Albertini et al. "Homoeopathic treatment of neuralgia using Arnica and Hypericum: a summary of 60 observations," Journal of the American Institute of Homoeopathy. 78 (September 1985): 126-128].

Vertigo and Nausea Studies

A study demonstrated a statistically significant improvement in reducing vertigo and nausea with a homoeopathic remedies. [C. F. Claussen, J. Bergmann. G. Bertora and E. Claussen. "Homoeopathische Kombinatlon bel Vertigo and Nausea," Arzneim. Forsch/drug res., 34(1984) 1791-98].

Merits of The New Concepts

They are able to surpass the restrictions set by Avogadro's Law. Viewing in light of Avogadro's law a potency above 12C or 24x will not have any original drug molecules. Therefore it becomes impossible for high potencies to have medicinal value. This is overruled by the new concept, which shows that an imprint of original drug molecules could be made upon vehicle molecules. So even in the absence of original drug molecules vehicle molecules bear the properties of drug molecules.

Limitations

Some of the new concepts still have a hypothetical base and are backed by indirect evidences. These concepts could explain only the action of potentised medicines, some could be extended to explain drug providing and dynamics of health and disease but they fail to explain other phenomena like susceptibility, primary and secondary actions of medicines, idiosyncrasy etc. They also fail to explain and define the vital force, except may be the bioinformatics/genome theory. One wonders at the necessity of having such an explanation for homoeopathy. But, surely the advantages of having a firm scientific basis weighs much. The scientific community will have to turn their attention to this relatively new system of healing. Subsequently, the amount of research in this field will increase, which, in turn, will expand our horizon.

Latest Research in Chemistry Laboratory under CCRH

1. **Pharmacopoeia:**
   (i) Homoeopathic Pharmacopoeia of India (HPI) revision and updating work (Volume I to X): About 60 monographs from plants and chemicals have been updated so far as advance analytical method in HPL.
   (ii) Preparation of monographs for HPI Volume XI: About 11 monographs from plants and chemicals have been incorporated in HPI Volume XI from Dr D. P. Rastogi Central Research Institute for Homoeopathy (DDPRCRIH), Noida. The publication work of HPI Volume XI is under progress.
   (iii) HPI-HPUS Harmonisation Work: 50 monographs of both pharmacopoeias have been harmonise so far in order to duplication of work.
2. **Chemical Profiling and Screening:** Chemical profiling of 7 exotic (foreign) plants cultivated in Indian conditions have been performed by chemical analytical method HPTLC in physico-chemical laboratory.
3. **Essential Pharmacognosy:** Phytochemical Screening: Estimation of phytochemical content, HPTLC (High Performance Thin Layer Chromatography) Analysis and evaluation of antioxidant potential of *Coffea cruda, Pyrus malus, Hydrastis canadensis, Thea chinensis* and *Thuja occidentalis* mother tinctures and their dilutions (6C, 12C, 30C and 200C) by Ultra-violet Visible (UV-Vis) Spectroscopy method.

Recent Advances in Homoeopathic Pharmacy

1. **New addition of drug source**
   (a) Allersodes
   (b) Isodes
2. **Advances in pharmaceutics**
   (a) Pharmaceutical Dosage Forms
   (b) Extra-neutral Alcohol (ENA)
   (c) Manufacturing Techniques
   Automatic Potentiser
   Mechanical Triturators
   (d) Standardising safe lower limit for Trituration.
3. **Essential pharmacognosy**
   (a) Microscopical examination of plant drugs
   (i) Leaf constants or diagnostic characters of leaves
   (ii) Stomata
   (iii) Trichome
   (iv) Quantitative Microscopy
   (b) Preliminary Phytochemical Screening
   (i) Successive Solvent Extraction (Quantitative)
   (ii) Qualitative Chemical Examination
4. **Pharmaceutical analysis**
   Chromatography
   Spectrometric/Spectroscopic Analysis
   Electro-chemical Techniques
5. **Experimental pharmacology**
6. **Recent advances in drug proving (human pathogenetic trial-HPT**
7. **Good Manufacturing Practices (GMP)**

8. Fundamental Research in this field

Basophilic Degranulation Test (- Jacques Benveniste)

Water-Memory Theory (- Jacques Benveniste)

Theory of IE Crystals (Ice Electrical Field Crystals) (- Dr. Shui Yi Lo)

Theory of High Dilutions (- Rolland R Conte, Henri Berliocchi, Yves Lasne)

Nuclear Magnetic Resonance (NMR) Spectroscopic Study (- Adam Sacks)

Positronium Complex Formation

Laboratory Evidence

Hydroxyl Ion Theory (- Davenas, E.)

Resonant Promotion Theory (- Smith R. B. Jr. & Boericke G. W.)

Light Isotopic Model (- Dr A. C. Dutta)

Biological Specificity and Resonant Promotion of Lone Pair Electrons (-Dr. Rati Ram Sharma.)

Forward and Reverse Reaction of Biomolecules/Biotemplates on Water (-Dr. Mahata)

Bioinformatics (- Dr. P. N. Va5rma)

Stimulating Homeostatic Mechanism

Molecular Clusters

Transient Localised Regions

Matching Wavelength

Study of Thyroxin in Tadpoles

Histamine dilutions and Basophil activation (- P. Belon, J. cumps)

Antiviral studies (- L. M. Singh and G. Gupta)

Allergy studies (- Lyon: Boiron, 1983)

Rheumatoid Arthritis studies (- P. G. Gibson)

Dental Neuralgia studies (- Henry Albertini)

Vertigo and Nausea studies (- C. F. Claussen, J. Bergmann. G. Bertora and E. Claussen).

Chapter 40

Computer-based Management Information System (MIS) in Homoeopathic Pharmacy

Introduction

With the advances in homoeopathic pharmacy, small homoeopathic pharmaceutical laboratories gradually takes the shape of an industry and constructed as per Rule 85-E(2) For proper monitoring of **manufacture** of standard quality homoeopathic medicines and their **distribution** in the market, a definite management information system is essential in homoeopathic pharmaceutical laboratory.

In manufacturing environments, the homoeopathic laboratory operation must support the production business by providing timely and accurate information about production processes and product quality. The homoeopathic laboratory is a critical part of the business, as it helps ensure that the manufacturing process works efficiently and that the products meet defined specifications, safety requirements and quality standards. In addition, the homoeopathic laboratory often provides an analytical service to the business, facilitating process optimisation, process troubleshooting and method or manufacturing process development.

In the context of rising globalisation and increased competition, today's homoeopathic manufacturing industries are under continual pressure to control costs and increase efficiency. In recent years, this has been accompanied by increasing safety and environmental regulation of the industry driven by both government and public concerns.

Maintaining a competitive edge in the industry requires efficient management of data and information generated by the laboratory, together with the automation of processes. Homoeopathic pharmaceutical laboratory information management systems require effective integration of data sources and information systems such as Enterprise Resource Planning (ERP), Manufacturing Resource Planning (MRP) and Process Control Systems.

Five main Resources of Information Management

A manager is required to manage five main types of resources effectively:

(a) **Physical:** (i) Personnel, (ii) Material, (iii) Machines (including facilities and energy).

(b) **Conceptual:** (i) Money, (ii) Information (including data).

Interest in Information Management

1. **Increasing complexity of business activity**

   (i) **International economy:** Firms of all sizes are subject to economic influences that can originate anywhere in the world. Such influences can be seen in the relative values of the currencies of each nation, where purchases are made in those countries with the highest currency value.

   (ii) **Worldwide competition:** Competition exists on a worldwide scale. Its effects can be seen in the imports from foreign countries.

   (iii) **Increasing complexity of technology:** Technology is used everywhere in business. Examples are bar code scanners, computer based airline reservation systems, automated teller machines, factory robots etc.

   (iv) **Shrinking time frames:** All phases of business operations are performed more rapidly than ever before (telemarketing, electronic sales orders, "just in time" delivery of raw materials etc).

   (v) **Social constraints:** Some products and services are found undesirable by society. Therefore, business decisions must be based on economic factors, but social costs and payoffs must be considered as well. Plant expansion, new products, new sales outlets and similar actions must all be weighed in terms of their environmental impact.

2. **Improved computer capabilities**

   —Size

   —Speed

Today's users have keyboard terminals or microcomputers in their offices.

Many of the micros are connected to other computers in a network and users know how to use them.

Who are the Information Users?

(a) **Managers:** The idea of using the computer as a management information system was a breakthrough because it recognised managers' need for problem solving information. Embracing the MIS concept made several firms develop applications specifically aimed at management support.

(b) **Non-managers:** Non-manages and staff specialists also use the MIS output.

(c) **Persons and organisations in the firm's environment** Users outside the company benefit from the MIS as well. They can be customers receiving invoices, stockholders getting dividend checks, and the federal government checking tax reports.

Management Levels

1. **Strategic Planning Level:** The strategic planning level involves managers at the top of the organisational hierarchy. The term *strategic* indicates the long-term impact of top managers' decisions on the entire organisation. The term *executive* is often used to describe a manager on the strategic planning level.
2. **Management Control Level:** Middle-level managers include regional managers, product directors, and division heads. Their level is called "management control level" due to their responsibility of putting plans into action and ensuring the accomplishment of goals.
3. **Operational Contro Level:** Lower level managers are persons responsible for carrying out the plans specified by managers on upper levels. Their level is called the "operational control level" because this is where the firm's operations occur.

Types of Information Systems

Organisations and individuals use different types of systems for different purposes. Here are some of the main types of information systems and their uses:

1. **Transaction Processing System (TPS)**

A TPS collects and stores information about transactions, and contols some aspects of transactions. A transaction is an event of interest to the organisation, e.g., a sale at a store.

A TPS is a basic business system. It is often tied to other systems such as the inventory system which tracks stock supplies and triggers reordering when stocks get low; serves the most elementary day-to-day activities of an organisation; supports the operational level of the business; supplies data for higher-level management decisions (e.g., MIS, EIS); is often critical to survival of the organisation; mostly for predefined, structured tasks; can have strategic consequences (e.g. airline reservation system); usually has high volumes of input and output; provides data which is summarised into information by systems used by higher levels of management; need to be fault-tolerant.

On-line transaction processing: A transaction processing mode in which transactions entered on-line are immediately processed by the CPU.

Sub-species of TPS

(a) **Manufacturing and Production System:** Systems that supply data to operate, monitor and control the production process. e.g. purchasing, receiving, shipping, process control, robotics, inventory systems, scheduling, engineering, operations, quality control, resource management etc.

Examples: A system in a factory that gets information from measuring samples of products does statistical analysis of samples shows when operators should take corrective action.

(b) **Sales and Marketing System:** Systems that support the sales and marketing function by facilitating the movement of goods and services from producers to customers. e.g.,

Sales support—keep customer records, follow-up;

Telemarketing—use phone for selling;

Order processing—process orders, produce invoices, supply data for sales analysis and inventory control;

Point-of-sale—capture sales data at cash register often by scanner;

Customer credit authorisation—advise on credit to be allowed to customer.

Examples: A Store's Sales System would automatically record total purchase transactions and prints out a packing list improve customer service maintain customer data

(c) **Finance & Accounting System:** Systems that maintain records concerning the flow of funds in the firm and produce financial statements, such as balance sheets and income statements. e.g., for budgeting, general ledger, billing, cost accounting, accounts receivable/payable; funds management systems, pay roll. They were among the earliest systems to be computerised.

Examples: Cash management, loan management, check processing, securities trading, visa's credit card payment system.

(d) **Human Resource System:** Systems that deal with recruitment, placement, performance evaluation, compensation, and career development of the firm's employees.

Examples: Personnel record keeping, applicant tracking, positions, training and skills, benefits.

2. Management Information System (MIS), 1964

IBM promoted the concept as a means of selling disk files and terminals. The MIS concept recognised that, computer applications should be implemented for the primary purpose of producing management information. Transactions recorded in a TPS are analysed and reported by an MIS. They have large quantities of input data and they produce summary reports as output. Used by middle managers. An example is an annual budgeting system.

3. Decision Support System (DSS), 1971

Helps strategic management staff (often senior managers) make decisions by providing information, models, or analysis tools. For support of semistructured and unstructured decisions (structured decisions can be automated). Used for analytical work, rather than general office support.

They are flexible, adaptable and quick. The user controls inputs and outputs. They support the decision process and often are sophisticated modelling tools so managers can make simulations and predictions.

Their inputs are aggregate data, and they produce projections. An example job for a DSS would be a 5 years operating plan.

4. Office Automation System (OAS), 1964

OAS provides individuals effective ways to process personal and organisational data, perform calculations, and create documents, e.g., word processing, spreadsheets, file managers, personal calendars, presentation packages.

They are used for increasing personal productivity and reducing "paper warfare". OAS software tools are often integrated (e.g., word processor can import a graph from a spreadsheet) and designed for easy operation.

Sub-species of OAS

(a) **Communication System:** helps people work together by sharing information in many different forms Teleconferencing (including audio-conferencing, computer conferencing, video-conferencing), electronic mail, voice mail, fax etc.

(b) **Groupware System:** helps teams work together by providing access to team data, structuring communication, and making it easier to schedule meetings. For sharing information, controlling work flows, and communication/integration of work.

5. Executive Information System (EIS)

Also known as an Executive Support System (ESS), it provides executives information in a readily accessible, interactive format. They are a form of MIS intended for top-level executive use. An EIS/ESS usually allows summary over the entire organisation and also allows drilling down to specific levels of detail. They also use data produced by the ground-level TPS so, the executives can gain an overview of the entire organisation.

Used by top level (strategic) management. They are designed to the individual. They let the CEO of an organisation tie-in to all levels of the organisation. They are very expensive to run and require extensive staff support to operate.

6. Knowledge Work System (KWS)

They are used by technical staff. KWS use modelling functions to convert design specifications into graphical designs. They may include computer-aided design/manufacture (CAD/CAM).

Examples: Research laboratory, Drug-proving unit.

7. Artificial Intelligence (AI)/ Expert System (ES) 1990S

AI is an application that enables the computer system to perform some of the same logical reasoning tasks as humans. An expert system is a special subclass of AI that functions as a specialist in a certain field. For example, it can provide management consultancy.

Limitation of ES: It doesn't improve its intelligence over time. One way to overcome this limitation is to use neural networks, electronic and mathematical analogs of the human brain.

Advantages of ES

The computer can store far more information than a human.

The computer does not 'forget', make silly mistakes or get drunk when it is most needed! Data can be kept up-to-date.

The expert system is available 24 hours a day and will never 'retire'.

The system can be used at a distance over a network.

> *Note:* Expert System (noun): "A computer system or program that uses artificial intelligence techniques to solve problems that ordinarily require a knowledgeable human. The method used to construct such systems, knowledge engineering, extracts a set of rules and data from an expert or experts through extensive questioning. This material is then organised in a format suitable for representation in a computer and a set of tools for inquiry, manipulation, and response is applied. While such systems do not often replace the human experts, these can serve as useful adjuncts or assistants. Among some of the successful expert systems developed are internist, a medical diagnosis tool that contains nearly 100,000 relationships between symptoms and diseases, and prospector, an aid to geologists in interpreting mineral data."

Chapter 41

Nomenclature and Classification of Homoeopathic Medicinal Plants and Animals in Respect of Botany and Zoology

It has been estimated that about two million different kinds of living organisms—**plants** and **animals**—are present in the world. Of this number, about 3,50,000 (17.5%) are plants and the remaining (82.5%) are all animals of all kinds. It is not possible to obtain a satisfactory knowledge of such a diverse multitude of plants and animals without arranging them systematically according to some definite rules or plans.

Systematics, i.e., Systematic Botany and Systematic Zoology: The term 'systematics' is interpreted more widely in a much wider sense to include the practice of classification, identification and nomenclature.

Historical Background

1. **Aristotle (384-322 B.C.)**, the Father of Biology, first indicated how animals might be grouped scientifically according to their characteristics.
2. **Theophrastus (370-285 B.C.)**, a disciple of Aristotle, is regarded as the Father of Botany. Though he made a more intelligent approach to the groupings of plants, yet he could not tide over the influence of the philosophy of his teacher.
3. **John Ray (1628-1705)**, an English philosopher and naturalist, propounded a system of plant classification. In this system, no doubt he gave much importance to the habits of plants, yet he laid the first foundation of the natural system. He was the first biologist to have a modern concept of species and to make classification of few groups of animals.
4. **Carolus Linnaeus or Carl Linne (1707-1778)**, a Swedish naturalist, is the Father of Taxonomy. He wrote about 180 books, some of which were published after his death in 1778. The three books that interest the biologists most are: (i) The *Systema Naturae*, first published in 1735, in which large number of plants and animals were classified and named according to the binomial system of nomenclature evolved by him; (ii) *Genera plantarum*—first appeared in 1737, and (iii) *Species plantarum*—first published in 1753.
5. **Cuvier (1769-1832)**, in 1829 proposed a division of animals into four branches: Vertebrata, Mollusca, Articulata and Radiata.
6. **Augustus Pyrame de Candolle (1778-1841)**, the French botanist who first proposed the term 'Taxonomy' for the classification of plants.

7. **George Bentham (1800-1884) and Joseph Dalton Hooker (1817-1911)**, two Englishmen, devise the Natural System of Classification. They jointly produced the monumentous work *Genera plantarum* (1862-1883) published in three volumes.

8. **Adolf Engler (1844-1930)**, Professor of Botany in the University of Berlin. He divided the plant kingdom into 13 Divisions.

Classification

It is the placing of a plant or animal or a group of plants and animals in categories according to a particular system and in conformity of the nomenclatural system.

Classification of Plants

1. **Systems of Classification of Plants**

   (a) ***Artificial System:*** Carolus Linnaeus, a Swedish naturalist, classified plants on the basis of number and conditions of the stamens and carpels. This System may be called Linnean System or Sexual System. The plants were principally grouped together into 24 Classes according to their number of stamens. The Classes were further divided into orders, according to their number of styles and stigmas in most cases. This system has never been recognised as an ideal system and has been superseded by the Natural Systems.

   (b) ***Natural System:*** This system is based on the natural relationships of plants. In this system, plants are primarily grouped into a few bigger divisions based only on the important morphological characters. The bigger divisions are then further classified into smaller and smaller groups.

   The natural system which is now followed in India and England was devised by **George Bentham and Joseph Dalton Hooker**. According to this system the plant kingdom is primarily divided into two subkingdoms—Cryptogamia and Phanerogamia. The phanerogamia are further grouped into two divisions—Gymnospermia and Angiospermia.

   The divisions are further divided into Classes, the Classes into Subclasses, the Subclasses into Natural orders (Families), the Families into Genera, and the Genera into Species.

   (c) ***Phylogenetic system:*** This system developed after the publication of Darwin's *Origin of Species* in 1859. This system of classification can be framed on the basis of evidences from fossil records, geographic distribution, and comparative studies of living plants including chromosomal characteristics and genetic constitution. Several phylogenetic systems have been proposed from time to time by different botanists, namely Adolf Engler and Hutchison. The Cronquist System, recently proposed jointly by Cronquist (1919-1992), an American, Zimmerman, a German, and Takhtajan, a Russian, is considered quite good. Adolf Engler divided the plant Kingdom into 13 Divisions. The 13th division is known as Embryophyta Siphanogama, which is divided into two classes—monocotyledonae and Dicotyledonae.

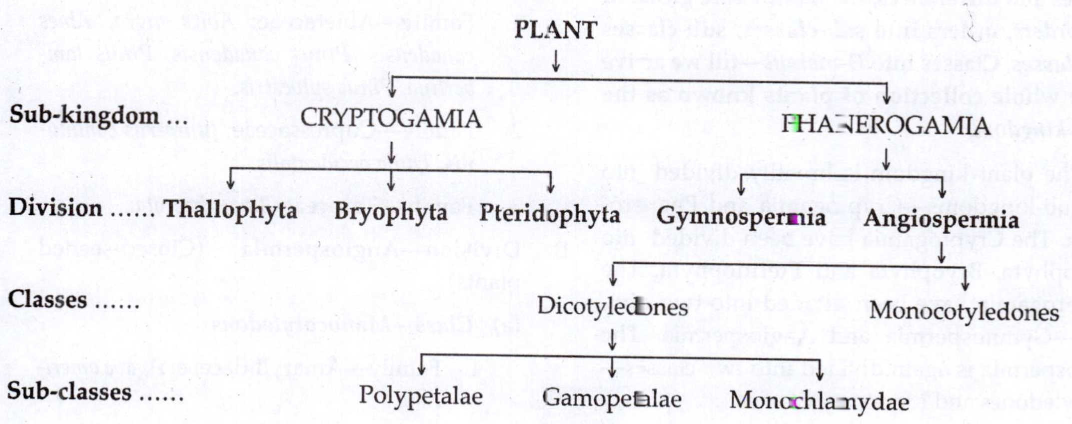

2. **Units of Classification of Plants**

(a) ***Species:*** A species may be defined as a kind of organisms which resemble one another in all their important characters apart from distinctions depending on age and sex.

Examples:

(i) All banyan trees form one species—*Ficus benghalensis;* all mango trees form one species—*Mangifera indica.* Sometimes variations are observed within the individuals of a species.

(ii) Within the species of mango, *Mangifera indica,* there are many variations, e.g., Langra, Bombai, etc. but all of them have the same specific characteristics of mango.

(b) ***Genus:*** A genus is a group of species which resemble one another in the structure of the reproductive organs.

Examples: *Rhus toxicodendron, Rhus venenata* and *Rhus aromatica.* No doubt they are different types of plants, that is, belonging to different species, but belong to the same genus 'Rhus'. Similarly, *Allium cepa* (onion) and *Allium sativa* (garlic) are of different species but belong to the same genus 'Allium'.

(c) ***Family:*** Genera (*Sing. Genus*) which are more or less similar to one another are grouped into a family. An assemblage of genera which have many characteristics in common constitutes a family.

Following the same principle of resemblances and differences, the *families* are grouped into *orders,* orders into *sub-classes,* sub-classes into *classes,* Classes into *Divisions*—till we arrive at the whole collection of plants known as the *Plant kingdom.*

The plant kingdom is broadly divided into two sub-kingdoms—Cryptogamia and Phanerogamia. The Cryptogamia have been divided into Thallophyta, Bryophyta and Pteridophyta. The Phanerogamia have been divided into two divisions—Gymnospermia and Angiospermia. The Angiospermia is again divided into two classes—Dicotyledones and Monocotyledones.

PLANT KINGDOM

↓

Cryptogamia	**Phanerogamia**
1. Thallophyta	1. Gymnospermia
2. Bryophyta	2. Angiospermia
3. Pteridophyta	(a) Dicotyledones
	(b) Monocotyledones

Systemic position of different Homoeopathic Medicines in plant kingdom are discussed next.

Sub-Kingdom: Cryptogamia

A. Thallophyta

(a) Algae, e.g., *Fucus vesiculosus*

(b) Fungi, e.g., *Agaricus emeticus, Agaricus muscarius, Agaricus phalloides, Boletus laricis (Polyporus officinalis), Boletus piniculate, Boletus satanas, Secale cornutum, Ustilago.*

(c) Lichens, e.g., *Cetraria islandica, Sticta pulmonaria, Usnea barbata.*

B. Bryophyta

Family—Polytrichaceae: *Polytrichum juniperinum.*

C. Pteridophyta

1. Family—Lycopodiaceae: *Lycopodium clavatum.*
2. Family—Equisetaceae: *Equisetum hyemale.*
3. Family—Aspidiaceae: *Filix mas.*

Sub-Kingdom: Phanerogamia

A. Division—Gymnospermia (Naked-seeded plants)

1. Family—Abietaceae: *Abies nigra, Abies canadensis, Pinus canadensis, Pinus lambertina, Pinus sylvestris.*
2. Family—Cupressaceae: *Juniperus communis, Thuja occidentalis.*
3. Family—Taxaceae: *Taxus baccata.*

B. Division—Angiospermia (Closed-seeded plants)

(a) ***Class—Monocotyledons***

1. Family—Amaryllidaceae: *Agave americana.*

2. Family—Araceae: *Arum dracontum, Arum maculatum, Arum triphyllum, Caladium seguinum, Pothos foetidus.*
3. Family—Cannabaceae: *Cannabis indica.*
4. Family—Cyperaceae: *Cyperus rotundus.*
5. Family—Gramineae: *Anthoxanthum odoratum, Avena sativa, Cynodon dactylon, Saccharum officinarum, Secale cornutum.*
6. Family—Lemnaceae: *Lemna minor.*
7. Family—Liliaceae: *Aletris farinosa, Allium cepa, Allium sativa, Aloe socotrina, Asparagus officinalis, Colchicum autumnale, Convallaria majalis, Lilium tigrinum, Paris quadrifolia, Sabadilla, Sarsaparilla, Veratrum album, Yucca filamentosa.*
8. Family—Zingiberaceae: *Curcuma longa, Zingiber officinale.*

(b) ***Class—Dicotyledons***

1. Family—Acanthaceae: *Andrographis paniculata, Hygrophila spinosa, Justicia adhatoda.*
2. Family—Amaranthaceae: *Achyranthes aspera.*
3. Family—Anacardiaceae: *Anacardium occidentale, Anacardium orientale, Comocladia dentata, Mangifera indica, Rhus toxicodendron, Rhus venenata.*
4. Family—Apocynaceae: *Alstonia scholaris, Apocynum cannabinum, Holarrhena antidysenterica, Rauwolfia serpentina, Strophanthus hispidus, Vinca minor.*
5. Family—Aristolochiaceae: *Aristolochia clematitis, Asarum canadense, Asarum europaeum.*
6. Family—Asclepiadaceae: *Calotropis gigentia, Condurango, Gymnema sylvestris, Hemidesmus indicus.*
7. Family—Berberidaceae: *Berberis vulgaris, Caulophyllum thalictroides, Podophyllum peltatum.*
8. Family—Caesalpinieae: *Caesalpinia bonducella, Cassia sophera, Janosia asoka.*
9. Family—Caprifoliaceae: *Sambucus nigra, Symphoricarpus racemosus, Viburnum opulus, Viburnum prunifolium.*
10. Family—Chenopodiaceae: *Beta vulgaris, Chenopodium anthelminticum.*
11. Family—Combretaceae: *Terminalia arjuna.*
12. Family—Compositae: *Abrotanum, Absinthium, Arnica montana, Artemisia maritima (Cina), Artemisia vulgaris, Bellis perennis, Blumea odorata, Brachyglottis repens, Calendula officinalis, Carduus marianus, Chamomilla, Cineraria maritima, Echinacea angustifolia, Erigeron canadense, Eupatorium perfoliatum, Gnaphalium uliginosum, Helianthus annus, Millefolium, Senecio aureus, Solidago virgaurea, Tanacetum vulgare, Tussilago farfara, Tussilago petasites.*
13. Family—Crassulaceae: *Bryophyllum calycinum.*
14. Family—Cruciferae: *Brassica nigra, Iberis amara, Raphenus sativus, Thlaspi bursa pastoris.*
15. Family—Cucurbitaceae: *Bryonia alba, Cephalandra indica, Colocynthis, Cucurbita pepo, Elaterium, Luffa amara, Momordica charentia, Trichosanthes dioica.*
16. Family—Ericaceae: *Chimaphila umbellata, Gaultheria procumbens, Kalmia latifolia, Ledum palustre, Rhododendron chrysanthum.*
17. Family—Euphorbiaceae: *Acalypha indica, Croton tiglium, Euphorbia corollata, Jatropha curcas, Mancinella, Mercurialis perennis, Ricinus communis.*
18. Family—Gentianaceae: *Gentiana chirata, Gentiana cruciata, Gentiana lutea, Menyanthes trifoliata.*
19. Family—Geraniaceae: *Geranium maculatum.*
20. Family—Iridaceae: *Crocus sativus, Iris versicolour.*
21. Family—Labiatae: *Coleus aromaticus, Collinsonia canadensis, Leucus aspera,*

Lycopus virginicus, Mentha piperita, Ocimum sanctum, Salvia officinalis, Teucrium marum varum, Thymus serpyllum.

22. Family—Lauraceae: *Cinnamomum zeylanicum.*

23. Family—Leguminosae: *Alfalfa, Baptisia tinctoria, Lathyrus sativus, Melilotus alba, Physostigma venenosum, Psoralea corylifolia, Ratanhia, Robinia pseudocacia, Trifolium pratense.*

24. Family—Loganiaceae: *Gelsemium sempervirens, Ignatia amara, Nux vomica, Spigelia anthelmintica.*

25. Family—Loranthaceae: *Viscum album.*

26. Family—Malvaceae: *Abelmoschus, Gossypium herbaceum.*

27. Family—Meliaceae: *Amoora rohituka, Azadirachta indica, Guarea trichiloides.*

28. Family—Moraceae: *Ficus indica, Ficus religiosa, Ficus venosa, Humulus lupulus.*

29. Family—Myristicaceae: *Myristica sebifera, Nux moschata.*

30. Family—Myrtaceae: *Eucalyptus globulus, Eugenia jambos, Myrtus communis, Syzigium jambolanum.*

31. Family—Papavaraceae: *Chelidoneum majus, Papaver somniferum* (Opium), *Sanguinaria canadensis.*

32. Family—Papilionaceae: *Desmodium gangeticum, Dolicosh, Melilotus alba, Psoralea corylifolia.*

33. Family—Passifloraceae: *Passiflora incarnata.*

34. Family—Pinaceae: *Abies canadensis.*

35. Family—Polygonaceae: *Fagopyrum esculentum, Polygonum punctatum, Rheum, Rumex crispus, Senega.*

36. Family—Primulaceae: *Anagalis arvensis, Cyclamen europaeum.*

37. Family—Ranunculaceae: *Aconitum napellus, Actaea racemosa, Actaea spicata, Adonis vernalis, Caltha palustris, Clematis erecta, Helleborus niger, Hydrastis canadensis, Paeonia officinalis, Pulsatilla nigricans, Ranunculus acris, Ranunculus bulbosus, Ranunculus flammula, Ranunculus repens, Ranunculus sceleratus, Staphysagria.*

38. Family—Rosaceae: *Crategus oxyacantha, Laurocerasus, Prunus americana, Prunus padus, Prunus spinosa.*

39. Family—Rubiaceae: *Anthocephalus kadamba, Cinchona officinalis, Coffea cruda, Ipecacuanha, Rubia tinctoria.*

40. Family—Rutaceae: *Aegle folia, Aegle marmelos, Barosma crenata, Jaborandi, Ptelea trifolia, Ruta graveolens, Xanthoxylum fraxineum.*

41. Family—Scrophulariaceae: *Chelone glabra, Digitalis purpurea, Euphresia officinalis, Gratiola officinalis, Verbascum thapsus.*

42. Family—Simaraubaceae: *Ailanthus glandulosus, Cedron.*

43. Family—Solanaceae: *Belladonna, Capsicum annum, Dulcamara amara, Duboisia myoporides, Hyoscyamus niger, Lycopersicum esculentum, Solanum carolinense, Solanum nigrum, Solanum tuberosum aegrotans, Solanum xanthocarpum, Tabacum, Withania somnifera.*

44. Family—Sterculiaceae: *Abroma augusta, Abroma radix, Sterculia accuminata.*

45. Family—Thymelaceae: *Daphne indica, Mezereum.*

46. Family—Umbelliferae: *Aethusa cynapium, Apium graveolens, Asafoetida, Branca ursina, Cicuta virosa, Conium maculatum, Erygium aquaticum, Hydrocotyle asiatica, Oenanthe crocata, Pastinaca sativa, Petroselinum, Phellandrium aquaticum, Sumbul.*

47. Family—Urticaceae: *Urtica urens.*

48. Family—Verbenaceae: *Agnus castus, Verbena officinalis, Vitex negundo.*

49. Family—Violaceae: *Viola odorata, Viola tricolor.*

50. Family—Vitaceae: *Ampelopsis quinquefolia.*

Classification of Animals

A. Systems of Classification of Animals

The biological classification may be defined as the grouping and arrangement of animals in such a way as to provide easy reference to them:

1. ***Artificial system:*** When the arrangement of animals are based only upon the place where the organisms live or upon their forms and structures, without any regard to relationship that may exist.
2. ***Natural system:*** This is an arrangement of animals considering the degree of relationship and have evolved from the living matter first developed upon this earth.
3. ***Phylogenetic system:*** This is an arrangement of animals which have endeavoured to establish the genetic and ancestral relationship of the biological objects.

B. Units of Classification of Animals

1. ***Species:*** It is the basic or smallest unit. It is a group of individual animals that constantly resemble each other to a greater degree than members of other groups.

Examples: The common bird, House Sparrow—wherever they are found—form one species, *Passer domesticus;* all tigers form the species *Panthera tigris.*

2. ***Genus:*** It is a group of species which resemble one another on the basis of their special body features.

Examples: *Tarentula cubensis* and *Tarentula hispanica.* No doubt they are different types of spiders, that is, belonging to different species, but both belong to the same genus 'Tarentula'. Similarly, *Aranea avicularis, Aranea diadema* and *Aranea scinencia* are of different species but belong to the same genus, 'Aranea.'

3. ***Family:*** A few genera (*sing.* Genus) which are more or less similar are grouped together to constitute a family. A number of families may form a super-family.

Following the same principle of resemblances and differences, the *families* are grouped into *orders,* Orders into *sub-classes,* Sub-classes into *Classes,* Classes into *Phyllum*—till we arrive at the whole collection of animals, known as the ***Animal kingdom.***

Non-Vertebrate

A. Phyllum—Arthropoda

1. Class: Crustacea (L. *rusta,* a hard shell) e.g., *Armadillo officinarum, Astacus fluviatilis, Homarus*
2. Class: Insecta (L. *Insectum,* having been cut into) e.g., *Apis mellifica, Blatta americana, Blatta orientalis, Bombyx chrysorrhoea, Bombyx processionae, Cantharis, Chenopodium glauci, Cimex lactularius, Coccinella indica (Coccus cacti), Coccinella septempunctata, Culex musca, Doryphora decemlineata, Formica rufa, Pediculus capitis, Pulex irritans, Vespa crabro.*
3. Class: Arachnida (G. *Arachne,* Spider; *Oid,* like) e.g., *Aranea avicularis, Aranea diadema, Aranea scinencia, Aranea tela, Cetruroides elegans, Latrodectus hasselti, Latrodectus katipo, Latrodectus mactans, Limulus (Xiphusura americana), Mygale lasiodora, Scorpio europus, Tarentula cubensis, Tarentula hispanica, Theridion curassavicum, Trombidium.*
4. Class: Myriapoda (G. *Myriad,* ten thousand; *podos,* foot) e.g., *Millepedes (Oniscus asellus).*

B. Phyllum—Porifera

Class: Calcarea or Calcispongiae e.g., *Badiaga, Spongia tosta.*

C. Phyllum—Coelenterata

1. Class: Anthozoa e.g., *Corallium rubrum.*
2. Class: Scyphozoa e.g., *Aurelia medusa.*
3. Class: Hydrozoa e.g., *Physalia.*

D. Phyllum—Annelida

Class: Hirudinea (L. *Hirudo,* Leech) e.g., *Sanguisuga officinalis.*

E. Phyllum—Mollusca

1. Class: Cephalopoda (G. *Kehalo,* head; *podos,* foot) e.g., *Sepia.*
2. Class: Gastropoda (G. *Gastros,* stomach; podos, foot) e.g., *Helix tosta, Murex purpurea.*

3. Class: Bivalvia e.g., *Calcarea calcinata, Pecten.*

F. **Phyllum — Echinodermata**

Class: Astroidea (G. *Aster*, star; *oidos*, form) e.g., *Asterias rubens* (Starfish).

Vertebrates

1. Class: Osteichthes (Bony fishes) e.g., *Gadus lata, Gadus morrhua, Pyrara.*
2. Class: Amphibia e.g., *Bufo rana.*
3. Class: Reptila e.g., *Ancistrodon contortrix, Bungarus fasciatus, Chelone, Crotalus horridus, Elaps corallinus, Lacerta agilis, Lachesis lanciolatus, Lochesis trigonocephalus, Naja tripudians, Toxicophis, Vipera berus.*
4. Class: Aves (Bird) e.g., *Calcarea ova testa (ova testa), Ovi gallinae pellicula.*
5. Class: Mammalia e.g., *Carbo animalis, Castoreum, Cervus braziliens, Castor equi, Fel piscinum, Fel tauri, Hippomanes, Ingluvin, Lecithin, Mephitis mephitica, Moschus moschiferus, Oleum animale, Oophorinum, Orchitinum, Sphingurus maritini, Typho-febrinum, Vulpis hepar, Vulpis pulmo.*

Nomenclature

Nomenclature or naming of plants and animals is a part of Taxonomy. It deals with the determination of the correct name of a plant or an animal. Botanical and zoological nomenclatures are in Latin. The reason why Latin is used and not Greek, Sanskrit or Hebrew is because Latin was the written language of all branches of learning in all the developed countries even about a century ago.

Binomial system of nomenclature—The scientific name of a plant or animal consists of two parts—the first part refers to the genus and the second part refers to the species, e.g., the scientific name of honey-bee is *Apis mellifica,* and of the tulsi *Ocimum sanctum*. The system of giving animals or plants a name consisting of two parts or words is called the **binomial system of nomenclature**. The great Swedish botanist Linnaeus is responsible for adopting this system.

In the binomial system, the first name or the generic name is a substantive (noun), nominative case and singular number; the name is usually taken from Greek or Latin language, e.g., *Rhus, Aloe, Apis.*

The second part—the specific epithet—is usually an adjective modifying the substantive; it must agree in gender with the generic name; sometimes the specific names are not common adjectives, but they may be proper nouns, name of a person or name of a country, e.g., *Acalypha indica, Blatta americana, Hydrastis canadensis, Hura brasiliensis.* By means of the binomial nomenclature all plants and animals are known by people in all countries.

By convention, generic and specific names are written in italics, while the names of families, orders, classes, etc. are not so written.

Previously the first letter of a specific name—which was after a person or a country—was in capital. According to the **International Codes of Nomenclature**, the first letter of such specific epithets should now be in small letter, e.g., *Cephalandra indica*—and not Cephalandra Indica.

The name of each species is to be followed by the name of the author who first described the species, e.g., *Cinchona officinalis* Linn or *Rhus toxicodendron* Mitch.

International Codes of Botanical and Zoological nomenclature—In view of the large number of plants and animals, and also in the absence of suitable agencies of publication in earlier times, often the same plant or animal was given two or more different names by the scientists of different countries, such names may be called **Synonyms**; or, the same name was given to two or more different plants or animals, such names may be called **Homonyms**. As a result there had been some confusion with regard to the names of many plants and animals. Biologists felt the need for framing special laws for the correct naming of plants and animals. The **International Codes of Zoological Nomenclature** was first accepted in the International Zoological Congress held in 1901 and published in 1905. After the 5th International Botanical Congress held in 1930, the **International Codes of Botanical Nomenclature** was framed and published in 1935. Later, these Codes have been discussed at the successive sessions of the International Zoological Congress and at the International Botanical Congress every four or five years changes in the laws of nomenclature, wherever felt necessary, have been made.

Some Botanical Terms Used

Common Name

Vernacular or common names are made up of words from native language of the country or the region and varies in different countries or regions of same country, e.g., Portuguese, Spanish, English, Hindi, Bangali, Kannada etc

Synonyms

A name rejected due to misuse or difference in taxonomic judgement is called synonym:

1. Taxonomic ('Facultative') synonym: names for contaxic taxa, based on different types.
2. Nomenclatural ('Obligate') synonym: two or more names based on one type, e.g., Atropa belladonna: A. lethalis, Belladonna baccifera, B. trichotoma, S. fluriosum, Azadirachta indica: M. azadirachta

Hyponyms

A name not assignable to a definable taxon (by lack of adequate circumscription or type; a genus without species etc). A name is rejected when the natural group to which it applies is undetermined, e.g., Adodendrum Necker and Calesian Adams are examples of generic hyponyms and *Gentiana hybrida* Raf. and *Lechea furfurca* Raf. of specific hyponyms.

Mercurialis perennis (Dogs mercury), *Lobelia inflata* (Indian tobacco) donot actually explain the nature of the plant.

Typonyms

A name based on the same type as another name and thus an illegitimate superfluous name (cf. isonym; metonym).

A name is rejected when there is an older valid name based on the same type. [The specific epithet *Asplenium vincentis* given by Herman Christ in 1897 is a typonym of *Asplenium guildangii* given by G. S. Jenman to the same species in 1894]

Examples:

1. *Miegia pers.* Syn 1:101(1805), is a typonym of *Arundinaria michx.* Fl. Bor. Am. 1 : 73 (1803) both being based on the same species.
2. *Asplenium vincentis* Christ, Bot. Jahrb. 24 : 109 (1897), is a typonym of *A. guildangii* Jenm. Gard Chron. III. 15 : 70 (1894), both being based on H. H. Smith's no. 1346 from St. Vincent.

Invalid Names

Old names changed with new nomenclature are considered as invalid names.

Examples:

1. *Banksia prostrata* became *Banksia gardneri*.
2. *Hibiscus rhodopetalus* became *Abelmoschus moschatus*.

Advantages/Disadvantages of Commercial Name

– Local name used by traders/cultivators/collectors who are illiterate

– Different plants known by same names at different locations

– Different species of Cinchona are known as Cinchona bark irrespective of species

– Different species of Aloes with different composition known in commerce as Aloe

Demerits of Common Names

1. More than one name used in one place.
2. Two or more names in different languages.
3. The same name used for different species of plants.
4. They may be quite indefinite.
5. They are restricted to the people of one language or even one section of the country.
6. They are not regulated by any constituted authority.
7. They are too vague for scientific usage.
8. A person will have to learn many sets of names of a single plant or animal.

Advantages of Scientific or Botanical Names

Some points on the advantages of scientific names are:

1. It is recognised and documented worldwide by international rules of nomenclature.
2. The names are same in any language.

3. The names are uniformly binominal, i.e., consisting of two parts, one generic name and one specific name.
4. Scientific names greatest advantage is its exactness.
5. Scientific names may be fairly descriptive but in Latin. Scientists around the world are familiar with Latin, the universal language.

Disadvantages of Scientific or Botanical Names

1. They are more difficult to remember and pronounce the Latin format.
2. The name is unfamiliar, not as commonly known.

Advantage of Using Scientific Name instead of Common Names

There is no confusion as to what people are referring to. Many common names vary from region to region and country to country. The use of a single standard Latin name for each species avoids any chance of confusion.

Anomalies and Erros in the Nomenclature of Homoeopathic Medicines

The errors, anomalies, irresponsibility, irregularities, negligence, ignorance, by whatever name may we call it, the fact is that homoeopathic authors, teachers and publishers have committed and allowed to exist serious defects in the nomenclature of homoeopathic medicines.

The leading manufacturing companies, the authors and teachers of the subject, never brought this matter to the notice and attention of the profession. The most painful thing is that three important institutions such as Homoeopathy Pharmacopoeia Laboratory (HPL), Ghaziabad, Central Council of Research in Homoeopathy (CCRH) and Homoeopathic Pharmacopoeia Committee (HPC) could have solved the problem better but they did not attempt or is it they could not solve or they did not consider it important. It is not very difficult to understand the gravity of such irregularities. The normal and standard thing would have been to use the same nomenclature or name of the drug which the earlier authors had used.

The errors and anomalies related to the names of the medicines can be grouped as:

A. Medicines described under Incomplete Names

Hahnemann's Mat Med Pura and The Chronic Diseases, Their Peculiar Nature and Homoeopathic Cure are no exceptions to these anomalies and lack of uniformity in nomenclature of medicines:

(i) **Hahnemann's *Mat. Med. Pura.*** has Arsenicum (Vol. I, p. 113), Digitalis (Vol. I, p. 550), Guaiacum (Vol. I, p. 619), Manganum aceticum (Vol. II, p. 114) but the same has been written in his ***The Chronic Diseases*** respectively as Arsenicum album, Digitalis purpurea, Guajacum, Manganum.

Unfortunately, the contents of *The Chronic Diseases* (p. iv) by Hahneman also is not in alphabetical order, e.g., Phosphorus is mentioned before Phosphoricum acidum.

The contents of Vol. I of Mat Med Pura have incomplete names, like Aconitum, Arnica, Bryonia, Cannabis, Capsicum, Cicuta, Cyclamen, Drosera, Euphrasia, Hyoscyamus, but they are written in complete form in the text of the same book. Similarly, in Vol. 1, some medicines are described under their complete names, but in some other cases the complete names are given underneath the heading of incomplete names. Examples of such medicines are Ledum (p. 43), Moschus (p. 200), Oleander (p. 270), Opium (p. 284), Pulsatilla (p. 344), Rhus (p. 400), Sambucus (p. 452), Sarsaparilla (p. 459), Scilla (p. 467), Spigelia (p. 478), Spongia (p. 508), Staphysagria (p. 554), Stramonium (p. 586), Taraxacum (p. 638), Thuja (p. 649) and Verbascum (p. 702).

(ii) **Constantine Hering's *The Guiding Symptoms*** has Aconitum napellus (Vol. I, p. 28), Ambra grisea (Vol. I, p. 211), Apis (Vol. I, p. 415), Borax (Vol. II, p. 473), Cantharides (Vol. III, p. 307), Guaiacum (Vol. V, p. 488), Silicea (Vol. IX, p. 362), but the same has been written in his ***Condensed Mat. Med.*** respectively as Aconitum (p. 9), Apis mellifica (p. 95), Borax veneta (p. 201), Cantharis (p. 262), Guajacum (p. 451), Silicea (p. 682).

(iii) **Boger's *Boenninghausen's Characteristics and Repertory*** has Aconite (p. 1 and 1154), Ambra (p. 6 and 1156), Argentum metallicum (p. 15 and 1160), Arsenicum (p. 19 and 1162), Aurum (p. 23

and 1163), Cannabis (p. 37 and 1170), Cicuta virosa (p. 49 and 1176), Glonoin (p. 70; the medicine is not mentioned in the list of concordances), Guaiacum (p. 73 and 1186), Hepar sulphuris calcareum (p. 75 and 1188; mark the 'ph' in sulphuris), Iodum (p. 81), but Iodium on p. 1190, Marum (p. 101 and 1199), Mercurius (p. 103 and 1200), Paris quadrifolia (p. 124 and 1207), Ruta graveolens (p. 147 and 1214), Silicea (p. 100 and 1220), Scilla (p. 153 and 1217) but the same has been written in his **Boenninghausen's** ***Therapeutic Pocket Book*** respectively as Aconitum (p. 322), Ambra grisea (p. 330), Argentum (p. 338), Ars. album (p. 342), Aurum foliatum (p. 346), Cannabis indica (p. 362), Cicuta (p. 374), Glonoine (p. 395), Guaiacum (p. 398), Hepar sulfuris calcareum (p. 400; mark 'f' in sulfuris), Iodium (p. 403), Marum verum (p. 420), Merc. vivus (p. 421), Paris (p. 434), Ruta (p. 450), Silicea (p. 462), Squilla (p. 465).

(iv) **Boenninghausen's** ***Characteristics and Repertory*** has as Anacardium (p. 9), Arsenicum (p. 19), Aurum (p. 23), Baryta carbonica (p. 23), Belladonna (p. 25), Bovista (p. 29), Dulcamara (p. 63), Euphorbium (p. 65), Guaiacum (p. 73), Magnesiamuriatica (p. 100), Mercurius (p. 103), Mezereum (p. 107), Rhododendron (p. 144), Sarsaparilla (p. 153), Senega (p. 157), Silicea (p. 160), Strontium (p. 169) was written in his *Repertory of Antipsorics* respectively as Semecarpus anacardium, Arsenicum album, Aurum foliatum, Baryta, Atropa belladonna, Lycoperdon bovista, Solanum dulcamara, Euphorbia officinarum, Guaiacum officinale, Magnesium muriate, Mercurius vivus, Daphne mezereum, Rhododendron chrysanthemum, Smilax sarsaparilla, Polygala senega, Silicea terra and Strontiana carbonica.

B. Same Medicine described under Different Names

The same medicines have been described under different names by different authors of Materia Medicas and Pharmacopoeias.

Examples in Materia Medica

(i) **Cenchris contortrix** of J. H. Clarke's Dictionary (Vol. 1, p. 446), Kent's Repertory and Boericke's Mat. Med., is named Agkistrodon contortrix in Allen's Encyclopedia (Vol. 10. p. 281).

(ii) **Coca** of Allen's Encyclopedia (Vol. 3, p. 369 & Vol. 10, p. 470) and J. H. Clarke's Dictionary (Vol. 1, p. 539) is Erythroxylon coca in Hering's Guiding Symptoms (Vol. 4, p. 244).

(iii) **Daphne indica** of J. H. Clarke's Dictionary (Vol. 1, p. 655) is Daphne odora in Hering's Guiding Symptoms (Vol. 5, p. 80).

(iv) **Eriodictyon californicum** of Allen's Encyclopedia (Vol. 4, p. 218) is Eriodictyon glutinosum in J. H. Clarke's Dictionary (Vol. 1, p. 172).

(v) **Fel bovis** of A. C. Blackwood's Mat. Med. (p. 345) is Fel tauri in T. F. Allen's Encyclopedia (Vol. 4, p. 302), Boericke's Mat. Med. (p. 282) and J. H. Clarke's Dictionary (Vol. 1, p. 752).

(vi) **Galium** of J. H. Clarke's Dictionary (Vol. 1, p. 795) is Galium aparine in Hale's New Remedies (Vol. 1, p. 317).

(vii) **Illicium anisatum** of J. H. Clarke's Dictionary (Vol. 2, p. 16) is named Illicium in Allen's Encyclopedia (Vol. 5, p. 91) and Boericke's Mat. Med. (p. 344) but is Anisum stellatum in Hering's Guiding Symptoms (Vol. 1, p. 334).

(viii) **Jambos eugenia** of Hering's Guiding Symptoms (Vol. 6, p. 291) is Eugenia jambos in Allen's Encyclopedia (Vol. 4, p. 231) and also in J. H. Clarke's Dictionary (Vol. 1, p. 722).

(ix) **Pothos foetidus** of Allen's Encyclopedia (Vol. 8, p. 154) has become Ictodes foetida in J. H. Clarke's Dictionary (Vol. 3, p. 4). There are endless examples but no record of any Homoeopathic teacher or author trying to correct it.

(x) **Prunus virginiana** in J. H. Clarke's A Dictionary of Practical Materia Medica, (Vol. 3, p. 891) is describe under E. M. Hale [New Remedies Vol. 1, p.177] it as Cerasus virginiana.

(xi) **Viola tricolor** in J. H. Clarke's Dictionary (Vol. 3, p. 1550) is described as Jacea in Hering's Guiding Symptoms (Vol. 7, p. 285).

Examples in Pharmacopoeias

Pharmacopoeias are standard books which are supposed to regularise and correct the anomalies but we find that such anomalies are abundant in pharmacopoeias.

(i) **Arctium lappa:** HPUS (1964, p. 360) describes it as Lappa major but B & T's AHP (1920) as Arctium lappa on p. 91 and E. P. Anshutz in Sexual Ills and Diseases, p. 110 I writes it as Lappa officinalis.

(ii) **Aristolochia serpentaria** of American Homoeopathic Dispensatory (p. 202) and HPUS (1964, p. 122) is only Serpentaria in Schwabe's Pharmacopoeia Homoeopathica Polyglotta and in the H.P.U.S of 1882 (p. 233).

(iii) **Branca ursina** in HPUS, 6th edition, (1941, p. 163), 7th edition (1964, p. 163) and 8th edition (1979 and 1981), p. 142, Boericke & Tafel's AHP, 5th edition (1896), p. 127, 6th edition (1899), p. 127, 7th edition (1904), p. 127, 9th edition (1920), p. 127 and 10th edition (1928), p. 127, in M. Bhattacharya's Pharmacopoeia, 12th & 13th editions p. 131 and 14th edition p. 113, Dr. N. Nundie's A Short Sketch of States Homoeopathic Pharmacopoeia p. 35 is described as Branca ursina, but BHP (1882, p. 375) and Jahr & Hempel's New Pharmacopoeia (1850), p. 119 describe as Heracleum spondylium. As if these were not enough, American Homoeopathic Dispensatory described it as Acanthus mollis on p. 118 but as Heracleum spondylium on p. 395 and Willmar Schwabe's Pharmacopoeia Homoeopathica Polyglotta p. 35 as Acanthus mollis and as Heracleum spondylium on p. 194. M. Bhattacharya's Pharmaceutists Manual or Pharmacopoeia, 10th edition (1944) also describes it twice under two names of Branca ursina on p. 241 and Heracleum spondylium on p. 435.

(iv) **Kousso** is described on p. 212 of Willmar Schwabe's Pharmacopoeia Homoeopathica Polyglotta, on p. 437 of Theo. D. William's The American Homoeopathic Dispensatory and as Koosso in HPUS (1882) p. 167, but it is described as Brayera anthelmintica on p. 447 of M. Bhattacharya's Pharmacopoeia, 14th edition, on p. 242 of its 10th edition, on p. 127 of B & T's AHP, 9th edition.

(v) **Linaria vulgaris** of Aurand's Pharmacological and Botanical Mat. Med. (p. 233), The Homoeopathic Pharmacopoeia of the United States (1964, p. 365), M. Bhattacharya's Pharmacopoeia (14th edition, p. 270) and Schwabe's Pharmacopoeia Homoeopathica Polyglotta (p. 220) is described as Antirrhinum linarium in Boericke & Tafel's AHP (1920, p. 868) and in American Homoeo. Dispensatory (p. 202).

(vi) **Psorinum** in AHP (1920, p. 380) is described as Psorinum in HPUS (1882, p. 216).

(vii) HPUS (1882, p. 224) describes as **Rumex obtusifolius** which is described as Lapathum acutum in Boericke & Tafel's AHP (1904, p. 286), Willmar Schwabe's Pharmacopoeia Homoeopathica Polyglotta (p. 21) and M. Bhattacharya's Pharmaceutists Manual (p. 488).

(viii) **Thymus serpyllum** in HPUS (1964, p. 156), was described as Thymus in AHP (1920, p. 439) and in American Homoeopatic Dispensatory (p. 620) but as Serpyllum in Schwabe's Pharmacopoeia Homoeopathica Polyglotta (p. 518).

C. Same Medicine described under Different Names in the same Book

Many authors or editors of materia medica and pharmacopoeia have described the same medicine in the same book under different names indifferent places. The impression of the innocent reader is that he is reading not one but more than one medicine.

Examples in Materia Medica

(i) **Wm. Boericke's A Manual of Homoeopathic Mat. Med.:**

Physalis solanum is written on p. 511 as Physalis solanum vesicarium, as only Solanum vesicarium on p. 598, but only as Physalis on p. 1001 in the Therapeutic Index under Enuresis, in Repertory of Urinary System under rubric acid (p. 818) and of Face, under rubric muscles, sub-rubric, Paralysis (p. 745).

Paullinia sorbilis under this name in Boericke's same Mat. Met. on p. 499 in the Repertory of Migraine, p. 702, is mentioned by its common name of Guarana.

Antimonium tartaricum is written on p. 58 and in the Repertory but written as Tartar emetic on p. 997 and 999 in the chapter on Therapeutic Index.

(ii) **E. M. Hale in his Mat. Med. and Special Therapeutics of the New Remedies:** Paullinia sorbilis described on p. 484 but adds more symptoms in it on p. 697 under its common name of Guarana.

(iii) **M. E. Douglas's Characteristics of the Homoeopathic Mat. Med.:** The symptoms of Abrotanum has been described on p.10, and its symptoms have been again described as Artemisia abrotanum on p. 122.

The symptoms of Actaea racemosa have been described on p. 21 and again as Cimicifuga on p. 283 and so on.

(iv) **M. E. Douglas's Pearls of Homoeopathy:** The symptoms of Abrotanum has been described on (p. 1) and also under Artemisia abrotanum (p. 36), symptoms of Chininum sulphuricum on p. 74 and again Quinia sulphate on p. 19.

Examples in Pharmacopoeias

(i) **M. Bhattacharya's Pharmaceutists' Manual** (10th Ed., 1944) describes as Thymus serpyllum on p. 755 and as Serpyllum on p. 704; as Guarana on p. 420 and as Paullinia sorbillis on p. 602.

It describes Cacao on p. 246 and again under its scientific name Erythroxylon coca on p. 369, Asoka on p. 211 and again Jonosia asoka on p. 458, Cyperus rotundus on p. 341 and again by its Bangla common name Mutha on p. 552.

The 12th, and 13th editions include both Cyperus rotundus (p. 204) and also Mutha (p. 360) and so does its latest 14th edition (1980) on p. 177 and on p. 304. There are many such examples.

(ii) **Willmar Schwabe's Pharmacopoeia Homoeopathica Polyglotta** describes Acanthus mollis on p. 34 and under its synonym Heracleum spondylium on p. 194.

This is the condition of the Pharmacopoeia which is the court of last appeal in the matters of standardisation of drugs, its preparation, nomenclature, identification, etc.

D. One and the same Medicine described as two Medicines or two different Medicines described as one and the same

Some names of medicines are stated as synonyms by a few authors while others describe them as different medicines. It is difficult to consider them as different medicines but it is more difficult to dismiss them as only one or as synonyms to each other.

Rhus radicans has been stated as a synonym of Rhus toxicodendron in HPUS, 6th (1941), 7th (1964) and 8th (1979) editions, in the HPI, Vol. 1 (1971), p. 166, M. Bhattacharya's The Pharmacopoeia, 12th (1962), 13th (1970) and 14th (1980) editions, in Willmar Schwabe's Pharmacopoeia Homoeopathica Polyglotta, p. 302, and in Carrol Dunham's Lectures on Hom. Mat. Med, Vol. 1, p. 121. But American Hom. Dispensatory (p. 571) mentions it as Synonym of Rhus tox. and as separate medicines. They are described as separate medicines also in BHP(1882), p. 261, Boericke and Tafel's AHP, 6th ed. (1899), p. 390, 7th edition (1904), p. 390, 9th ed. (1920), p. 390, 10th ed. (1928), p. 390 and in M. Bhattacharya's The Pharmaceutics Manual or Pharmacopoeia, 10th ed., p. 667.

The same errors were present in the Repertories and Mat. Med. Jahr's Symptom en Codex, Vol. 2, serial no. 216, p. 645, William D. Gentry's The Concordance Repertory, Vol. 5, p. xii, William Boericke's A Pocket Manual of Mat. Med., p. 555, Richard Hughes A Cyclopaedia of Drug Pathogenesy, Vol. 3, p. 720 and C. Hering's Analytical Repertory of the Symptoms of the Mind, p. 63.

Cinchona rubra is mentioned as a separate medicine in the price list of 1981 (p. 32) of Hahnemann Publishing Co., Boericke & Tafel's catalogue and price list of 1951 (p. 19) and in J. H. Clarke's The Prescriber, but HPUS of 1964 (p. 213), of 1981 (p.196) and The Amer. Hom. Dispensatory (p. 299) mention it as a synonym of Cinchona officinalis or China.

Similarly, **Tinctura acris sine kali** has been described by HPUS of 1964 (p. 193) and the American Hom. Dispensatory (p. 291) as a synonym of Causticum while the New Homoeopathic Pharmacopoeia of Buchner, Gruner and Jahr compiled by C. J. Hempel (1850) and Homoeopathic Pharmacopoeïa and Posology by C. J. Hempel (p. 233) described its preparation separately from Causticum (p. 211) and Pharmacopoeia Homoeopathica of F. F. Quin (1834), in Latin, describes the preparation of Causticum (p. 63) and of Tinctura acris sine kali (p. 138) separately and independently.

E. The same Medicine described under different names in different Editions of the same Book

M. Bhattacharya's *Pharmaceutics Manual* or *Pharmacopoeia* (10th ed., 1944) describes Leucas aspera on p. 503, but its 14th edition describes it under its common name (in Sanskrit and Bangla) of Drone on p. 183, but the book Manual of Mat. Med. (Vol. 3, p. 2262) by the same publisher describes the symptomatology, rather clinical indications, under the name of Leucas aspera.

M. Bhattacharya & Co.'s *Pharmacopoeia,* 10th edition, describes Embelica on p. 358, but on p. 54 in the 14th edition of the same book, the correct Latin name has been changed to its Bangla common name Amloki.

F. Different spellings for same name

Another painful aspect of the nomenclature of homoeopathic medicines is that different spellings for the same name have been used by different authors, by the same author in his different books or in his same book.

(i) **Amyl nitrosum** in HPUS (1964, p. 101) and Boericke's Mat. Med. (p. 47), is Amyl nitris in A. L. Blackwood's *Mat. Med.* (p. 119) is is Amyl nitrit in *Allen's Encyclopedia* (Vol. 1, p. 309), in Cowperthwaite's *A Text book of Mat. Med.* (p. 49) and Hale's *Mat. Med.* and *Special Therapeutics* of the New Remedies (Vol. 1, p. 20), Amylenum nitrosum in Hering's *Guiding Symptoms* (Vol. 1, p. 269), Clarke's *Dictionary of Mat. Med.* (Vol. 1, p. 98) and Amyl nitritum in Wm. Burt's *Physiological Mat. Med.* (p. 64).

(ii) **Aranea diadema** in Clarke's Dictionary (Vol. 1, p. 152), Allen's *Encyclopedia* (Vol. 1, p. 433), and Hughes *Cyclopaedia of Drug Pathogenesy* (Vol. 1, p. 330) is Diadema aranea in *Hering's Guiding Symptoms* (Vol. 5, p. 88).

(iii) **Cobaltum** in Clarke's Dictionary (Vol. 1, p. 537), T. F. Allen's Encyclopedia (Vol. 3, p.361) and H. C. Allen's Keynotes (p. 310) is Kobaltum in Hering's Guiding Symptoms (Vol. 6, p. 489), and Lippe's Text book of Mat. Med. (p. 342).

(iv) **Condurango** in Hering's Analytical Repertory (p. 59), Blackwood's Mat. Med. (p. 204) is Cundurango in Hering's Guiding Symptoms (Vol. 5, p. 1), Clarke's Dictionary (Vol. 1, p. 630), T. F. Allen's Encyclopedia (Vol. 4, p. 1; Vol. 10, p. 499) and Hughes Cyclopaedia of Drug Pathogenesy (Vol. 2, p. 463).

(v) **Copaiva** in Allen's Encyclopedia (Vol. 3, p. 554; Vol. 10, p. 491), Hering's Guiding Symptoms (Vol. 4, p. 447), Clarke's Dictionary (Vol. 1, p. 592), Hughes Cyclopaedia of Drug Pathogenesy (Vol. 2, p. 395) is Copaivae in Jahr's Symptomen Codex (Vol. 1, p. 602) and is Copaiba in, Clarke's The Prescriber, H. C. Allen's Keynotes (p. 310), Richard Hughes A Manual of Pharmacodynamics (p. 465) and Blackwood's Mat. Med. (p. 266).

(vi) **Cubeba** in Lippe's Key notes and Red Line Symptoms of the Mat. Med. (p. 317) and in A. L. Blackwood's Mat. Med., Therapeutics and Pharmacology (p. 273) is Cubebae in Lippe's Text book of Mat. Med. (p. 199), C. J. Hempel's Mat. Med. (Vol. 2, p. 35), and Jahr's Symptomen Codex (Vol. 1, p. 626).

(vii) **Fuchsin** in T. F. Allen's Encyclopedia (Vol. 10, p. 529) is Fuschisinum in Hughes

Cyclopaedia of Drug Pathogenesy (Vol. 4, p. 485), Fuchsine in M. Bhattacharya's Mat. Med. (Vol. 3, p. 2178), Fuchina in Wm. Boericke's Mat. Med. (p. 166) and Fuchsina on p. 296 of the same book.

(viii) **Guaiacum** in Hahnemann's Mat. Med. Pura (Vol.1, p. 619), Hering's Guiding Symptoms (Vol. 5, p. 488) and Allen's Keynotes (p.312) is Guajacum in Hahnemann's Chronic Diseases (Vol. 1, p. 755).

(ix) **Hekla lava** in C. B. Knerr's Repertory, Hering's Guiding Symptoms (Vol. 5, p. 525) and Hering's Analytical Repertory (p. 61) is Hecla in Clarke's Dictionary (Vol. 1, p. 870) and H. C. Allen's Keynotes (p. 312).

(x) **Iodum** in Hughes Cyclopaedia (Vol. 2, p. 691), Allen's Encyclopedia (Vol. 5, p. 119), Hering's Condensed Mat. Med. (p. 498) and Hering's Guiding Symptoms (Vol. 6, p. 205) is Iodium in Clarke's Dictionary (Vol. 2, p. 127), Hahnemann's Chronic Diseases (Vol.1, p.783), Allen's Keynotes (p. 146), Hering's Condensed Mat. Med. (p. 420, 176) and Hering's Guiding Symptoms (Vol. 4, p. 202), is Iodine in Allen's Keynotes (p. 312) but is Jodum in C. J. Hempel's Mat. Med. (Vol. 2, p. 217) and Hering's Guiding Symptoms (Vol. 4, p. 290).

(xi) **Kreasotum** in Clarke's The Prescriber, C. J. Hempel's Mat. Med. (Vol. 2, p. 267) is Creosotum in P. P. Well's Intermittent Fever (p. 45) and in Lippe's Text book of Mat. Med. (p.188), is Kreosotum in Clarke's Dictionary (Vol. 2, p.176), Hering's Guiding Symptoms (Vol. 6, p. 495) and Allen's Keynotes (pp. 155, 313) but is Kreasota in A. Teste's The Homoeo. Mat. Med. (pp. 119-124).

(xii) **Silicea** in Allen's Encyclopedia Vol. 9, p. 1) and Hering's Analytical Repertory, is Silica in Clarke's Dictionary (Vol. 3, p. 1175) and Hering's Guiding Symptoms (Vol. 9, p. 362)

(xiii) **Sulphur** in Hughes Cyclopaedia of Drug Pathogenesy (Vol. 4, p. 171), Hering's Guiding Symptoms (Vol.10, p. 96) and H.C. Allen's Keynotes (p. 317) is Sulfur in Allen's Encyclopedia (Vol. 9, p. 276).

(xiv) **Thuja** in Hering's Guiding Symptoms (Vol. 10, p. 30-), Hering's Condensed Mat. Med. (p. 105), Allen's Encyclopedia (Vol. 9, p. 596), H.C. Allen's Keynotes (p. 318), Clarke's Dictionary (Vol. 3, p. 1419) is Thuya in Knerr's Repertory, Hering's Analytical Repertory (p. 64), and Hering's Guiding Symptoms (vol. 4, p. 213). Wm. Boericke in his Mat. Med. used both the spellings.

G. Additions and Omissions of Medicines

There are many medicines which were described in the earlier editions of a pharmacopoeia but have been omitted in its later editions. This was done in most of the pharmacopoeias which had more than one edition.

M. Bhattacharya's Pharmaceutics Manual, 10th edition (1944) contained 1193 medicines (with many double entries) but the 12th, 13th and 14th editions has 744 medicines only.

Chapter 42

Anomalies or Errors Exist in Parts used in Homoeopathic Pharmacy

The worst and most harmful of the anomalies relate to gross difference in the statement of the part of the plant, used in preparation of the medicine.

It is well-known that the different parts of the same plant will produce different kinds of action. There are examples where different same plant—whether used as medicine or food—have almost diametrically opposite effects.

There is hardly any plant in the world whose seed, leaves, bark, or fruits do not differ in their actions; e.g.,

1. **Solanum tuberosum (*Potato*):** Potato contains more or less 100% carbohydrate while its leaves contain more or less 100% protein.
2. **Cassia fistula (*Bandar-lathi*):** Pulp, root-bark, seeds and leaves possess purgative properties, roots act as purgative, tonic and febrifuge and fruit is cathartic.
3. **Dolichos pruriens (*Mucana*):** Is a nerve tonic and diuretic, seeds are astringent, anthelmintic and hairs are locally stimulant and vesicant.

Thus, it is evident that whatever part of the plant has been used in the proving of a medicine, the same part should be used in the manufacture of the medicine and used in the treatment of patients. The properties, symptoms or action of the drug substance in the proving during treatment can never be different. This is why, in all the monographs of the proving, the authors have mentioned *"the part of the plant from which the medicine was prepared for proving"*. Even if different parts of a plant possess same chemical properties or produce same symptoms, the intensity of the symptom and its modification etc. will vary and does vary.

If we compare the monographs of proving, various materia medicas, and pharmacopoeias we can see that there are serious differences about the instructions regarding, *"the part used"* in the preparation of medicine.

The following abbreviations have been used:

W.S.P.	=	Willmar Schwabes pharma
A.E.	=	Allen's Encyclopaedia
A.D.	=	American Dispensatory
B.T.H.P.	=	Boericke and Taffel's Hom. Pharma
C.M.M.	=	Clarke's Materia Medica
H.N.R.	=	Hale's New Remedies
H.M.M.	=	Hempel's Materia Medica
H.P.U.S.	=	Homoeopathic Pharmacopoeia of United States
H.P.I.	=	Homoeopathic Pharmacopoeia of India

B.H.P. = British Homoeopathic Pharmacopoeia
H.G.S. = Hering's Guiding Symptoms
H.C.D. = Hahnemann's Chronic Diseases
H.M.M.P. = Hahnemann's Materia Medica Pura
G.J.P.P. = Gruner and Jahr's Pharmacopoeia and Posology
C.P.P. = Cooper's Materia Medica.

1. **Abies canadensis:** Bark (H.P.I.); Fresh bark and young buds (B.T.H.P., C.M.M.); The bark and young buds (A.E.); Fresh buds and young twigs (A.D.); Fresh shoots for essence (W.S.P.); Bark and buds (H.N.R.; H.M.M.).
2. **Absinthium:** Fresh young leaves and flowers (A.E.); Leaves and flowers (C.M.M., H.P.I.).
3. **Aesculus hippocastanum:** Fresh fruit without shell (A.E.); Fruit and young bark (A.D.); Ripe, fresh hulled nut (B.T.H.P.; W.S.P.); Fruit with capsule, tree dry kernel (C.M.M.); Root, bark, leaves and seeds (H.M.M.); Both fruit and capsule (H.G.S.); Fresh ripe nut (H.P.U.S.); Ripe nut excluding the outer shell (H.P.I.).
4. **Agaricus muscarius:** Entire fresh fungus (B.H.P.); Whole fresh fungus with the exception of the outer skin (H.P.U.S.); The fresh fungus (A.E., H.M.M., W.S.P.); Whole plant except the epidermis of stem and cap (B.T.H.P.); Dried up cap, fresh fungus (C.M.M.); Fresh plant and grains or dried toad stool 1 grain (H.C.D.); Dried cap (H.G.S.); Whole young fungus except the outer skin (H.P.I.).
5. **Agnus castus:** Recently dried leaves and berries (A.D.); Fresh ripe berries (B.T.H.P.); Fresh ripe fruit (W.S.P.); Ripe berries (A.E., B.H.P., C.M.M.); Berries (H.P.I.); Recently dried berries (H.P.U.S.); Seeds (H.M.M.).
6. **Agave americana:** Fresh root and leaves (A.D.); Fresh leaves (H.P.U.S., B.T.H.P., W.S.P., C.M.M.); Plant, leaves (H.M.M.).
7. **Ailanthus glandulosus:** Dried bark from the root and young shoots, freshly dried leaves and flowers (A.D.); Fresh shoots, leaves, blossoms and the young bark (B.T.H.P., W.S.P.); Flower beginning to blossom (A.E., C.M.M.); Fresh well-developed flowers and the fresh bark of young shoots and roots or dry bark of branches and root and fresh bark of the young shoots and root (B.H.P.); Stalk (H.M.M.); Fresh bark of young shoots and the fresh well-developed flowers (H.P.U.S.); Stem bark of young shoots and well-developed flowers (H.P.I.).
8. **Aletris farinosa:** Recently dried root (A.D.); Fresh bulb (B.T.H.P., W.S.P.); Roots (A.E., C.M.M.; H.M.M.); Fresh root, dried root (H.N.R.); Rhizome and root (H.P.I.); The fresh root (H.P.U.S.).
9. **Allium cepa:** Red onion (A.E., H.G.S.); Mature bulb (B.H.P.); Onion or whole fresh plant (C.M.M.; H.M.M.); Fresh mature bulb or red onion (H.P.U.S.); Fresh red bulb (W.S.P.).
10. **Alstonia constricta:** Alkaloid of the bark (A.D.); Bark (A.E., B.T.H.P., C.M.M.); Bark (H.P.I.).
11. **Ambrosia artemisaefolia:** Whole fresh plant (H.P.U.S.); Flower heads and young shoots (C.M.M.); Fresh leaves and flowers (B.T.H.P.); Recently dried herb (A.D.).
12. **Amygdala amara:** Kernel of ripe seeds (H.P.I.); The dried ripe seed kernels (H.P.U.S.); Ripe kernel (B.T.H.P.); Bitter almond (A.D., A.E.); Kernel (W.S.P.).
13. **Anacardium orientale:** Resinous juice of the seeds (H.P.I.); Seed the resinous juice contained in the seed (H.P.U.S., B.T.H.P.); Juice of seed (H.C.D.); Soft resin contained in the fruit (W.S.P.); Whole nut (H.G.S.); Cashew nut without the kernel (A.D.); Kernel (H.M.M.); The Layer of the nut between the shell and kernel (A.E., C.M.M.).
14. **Argimone mexicana:** Seeds (A.D.); Fresh plant just coming into bloom (B.T.H.P.).
15. **Arnica montana:** Whole plant (H.P.I.); Entire fresh plant including the root (B.H.P., H.P.U.S.); Fresh dried pulversed root (W.S.P.); Root (C.M.M., H.M.M.P., H.G.S.); Whole plant when in blossom (A.E.); Flowers and roots (H.M.M.).
16. **Artemisia vulgaris:** Root, the root gathered in dry weather, taking care not to wash it (H.P.I., H.P.U.S., H.M.M., A.E.); Fibrillae of root (H.G.S.); Root which is dug up in November

in dry weather (G.J.P.P.); Fresh root (B.T.H.P., C.M.M., W.S.P.); Recently dried whole plant (A.D.).

17. **Asarum europaeum:** Whole plant (H.P.I.); The fresh plant and the root (H.P.U.S.); Root (H.M.M.P., H.G.S.); Root and whole fresh plant (C.M.M.); Root and the whole plant (A.E.); Recently dried whole plant (A.D.); Entire fresh plant gathered when in blossom (B.T.H.P.); Leaves and root (H.M.M.).

18. **Baptisia tinctoria:** Bark of root (H.P.I.); Fresh root with its bark (W.S.P.); Fresh plant or bark of the root (H.N.R.); Recently dried root (A.D.); Fresh root with its bark (B.T.H.P., C.M.M.); Bark of the fresh roots (B.H.P., H.P.U.S., H.N.R.).

19. **Belladonna:** Whole plant (H.P.I., H.M.M.P.); Fresh plant (B.H.P.); Fresh plant when in blossom (W.S.P.); Recently dried leaves (A.D.); Whole plant when beginning to blossom (A.E., B.T.H.P., C.M.M., H.P.U.S.); Berries, leaves and roots (H.G.S.).

20. **Cactus grandiflorus:** Flowering stems (H.P.I.); The fresh stems (H.P.U.S.); Flowers and young twigs (A.E.); Fresh flowers and the youngest and tenderest stem (B.T.H.P.).

21. **Calendula officinalis:** Fresh flowering tops and leaves (H.P.I.); Fresh flowering tops (H.N.R.); Flowers (H.M.M.); Recently dried flowers (A.D.); Fresh leaves at the top of the plant with blossoms and buds (B.T.H.P.); Herb in bloom (W.S.P.).

22. **Cannabis indica:** Leaves (H.P.I.); Young leaves and twigs (C.M.M.); Recently dried plant (A.D.); Resin (B.H.P.); Dried herb-tops (B.T.H.P., W.S.P.).

23. **Capsicum annum:** Recently dried ripe fruit (A.D.); Ripe dried fruit (B.T.H.P., W.S.P.); Dry capsules and seeds (B.H.P.); Dried pods (C.M.M.); Ripe seed capsules along with the seeds (H.M.M.P.); Ripe fruit with seeds (H.P.I.); The ripe capsule and seeds (H.P.U.S.).

24. **Carduus marianus:** Seeds (H.P.I., C.M.M.); Whole ripe seeds (B.T.H.P.); Root and seeds (H.N.R.); Ripe ungrinds seed (W.S.P.).

25. **Chelindonium majus:** Whole plant (H.P.I.); Fresh plant (B.T.H.P.); Entire fresh plant including the roots (B.H.P., H.P.U.S.); Entire fresh plant at the time of blooming (C.M.M.); Whole plant when in blossom (A.D.). Whole plant (H.N.R.); Roots (H.M.M.P., H.M.M.); Fresh root (W.S.P.).

26. **Cicuta virosa:** Fresh root at the time of blooming (A.E., B.T.H.P., W.S.P.); Fresh root (B.H.P., H.P.U.S.; C.M.M.); Root (H.P.I.; H.M.M.P.); Root before blooming time (H.M.M.); Fresh root gathered at blooming time (C.M.M.); Recently dried plant (A.D.).

27. **Cina:** Flower heads (H.P.I.; A.E.; H.P.U.S.); Unexpanded flower heads (C.M.M.); Recently dried flowers (A.D.); Dried flowers (B.T.H.P., W.S.P.); Unpowdered buds (H.M.M.P.); Seeds (H.M.M.).

28. **Cocculus indicus:** Seeds (H.P.I., A.E., H.P.U.S.); powdered seeds (C.M.M.); Dried fruits (A.D., B.T.H.P., H.P.U.S.); Berries (B.H.P., H.M.M.).

29. **Coffea cruda:** Seeds (H.P.I., H.P.U.S.); Raw berries (A.E.); Green coffee berries (A.D.); Raw unroasted bean (H.G.S.); Coffee beans, unroasted (B.t.H.P., W.S.P.).

30. **Collinsonia canadensis:** Rhizome (H.P.I.); Roots (B.H.P.); Fresh roots (C.M.M., H.P.U.S.); Recently gathered fresh roots (A.D.); Roots and plant (A.E.); Whole plant (H.M.M.); Fresh plant (W.S.P.); Whole plant and fresh roots (H.N.R.).

31. **Condurango:** Dried bark (B.T.H.P., H.G.S. W.S.P.); Recently dried bark (A.D.); Bark of the stem (A.E.).

32. **Crocus sativus:** Dried stigmas of flowers (H.P.I. B.T.H.P); Dried stigmata (A.E., B.H.P., H.P.U.S., W.S.P., C.M.M.); Recently dried flowers (A.D.); Fresh young shoots (C.M.M.); Stigmata and style of flower (H.M.M.).

33. **Dulcamara:** Whole plant (H.P.I.); Stems (H.M.M.); The whole plant before blooming (H.P.U.S.); Fresh green stem and the leaves before blooming (C.M.M.); Fresh twigs and leaves of the plant before blooming (W.S.P.); Recently dried twigs (A.D.); Young stalks and leaves (H.M.M.P.).

34. **Gelsemium sempervirens:** Rhizome (H.P.I.);

Roots (B.H.P., H.G.S.); Fresh roots (B.T.H.P., H.P.U.S., W.S.P.); Green roots (H.M.M.); Bark of the roots (A.E., C.M.M.); Fresh bark of the roots (H.N.R.); Fresh young rootlets (A.D.).

35. **Grindelia squarrosa:** Recently dried leaves (A.D.); Fresh herb in blossom (B.T.H.P.); The leaves and unexpanded flower heads (H.P.U.S.).

36. **Hamamelis virginica:** Stem bark and also bark of the root (H.P.I.); The fresh bark including bark of the roots (H.P.U.S.); Bark and leaves (H.M.M.); Bark (H.N.R., B.H.P.); Fresh bark of the twigs and root (B.T.H.P., W.S.P., C.M.M., H.G.S.); The fresh bark of the twigs (A.D.); Leaves and twigs (A.E.).

37. **Ranunculus scleratus:** Whole plant including root (H.P.I.); Whole plant (A.E., C.M.M., H.M.M.); Fresh whole plant (A.D., B.H.P., H.P.U.S., W.S.P.); Fresh herb gathered in October (B.T.H.P.).

38. **Rhododendron chrysanthemum:** Leaves and flower buds gathered when the buds are well developed but not bloomed (H.P.I.); Leaves (A.E., G.J.P.P.); Recently dried leaves (A.D.); Dried leaves (B.T.H.P.); Dried leaves and flower buds (B.H.P.).

39. **Rumex acetosella:** Fresh leaves (A.E., H.P.U.S.); Leaves (C.M.M.); Fresh root gathered in June (W.S.P.).

40. **Ruta graveolens:** Whole plant (H.P.I., A.E.); Whole fresh plant (H.M.M.P., C.M.M., H.P.U.S.); Fresh leaves (A.D.); Fresh herb before blooming (B.T.H.P.); Herbaceous parts (B.H.P.); Fresh herb gathered shortly before blooming (H.G.S., W.S.P.); Leaves together with buds while these are not yet bloomed (G.J.P.P.).

41. **Sabina:** Stems and leaves (H.P.I.); The fresh stems and leaves (H.P.U.S.); Recently dried leaves and stems (A.D.); Tops of the plant (H.N.R.).

42. **Sambucus nigra:** Fresh leaves and flowers (B.T.H.P., C.M.M. H.G.S., H.P.U.S., W.S.P.); Leaves and flowers (H.M.M.P., A.E.); Recently dried inner bark (A.D.).

43. **Stramonium:** Whole plant (H.P.I.); Fresh plant (H.M.M.P.); Herb in flower and fruits (A.E.); Recently dried ripe seeds (A.D.); Ripe seed (B.T.H.P., H.G.S.); Entire herb (B.H.P.); Fresh plant in flower and flower and fruits (C.M.M., H.M.M.); Seeds (G.J.P.P., H.M.M.).

44. **Symphytum officinale:** Root (H.P.I.); Fresh root (H.G.S., H.P.U.S.); Fresh root before the plant blooms (B.T.H.P., W.S.P.); Recently dried root (A.D.).

45. **Thuja occidentalis:** Leaves and twigs (H.P.I.); Green leaves (H.M.M.P.); Fresh leaves (A.D.); Fresh leaves and twigs (H.P.U.S.); Green twigs just at the time of blooming (B.T.H.P., W.S.P.); Green twigs (A.E., C.M.M., H.G.S.); Fresh bark and berries (H.E.H.S.).

46. **Viburnum prunifolium:** Bark (H.P.I., H.N.R.); Fresh fruits (A.D. W.S.P.); Fresh bark (C.M.M.).

47. **Xanthoxylum fraxineum:** Bark (A.E.); Fresh bark (B.T.H.P., C.M.M., H.G.S.); Recently dried bark (A.D.); Bark and berries (B.H.P., H.N.R.).

Chapter 43

Practical Pharmacy

Q. 1. Determine the percentage of moisture of a sample of leaves.

Q. 2. Find out the specific gravity of the given sample of alcohol.

Q. 3. Justify the purity of a sample of water.

Q. 4. Medicate Belladonna 30 in globules No. 20.

Q. 5. Find out the number of globules.

Q. 6. Justify the purity of a sample of sugar of milk.

Q. 7. Test the sample of alcohol to detect any impurity.

Q. 8. Prepare Cantharis ointment 10 gm.

Q. 9. prepare Phytolacca glycerole 10 ml.

Q. 10. Prepare Argentum nitricum lotion 10 ml.

Q. 11. Prepare Rhus tox liniment 10 ml.

Q. 12. Prepare Cephalandra indica-θ, 15 ml (Class I).

Q. 13. Prepare Allium cepa-θ, 15 ml (Class II).

Q. 14. Prepare Zingiber-θ, 15 ml (Class III).

Q. 15. Prepare Capsicum-θ, 12 ml (Class IV).

Q. 16. Prepare Nitric acid θ soln. 10 ml (Class VA).

Q. 17. Prepare Borax θ soln. 50 ml (Class VB).

Q. 18. Prepare Camphor θ soln. 50 ml (Class VIA).

Q. 19. Prepare Iodine θ soln. 50 ml (Class VIB).

Q. 20. Prepare Calcarea carb. IX. 20 gm (Class VII).

Q. 21. Prepare Petroleum IX. 10 gm (Class VIII).

Q. 22. Prepare Allium cepa IX. 10 gm (Class IX).

Q. 23. Convert Calcarea carb. 6X (Trit.) into its next higher potency in liquid form.

Q. 24. Potentise Calcarea phos. 6X (Trit.) into its corresponding higher potency.

Q. 25. Prepare Bryonia 30th potency from 29th potency—1 drachm.

Q. 26. Write and serve a prescription in liquid form for internal use only.

Q. 1. Determine the percentage of moisture of a sample of leaves

Requirements

1. Sample of leaves.
2. Water-bath.
3. Chopping board.
4. Chopping knife.
5. Empty porcelain crucible.
6. Balance with measuring weights.
7. Tripod stand with wire gauze.
8. Bunsen burner.
9. Glass rod.

10. Watch.
11. Pen, paper etc.

Procedure

1. The fresh leaves are at first chopped on the chopping board with a chopping knife.
2. The chopped leaves are weighed and weight is recorded. It is found that it is 5.4 gram.
3. Then this substance is taken in a crucible, which is then placed on a water-bath. Then it is heated by means of a Bunsen burner from below so that the juice of the plant is evaporated.
4. The chopped substance should be kept on the water-bath, until the weight scale shows no further reduction of weight.
5. The substance is weighed every 15 minutes after cooling, for a minute, until a constant weight is obtained.
6. On obtaining a constant weight (which means there is no more water vapour left) the final weight that is found is 3 grams.
7. Now comparing the final weight with that which is taken before, will give the amount of moisture present in the leaves.

Calculations

The initial weight of the fresh leaves = 5.4 gms.

at 12.30 P.M. = 5 gms

at 12.45 P.M. = 4.6 gms

at 1 P.M. = 4 gms

at 1.15 P.M. = 3.40 gms

at 1.30 P.M. = 3 gms

at 1.45 P.M. = 3 gms

The final weight of the leaves = 3 gms.

Difference of weight = (5.4 – 3) gms = 2.4 gms.

So, in 5.4 gms of leaves, moisture is 2.4 gms.

In 1 gram of leaves, moisure is $\frac{2.4}{5.4}$ gms.

In 100 gms of leaves, moisture is $\frac{2.4 \times 100}{5.4}$

= 44.44%.

Hence, the percentage of moisture of the given sample is 44.44%.

Q. 2. Find out the specific gravity of the given sample of alcohol

Requirements

1. A big glass-cylinder.
2. Hydrometer.
3. The liquid in question.

Procedure

The given liquid is taken in a glass-cylinder and a hydrometer is slowly and carefully inserted into it.

It is seen that the upper level of liquid corresponds to the mark of hydrometer expressing 0.816.

Conclusion

The specific gravity of the given liquid is 0.816 and it may be strong alcohol.

Q. 3. Justify the purity of a sample of water

Requirements

1. Water to be tested.
2. Test tubes with holder.
3. Ammonium oxalate.
4. Ammonium hydroxide.
5. Ammonium chloride.
6. Nitric acid.
7. Sodium hydrogen phosphate.
8. Silver nitrate.
9. Barium chloride.
10. Hydrochloric acid.

Procedure

Experiment	*Observation*	*Inference*
1. Ammonium oxalate is added to the sample of water in a clean test tube	1. No white ppt. is formed	1. Calcium absent
2. Sample of water is boiled with dilute HNO_3 and NH_4Cl added. It is warmed and NH_4OH added	2. No brown ppt. is formed	2. Iron absent
3. The sample of water + Ammonium hydroxide and Sodium hydrogen phosphate	3. No white ppt. is formed	3. Magnesium absent

Contd.

4. $AgNO_3$ is added to the sample of water in a clean test tube	4. No white ppt. is formed	4. Chloride absent
5. $BaCl_2$ solution is added to the sample of water in a clean test tube	5. No white ppt. is formed	5. Sulphate absent

Conclusion

The supplied sample of water is pure and not adulterated.

Q. 4. Medicate Belladonna 30 in globules no. 20

Theory

In this experiment medication of the supplied globules is to be done with Belladonna-30 medicine.

The medicines in the globule form possess the virtues for a longer period than those preserved in liquid form.

Requirements

1. A perfectly cleansed phial.
2. A new non-porous velvet cork.
3. Supplied Belladonna-30 in liquid form.
4. Supplied globules.
5. Labelling paper, gum, pen, scissors etc.

Procedure

1. A perfectly dry, clean round phial and a new non-porous velvet cork is taken after it is carefully cleansed.
2. Name of the medicine and its potency (here, Bell-30) is written over the top of the cork.
3. The fresh non-medicated globules no. 20, are poured in the filling up to ¾ part of it.
4. Then a few drops of Belladonna-30 liquid (medicinal substance) is poured upon the globules so that the globules are uniformly moistened. Then the phial is closed by the cork and kept standing on the cork for 8 hours.
5. After this period excess liquid medicine (if any) is drained out by loosening the cork a little.
6. Then the cork is again closed. A label is pasted over the body of the phial, writing the name of the medicine and the potency.
7. These medicated globules are kept for 48 hours and then they become ready for use.

Q. 5. Find out the number of globules

Theory

The space of a scale (mm) occupied by ten unknown size of globules is the number of these globules.

Requirements

1. A millimetre measuring scale.
2. The globules of equal size which are to be measured.
3. A clean piece of paper sheet.
4. Paste or gum.
5. Stationery goods—pen, paper etc.

Procedure

(a) **Pre-process**

1. The supplied instruments are checked.
2. These are arranged properly.

(b) **Process-proper**

1. The paper sheet is folded.
2. Gum is attached along the folded line of paper.
3. Then ten given globules of uniform size are attached in such a way as to avoid interglobular spaces.
4. Then a milimetre scale is kept and the space occupied by the globules is measured.
5. The process is repeated for three times.
6. The average of the reading is noted.

Calculations

No.	*Space occupied by globules (in mm. scale)*	*Mean*
1.	22	
2.	23	22
3.	21	

Hence, the number of globules is 22.

(c) **Post-process**

The utensils are cleaned and handed over to the laboratory attendants.

Q. 6. Justify the purity of a sample of sugar of milk

Theory

Sugar of milk use for homoeopathic purpose must be pure and unadulterated.

Requirements

1. Sample of sugar of milk.
2. Blue litmus paper.
3. Iodine solution.
4. Purified water.
5. NaOH solution.
6. Potassium ferrocyanide solution.
7. $AgNO_3$ solution.
8. Test tubes with holder.

Procedure

A. **Physical Test**

Experiment	*Observation*	*Inference*
1. Sample is taken in between the finger and smelt	1. Sandy or gritty feeling; odourless	1. May be pure
2. Taste	2. Faintly sweet in taste	2. May be pure
3. Colour and consistency	3. Milky-white, hard, crystalline substance	3. May be pure

B. **Chemical Test**

Experiment	*Observation*	*Inference*
1. **Litmus Test:** In a test tube containining aqueous solution of sugar of milk—a blue litmus paper is added	1. Blue litmus paper remains unchanged	1. Absence of acid
2. **Iodine Test:** In a test tube solution of iodine is prepared. A few drops of iodine solution is added to the sugar of milk solution	2. The colour not changed into blue	2. Starch absent
3. A weak solution of sugar of milk is prepared in a clean test tube with purified water	3. The colour remains	3. Starch absent

Conclusion

The supplied sample of sugar of milk is pure and not adulterated.

Q. 7. Test the sample of alcohol to detect any impurity

Requirements

1. The alcohol to be tested.
2. Purified water.
3. Conc. H_2SO_4.
4. $AgNO_3$ solution.
5. White anhydrous $CuSO_4$.
6. Blue litmus paper.
7. Salicylic acid.
8. Test tubes with holder.

Procedure

See top of the next page.

Q. 8. Prepare Cantharis ointment 10 gm

Principle

One part by weigh or volume of mother tincture is mixed with nine parts by weight or volume of vaseline.

Requirements

A. **Ingredients**

1. Cantharis θ.
2. White vaseline.

Procedure

Experiment	*Observation*	*Inference*
1. The given sample of alcohol is soaked with blue litmus paper	1. It turns red	1. Presence of acid
2. The purified water is added to the sample of alcohol in equal volume	2. A foreign smell is found	2. Impure alcohol
3. A few drops of $AgNO_3$ solution is added to the sample of aochol in a test tube and exposed to bright light	3. A reddish colour appears	3. Presence of fusel oil
4. Conc. H_2SO_4 is added to the sample of alcohol in equal weight in a test tube and exposed to bright light	4. A reddish colour noticed $C_2H_5OH + H_2SO_4 = C_2H_5HSO_4 + H_2O$	4. Presence of fusel oil
5. Alcohol is made to evaporate from a porcelain dish, protected from dust	5. After evaporation no foreign odour is issued	5. Absence of fusel oil
6. (i) White anhydrous $CuSO_4$ is added to the sample of alcohol, or (ii) Calcium carbide is added to the sample of alcohol	6. (i) Turns blue (ii) Produces Acetylene gas $CaC_2 + 2H_2O = Ca(OH)_2 + C_2H_2$	6. Presence of water
7. To the given sample salicylic acid is added and conc. H_2SO_4 added and warm	7. Smell of oil of wintergreen	7. Presence of CH_3OH.

B. **Appliances**

1. Ointment slab.
2. Spatula.
3. Ointment phial.
4. Balance with weight box.
5. Pen, paper, gum, scissors etc.

Calculations

Ointment is prepared in the ratio of 1 : 9, 1 part medicinal substance and 9 parts white vaseline.

We have to prepare 10 gms, so 1 gm Cantharis mother tincture and 9 grams white vaseline is required.

Procedure

1. 9 grams of white vaseline is weighed on the balance and placed on the clean slab.
2. 1 gram of Cantharis mother tincture is poured on the slab containing white vaseline.
3. It is thoroughly mixed with the help of spatula till the colour of the whole solution becomes uniform.
4. It is then poured in a clean ointment phial. A labelling paper is pasted on the wall of the phial, writing **'Cantharis ointment-10 gms'** (for 'External Use Only').

Q. 9. Prepare Phytolacca glycerole 10 ml

Principle

One part by weight or volume of mother tincture is mixed with nine parts by weight or volume of glycerine.

Requirements

A. **Ingredients**

1. Phytolacca θ.
2. Glycerine.

B. **Appliances**

1. A perfectly clean round phial.
2. A new non-porous velvet cork.
3. Balance with weight box.
4. Weighing bottles.
5. Pen, paper, gum, scissors etc.

Calculations

Glycerole is prepared in the ratio of 1 : 9, 1 part of medicinal substance and 9 parts of glycerine. We have to prepare 10 ml, so, 1 ml Phytolacca mother tincure and 9 ml glycerine is required.

Procedure

1. 9 ml of glycerine is taken in a clean round phial.
2. 1 ml of Phytolacca mother tincture is poured in the phial containing glycerine.
3. The cork is fixed and a homogeneous mixture is prepared by vigorous shaking.
4. A labelling paper is pasted on the wall of the phial, writing, **'Phytolacca glycerole-10 ml'** and mentioned **'for External Use Only.'**

Q. 10 Prepare Argentum nitricum lotion 10 ml

Principle

One part of the requisite mother tincture is mixed with nine parts of purified water.

Requirements

A. **Ingredients**
   1. Argentum nitricum-θ.
   2. Purified water.

B. **Appliances**
   1. One clean round phial.
   2. One new non-porous velvet cork.
   3. Balance with weight box.
   4. Weighing bottle.
   5. Pen, paper, pasting gum, scissors etc.

Calculations

Lotion is prepared in the ratio of 1 : 9, 1 part medicinal substance and 9 parts of purified water. We have to prepare 10 ml, so 1 ml Argentum nitricum mother tincture and 9 ml of purified water are required.

Procedure

1. 9 ml of purified water is taken in a clean round phial.
2. 1 ml of Argentum nitricum mother tincture is poured in the phial containing purified water.
3. The phial is corked and shaken well. The mixture is shaken vigorously till its colour becomes uniform.
4. A labelling paper is pasted on the wall of the phial writing 'Argentum nitricum lotion-10 ml' and mentioned for 'External Use Only.'

Q. 11. Prepare Rhus tox liniment 10 ml

Principle

One part by weight or volume of mother tincture is mixed with nine parts by weight or volume of olive oil.

Requirements

A. **Ingredients**
   1. Rhus tox θ.
   2. Olive oil.

B. **Appliances**
   1. A clean round phial.
   2. A new non-porous velvet cork.
   3. Balance with weight box.
   4. Weighing bottle.
   5. Pen, paper, gums, scissors etc.

Calculations

Liniments is prepared in the ratio of 1 : 9, 1 part medicinal substance and 9 parts of olive oil. We have to prepare 10 ml, so 1 ml Rhus tox. mother tincture and 9 ml of olive oil are required.

Procedure

1. 9 ml of olive oil is taken in the phial.
2. 1 ml of Rhus. tox mother tincture is poured in the phial containing olive oil.
3. The cork is fixed and a homogenous mixture is prepared by vigorous shaking.
4. A labelling paper is pasted over the wall of phial writing, 'Rhus tox liniment 10 ml' and mentioned for 'External Use Only'.

Q. 12. Prepare Cephalandra indica-θ, 15 ml (Class I)

Part used: Fresh green leaves.

Requirements

A. **Ingredients**

1. Leaves of Cephalandra indica (fresh plant).
2. Strong alcohol.

B. **Applicances**

1. Wooden chopping board and knife.
2. Porcelain mortar and pestle.
3. Horn-made spatula.
4. Linen cloth—new and sterilised.
5. A clean small beaker.
6. Glass-stoppered phial; weighing bottle or minim glass.
7. Glass funnel with stand.
8. Filter paper.
9. Another clean phial with a new non-porous velvet cork.
10. Balance with weight box.
11. Pen, paper, gum, scissors etc.

Calculations

Prepared under Class I, where ratio 1 : 1.

Drug power = ½; Residue—Nil or negligible.

Amount to be prepared = 15 ml.

To prepare 2 ml required drug substance = 1 ml

" " 1 ml " " " = ½ ml

" " 15 ml " " " = 7.5 ml (½ × 15 ml)

Here, required drug substance = 7.5 ml and required strong alcohol = (15 – 7.5) ml = 7.5 ml.

Procedure

A. **Pre-process**

The utensils that are to be used are to be thoroughly washed, then checked up and arranged properly.

B. **Process-proper**

1. The fresh leaves are cut into small pieces with well-polished steel-knife on a clean chopping board and pounded to a pulp with mortar and pestle.
2. The pulp is now enclosed in a new linen cloth and the juice is squeezed out.
3. 7.5 ml of juice is measured with minim glass and kept in a glass-stoppered bottle.
4. An equal quantity (i.e., 7.5 ml) of strong alcohol is added to it.
5. The mixture is shaken vigorously for some time and then put into a well-stoppered bottle and allowed to stand for 8 days, in a cool dark place and is then filtered.
6. Then it is poured in a clean phial provided with velvet cork.

C. **Post-process**

1. A label is pasted on the body of the phial writing. 'Cephalandra indica-θ; 15 ml'.
2. All utensils are cleaned and handed over to laboratory attendant.

Q. 13. Prepare Allium cepa-θ, 15 ml (Class II)

Part used: Fresh bulb of the red onion.

Requirements

A. **Ingredients**

1. Onion.
2. Strong alcohol.

B. **Appliances**

1. Wooden chopping board and knife.
2. Porcelain mortar and pestle.
3. Horn-made spatula.
4. Linen cloth—new and sterilised.
5. A clean small beaker.
6. A glass-stoppered phial.
7. Glass funnel with stand.
8. Another clean phial provided with best quality of new non-porous velvet cork.

9. Filter paper.
10. Balance with weight box.
11. Weighing bottle.
12. Pen, paper, gum, scissors etc.

Calculations

Prepared under Class II, where ratio of medicinal substance and vehicle = 3 : 2; Drug power = ½

But medicinal sub., in 1 ml loss = ⅓ ml

" " " " 3 ml loss = ⅓ × 3 ml

= 1 ml

∴ Net medicinal substance = (3 – 1) ml = 2 ml

Net medicinal substance	Strong alcohol	Mother tincture
2 ml	2 ml	4 ml

Final ratio,

Medicinal substance	Strong alcohol	Mother tincture
3 ml	2 ml	4 ml

∴ To prepare 4 ml mother tincture, req. medicinal subst.= 3 ml

∴ " " 1 ml " " " " " = ¾ ml

∴ " " 15 ml " " " " " =¾×15

= 11.25 ml

To prepare 4 ml mother tincture required vehicle= 2 ml

" " 1 ml " " " " " = ½ ml

" " 15 ml " " " " " = ½×15

= 7.5 ml

So, 11.25 ml medicinal juice and 7.5 ml of strong alcohol is required for 15 ml of mother tincture.

Procedure

A. **Pre-process**

1. Utensils are checked properly.
2. These are arranged systematically.

B. **Process-proper**

1. Red onion is taken and dry scales are removed.
2. The bulb of the onion is cut into small pieces with well-polished steel-knife on a clean chopping board and pounded to a pulp with mortar and pestle.
3. The pulp is then squeezed and the juice taken out. Now the residues are taken in a beaker and a few drops of alcohol added and again squeezed.
4. Now 11.25 ml of juice is taken in a macerating jar. To it, 7.5 ml of strong alcohol is added and gently shaken and then kept in a dry cool place for 8 days.
5. After 8 days the mixture is decanted off and filtered in a clean glass phial. This is Allium cepa-θ.

C. **Post-process**

1. A label is pasted on the body of the phial writing 'Allium cepa-θ, 15 ml'.
2. All utensils are cleaned and handed over to the laboratory attendant.

Q. 14. Prepare Zingiber-θ, 15 ml (Class III)

Part used: Fresh roots.

Common name: Ginger.

Requirements

A. **Ingredients**

1. Dried, modified fresh (as far practicable) stem of ginger, about 10 gms.
2. Strong alcohol—20 ml.

B. **Appliances**

1. Wooden chopping board and knife.
2. Porcelain mortar and pestle.
3. Horn-made spatula.
4. Linen cloth—new and sterilised.
5. A clean small beaker.
6. A glass-stoppered phial.
7. Another clean phial with new non-porous velvet cork.
8. Glass funnel with stand.
9. Filter paper.
10. Balance with weight box.
11. Pen, paper, gum, scissors etc.

Calculations

Prepared under Class III, where ratio of medicinal substance and vehicle = 1 : 2.

Drug power = $\frac{1}{6}$

Amount to be prepared = 15 ml

But medicinal substance in 1 ml loss = $\frac{2}{3}$ ml

$\therefore$ Net medicinal substance = $(1 - \frac{2}{3}) = \frac{1}{3}$ ml

Vehicle total loss in 2 ml = $\frac{1}{3}$ ml

$\therefore$ Net vehicle = $(2 - \frac{1}{3})$ml = $\frac{5}{3}$ ml

Net medicinal substance	Net vehicle (Strong alcohol)	Mother tincture
$\frac{1}{3}$ ml	$\frac{5}{3}$ ml	$\frac{1}{3} + \frac{5}{3}$ ml = 2 ml

Final ratio,

Medicinal substance	Strong alcohol	Mother tincture
1 ml	2 ml	2 ml

$\therefore$ To prepare 2 ml mother tincture, req. medicinal subst.= 1 ml

$\therefore$ " " 1 ml " " " " " = $\frac{1}{2}$ ml

$\therefore$ " " 15 ml " " " " " = $\frac{15}{2}$ ml = 7.5 ml

To prepared 2 ml mother tincture required vehicle= 2 ml

" " 1 ml " " " " = 1 ml

" " 15 ml " " " " = 15 ml

$\therefore$ 7.5 ml of juice and 15 ml of strong alcohol are required to prepare 15 ml mother tincture.

Procedure

A. **Pre-process**

The utensils are checked and arranged systematically.

B. **Process-proper**

1. The selected roots of Zingiber are taken and cut into small pieces with a well-polished steel knife on a clean chopping board and pounded to a pulp with mortar and pestle.
2. The pulp is then squeezed with linen cloth and the juice is taken out. Now the residue is taken in a beaker and a few drops of alcohol is added and again squeezed.
3. Now, 7.5 ml of juice is taken in a macerating jar. To it, 15 ml of strong alcohol is added and gently shaken and kept in a dry cool place for 8 days.
4. After 8 days, the mixture is decanted off and filtered in a clean glass phial. This is Zingiber-θ.

C. **Post-process**

1. A label is pasted on the body of the phial writing 'Zingiber-θ, 15 ml'
2. All utensils are cleaned and handed over to the laboratory attendant.

Q. 15. Prepare Capsicum-θ, 12 ml (Class IV)

Part used: The ripe capsule and seeds.

Requirements

A. **Ingredients**

1. Ripe, dried fruits and seeds—3 gm.
2. Strong alcohol—15 ml.

B. **Appliances**

1. Wooden chopping board and knife.
2. Porcelain mortar and pestle.
3. Horn-made spatula.
4. A linen cloth—new and sterilised.
5. A clean small beaker.
6. A glass-stoppered phial.
7. Another clean phial with new non-porous velvet cork.
8. Glass funnel with stand.
9. Filter paper.
10. A glass rod.
11. Balance with weight box.
12. Pen, paper, gums, scissors etc.

Calculations

Prepared under Class IV, where ratio of medicinal substance and vehicle = 1 : 5

Drug power = $\frac{1}{10}$

Amount to be prepared = 12 ml

But medicinal substance in 1 ml loss = $\frac{1}{2}$ ml

$\therefore$ Net medicinal substance = $(1 - \frac{1}{2})$ ml = $\frac{1}{2}$ ml.

Vehicle in 1 ml loss = $\frac{1}{10}$ ml

" " 5 ml " = $\frac{1}{2}$ ml

$\therefore$ Net vehicle = $(5 - \frac{1}{2})$ ml = $\frac{9}{2}$ ml.

Net medicinal substance	Net vehicle (Strong alcohol)	Mother tincture
½ ml	9/2 ml	½ + 9/2 ml = 5 ml

Final ratio,

Medicinal substance	Strong alcohol	Mother tincture
1 ml	5 ml	2 ml

∴ To prepare 2 ml q, req. medicinal subst.= 1 ml.

∴ " " 1 ml q, " " " = ⅕ ml.

∴ " " 12 ml q, " " " = ⅕ × 12 = 2.4 ml.

To prepare 5 ml q, required vehicle = 5 ml.

" " 12 ml q, " " = 12 ml.

So, to prepare 12 ml of Capsicum θ, 2.4 ml (or gram) medicinal substance and 12 ml of strong alcohol are required.

Procedure

A. **Pre-process**

The utensils are checked and arranged properly.

B. **Process-proper**

1. The red, dried fruits and seeds of Capsicum are pulverised into fine powder.
2. 2.4 gms of powdered drug substance is taken in a glass jar.
3. 12 ml of strong alcohol is added to it and the same mixed with the powder.
4. After thoroughly mixing, the whole mass is kept in a glass-stoppered bottle in cool dark place for 15 days.
5. The mixture is shaken well, twice daily.
6. After this period, the clear part is decanted, the residual substance is strained by a new linen cloth and is added to the previously decanted tincture. This is again filtered by a filter paper and stored in a glass-stoppered bottle. It is Capsicum θ.

C. **Post-process**

1. A label is pasted on the body of the phial writing '**Capsicum-θ, 12 ml.**'
2. All utensils are cleaned and handed over to the attendant.

Q. 16. Prepare Nitric acid θ solution 10 ml (Class VA)

Chemical Symbol: HNO_3; Mol. wt.: 63.013

Synonyms: Acidum nitri; Aqua fortis. Hydrogen nitricum.

Requirements

A. **Ingredients**

1. Nitric acid.
2. Purified water

B. **Applicances**

1. Clean phial with cork.
2. Balance with weight box.
3. Labelling paper and gum.

Calculation

Prepared under Class V(A), where ratio of medicinal substance and vehicle (purified water) = 1 : 9

Drug power = 1/10

Amount to be prepared = 10 ml.

No loss of medicinal substance and vehicle.

Medicinal substance	Vehicle (Purified water)	Mother solution
1 ml	9 ml	10 ml

So, to prepare 10 ml of Nitric acid θ solution, 1 ml Nitric acid and 9 ml purified water are required

Procedure

A. **Pre-process**

All utensils are cleansed and arranged properly.

B. **Process-proper**

1. 1 ml of Nitric acid is taken in a clean glass phial.
2. 9 ml of purified water is poured into phial and mixed with the acid thoroughly. Thus, Nitric acid mother solution is prepared.

C. **Post-process**

1. A label is pasted on the body of the phial writing, '**Nitric acid θ solution-10 ml.**'

2. All the utensils are washed properly and handed over to the laboratory attendant.

Q. 17. Prepare Borax θ solution 50 ml (Class VB)

Chemical Symbol: $Na_2B_4O_7,10H_2O$; Mol. wt.: 381.373.

Synonyms: Borate of Sodium; Natrum boracicum.

Requirements

A. **Ingredients**

1. Borax.
2. Purified water.

B. **Appliances**

1. Clean porcelain basin.
2. Tripod stand with wire-gauge.
3. Burners.
4. Spatula.
5. Balance with weight box.
6. Weighing bottle.
7. A clean round phial and a new non-porous velvet cork.
8. Pen, paper, gum, scissors etc.

Calculations

Prepared under Class V(B), where ratio of medicinal substance and vehicle (purified water) = 1 : 99

Drug power = $\frac{1}{100}$

Amount to be prepared = 50 ml.

No loss of medicinal substance and vehicle.

Medicinal substance	Vehicle (Purified water)	Mother solution
1 gm	99 gm	100 ml

To prepare 100 ml of mother soln. req. medicinal subs. = 1 gm

" " 1 ml " " " " " = $\frac{1}{100}$ g

" " 50 ml " " " " " = 0.5 g

To prepare 100 ml of mother soln. required vehicle = 99 gm

" " 1 ml " " " " = $\frac{99}{100}$ gm

" " 50 ml " " " " = $\frac{99}{100} \times 50$

= 49.5 gm

So, to prepare 50 ml of Borax θ soln., 0.5 gram of Borax and 49.5 gram of purified water is required.

Procedure

A. **Pre-process**

All utensils are washed thoroughly and arranged properly.

B. **Process-proper**

1. About 1 gram of Borax is taken in a clean porcelain basin and heated strongly by a Bunsen burner. It is then allowed to cool. After cooling it is pulverised.
2. 0.5 gram of Borax is weighed from the pulverised powder and taken in a clean round phial.
3. 49.5 gram of purified water is weighed with weighing bottle and poured into the phial.
4. The phial is closed with the cork and a homogeneous solution is prepared by gentle shaking. It is Borax θ solution.

C. **Post-process**

1. A label is pasted on the wall of the phial writing, 'Borax θ solution-50 ml.
2. All the utensils are washed properly and handed over to the laboratory attendant.

Q. 18. Prepare Camphor θ solution 10 ml (Class VIA)

Chemical Symbol: $C_{10}H_{16}O$

Mol. wt.: 152, 238.

Requirements

A. **Ingredients**

1. Camphor.
2. Strong alcohol.

B. **Appliances**

1. Two porcelain basin.
2. Blotting paper.
3. Tripod stand and wire-gauge.
4. Bunsen burner.

5. Balance with weight box.
6. Weighing bottle.
7. Spatula.
8. A clean round phial and a new non-porous velvet cork.
9. Pen, label paper, gum, scissors etc.

Calculation

Prepared under Class VI(A), where the ratio of medicinal substance and vehicle (strong alcohol) = 1 : 9.

Drug power = 1/10

Amount to be prepared = 10 ml.

No loss of medicinal substance and vehicle.

Medicinal substance	Vehicle (Strong alcohol)	Mother solution
1 gm	9 gm	10 ml

So, to prepare 10 ml of Camphor θ soln., 1 gram of sublimed camphor and 9 gram of strong alcohol are required.

Procedure

A. Pre-process

All the utensils are washed thoroughly and arranged properly.

B. Process-proper

1. At first some amount of camphor is sublimated by the porcelain basin, covered by blotting paper, heated by Bunsen burner.
2. Then 1 gram of sublimed camphor is taken in a clean phial.
3. Then 9 gram strong alcohol is added to the phial.
4. The phial is closed tightly by the cork.
5. A homogeneous solution is prepared by gentle shaking. It is Camphor θ solution.

C. Post-process

1. A label is pasted on the wall of the phial writing **'Camphor θ solution-10 ml.'**
2. All utensils are cleansed properly and handed over to the laboratory attendant.

Q.19. Prepare Iodine θ solution 50 ml (Class VIB)

Chemical Symbol: I

Synonyms: Iodum; Iodinium

Requirements

A. Ingredients

1. Iodine crystals
2. Strong alcohol

B. Appliances

1. Porcelain basin-2.
2. Blotting paper.
3. Tripod stand and wire gauge.
4. Spatula (horn-made).
5. A clean phial and a new non-porous velvet cork.
6. Balance with weight box.
7. Weighing bottles.
8. Bunsen burner.
9. Pen, paper, gum, scissors etc.

Calculations

Prepared under Class VI(B), where ratio of medicinal substance and vehicle (strong alcohol) = 1 : 99.

Drug power = 1/100

Amount to be prepared = 50 ml.

No loss of medicinal substance and vehicle.

Medicinal substance	Vehicle (Strong alcohol)	Mother solution
1 gm	99 gm	100 ml

To prepare 100 ml of mother soln. req. medicinal subs. = 1 gm

" " 1 ml " " " " = 1/100 g

" " 50 ml " " " " = 0.5 g

To prepare 100 ml of mother soln. required vehicle = 99 gm

" " 1 ml " " " " = 99/100 gm

" " 50 ml " " " " = 99/100×50

= 49.5 gm

So, to prepare 50 ml of Iodine θ solution, 0.5 gram of Iodine and 49.5 gram of strong alcohol are required.

Procedure

A. **Pre-process**

All utensils are cleansed properly and arranged systematically.

B. **Process-proper**

1. At first some amount of Iodine is sublimated in porcelain basin, covered by blotting paper, heated by busen burner.
2. Then 0.5 gram of sublimed iodine is taken in a clean phial.
3. Then 49.5 gram of strong alcohol is added to the phial.
4. The phial is closed tightly by the cork.
5. A homogeneous solution is prepared by gentle shaking. It is Iodine θ solution.

C. **Post-process**

1. A label is pasted on the wall of the phial writing **'Iodine θ solution—50 ml.'**
2. All utensils are cleansed properly and handed over to the laboratory attendant.

Q. 20. Prepare Calcarea carb. IX, 20 gm (Class VII)

Chemical Symbol: $CaCO_3$

Requirements

A. **Ingredients**

1. Oyster shell.
2. Sugar of milk.

B. **Appliances**

1. Iron mortar and pestle.
2. Porcelain mortar and pestle.
3. Spatula.
4. Balance and weight box.
5. Stop-watch.
6. A clean round phial and a new non-porous velvet cork.
7. Pen, paper, gum, scissors etc.

Calculations

Prepared under Class VII, where ratio of medicinal subtance and vehicle (sugar of milk) = 1 : 9 (under decimal scale).

Drug power = $\frac{1}{10}$

Amount to be prepared = 20 gram.

No loss of medicinal substance and vehicle.

Medicinal substance	Vehicle (Sugar of milk)	Mother solution
1 gm	9 gm (3 + 3 + 3) gm	10 gm

So, to prepare 20 grams mother substance, 2 grams medicinal substance and 18 grams (6+6+6) of sugar of milk are necessary.

Procedure

A. **Pre-process**

All the required utensils are washed thoroughly and arranged systematically.

B. **Process-proper**

1. The oyster shell is at first cleaned by rubbing. Then it is grinded by iron mortar and pestle, and finally with porcelain mortar and pestle. The powder is shifted by a sieve and only the very fine powders are taken as the medicinal substance.
2. 2 grams of fine powder is taken in a clean porcelain mortar. Then 6 grams ($\frac{1}{3}$ of 18 grams) sugar of milk is added to it and triturated as:

(a) The sugar of milk is mixed with the medicinal substance for one minute. Then it is grinded for six minutes in one direction and with uniform pressure by a pestle, and scraped in four minutes time. Again, this process is repeated for ten minutes.

(b) Second part of sugar of milk (i.e., 6 grams) is added to the triturated substance in the mortar, mixed for one minute, grinded for six minutes in one direction and with uniform pressure, scraped, collected and stirred for three minutes.

Again, grinded for six minutes and scraped, collected and stirred and scraped for four minutes. Thus, the second step of trituration is completed.

(c) Now, the 3rd part of sugar of milk (i.e., remaining 6 grams) is added to the triturated substance and the same procedure is adopted for another twenty minutes and thus the third and last part of trituration is completed.

In this way, trituration process is completed in one hour's time.

3. Now, the prepared medicine is poured in a clean phial which is closed by a new non-porous velvet cork.

C. **Post-process**

1. A label is pasted on the wall of phial writing, **'Calcarea carb. IX-20 gram'**.
2. All the used utensils are washed properly and handed over to the laboratory attendant.

Q. 21. Prepare Petroleum IX, 10 gm (Class VIII)

Synonyms: Rock oil; Coal oil

Requirements:

A. **Ingredients**

1. Petroleum oil.
2. Sugar of milk.

B. **Appliances**

1. Porcelain mortar and pestle.
2. Horn-made spatula.
3. Balance with weight box.
4. Weighing bottles.
5. A clean phial and a new non-porous velvet cork.
6. Pen, paper, gum, scissors etc.
7. Wrist-watch.

Calculations

Prepared under Class VIII, where ratio of medicinal substance and vehicle (sugar of milk) = 1 : 9 (under decimal scale).

Drug power = $\frac{1}{10}$

Amount to be prepared = 10 gram.

No loss of medicinal substance and vehicle.

So, to prepare 10 grams of petroleum IX, 1 gram petroleum oil and 9 grams of milk are necessary.

Procedure

A. **Pre-process**

All the utensils are washed thoroughly and arranged systematically.

B. **Process-proper**

1. 9 grams sugar of milk is taken first in a clean porcelain mortar. Then 1 gram of petroleum oil (pure) is poured over it and triturated for thrice twenty minutes as shown:

(a) The petroleum oil is mixed with the sugar of milk by a spatula in one minute, it is grinded for six minutes in one direction and with uniform pressure, then it is scraped, collected and stirred for four minutes. It is again grinded for six minutes and scraped for four minutes. During this twenty minutes the first step of trituration is completed.

(b) As the whole quantity of sugar of milk is taken at a time, no more sugar of milk is to be added and the same triturated material is again triturated as stated above for another twenty minutes. Thus, second step of trituration is completed.

(c) Again the triturated material is triturated for twenty minutes as stated above and thus the third step of trituration is completed.

In this way, trituration process is completed in one hour.

2. Now, the prepared medicine is poured in a clean phial which is closed by a new non-porous velvet cork.

C. **Post-process**

1. A label is pasted on the wall of the phial, writing **Petroleum IX, 10 gram'**.

2. All the used utensils are washed properly and handed over to the laboratory attendant.

Q. 22. Prepare Allium cepa IX, 10 gm (Class IX)

Synonyms: Onion; Piyaj.

Requirements

A. **Ingredients**

1. Red onions.
2. Sugar of milk.

B. **Appliances**

1. Porcelain mortar and pestle.
2. Spatula; weighing bottle.
3. Balance and weight box.
4. A clean phial and a new non-porous velvet cork.
5. Wrist-watch.
6. Pen, paper, gum, scissors etc.

Calculations

Prepared under Class IX, where ratio of medicinal substance and vehicle (sugar of milk) = 2 : 9 (under decimal scale).

Drug power = $\frac{1}{10}$

Amount to be prepared = 10 gram.

No loss of sugar of milk but some loss of medicinal substance by evaporation.

To prepare 10 grams of mother substance, 2 grams medicinal substance and 9 grams of sugar of milk are necessary.

Procedure

A. **Pre-process**

All utensils are washed properly and arranged systematically.

B. **Process-proper**

1. The red onions are cleansed and chopped by chopping knife.
2. Then it is pulversied very finely by porcelain mortar and pestle.
3. Then 2 grams of the fine pulp is taken in a perfectly clean porcelain mortar. $\frac{1}{3}$ of 9 grams (i.e., 3 grams) of sugar of milk is added to it and triturated as shown:
   (a) The sugar of milk is mixed with the medicinal substance for one minute. Then it is grinded for six minutes in one direction and with uniform pressure by pestle, and scraped in four minutes time. Again, this process is repeated for ten minutes.
   (b) Second part of sugar of milk (i.e., 3 gms) is added to the triturated substance in the mortar, mixed for one minute, grinded for six minutes in one direction and with uniform pressure, scraped, collected and stirred for three minutes. Again, grinded for six minutes and scraped, collected and stirred for four minutes. Thus, the second step of trituration is completed.
   (c) Now, the third part of sugar of milk (i.e., remaining 3 grams) is added to the triturated substance and the same procedure is adopted for another twenty minutes and thus the third and last part of trituration is completed.
   In this way, trituration process is completed in one hour's time.
4. Now, the prepared medicine is poured in a clean phial which is closed by a new non-porous velvet cork.

C. **Post-process**

1. A label is pasted on the wall of the phial writing. **'Allium cepa IX, 10 gram'**.
2. All the used utensils are washed properly and handed over to the laboratory attendant.

Q. 23. Convert Calcarea carb. 6X (Trit.) into its next higher potency in liquid form

Requirements

A. **Ingredients**

1. Calcarea carb. 6X (trituration).
2. Purified water.
3. Strong alcohol.

B. **Appliances**

1. Balance with weight box.
2. Weighing bottles.
3. A clean round phial and a new non-porous velvet cork.
4. Pen, paper, gum, scissors etc.

Calculations

This is prepared by taking one part of medicinal substance and 50 parts by weight of purified water and 50 parts by weight of strong alcohol.

Procedure

A. **Pre-process**

All utensils are washed and arranged systematically.

B. **Process-proper**

1. 5 grains Calcarea carb. 6X (trit.) is taken in a clean phial.
2. 250 grains (5 × 50 grains) purified water is added to it.
3. A homogeneous solution is prepared by gently shaking the phial.
4. Then 250 grains (5 × 50 grains) of strong alcohol is added to it taking care that at least $^1/_4$th part of the phial remains vacant.
5. The phial is closed by the above cork and ten forceful downward strokes are given by holding the phial firmly, so that each stroke may terminate in a jerk. Now, it is Calcarea carb. 7X.

C. **Post-process**

1. A label is pasted on the wall of the phial, writing 'Calcarea carb 7X'.
2. All used utensils are washed properly and handed over to the laboratory attendant.

Q. 24. Potentise Calcarea phos. 6X (Trituration) into its corresponding higher potency

Requirements

A. **Ingredients**

1. Calcarea phos. 6X (Trituration).
2. Sugar of milk.

B. **Appliances**

1. Porcelain mortar and pestle.
2. Balance with weight box.
3. Spatula
4. A clean phial provided with new non-porous velvet cork.
5. Wrist watch
6. Pen, paper, gum, scissors etc.

Calculations

The potentisation in this case is done under decimal scale, i.e., ratio is 1 : 9.

Say, amount to be prepared = 10 grams.

So 1 gram Calcarea phos. 6X (Trit.) and 9 grams of sugar of milk are necessary.

Procedure

A. **Pre-process**

All utensils are washed properly and arranged systematically.

B. **Process-proper**

1. 1 gram Calcarea phos. 6X. (Trit.) is taken in a clean porcelain mortar and ⅓ of 9 grams (i.e., 3 grams) of sugar of milk is added to it and triturated as shown:

(a) The sugar of milk is mixed with the medicinal substance for one minute. Then it is grinded for six minutes in one direction and with uniform pressure by pestle and scraped in four minutes time. Again, this process is repeated for ten minutes.

(b) Second part of sugar of milk (i.e., 3 grams) is added to the triturated substance in the mortar mixed for one minute, grinded for six minutes in one direction and with uniform pressure, scraped, collected and stirred for three minutes.

Again, grinded for six minutes and scraped, collected and stirred for four minutes. Thus, the second step of trituration is completed.

(c) Now, the third part of sugar of milk (i.e., remaining 3 grams) is added to the triturated substance and the same procedure is adopted for another twenty minutes and thus the third and last part of trituration is completed. In this way, trituration process is completed in one hour's time.

2. Now, the prepared medicine is poured in a clean phial which is closed by a new non-porous velvet cork.

C. **Post-process**

1. A label is pasted on the wall of the phial writing 'Calcarea phos-7X'.
2. All the used utensils are washed thoroughly and handed over to the laboratory attendant.

Q. 25. Prepare Bryonia 30th potency from 29th potency—1 drachm

Requirements

A. **Ingredients**

1. Bryonia 29th potency
2. Dispensing alcohol.

B. **Appliances**

1. Minim glass
2. Graduated minim pipette
3. Clean phial with cork
4. Pen, paper, gum, scissors etc.

Calculations

To prepare 30th potency from 29th potency, one minim is to be taken from 29th potency and mixed with 99 minims of dispensing alcohol in centesimal scale.

But here only one drachm, i.e., 60 minims, is to be prepared.

So, in 100 minims of dispensing alcohol, 1 minim of 29th potency is taken.

So, in 60 minims of dispensing alcohol $\frac{1}{100} \times 60 = 0.6$ minims of 29th potency will be taken.

The required dispensing alcohol = (60 – 6) minims = 59.4 minims.

Procedure

A. **Pre-process**

All utensils are washed properly and arranged systematically.

B. **Process-proper**

1. A clean phial with new velvet cork is taken.
2. 59.4 minims of dispensing alcohol is poured by a minim glass into the phial.
3. Then 0.6 minim of 29th potency of Bryonia is poured with the help of graduated minim pipette and the phial is corked.
4. Then ten downward uniform strokes are given holding the phial with the right hand thumb upon the cork and the bottom of the phial inside the first, then on the left hand palm.

C. **Post-process**

1. A label is pasted on the wall of the phial writing. **'Bryonia-30°'**
2. All used utensils are washed properly and handed over to the laboratory attendant.

Q. 26. Write and serve a prescription in liquid form for internal use only

For

Baby Mukut

R_x

Phytolacca 30

Gtt. IV

Aqua. dest. 1Oz.

M. Ft. Mist.

Div. in 6D.

To be taken B.D.

Sd/-

B. Mandal

21.8.92

Requirements

A. **Ingredients**

1. Phytolacca 30 liquid.
2. Purified water.

B. **Appliances**

1. A clean round phial.

2. A new non-porous velvet cork.
3. Measuring glass.
4. Pen, paper, gum, scissors etc.

Procedure

A. **Pre-process**

The phial and the cork are properly cleaned with purified water.

B. **Process-proper**

One ounce purified water is taken in the phial and four small drops of phytolacca-30 are added to it. The phial is closed with the cork and shaken very gently.

C. **Post-process**

1. A label is pasted on the body of the phial writing **'For, Baby Mukut, 6 doses to be taken twice daily.'**
2. All used utensils are washed properly and handed over to be laboratory attendant.

Chapter 44

Plant Collection and Preparation of Herbarium

Introduction

In botany, a **herbarium** (plural: **herbaria**)— sometimes known by the Anglicised term **herbar**—is a collection of preserved plant specimens. These specimens may be whole plants or plant parts: these will usually be in a dried form, mounted on a sheet, but depending upon the material may also be kept in alcohol or other preservative. The same term is often used in mycology to describe an equivalent collection of preserved fungi.

The term can also refer to the building where the specimens are stored, or the scientific institute that not only stores but researches these specimens. The specimens in a herbarium are often used as reference material in describing plant taxa; some specimens may be types.

Some Important Herbaria of India

1. The Madras Herbarium (MH), Botanical Survey of India, Southern Circle, TNAU Campus, Coimbatore 641 003, Tamil Nadu Madras: It was started by Lawson (1873). It has approximately 150,000 specimens.
2. Central National Herbarium, Botanical Survey of India, P.O. Botanic Garden, Howrah 711103: It was started in 1800 by some plant collector. There are approximately 2,000,000 specimens. It is the largest herbarium in India.
3. Botanical Survey of India, Western Circle, 7 Koregaon Road, Pune 411001, Maharashtra: It was started in Poona. It has. approximately 120,000 specimens.
4. Regional Herbarium at Shillong: It has approximately 86,000 specimens. It was started under the control of Forest Department.
5. Herbarium, National Botanical Research Institute, Rana Pratap Marg, Lucknow 226001, Uttar Pradesh: Started in 1948 and possess about 80,000 specimens.
6. Herbarium of Forest Research Institute (FRI), Dehradun: It was started in 1830 and has about 300,000 specimens

Purposes of Herbaria

1. Herbaria are essential for the study of plant taxonomy, the study of geographic distributions, and the stabilising of nomenclature. Thus it is desirable to include in a specimen as much of the plant as possible (e.g., flowers, stems, leaves, seed, and fruit).
2. Specimens housed in herbaria may be used to catalogue or identify the flora of an area.

A large collection from a single area is used in writing a field guide or manual to aid in the identification of plants that grow there.

3. Herbaria also preserve an historical record of change in vegetation over time. In some cases, plants become extinct in one area, or may become extinct altogether. In such cases, specimens preserved in an herbarium can represent the only record of the plant's original distribution. Environmental scientists make use of such data to track changes in climate and human impact.

4. Many kinds of scientists use herbaria to preserve voucher specimens; representative samples of plants used in a particular study to demonstrate precisely the source of their data.

5. They may also be a repository of viable seeds for rare species.

Plant Collection and Herbarium Techniques

The collection of plants began in the 16th century. Later, J. P. Tourefort (ca 1700, France) used the term herbarium for plants (Bridson and Forman 1999). Plant collections are essentials for taxonomic researches because they serve as voucher specimens. They also help to identify the family, genus and species. So a herbarium is basically a storehouse of botanical specimens, which are arranged in the sequence of an accepted classification system, and available for reference or other scientific study. Once mounted and deposited in the herba-rium, the collections are referred to as herbarium specimens. Such herbarium specimens can be stored for many years.

1. Materials required for plant collection

(i) Plant cutter (secateur), pruner, digger, knife, leather gloves.

(ii) Field note book, pencil, permanent ink pens, magnifying glass, digital camera, flora book (colorful), forceps.

(iii) Flimsies or newspaper, blotters, corrugated plates, herbarium pressure, straps, tissue paper, plastic (poly) bags, herbarium bags.

(iv) Drying table, mountain survival blanket, clipper, heater.

(v) First aid box, topographic maps, computer, binocular.

2. Collection procedure

Twig with good flowers need to be collected for the specimen. The portion of the specimen should have to contain clear phyllotaxy and the branching system. For small herb, collection of more specimens as could fix on the herbarium sheet (up to six) is desirable. In general, secateurs are used to cut the twigs, while for a bit height or down, pruner is used and for spiny specimens, such as Berberis mucrifolia, leather glove is required. For ferns and herbs, digger is applied to take out underground portion. Some plants stem lies horizontally under the ground; for example, some Salix and Myricaria species. In such cases, the underground portion should be cleaned from the soil particles, etc. If it is stem, then, specimens have be contained branching manner.

Aquatic plants are filmy or somewhat filamentous and are difficult to be arranged on the sheet. A sheet of mounting paper is placed under a floating or submerged minute plants, and then slowly raising the paper until the specimen is lying on the paper and out of the water. Then paper is lifted making a slope carefully, so that it facilitates water runoff. These plants need to be shaken well before putting in flimsies. Some plants can be put in plastic bags. The plants that easily damage or can be lost among larger plants from the same collection site can be placed in small bags within the larger bag. Diseased plants, depauperate specimens, infected twigs, etc. should be avoided.

At the time of collection, it is usually not possible to identify many specimens in the field. Therefore, botanists identify the specimens that have been pressed and dried. The specimens are grouped into bundles according to location. The confirmed specimens should contain their botanical name, including author. The collection number can be used as a specimen tag. These number usually begin with 1, 2, 3, etc. and continue indefinitely. Plant collectors sometimes use a modified system, beginning each new year. Instead of tags, collection number also can be written in flimsies by marker.

3. Field Note

After specimen collection, a field record is noted in small pocket sized notebook. Date of collection, location (name of place or distance from definite point), collection number, if possible, name of the specimen, and description of the floral parts that may change after drying are noted down. The good quality specimens also become worst if it does not have good field record. Topographic map is essential for the location. It needs to examine the floral parts carefully, if small by using magnifying lens. The characters should tally with the literature and pictures of the books. From various angles, the flower photos require to be taken.

Dorsal and ventral leaf view photos are also essential for the further identification confirmation. Digital camera should have at least 5-mega pixels so that close up image can be taken even if the flower is too small. The range, latitude and longitude as well ecology of plant need to be noted down by GPS (Global Positioning System) and eyesight vision. Likewise specimen's micro-habitat; means associated species should be mentioned, at least five species. Finally, the distribution status of plant also needs to be mentioned, either the collected species is rare, frequent, common, locally common or occasional. Duplicate specimens of one species that are collected on the same date and same locality should be given the same collection number.

4. Pressing

When time and carrying facilities permit, the most usual method is to press each specimen as it is collected. Another method is to accumulate the specimens in vasculum (also black colored plastic bags can be used for short duration, especially in high altitude) and pressed later. Specimens should be of good quality with good field note. Collection numbers have also to be written in the flimsies (newspaper or blank newspaper). The specimens are kept gently within newspaper. Parts of flower are much carefully spread without overlapping in original shape. If the specimens are long, then it needs to be folded in V and N or Z shape. Unnecessary overlapping leaves and other parts must be avoided. Large leaf, if palmately compound, split in half lengthwise and one half is discarded. If pinnately compound, a branch is only kept. A few leaves may be turned over to show lower and upper view. If there is bulgy Rhizome, needs to cut or dissect longitudinally by knife, so that moisture evaporates through there. If the specimen is Gymnosperms, like Abies spectabilis (leaves fall before dry), the specimens needs to deep in the glycerin before pressing. Flowers with gamopetalous corollas should have to be pressed a few flowers separately and some of these split open and spread. If flower is large, cotton padding is often helpful to dry quickly.

The specimens thus kept inside flimsies, are covered by on either side by blotters and then it is put herbarium pressure. After press is filled or all the specimens pressed, the plant press is closed and pressure applied by means of tightening the straps. Hard and dried fruits and cones need not preserve and press, but have to keep in special boxes. The final appearance of the specimen depends on how it is pressed and dried (Jones and Luchsinger 1986).

5. Re-pressing

The specimens are repressed in the evening in the camp. The blotters are changed, if they are moistened. But flimsies need not change. The specimens are kept with the new blotters. After blotter, for ventilation and equal heat diffusion, aluminum plates (corrugates 12 × 18 in) are placed. The process is repeated for each specimen. Thus racked specimens are designated as corrugated-blotter-flimsies with specimen-blotter-corrugated. Then it is tied up inside the herbarium pressure or plant pressure by two straps or belts around the outside. It is usually constructed of a sturdy metal, plywood, or wooden grid frame 30 × 46 cm or 12 × 18 in. (Woodland 1997). The herbarium pressure equipment can be inexpensively made from wood scraps, old cardboard boxes, old newspaper, and small rope. The final data is recorded in the computer using Microsoft Excel program, before specimens repressed for drying in the field. Thus prepared database is helpful in future.

6. Drying Techniques

Drying techniques are of two types; those accomplished without heat, and those with the aid of artificial heat. **Drying with the aid of artificial heat is the prevalent method.** It is accomplished by means of heated dry air passing up and through the canal of the corrugate. Corrugates, often referred to as ventilators, are used in presses when plants are dried by means of artificial heat (Lawrence 1951). It is a sheet of paste board or thin aluminum metal, with fluted ducts. It provides air passages through the press for movement of dry heated air.

The dryer with the herbarium pressure is covered by mountain survival blanket. It is heat resistant blanket that is attached to stand with clips. At the base (single) for coming and at the tip, for out going air, series ventilations need to keep. The best heat source is heater. Stove can be used as an alternative source. The usual time period for drying specimens is 12 hours. But it depends upon the material; and also dryer set, humidity, the type of heat source, climate, and temperature affect the drying period. Too high temperature for too long time period will cause a specimen to become brittle and discolored. Too short a drying period or too low a temperature will keep the specimens, moist to touch, and possibly cause mildew. Specimens will need to be checked regularly until dry. A specimen is not dry if it is still limp when picked up and cool and moist to the touch. The pressures become loose when the plants are dry.

The most common method of drying is without applying heat. Plants are placed in pressing papers between the blotters of the plant press. No corrugates are used. The press is locked up for about 24 hours, this is known as the sweating period. It is then opened, and as blotters are removed each pressing sheet is turned back, the specimens are examined, and parts rearranged as the situation demands. The difference between a poorly and a well arranged specimen usually results from the attention given at this stage of the process.

After rearrangement the folder sheet is lifted on to a fresh dry blotter and covered by another dry blotter. The new pile of blotters and specimens is then locked up in the press and allowed to stand for another 24 to 36 hours, when the process of replacing wet blotters with dry one is repeated.

A third change of blotters follows usually after 2 to 3 days. Blotters must be changed 3-4 times; every wet blotter removed must be dried, usually by placing in the sun and reused. About a week is required for completion of drying. Dried specimens are packed with much care. Fungi as well as insects damage if proper care is not given till the permanent storage.

7. Mounting of herbarium specimens

Mounting is the process by which a specimen is attached to a herbarium sheet and a label affixed at the lower right corner. Specimens are mounted on sheets of standard size herbarium paper (29 × 43 cm). North American standard size sheets are 29 × 41.5 cm or 11.5 × 16.5 in (Woodland 1997). Most herbaria use a glue or paste to fasten specimens to the sheets. The specimen may be attached by various methods. A common method involves smearing a glass plate with a water-soluble paste, placing the specimen on the paste, and then transferring the glued plant to the mounting sheet. Small paper envelopes called fragment packets are attached to the sheet to hold seeds, extra flowers, or any part of the specimen.

8. Protection of herbarium sheet against insects and moulds

Precaution should be taken to protect herbarium specimens from damage by insect pests. The most destructive insects are herbarium beetle, cigarette beetle, booklice, and silverfish. Insect repellants such as naphthalene ball or Para dichlorobenzene are sometimes placed in small quantities in herbarium cabinet. Although dangerous and hazardous to health, mercuric chloride is believed to be valuable because it provides long-term protection against insect attack. Besides the insect pest, the moulds and mildew are constant threat to material stored in damp condition or in areas of high humidity. Naphthalene and LPCP are believed to have fungicidal properties, however, Thymol is quite effective as a fungicide.

9. Labelling of herbarium specimen

Herbarium label is an important and essential part of permanent plant specimens. The size and shape of label may vary slightly but will usually be a rectangular and range between 10 × 15 cm (4 × 6 in). The best position for the main label is generally thought to be the bottom right; this makes the label easier to read when kept in genus covers which open on the right hand side. Ideally a space should be left above the label to allow for the future attachment of determination slips. Generally herbarium label should contain the following information:

1. Heading: name of the institution in which the specimens originated/deposited.
2. Scientific name: Genus, specific epithet, author, or authors
3. Family
4. Localilty of collection
5. Range, latitude and longitude
6. Habitat
7. Date of collection
8. Name of collector(s)
9. Determined by
10. Remarks

List of Drugs for Herbarium Sheet

Common name: ADA
Synonym: Ginger
Drug name: **Zingiber officinale**
Natural order: Zingiberaceae
Part used: Dried rhizome
Class: IV
Drug power: 1/10
Ratio: 1: 5

Common name: AKANDA
Synonym: Madar
Drug name: **Calotropis gigantia**
Natural order: Asclepiadaceae
Part used: Dried roots
Class: IV
Drug power: 1/10
Ratio: 1 : 5

Common name: AAM
Synonym: Mango
Drug name: **Mangifera indica**
Natural order: Anacardiaceae
Part used: Green fresh leaves
Class: III
Drug power: 1/6
Ratio: 1 : 2

Common name: AMLAKI
Synonym: Emblic myrobalan
Drug name: **Embelica officinalis**
Natural order: Euphorbiaceae
Part used: Dried fruits
Class: IV
Drug power: 1/10
Ratio: 1 : 5

Common name: ARJUN
Synonym: White murdah
Drug name: **Terminalia arjuna**
Natural order: Combretaceae
Part used: Bark of the tree
Class: IV
Drug power: 1/10
Ratio: 1 : 5

Common name: ASWATHA
Synonym: Peepal
Drug name: **Ficus religiosa**
Natural order: Moraceae
Part used: Tender leaves
Class: III
Drug power: 1/6
Ratio: 1: 2

Common name: BABLA
Synonym: Gum tree
Drug name: **Acacia arabica**
Natural order: Mimosae
Part used: Dried bark
Class: IV
Drug power: 1/10
Ratio: 1 : 5

Common name: BASAK
Synonym: Malabar nut
Drug name: **Justicia adhatoda**
Natural order: Acanthaceae
Part used: Fresh leaves
Class: III
Drug power: 1/6
Ratio: 1 : 2

Common name: **BOT**

Synonym: Banyan tree

Drug name: **Ficus indica**

Natural order: Moracea

Part used: Leaves and aerial roots

Class: III

Drug power: 1/6

Ratio: 1 : 2

Common name: **BETHOSHAK**

Synonym: Goose foot

Drug name: **Chenopodium anthelminticum**

Natural order: Chenopodiaceae

Part used: Whole plant

Class: III

Drug power: 1/6

Ratio: 1 : 2

Common name: **BILATI ANARAS**

Synonym: Century plant

Drug name: **Agave americana**

Natural order: Amaryllidaceae

Part used: Fresh leaves

Class: III

Drug power: 1/6

Ratio: 1 : 2

Common name: **BILWA PATRA**

Drug name: **Aegle folia**

Natural order: Rutaceae

Part used: Fresh leaves

Class: III

Drug power: 1/6

Ratio: 1 : 2

Common name: **BRAHMI**

Drug name: **Bacopa monnieri**

Natural order: Scrophulariaceae

Part used: Whole plant

Class: III

Drug power: 1/6

Ratio: 1 : 2

Common name: **CHANDRAMALLIKA**

Synonym: Chrysanthemum

Drug name: **Chrysanthemum coronarium**

Natural order: Compositae

Part used: Flower buds and leaves

Class: III

Drug power: 1/6

Ratio: 1 : 2

Common name: **CHATIM**

Synonym: Devil tree

Drug name: **Alstonia scholaris**

Natural order: Apocynaceae

Part used: Dried bark

Class: IV

Drug power: 1/10

Ratio: 1 : 5

Common name: **DALIM**

Synonym: Pomegranate

Drug name: **Punica granatum**

Natural order: Granateae

Part used: Dried bark of the root

Class: IV

Drug power: 1/10

Ratio: 1 : 5

Common name: **DARUCHINI**

Synonym: Cinnamon

Drug name: **Cinnamomum zeylanicum**

Natural order: Lauraceae

Part used: Dried bark of shoots

Class: IV

Drug power: 1/10

Ratio: 1 : 5

Common name: **DATURA**

Synonym: Thorn-apple

Drug name: **Datura stramonium**

Natural order: Solanaceae

Part used: Plant in flowering; fruit

Class: IV

Drug power: 1/10

Ratio: 1 : 5

Common name: **DURBA**
Synonym: Doob grass
Drug name: **Cynodon dactylon**
Natural order: Loganiaceae
Part used: Dried herbs
Class: III
Drug power: $\frac{1}{6}$
Ratio: 1 : 2

Common name: **EUCALYPTUS**
Synonym: Blue Gum Tree
Drug name: **Eucalyptus globulus**
Natural order: Myrtaceae
Part used: Leaves
Class: III
Drug power: $\frac{1}{6}$
Ratio: 1:2

Common name: **GANDHA**
Synonym: Marigold
Drug name: **Calendula officinalis**
Natural order: Compositae
Part used: Fresh leaves
Class: I
Drug power: $\frac{1}{2}$
Ratio: 1 : 1

Common name: **GHRITAKUMARI**
Synonym: Indian aloe
Drug name: **Aloe socotrina**
Natural order: Liliaceae
Part used: Inspissated juice of leaves
Class: IV
Drug power: $\frac{1}{10}$
Ratio: 1 : 5

Common name: **GULANCHA**
Drug name: **Tinospora cordifolia**
Natural order: Menispermaceae
Part used: Dried stem with bark
Class: IV
Drug power: $\frac{1}{10}$
Ratio: 1 : 5

Common name: **HALUDA**
Synonym: Turmeric
Drug name: **Curcuma longa**
Natural order: Zingiberaceae
Part used: Rhizome
Class: IV
Drug power: $\frac{1}{10}$
Ratio: 1 : 5

Common name: **HING**
Drug name: **Ferula asafoetida**
Natural order: Umbelliferae
Part used: Gum resin from root
Class: IV
Drug power: $\frac{1}{10}$
Ratio: 1 : 5

Common name: **JAM**
Synonym: Jambol seeds
Drug name: **Syzygium jambolanum**
Natural order: Myrtaceae
Part used: Fresh seeds
Class: IV
Drug power: $\frac{1}{10}$
Ratio: 1 : 5

Common name: **JHAU**
Synonym: Arbor-vitae
Drug name: **Thuja occidentalis**
Natural order: Coniferae
Part used: Fresh leaves
Class: II
Drug power: $\frac{1}{2}$
Ratio: 3 : 2

Common name: **KALMEGH**
Synonym: Creat
Drug name: **Andrographis paniculata**
Natural order: Acanthaceae
Part used: Whole plant
Class: III
Drug power: $\frac{1}{6}$
Ratio: 1 : 2

Common name: **KANCHAN**
Synonym: Orchid tree
Drug name: **Bauhinia variegata**
Natural order: Fabaceae
Part used: Fresh leaves
Class: I
Drug power: $1/2$
Ratio: 1 : 1

Common name: **KAPAS**
Synonym: Cotton plant
Drug name: **Gossypium herbaceum**
Natural order: Malvaceae
Part used: Dried bark of root and seed
Class: III
Drug power: $1/6$
Ratio: 1 : 2

Common name: **KARELA**
Synonym: Bitter guard
Drug name: **Momordica charantia**
Natural order: Cucurbitaceae
Part used: Fruits
Class: IV
Drug power: $1/10$
Ratio: 1:5

Common name: **KOROBI**
Synonym: Rose-laurel
Drug name: **Nerium oleander**
Natural order: Apocynaceae
Part used: Fresh leaves
Class: II
Drug power: $1/2$
Ratio: 3 : 2

Common name: **KUCHILA**
Synonym: Poison nut
Drug name: **Nux vomica**
Natural order: Loganiaceae
Part used: Seeds
Class: IV
Drug power: $1/10$
Ratio: 1 : 5

Common name: **KURCHI**
Synonym: Easter tree
Drug name: **Holarrhena antidysenterica**
Natural order: Apocynaceae
Part used: Dried bark
Class: IV
Drug power: $1/10$
Ratio: 1 : 5

Common name: **LANKA**
Synonym: Red pepper
Drug name: **Capsicum annuum**
Natural order: Solanaceae
Part used: **Ripe fruit with seeds**
Class: IV
Drug power: $1/10$
Ratio: 1 : 5

Common name: **LEBU**
Synonym: **Lemon**
Drug name: **Citrus limon**
Natural order: Rutaceae
Part used: Leaves and fruits
Class: New method (Maceration)
Drug power: $1/10$
Ratio: 1 : 9

Common name: **MULA**
Synonym: **Radish**
Drug name: **Raphanus sativus**
Natural order: Cruciferae
Part used: Fresh root
Class: III
Drug power: $1/6$
Ratio: 1 : 2

Common name: **MUTHA**
Synonym: Common sedge
Drug name: **Cyperus rotundus**
Natural order: Cyperaceae
Part used: Whole plant
Class: IV
Drug power: $1/10$
Ratio: 1 : 5

Common name: **NAGDONA**
Synonym: Mugwort
Drug name: **Artemisia vulgaris**
Natural order: Compositae
Part used: Roots
Class: III
Drug power: $\frac{1}{6}$
Ratio: 1 : 2

Common name: **NAYANTARA**
Synonym: Periwinkle
Drug name: **Vinca rosea**
Natural order: Apocynaceae
Part used: Leaves
Class: III
Drug power: $\frac{1}{6}$
Ratio: 1 : 2

Common name: **NIM**
Synonym: Margosa bark
Drug name: **Azadirachta indica**
Natural order: Meliaceae
Part used: Fresh bark of the tree
Class: III
Drug power: $\frac{1}{6}$
Ratio: 1 : 2

Common name: **PAPAY**
Synonym: Melon tree
Drug name: **Carica papaya**
Natural order: Passifloraceae
Part used: Fresh leaves
Class: III
Drug power: $\frac{1}{6}$
Ratio: 1 : 2

Common name: **PATHARKUCHI**
Synonym: Sprout-leaf plant
Drug name: **Bryophyllum calycinum**
Natural order: Labiatae
Part used: Fresh leaves
Class: I
Drug power: $\frac{1}{2}$
Ratio: 1 : 2

Common name: **PAYAJ**
Synonym: Onion
Drug name: **Allium cepa**
Natural order: Liliaceae
Part used: Red, mature bulb
Class: III
Drug power: $\frac{1}{6}$
Ratio: 1 : 2

Common name: **RASUN**
Synonym: Garlic
Drug name: **Allium sativum**
Natural order: Liliaceae
Part used: The mature bulb
Class: III
Drug power: $\frac{1}{6}$
Ratio: 1 : 2

Common name: **REHRI**
Synonym: Castor oil plant
Drug name: **Ricinus communis**
Natural order: Euphorbiaceae
Part used: Fresh seeds
Class: IV
Drug power: $\frac{1}{10}$
Ratio: 1:4

Common name: **SHATAMULI**
Synonym: Asparagus
Drug name: **Asparagus officinalis**
Natural order: Liliaceae
Part used: Young root
Class: III
Drug power: $\frac{1}{6}$
Ratio: 1 : 2

Common name: **SHIALKANTA**
Synonym: Mexican poppy
Drug name: **Argemone mexicana**
Natural order: Papaveraceae
Part used: Fresh plant in flower
Class: III
Drug power: $\frac{1}{6}$
Ratio: 1 : 2

Common name: **SURYAMUKHI**
Synonym: Sunflower
Drug name: **Halianthus annus**
Natural order: Compositae
Part used: Flowering heads
Class: IV
Drug power: $\frac{1}{10}$
Ratio: 1 : 5

Common name: **TEJPATA**
Synonym: Indian bay leaf
Drug name: **Cinnamomum tamala**
Natural order: Lauraceae
Part used: Leaves
Class: IV
Drug power: $\frac{1}{10}$
Ratio: 1:5

Common name: **TELAKUCHA**
Synonym: Scarlet gourd
Drug name: **Cephalandra indica**
Natural order: Cucurbitaceae
Part used: Fresh green leaves
Class: I
Drug power: $\frac{1}{2}$
Ratio: 1 : 1

Common name: **TETUL**
Synonym: Imli
Drug name: **Tamarindus indica**
Natural order: Fabaceae
Part used: Fruits
Class: IV
Drug power: $\frac{1}{10}$
Ratio: 1 : 5

Common name: **THANKUNI**
Synonym: Indian pennywort
Drug name: **Hydrocotyle asiatica**
Natural order: Umbelliferae
Part used: Dried leaves
Class: IV
Drug power: $\frac{1}{10}$
Ratio: 1 : 5

Common name: **TULSI**
Synonym: Sacred basil
Drug name: **Ocimum sanctum**
Natural order: Labiatae
Part used: Fresh leaves
Class: III
Drug power: $\frac{1}{6}$
Ratio: 1 : 2

Name of Plants	Common name	Parts used	Class	Drug power	Ratio
Acacia arabica	Babla/Gum tree	Dried bark	IV	$\frac{1}{10}$	1 : 5
Aegle folia	Bilwa patra	Fresh leaves	III	$\frac{1}{6}$	1 : 2
Agave americana	Bilati anaras	Fresh leaves	III	$\frac{1}{6}$	1 : 2
Aloe socotrina	Gritakumari	Inspissated juice of leaves	IV	$\frac{1}{10}$	1 : 5
Allium cepa	Payaj/Onion	Red, mature bulb	III	$\frac{1}{6}$	1 : 2
Allium sativum	Rasun/Garlic	The mature bulb	III	$\frac{1}{6}$	1 : 2
Alstonia scholaris	Chatim/Devil tree	Dried bark	IV	$\frac{1}{10}$	1 : 5
Andrographis paniculata	Kalmegh/Creat	Whole plant	III	$\frac{1}{6}$	1 : 2

Contd.

Contd.

Name of Plants	Common name	Parts used	Class	Drug power	Ratio
Argemone mexicana	Shialkanta	Fresh plant in flower	III	$\frac{1}{6}$	1 : 2
Artemisia vulgaris	Nagdona/Mugwort	Roots	III	$\frac{1}{6}$	1 : 2
Asparagus officinalis	Shatamuli	Young root	III	$\frac{1}{6}$	1 : 2
Azadirachta indica	Nim/Margosa bark	Fresh of the tree	III	$\frac{1}{6}$	1 : 2
Bacopa monnieri	Brahmi	Whole plant	III	$\frac{1}{6}$	1 : 2
Bauhinia variegate	Kanchan/Orchid tree	Fresh leaves	I	$\frac{1}{2}$	1 : 1
Bryophyllum calycinum	Patharkuchi	Fresh leaves	I	$\frac{1}{2}$	1 : 2
Calendula officinalis	Gandha/Marigold	Fresh leaves	I	$\frac{1}{2}$	1 : 1
Calotropis gigantia	Madar/Akanda	Dried roots	IV	$\frac{1}{10}$	1 : 5
Capsicum annum	Lanka	Ripe fruits with seeds	IV	$\frac{1}{10}$	1 : 5
Carica papaya	Papay/Melon tree	Fresh leaves	III	$\frac{1}{6}$	1 : 2
Cephalandra indica	Telakucha	Fresh green leaves	I	$\frac{1}{2}$	1 : 1
Chenopodium anthelminticum	Bethoshak	Whole plant	III	$\frac{1}{6}$	1 : 2
Chrysanthemum coronarium	Chandramallika	Flower buds and leaves	III	$\frac{1}{6}$	1 : 2
Cinnamomum tamala	Indian bay leaf	Leaves	IV	$\frac{1}{10}$	1 : 5
Cinnamomum zeylanicum	Daruchini/Cinamon	Dried bark of shoots	IV	$\frac{1}{10}$	1 : 5
Citrus limon	Lemon	Leaves and fruits	Maceration	$\frac{1}{10}$	1 : 9
Curcuma longa	Turmeric	Rhizome	IV	$\frac{1}{10}$	1 : 5
Cynodon dactylon	Durba/Doob grass	Dried herbs	III	$\frac{1}{6}$	1 : 2
Cyperus rotundus	Mutha	Whole plant	IV	$\frac{1}{10}$	1 : 5
Datura stramonium	Datura/Thorn apple	Plant in flowering; fruits	IV	$\frac{1}{10}$	1 : 5
Embelica officinalis	Amlaki	Dried fruits	IV	$\frac{1}{10}$	1 : 5
Eucalyptus globulus	Blue Gum Tree	Leaves	III	$\frac{1}{6}$	1 : 2
Ferula asafoetida	Hing	Gum resin from root	IV	$\frac{1}{10}$	1 : 5
Ficus indica	Bot/Banyan tree	Leaves and aerial roots	III	$\frac{1}{6}$	1 : 2
Ficus religiosa	Aswatha/Peepal	Tender leaves	III	$\frac{1}{6}$	1 : 2

Contd.

Contd.

Name of Plants	Common name	Parts used	Class	Drug power	Ratio
Gossypium herbaceum	Kapas/Cotton plant	Dried bark of root and seed	III	$\frac{1}{6}$	1 : 2
Halianthus annus	Suryamukhi	Flowering heads	IV	$\frac{1}{10}$	1 : 5
Holarrhena antidysenterica	Kurchi	Dried bark	IV	$\frac{1}{10}$	1 : 5
Hydrocotyle asiatica	Thankuni	Dried leaves	IV	$\frac{1}{10}$	1 : 5
Justicia adhatoda	Basak	Fresh leaves	III	$\frac{1}{6}$	1 : 2
Mangifera indica	Mango	Green fresh leaves	III	$\frac{1}{6}$	1 : 2
Momordica charantia	Bitter guard	Fruits	IV	$\frac{1}{10}$	1 : 5
Nerium oleander	Korobi/Rose laurel	Fresh leaves	II	$\frac{1}{2}$	3 : 2
Nux vomica	Kuchila/Poison nut	Seeds	IV	$\frac{1}{10}$	1 : 5
Ocimum sanctum	Tulsi/Sacred basil	Fresh leaves	III	$\frac{1}{6}$	1 : 2
Punica granatum	Dalim	Dried bark of the root	V	$\frac{1}{10}$	1 : 5
Raphanus sativus	Mula/Radish	Fresh root	III	$\frac{1}{6}$	1 : 2
Ricinus communis	Castor oil plant	Fresh seeds	IV	$\frac{1}{10}$	1 : 4
Syzygium jambolanum	Jam/Jambol seeds	Fresh seeds	IV	$\frac{1}{10}$	1 : 5
Tamarindus indica	Imli	Fruits	IV	$\frac{1}{10}$	1 : 5
Terminalia arjuna	Arjun	Bark of the tree	IV	$\frac{1}{10}$	1 : 5
Thuja occidentalis	Jhau/Arbor vitae	Fresh leaves	II	$\frac{1}{2}$	3 : 2
Tinospora cordifolia	Gulancha	Dried stem with bark	IV	$\frac{1}{10}$	1 : 5
Vinca rosa	Nayantara/Periwinkle	Leaves	III	$\frac{1}{6}$	1 : 2
Zingiber officinale	Ginger	Dried rhizome	IV	$\frac{1}{10}$	1 : 5

Chapter 45

Word-meaning, History and Authority of some Drugs of Plant Kingdom

Aconite napellus

The word ACONITE is derived from ACONIS, a city of Bithynia (in Asia Minor). Also, ACON means 'odart', because the darts were poisoned with Aconite. Also, from Greek word *Aconitum* means without soil, as this plant grows on a stony ground.

The word NAPELLUS means 'little turnip', it refers to the shape of the root.

History and Authority: Hahnemann introduced it in homoeopathy in 1805. *Allen's Encyclopedia Materia Medica* Vol. I, 12. Hering's Guiding Symptoms Vol. I, 28.

Arnica montana

The name ARNICA is derived from *Arnakis* meaning 'lamb's skin' due to the woolly appearance of the leaf.

MONTANA from Latin word *Mountainous* from the place that it grows.

History and Authority: Hahnemann introduced it in homoeopathic practice in 1805. Allens' Encyclopedia Materia Medica, Vol I, 476.

Atropa belladonna

The word BELLADONNA is derived from two Latin words: *Bella* meaning 'fine or beautiful' and *Donna* meaning lady. Its generic name 'ATROPA' comes from the Greek word *Atropos*, 'The inflexible one'.

History and Authority: Hahnemann introduced this drug in homoeopathy in 1805. Allen's Encyclopedia Materia Medica, Vol. II, 67; X 373, 645.

Baptisia tinctoria

This plant was used officially in medicine from 1830 to 1840. It somewhat resembles asparagus. The INDIGO was used by the American Indians as an antiseptic and as a dressing for gangrenous wounds, especially when these wounds were accompanied by fever.

History and Authority: It was introduced by Dr. W. L. Thompson in 1857. Allen's Encyclopedia Materia Media, Vol II, 31; X, 372.

Bryonia alba

The word BRYONIA means 'growing rapidly', as the stem grows rapidly.

ALBA, from Latin word *Albus* means 'white' as the roots and flowers are yellowish or white.

History and Authority: Hahnemann introduced this drug in homoeopathic practice in 1816. Allen's Encyclopedia Materia Medica, Vol. II, 249.

Berberis vulgaris

It was used in Medicine by Galen, Pliny and Dioscorides. The bark of the root was official from 1860 to 1880. The fruit was official from 1830 to 1840.

History and Authority: This drug was introduced by Hesse in homoeopathic practice. Allen's Encyclopedia Materia Medica, Vol. II, 139.

Cactus grandiflorus

The name CACTUS was originally given by Theophrastus; to a spiny plant of Sicily in Italy.

History and Authority: Rubini introduced this drug in homoeopathic practice in 1864. Allen's Encyclopedia Materia Medica, Vol. II, 321.

Calendula officinalis

The word CALENDULA is derived from *Calendos*, the first day of the month. This plant flowers on the first of the month or at least once a month.

History and Authority: Dr. Franz introduced this drug in homoeopathic practice in 1838. Allen's Encyclopedia Materia Medica, Vol. II, 419.

Chamomilla

The word CHAMOMILLA is derived from *Chamaemelum* and MATRICARIA from *Matrix* means 'apple on the ground', because the plant grows to the ground and has an odour like that of apples. It has been used since long as a domestic remedy by the name of Chamomile.

History and Authority: Hahnemann introduced this drug in homoeopathic practice in 1805. Allen's Encyclopedia Materia Medica, Vol. III, 89.

Chelidonium majus

The word CHELIDONIUM is derived from *Cheledon*, which means 'a swallow', because its flowers were said to bloom and wither with the arrival and departure of the swallows. The word MAJUS means 'greater' or 'larger'.

History and Authority: Hahnemann introduced this drug in homoeopathic practice in 1819. Allen's Encyclopedia Materia Medica, Vol. III, 127.

Carduus marianus

The Word CARDUUS is the genus of this and other prickly plants known as thistles.

The word MARIANUS is related to Virgin Mary because according to the fables, portion of the Virgin Mary's milk fell on the leaves, producing the white veins.

History and Authority: Reil introduced this drug in homoeopathic practice in 1852. Allen's Encyclopedia Materia Medica, Vol. II, 635.

Caulophyllum thalictroides

The word CAULOPHYLLUM is derived from *Kavles*, meaning 'a stem', and *Phyllon*, 'leaf', as the stem appears to be a leaf stalk.

The word THALICTROIDES, derived from *Thalow*, meaning to 'grow green', and *Troides*, resembling 'green stem'.

History and Authority: E. M. Hale introduced this drug in homoeopathic practice. Allen's Encyclopedia Materia Medica, Vol. III, 34.

Chimaphila umbellata

The word CHIMAPHILA is derived from *Cheima*, meaning 'winter', and *Phileo*, 'to love'.

The word UMBELLATA is derived from the Latin word *umbellatus*, meaning umbellated.

History and Authority: S. A. Jones first introduced this drug in homoeopathic practice in 1875

Chionanthus virginica

The word CHIONANTHUS comes from Greek *Chion*, meaning 'white' and *anthos* meaning 'a flower', due to its snow-white flowers.

The word VIRGINICA is derived from *Virginia*, one of the States of U.S.A. in which it grows abundantly.

History and Authority: E. M. Hale introduced this drug in homoeopathic practice.

Cimicifuga racemosa

The word CIMICIFUGA is derived from *Cimex*, meaning, a 'bug', and *fugo* 'to drive away'. It was used in Siberia and Kamchatka to drive away the bugs.

The word RACEMOSA is derived from Latin *Racemosus* meaning 'full of clusters', racemes as the flowers are.

History and Authority: Houghton— N.A.J. of Hom. V. 27, 1856. Allen's Encyclopedia Materia Medica, Vol. X, 468.

Cina pauciflora

The word CINA comes from one of its common name CYNAE. PAUCIFLORA from the word *Pauses* meaning few and *florus* meaning flower, as it has few real blossoms and mostly only bud; it was first used as an antihelmintic.

In Europe, it was introduced by the Crusaders. After being isolated of its alkaloid SANTONINE, Cina was discontinued.

History and Authority: Hahnemann introduced this drug in homoeopathic practice in 1829. Allen's Encyclopedia Materia Medica, Vol. III, 307.

Cinchona officinalis

CINCHON, a place where the Countess Ann, wife of the 4th Count of CINCHON, lived. She was cured from tertian fever in 1638 by the use of cinchona bark. Its virtues were made known to Europe in 1640. It was identified by the botanists in 1717. This drug shows the pathway for the establishment of homoeopathy.

History and Authority: Allen's Encyclopedia Materia Medica, Vol. III, 182, X, 460.

Cocculus indicus

The word COCCULUS is derived from *Cocculin*, means Kermes berry. INDICUS, of India.

The berries were powdered and mixed with dough and used for stupefying the fishes for games. The berries have been used to prevent secondary fermentation of liquors and also by brewers to impart intoxicating properties to beer.

History and Authority: Hahnemann introduced this drug in 1805, in homoeopathic practice. Allen's Encyclopedia Materia Medica, Vol. III, 338.

Coffea cruda

The word COFFEA is derived from the Turkish *Qahveh* or the Arabic *Qahuah*, the name of a beverage.

The plant is indigenous to Abyssinia but is largely cultivated in tropical countries.

History and Authority: Stapf introduced this in homoeopathic practice in 1823.

Allen's Encyclopedia Materia Medica, Vol. III, 435.

Colchicum autumnale

The word COLCHICUM is derived from *Colchis*, an ancient province in Asia Minor, east of Black Sea, where this poisonous plant grows and flourishes.

AUTUMNALE, is the season in which it flowers.

+ and Authority: Stapf introduced this drug in homoeopathic practice in 1826. Allen's Encyclopedia Materia Medica, Vol. III, 448.

Colocynthis (Citrulus colocynthis)

The name CITRULUS COLOCYNTHIS is derived from the Latin word *Citrus*, means orange, as the colour of the fruit is yellow after cutting. It was known as early as the 11th century to the Greek, Roman and Arabian physicians.

History and Authority: Hahnemann introduced this drug in homoeopathic practice in 1821. Allen's Encyclopedia Materia Medica, Vol. III, 477.

Conium maculatum

The name CONIUM comes from the Greek '*Konas*', meaning 'to whirl about', because, when eaten, the plant causes great vertigo before death.

MACULATUM is French, *Macula* means 'spot'; Latin *Maculatus* means 'spotted', as the stem has small brownish/purple spots.

History and Authority: Hahnemann introduced this drug in homoeopathic practice in 1825. Allen's Encyclopedia Materia Medica, Vol. III, 519.

Croton tiglium

The word CROTON means dog tick, as the seeds resemble that of dog tick. This plant was introduced in 1818.

History and Authority: Joret introduced this drug in homoeopathic practice in 1834. Allen's Encyclopedia Materia Medica, Vol. III, 606.

Cinamomum camphora (or Camphora officinarum)

The word CINAMOMUM is derived from *Kaju manis* which means sweet wood, from its aromatic odour and taste.

The word CAMPHOR is derived from *Kafur*, means chalk or lime.

History and Authority: Hahnemann introduced this drug in homoeopathic practice. Allen's Encyclopedia Materia Medica, Vol. II, 422.

Cannabis sativa

The word CANNABIS is derived from Greek Kannabis, which is derived from sanskrit root canna, meaning cane. SATIVA means, 'cultivated'.

History and Authority: Hahnemann introduced this drug in homoeopathic practice in 1811. Allen's Encyclopedia Materia Medica, Vol. II, 492.

Capsicum annum

The word CAPSICUM is derived from *Capsa*, meaning *a chest, a box,* because the shape of the fruit is like chest or box which covers or conceals the seeds. On the other hand, it may be derived from Greek *Kapto* meaning *to bite*, because of its hot pungent properties.

History and Authority: Hahnemann introduced it in homoeopathic practice in 1805.

Digitalis purpurea

The word DIGITALIS is derived from *Digitus*, meaning *a finger*, due to its finger-shaped corolla.

The word PURPUREA is derived from the Latin word *Purpureus*, meaning *purple-coloured* because of its purple flowers.

History and Authority: Hahnemann introduced this drug in homoeopathic practice in 1805. Allen's Encyclopedia Materia Medica, Vol. IV, 92.

Drosera rotundifolia

The word DROSERA is derived from the Greek word *Droseros*, meaning *'dewy'*.

History and Authority: Hahnemann introduced this drug in homoeopathic practice in 1805. Allen's Encyclopedia Materia Medica, Vol. IV, 1701.

Dulcamara amara

The word DULCAMARA is derived from the Latin word *Dulces*, meaning *sweet*, and *Amarus* meaning *bitter*, owing to the transition of tastes which it yields.

History and Authority: Hahnemann introduced this drug in homoeopathic practice in 1811. Allen's Encyclopedia Materia Medica, Vol. IV, 178.

Eupatorium perfoliatum

The word *Eupatorium* means born of a noble father, after King Pontus who discovered one of the species. *Per* means through and *Folium* means leaves, i.e. a stem passing through the leaves.

History and Authority: Williamson introduced this drug in homoeopathic practice in 1845. Allen's Encyclopedia Materia Medica, Vol. IV, 178.

Euphrasia

The name EUPHRASIA is derived from the Greek *Euphrosyne*, one of the muses expressing joy or pleasure.

History and Authority: Hahnemann introduced this drug in homoeopathic practice in 1819. Allen's Encyclopedia Materia Medica, Vol. IV, 254.

Gelsemium sempervirens

The word GELSEMIUM is derived from Latin word *Gelsimino* meaning *Jasmine* and *Sempervirens* meaning *evergreen*.

History and Authority: Metcafe introduced this drug in homoeopathy in 1853. Allen's Encyclopedia Materia Medica, Vol. IV, 385.

Hamamelis virginica

The word HAMAMELIS is derived from the Greek word *Hama*, meaning at the *same time* and *Melles* meaning *a fruit*. VIRGINICA, from *Virginia*, one of the States of U.S.A.

History and Authority: Preston introduced this drug in homoeopathic practice in 1851. Allen's Encyclopedia Materia Medica, Vol. IV, 528.

Hyoscyamus niger

The word HYOSCYAMUS is derived from *Hyos*, meaning a hog and *Kyamos* meaning a bean, because bean acts as an intoxicant upon swine, but not on other animals. The word NIGER means black, as inside or throat of the flowers is purplish black.

History and Authority: Hahnemann introduced this drug in homoeopathic practice in 1805. Allen's Encyclopedia Materia Medica, Vol. V, 25.

Hypericum perforatum

The word HYPERICUM is derived from *Hyper* meaning *above*, and *Eicon* meaning *an image*, because the superior part of the flower represents a figure.

History and Authority: Mueller introduced this drug in homoeopathic practice in 1837. Allen's Encyclopedia Materia Medica, Vol. V, 53.

Hydrastis canadensis

The word HYDRASTIS is derived from *Hydro*, meaning *water*, and *Drao*, meaning *to act*, supposed to be thus named because of the active properties of the juice.

CANADENSIS is related to its habitat, *the northern limits of Canada*.

History and Authority: It was introduced in homoeopathic practice in 1866. Allen's Encyclopedia Materia Medica, Vol. IV, 613.

Ipecacuanha

The name IPECACUANHA is from the Portuguese word meaning, *'Roadside-sick-making plant'*, and mention of it as a remedy for 'the bloody flux' or dysentery; goes back as far as the late sixteenth century.

History and Authority: Hahnemann introduced this drug in homoeopathic practice in 1805. Allen's Encyclopedia Materia Medica, Vol. V, 137.

Iris versicolor

The word IRIS meaning *rainbow* due to bright and varying coloured flowers.

VERSICOLOR derived from Latin word *versare* meaning *to change*, because of changeable colour combination of flower.

History and Authority: Kitchen first introduced this drug in homoeopathic practice in 1851.

Lobelia inflata

The word LOBELIA derived from *Mathias lobel*, a flemish botanist. INFLATA, from the Latin word *Inflatus* meaning inflated, swollen, because the seeds are born in an egg-shelled inflated pod.

History and Authority: It was introduced in homoeopathic practice in 1841.

Lycopodium clavatum

The word LYCOPODIUM is derived from *Lykos* meaning *wolf* and pod meaning the *foot*, as the shoots have an appearance of the wolf's foot. CLAVATUM derived from Latin word *Clavatus* meaning *club-like*.

History and Authority: Hahnemann introduced it in homoeopathy in 1828. Allen's Encyclopedia Materia Medica, Vol. VI, I.

Mezereum (or Daphne mezereum)

The word MEZEREUM is derived from *Mazariyum*, which was then applied to *a species of daphane.*

The word DAPHNE, derived from *Daio*, meaning *burn* and *Phone*, meaning *noise* because of cracking noise it makes while burning.

History and Authority: Hahnemann introduced this in homoeopathic practice in 1805. Allen's Encyclopedia Materia Medica, Vol. VI, 330.

Millefolium

The word MILLEFOLIUM is derived from *Mille* meaning *thousand* and *Folium*, meaning *leaf* due to its numerous narrow painted leaves.

History and Authority: Hahnemann introduced this drug in homoeopathic practice in 1833.

Nux moschata (or Myristica fragrans)

The Latin word *Myristica* means *to anoint or be sprinkled with perfume*. It has a fragrant odour.

History and Authority: Dr. Helbig introduced this drug in homoeopathic practice in 1833. Allen's Encyclopedia Materia Medica, Vol. VII, 61.

Nux vomica

The word NUX VOMICA is derived from the Latin word *Nux* meaning *nut* and *Vomere* meaning *vomiting* because of the peculiar property of the nut.

History and Authority: Hahnemann introduced this drug in homoeopathic practice in 1805. Allen's Encyclopedia Materia Medica, Vol. VII, 83.

Opium (or Papaver somniferum)

The Latin word *Opium* meaning *juice of the poppy*. *Somnus* meaning *sleep*.

History and Authority: Hahnemann introduced this drug in homoeopathic practice in 1805. Allen's Encyclopedia Materia Medica, Vol. III, 173.

Passiflora incarnata

The word PASSIFLORA is derived from *Passio*, meaning *passion* and *Flos*, meaning *flower*.

The word INCARNATA is derived from the Latin word *Incarnatus* meaning *to clothe with flesh*, due to its purple and flesh-coloured flower-crown.

History and Authority: Hait first introduced it in homoeopathic practice.

Phytolacca decandra

The word PHYTOLACCA is derived from *Phyton*, meaning *plant* and *Lacca* meaning *ten stamens* because of the flowers have ten stamens.

History and Authority: Hahnemann introduced this drug in homoeopathic practice. Allen's Encyclopedia Materia Medica, Vol. VII, 502.

Podophyllum peltatum

The word 'PODOPHYLLUM' is derived from the Latin *'Podos'*, meaning 'foot' and *'Phyllon'* meaning 'leaf', as its leaves resembles the webbed feet of a duck; hence, also its nickname 'duck's foot'.

The word PELTATUM is derived from the Latin word *Peltatus* having a *pelta or tight shield* because the petioles are attached to the middle of lamina which gives it the appearance of a shield.

History and Authority: Williamson introduced it in homoeopathic practice in 1842. Allen's Encyclopedia Materia Medica, Vol. VIII, 130.

Pulsatilla nigricans

The word PULSATILLA is derived from *Pulsatus* meaning *to beat or to strike* as it pulsates from the blowing winds.

History and Authority: Hahnemann introduced this drug in homoeopathic practice in 1805. Allen's Encyclopedia Materia Medica, Vol. VIII, 20.

Rhus toxicodendron

The word RHUS means *red* because its flowers and leaves are red in colour. TOXICODENDRON means *poison tree*.

History and Authority: Hahnemann introduced this drug in homoeopathic practice in 1816.

Sanguinaria canadensis

The word SNAGUINARIA is derived from *Sanguis* meaning *blood* because when the plant is injured, it emits blood-like juice. CANADENSIS, related to its habitat *Canada*.

History and Authority: Bute introduced this drug in homoeopathic practice in 1837. Allen's Encyclopedia Materia Medica, Vol. VIII, 481.

Thuja occidentalis

The name 'THUJA' derives from the Greek *Thero* which means *'fumigate'* or *'sacrifice'*, for in ancient times this fragrant wood was burnt at sacrifices.

History and Authority: Hahnemann introduced this drug in homoeopathic practice in 1819. Allen's Encyclopedia Materia Medica, Vol. IX, 576.

Chapter 46

Common names in Indian Languages of Indigenous Homoeopathic Drugs

The following abbreviations have been used:

E. = English; S. = Sanskrit; B. = Bengali; H. = Hindi; T. = Tamil; Te. = Telegu; M. = Malayalam; Bom. = Bombay; A. = Assamese; O. = Oriya; P. = Punjabi; G. = Gujrati; Mar. = Marathi; C. = Canarease; U. = Urdu; Dec. = Deccan; Ar. = Arabic.

Abelmoschus esculentus

E. Lady's finger; S. Gandhamula; B. Dhenras; H. Bhindi; U. Bhendi; A. & O. Bhendi; G. Bhinda; M. vanta; T. vendi; Te. Benda; C. Bende.

Abroma augusta

E. Devil's cotton; B. & H. Ulat kambal; A. Gunakhiakarai; O. Pishachogonjali; G. Olat kambal; T. Sivaputtutti.

Abroma radix

B. Ulat kambal; H. Olat kambal; Mar. Olat kambol.

Abrus precatorius

E. Crab's eye; S. Ganja; B. Kunch; H. Rati; Bom. Gunja; Mar. Ganj; M. Kunni; C. Galaganji.

Acalypha indica

B. Mukta-jhuri; Bom. & H. Khokali; G. Vanchi kanto; M., T. & Te. Kuppamani; O. Indramaris; C. Kuppi; S. Arittamunjari.

Achyranthes aspera

E. Prickly chaff-flower; S. Apamarga; B. Apang; H. Laljiri; A. Ubtisath; P. Kutri; Bom. Aghada; Mar. Aghara; M. Katalati; T. Nayurivi; Te. Uttareni; C. Utranigida.

Aconitum napellus

E. Monk's hood; S. Bisha; B. Katbish, Mithabis; A. Bish; H. Mitha-zahar; G. Shangadio.

Aegle folia

B., Mar. & H. Bel; S. Bilva; T. Villuvum; Tel. Maredu.

Aegle marmelos

E. Wood apple, Bael tree; S. Sriphal; B. and A. Bel; H. Bili, Sriphal; U. Bel; O. Bela, Bilwa; P. Bil; G. Billy; Bom. Bela; Mar. Bel; M. Vilvam; T. Villuamaram; Te. Bilambu; C. Bilva.

Agaricus campestris

B. & H. Chhata; Bom. Alombe; P. Bleophre; S. Chhatra.

Alfalfa

G. Vilayati ghas; H. Wilayti gawuth, Lasun ghas; C. Villayati hullu.

Allium cepa

E. Onion; H. Piyaz; B. Pianj; S. Paladu; A. Ponoru; P. Peyaz; Bom. Puyaj; Mar. Kanda; M. Ulli; T. Irulli; Te & C. Nirulli.

Allium sativum

E. Garlic; S. Lashuna; B. Rasun; H. Lashun; U. Lehsun; O. Rasuna; G. Lasan; Bom. Lusoon; Mar. Lasun; M. Veluthulli; T. Vallipundu; Te. Tellagadda; C. Belluli.

Aloe socotrina

Ar. Musabar; B., M. & C. Ghritakumari; G. Kudvikunvar; H. Ghikumari, Ghikavar; Mar. Kunvarpata; T. Kattalai; Te. Manjikattali; U. Ghiqwara.

Alstonia scholaris

E. Devil tree; S. Saptaparni; B. Chatim; H. Chatium; P. Satona; Mar. Satvin; C. Hale; A. Chatian. AMOORA ROHITAKA S. Rohitaka; B. Taktaraj; H. Harinhara; G. Ragtarohido; Mar. Raktarohida; M. Sim; T. Vangul; Te. Rohitaka.

Amygdalus amara

H., P. & M. Badam; S. Badama; T. Vadumai; Tel. Badamu.

Anacardium occidentale

B. Hijli badam; Bom. & H. Kaju; M. Kashumavu; Tel. Mokkamamidi.

Anacardium orientale

H. Vilba, Bhilwa; B. Vela; S. Bhallika; M. Temprakku; T. Serangottai; Te. Bhallatamu.

Anagallis arvensis

G. Anagallide; H. Jonkmari; P. Dhabar.

Andrographis paniculata

B. Kalmegh; G. Kariyatu; H. Kiryat; M. Kiryat, Nelavepu; Mar. Olikirayat; S. Bhunimba; T. Nilavembu; Te. Nelavemu.

Apium graveolens

S. Ajmoda, Andha patrika; B. Chanu, Randhuni; H. Ajmod; E. Celery, Cultivated celery, Marsh parsley; A. Karaja, Karajs navali; U. Ajmod.

Artemisia vulgaris

E. & Bom. Nagadona; H. Nagadouna; P. Tarkha; S. Nagadamani; T. Mashibattiri; Te. Machipatri.

Asafoetida

H. Hing; Bom. Hinga; S. Hingu.

Asparagus officinalis

E. Asparagus; S. Shatavari; B. Satamuli; H. Satwar; U. Satavara; A. Shatmul; P. Satwar; G. & Bom. Satavari; Mar. Satmuli; M. Satavali.

Atista indica

E. Toothbrush plant; S. Ashvashakota; B. Ashshaora; H. Bannimbu; A. Chauldhoa; O. Chauladhua; Bom. Kirmira; M. Panal; T. Anam; Te. Gongugu.

Atropa belladonna

E. Deadly night shade; B. Yebruj; H. Sugangur; P. Suchi; Bom. Girbutta.

Avena sativa

E. Oat; B. Jai; H. Ganer; P. Ganerji; C. Togekoddi.

Azadirachta indica

E. Neem, Margosa; E & H. Nim; Bom. Balnimb, Nim; G. Limbado; Mar, Nimbay; O. Nimo; S. Nimba; T. Veppu; Te. Nimbamu.

Beta vulgaris

E. Sugar beet; B. Palangshak; H. Chukandar; U. Chakundar; A. Beet-palang; O. Palanga saga. G. & Mar. Beet; T. Chakunda.

Boerhaavia diffusa

B. Punarnaba; H. Thikri, Punarnava; G. Moto satodo; Mar. Vasu; S. Shothaghai, Punarnava; T. Mukkarattai, Tel. Punarnaba.

Brahmi or Herpestis monnieri

S. Brahmacharini; B. Brahmi; H. Barambhi; U. Jalanim; O. Krishnaparni; Bom. Bama; T. Brame; Te. Sambranichattu.

Brassica nigra

B. Sarsha; E. Black mustard, Mustard; G. & H. Rai, Kali rai; H. Kali sarson; C. Sasave; P. Banarsi rai; S. Asuri, Bimbati; T. Kadugu; Te. Avalu.

Bryophyllum calycinum

E. Sprout-leaf plant; S. Paranabija; B. pathar kuchi; A. Petegaza; O. Amarpoi; U. Chubehayat; P. Pathurchat; Bom. Ahirvana; Mar. Panphuti; T. Ranakalli.

Ceasalpinia bonducella

E. Fever nut; S. Kuberakshi; B. Nata; H. & P. Katkaranj; A. Letaguti; O. Gila; G. Kakachila; Bom. Gaja; Mar. Sagargota; T. Kalakkodi; Te. Gacha; C. Gajjiga.

Calotropis gigantea

E Madar; S. Arka; B. Akanda; Bom. Ak; G. Akado, Akro; H. AK. Mudar; Mar. Akanda; O. Arka; T. Errukku; Tel. Jilledu.

Cannabis sativa

B. Bhang, Ganja; M. Bhang; H. Bhung, Charas, Ganja; G. T. & Te. Ganja. S. Bhanga, Ganjika.

Capsicum annum

E. Chilli, Red pepper; B. Lanka; H. & P. Lalmircha; U. Lalmarach; A. Joloka; O. Lankamaricha; G. & Mar. Mirchi; Bom. Lalmirchi; M. & T. Mulagu; Te. Mirapakaya.

Carica papaya

B. Papay; H. Ambal; E. papaw; A. Amita; G. Papayi; C. Parangi; M. Murutha; O. Amrutabhanda; T. Papali; Te. Boppay.

Cassia sophera

S. Talapota; B. Kalkashunda; H. & P. Kasunda; A. Medelua; O. Kolokasunda; G. Kasundari; Mar. Kala-kasbinda; Te. Tegara.

Cephalandra indica

E. Scarlet gourd; S. Bimba; B. Telakucha; H. Bhimba; U.Kundaru; A. Belipoka; O. Kunduri; P. Kundru; G. Ghol; Bom. Bhimb; Mar. Tondale; M. Kovel; T. Kovarai; Te. Kakidonda.

Cinnamomum camphora

E. Camphor; S. & O. Karpura; B. & E. Karpur; H., G. & Mar. Kapur; P. Kafur; M. Karpuravriksham.

Citrus decumana

E. Shaddock; S. Madhukarkari; B. Batabilebu; H. & P. Chakotra; U. Chokutrah; O. Batapi; G. Obakotru; Bom. Papnas; T. Bambalmas; Mar. Papanas.

Clerodendron infortunatum

S. Bhantaka; B. Ghettl; H. Bhant; A. Bhettita; O. Kunti; P. Karu; Bom. & Mar. Kari; M. Pelluvallem; T. Karukanni; Te. Basavanapadu.

Cocculus indicus

B. & H. Kakmari; Bom. Kakphal; G. Kakaphola; S. Kakmari; T. Kaka; Te. Kakamari.

Coffea arabica

E. Coffee; B. Kafi; H. Kahwa; M. Kappi, Bannu; T. Kaddumallikal; Te. & C. Kapi.

Colchicum autumnale

H. Hirantutiya, Suringam; P. Surinjin talkh; S. Hiranya utha; Ur. Suranjane talkh.

Coleus aromaticus

B. Pather chur; Bom. & H. Pathorchur; S. Pashanbhedi; T. Karpurvalli.

Colocynthis

B. Indrayan, Makhal; Bom. Indrayan; P. Tumbi, Ghurumba; S. Mahendravaruni; T. Payk Kumutti; Tel. Etipuchchha.

Crocus sativus

E. Saffron; B. & A. Jafran; H. Zafran; G. & Mar. Keshar; T. Kungumapu; Te. Kunkumapave.

Croton tiglium

B. Jaypal; Bom. & H. Jamalgota; M. & T. Nirvalam; S. Jayapala; Te. Nepala.

Cubeba officinalis

B., M. & H. Kabab chini; S. Sugandha muricha.

Cucurbita pepo

B. Shada kumra; H. Kaddu;; Mar. Kaula; S. Kurkaru; T. Suraikayi.

Curcuma longa

B. & H. Haldi; G. Halada; S. Haridra; T. Mannjal; Tel. Pasupu.

Cynodon dactylon

E. Doob grass; B. Durba; S. & G. Durva; H. & P. Doob; U. Dub; A. Duboribon; O. Dubaghasa; Mar. Harali; M. & T. Arugampullu; Te. Gericha gaddi; C. Garikehulla.

Cyperus rotundus

A. Suad; B. Mutha, Motha; E. Indian cyperus; H. Nagar motha; S. Abda, Varida, Bhadra musta.

Datura metel

E. Thorn-apple; S. Dhutura; B.; H. & U. Dhutura; A. Dhotura; O. Dudura; P. & C. Dattura; G. Dhatoora; Mar. Dhotra; M. Ummam; T. Umathi; Te. Ummathi.

Desmodium gangeticum

S. Shaliparni; B. Shalpani; H. Salpan; U. Shalwan; O. Karsopani; P. Shalpurchi; G. Salvan; Bom. & Mar. Salparni; M. Pullati; T. Pulladi; Te. Gitanaram; C. Murelehonne.

Dolicosh

B. Alkusa; H.& P. Kawanch; M. Kuhili, Shoriyanam; S. Almagupta; T. Punaik kali; Tel. Dulagondi.

Embelia ribes

B. Biranga, Baibirang; G. Vavading; H. Kannad; T.&Tel. Vyuvilanga; M. Vaivarang, Vizhal; P. Babrung.

Emblica officinalis

A Amlaj, Ambliy, Amlag; B. Amlaki, Ambolaki, Aunlah; E. Emblic myrobalan; H. Amla; S. Amlika, Siva, Sriphala; U Anwala.

Eucalyptus globulus

E. Eucalyptus tree; T. Karpuram; Te. Karpuramu; C. Karpura.

Fagopyrum esculentum

A Doron; H. Koti; P. Ogal.

Ficus indica

E. Banyan; S. Vitapa; B. Bot; H. & P. Barh; U. Bargoda; A. Borgoch; O. Bara; G. & Mar. Wad; M. Vatam; T. Vadam; Te. Vitapi; C. Ala, Vata. FICUS RELIGIOSA B. Ashwattha; G. Jeri; H. Pipal; M. Areyal; S. Pippala; T. Arshemaran.

Gambogia

B. H.&T. Irevalsinni; M. Pinnarpuli; Mar., and S. Tamala; Tel. Pasupuvame.

Glycyrrhiza glabra

E. Liquorice root; B. Yashtimadhu; S. Yashtimadhuka; G. Jethimadh; H. Jethimadhu; T. Athimadhuram; Te. Atimadhuramu; M. Irattimadhuram; P. Jethimadh.

Gossypium herbaceum

E. Cotton; S. Karpasi; A. Kopah; B., H., Bom. & Mar. Kapas; O. Kapa; P. & g. Rui; M. Kuruparathy; T. Parathy; Te. Patti; C. Hatti.

Granatum

S. Darimba; B. & A. Dalim; H. & P. Anar; O. Dalimba; G. Dadam; Mar. Dalimb, M. Mathalam.

Gymnema sylvestris

B. & H. Mesasingi; Bom. Kavali; S. Meshashringi; T. Shiru Kuranja.

Helianthus annus

E. Sunflower; S. Adityabhakta; B. Suryamukhi; H. & P. Shuryamukhi; U. Suryamakkhi; A. Beliphul; G. Suryamukhi; Bom. Surajmaki; Mar. Suryaphul; M. & T. Suriyakanti; Te. Suriyakanta; C. Hottutirugana.

Hemidesmus indicus

E. Indian sarsaparilla; H. Salsa; S. & O. Anantamula; Bom. Upasara; B. & A. & Mar. Anantamul; P. Desisarva; G. & Mar. Upalasari; M. Narunari; T. Nannari; Tel. & C. Sugandipala.

Holarrhena antidysenterica

A. Dudcory; B. Kurchi; Bom. Kalakura; G. Dhowda; H. Kurchi, Kura; M. Kodagapala; O. Kherwa; S. Kutaja; T. Indrabam; Te. Palakodsa.

Hydrocotyle asiatica

A. Manimuni; B. Thankuni; Bom. Karinga; G. Barmi; S. Bramamanduki; H. & Mar. Mandukparni; T. Vallerai; Te. Bokkudu; U. Brahmi.

Hydrophila spinosa

S. Kakilaksha; B. Kyleykhara; U. Talimkhana; O. Kantakalia; P. Talmakhana; G. Ekharo; Bom. Kolsunda; Mar. Kolshinda; M. Vayal Chulli; T. Nirmulli; Te. Nirguvivera.

Hyoscyamus niger

E. Henbane; B. Khorasaniajayan; G. Khorasani ajmo; H. & U. Khurassani ajvayan; Mar. Khorasaniova; S. Parasikaya; T. Kurasaniyoman; Te. Kurashnivamam. HYPERICUM PERFORATUM H. Bassant; U. Balsana.

Indigofera tinctoria

E. Indigo; S. Nili; B., H. & A. Nil; U. & O. Nila; G. Gali; Bom. Nilaguli; Mar. Neel; Te. Aviri; C. Ajara.

Jatropha curcas

E. Purging nut; S. Parvateranda; B. Bagbharenda; H. Jangli-arandi; A. Bongliara; O. Baigaba; P. Jamalgota; G. Jepal; Bom. Irundi, Jepal; Mar. Mogali erand; M. Katalvanakku; T. Adalai; C. Adavijamudamu.

Jonosia asoka

B. Asok; G. Ashopalaya; H. Ashok; M. Asoka; Mar. Ashoka; O. Osoko; T. Asogam.

Justicia adhatoda

E. Malabar nut; B. Basak; G. Ardhsi; H. Adulasa, vasaka; Mar. Baksá; O. Basongo; P. Bhaikar; S. Vasaka; T. Adhatodai; V. Arusa.

Lathyrus sativus

B. & H. Khesari; Mar. Laka; P. Kisari; S. Sandika.

Leucas aspera

S. Dandakalash; B. Ghalghase; H. Barahalkhusa; A. Doron, Durumphul; O. Gaisa; Bom. Tampa; M. Thumpa; T. Tumbai; Te. Tummaehettu.

Luffa aegyptiaca

E. Sponge-gourd; S. Ghoshaka; B. Dhundul; H. & P. Ghiya-tori; U. Turi; A. Bhol; O. Pitatarada; G. Taria; Bom. Ghosali; Mar. Goshale; T. Tikku; Te. Guttibira.

Lycopersicum esculentum

E. Tomato; B. Bilati-begun; H. & P. Tamatar; A. Belahibengena; O. Bilatibaigana; G. Tameta; Mar. Tambeta, M. Thakkali.

Lycopodium clavatum

H. Bendarli; P. Walayati bagan.

Mangifera indica

B. Am; G. Amri; H. Am, Amb; C. Mavu; M. Amram, cutam, mavu; Mar. Amba; S. Amra, chuta; T. Mamaram, Mau; Tel. Mamidi, Mavi.

Melilotus alba

E. White melilot; S. Methika; B. Sadamethi; H. Safed methi.

Mentha piperita

H., B., Mar., T. & Tel. Pudina; A. Poduna; G. Phudino; M. Puthina; S. Putiha, Podinaka.

Momordica charantia

E. Bitter gourd; S. Karavella; B. Karala; H. Kareli; U. Karella; A. Titakerata; O. Kalara; G. Karelu; Bom. Karla; Mar. Karle; M. & T. Paval; Te. Kakara; C. Hagola.

Musa sapientum

B. Kala, Kalagach; E. Banana, Plantain, Kadali; H. Kela; C. Balehannu; M. Kadalivala, Vazha, Kshetrakadali; S. Kadali; T. Kadali vazhai; Tel. Ariti, Kadalamu

Myristica fragrans

S. Jatiphala; A. Jaiphal, Kanivish; B. Jaiphala, Jaitri; E. Nutmeg; G. Jaiphala, Jayfar; H. Jaiphal C. Jadikai, Jaykai, Jaidikai; Mar. Jaiphal; O. Jaiphal; P.Jaiphal; T. Sathikkai, Jathikkai, Jatikkai, Jadhikai, Jadhikkai; Tel. Jajikaya; U. Jauzbuwa, Jaiphal.

Myrtus communis

E. Myrtle; B. Bilati-mehedi; H. & P. Vilayatimehedi; U. Hubulas; T. Kulinaval.

Nux moschata

B. Jayphal; Bom; P. & H. Jaiphal; G. Jayephal; S. Jaiphata; T. Jadikkai; Te. Jaji Kava.

Nux vomica

B. Kuchila; Bom. Kaira; G. & H. Kuchla; M. Kanjhiram; Tel. Mushti; U. Kuchala; P. Kuchila; S. Kachchira; T. Ettikkottai.

Nyctanthes arbortristis

E. Night jasmine; S. Sephalika; B. Sheuli; H. Harishinagar; U. Gulejafari; A. Sewali; O. Singadhara; P. Harsanghar; G. Ratrase; Bom. Parijataka; Mar. Parijatak; M. Parizhamulla; T. Pavrelem; Te. parijatham; C. Harisringi.

Ocimum canum

T. Kukka-tulasi, Gunjamkorai; E.Rosary tulasi; Tel. Thulasi, Kuppatulasi; M. Kattu Ram tulasi; C. Nayitulasi; B. & H. Kala tulsi; S. Gramya, Thiksnamanu.

Ocimum sanctum

H. Tulsi; B. Tulasi; O. Tulasi; Bom., T., Te. & Mar. Tulasi; M. Shiva-tulsi, Krishna tulasi.

Oldenlandia herbacea

S. Parpata; B. Khet-papra; H. Daman-pappar; G. parpat; O. Gharpodia; Mar. Pitapada; T. parpadagaru; Te. Verinella-vamu.

Oleander

S. Karavira; H. & P. Kaner; B. Karabi; Bom. Kanhera; M. Lam; Te. Karavirum. OPIUM S. Ahiphena; H., B. & P. Afim; Bom. Aphim; M. & A. Afium; T. Abini; Te. Kosakosa; G. Aphina; Mar. Aphim.

Phyllanthus emblica

S. Amlika; B. & A. Amloki; H. & P. Amla; U. Anwala; O. Anala; G. Ambala; Bom. Avala; Te. Usiri; Mar. Awala; M. Amalakam; T. Amalgam; C. Amalaka

Piper nigrum

E. Pepper, Black pepper, Common pepper; G. Kala mari, Kalomirich; B. Gol morich, Kalomorich; H. & P. Kali mirch; C. Kare manasu; M. Karumulaku; Mar. Mire, Kali mirch; O. Gol maricha; T. Milagu; Te. Miriyalu; S. Maricha ushana, hopusha; U. Siah mirch.

Plantago major

H. Lahuriyai; M. Bartang.

Prunus amygdalus

E. Almond; B. Kath badam; H., Mar. & P. Badam; C. Badami; M. Vatam kotta; T. Vaadumai; Vaadamkottai; Tel. Badam vittulu.

Psoralea corylifolia

S. & O. Bakuchi; B. Lata kasturi; H. & P. Babchi; U. Babechi; G. Bavacha; Bom. Bawachi.

Punica granatum

S. Darimba; B. & A. Dalim; H. & P. Anar; O. Dalimba; G. Dadam; Mar. Dalimb.

Rauwolfia serpentina

B. Sarpagandha; S. Chandrika; H. Sarpagandh; M. Amalpariyan; T. Sovannamilbori; Te. Dumparasna.

Rheum emodi

S. Revatchini; B. Revanchini; H. Dolu; P. Atsu; U. Rewanchini.

Ricinus communis

S. Eranda; B. Rehri; H. Arand; U. Erenda; A.

Erigoch; O. Joda; P. Rendi; G & Bom. Erandi; Mar. Erand; M. & T. Avanakku; Te. Amidamu; C. Avudalu

Ruta graveolens

B. Ermul; Bom. Satap; H. Sadab; P. Sudab; S. Somalata; T. Arvada.

Santalum album

S. Chandanna; B. & A. Chandan; H. Sufed chandan; O. & P. Chandana; G. Sukhada; Bom. Chandan; Mar. Chandan; M. Chandanam.

Senna

B. Sanna-makki; H. Sana; M. Nilavaka; Mar. Sonamukhi; T. Nila varai; Tel. Nela-tangedu.

Sinapis nigra

H. Safed rai.

Solanum nigrum

B. Raisarisha; H. Asirai; Mar. Rai; S. Madhurika; T. Kadugu; Tel. Avalu.

Solanum xanthocarpum

B. Kantikari; H. Kateli; O. Ankaranti; P. Kandiali; G. Bhoyaringani; Bom. Bhuringni; Mar. Kateringani; Te. Nelavakudu.

Swertia chirata

B. & H. Chirata; Bom. Chiraita; M. Nelavappa; S. Kairata; T. & Tel. Nilavembu.

Syzygium jambolanum

A. Jamu; B. Jam; Bom. Jambhul; G. Jambu; H. Jaman; S. Jambu; T. Nagai; Tel. Jambuvu.

Tabacum

B. Tamak; B. & H. Tambaku; P. Tamaku; M. Pokala; S. Tamakhu; T. Pugaiyilay; Tel. Pogaku.

Taraxacum

H. Kanphul; Mar. Bathur; P. Kanphul.

Taxus baccata

B. Bhirmie; H. Kash; Mar. Barmi; P. Birmi.

Terminalia arjuna

A. Orjun; B., Bom. & H. Arjuna; G. Arjunasadra; M. Marutu; O. Orjuno; S. Arjuna; T. Maruda; Tel. Tellamaddi.

Terminalia chebula

S. & B. Haritaki; H. Harara; A. Shilikha; O. Harida; P. Harrar; G. Pilo-harda; Bom. Harada; Mar. Hirda; M. & T. Kadukkai; Te. Karaka; C. Harade.

Thea chinensis

B., H., Bom., & P. Cha, Chay; T. Thayilai; Tel. Theyaku.

Tribulus terrestris

B. Gokhru; G. Gokharu; H. Chota gokhru; M. Neringil; S. Gokshura; T. Nerunji.

Trichosanthes dioica

S. Patola; B. Patol; H. Parwal; U. Parawal; A. Patal; O. Patala; P. Palwal; G. Potala; M. Patolam; Mar. Parwar.

Tylophora indica

B. & H. Anantamul; Bom. Anthamul; M. Vallippala; T. Nayppalai; Tel. Vettipala.

Valeriana officinalis

H. Billiotan; M. Kalavala.

Vernonia athelmintica

S. Somraji; B. & H. Somraj; M. Karalye; T. Kattushiragam; Te. Advijilakara.

Viscum album

B. Banda; H. & P. Bhangara; U. Maizakeashi; T. Ottu; A. Roghumala; O. Malanga; Mar. Jalundar; M. Iththil.

Withania somnifera

B. Ashvagandha; H. & P. Asgandh; A. Lakhana; O. Ajagandha; G. Asundha; Bom. Asgund; Mar. Askandh; M. Peretti; T. Amukkiram; Te. Asvagandi.

Zingiber officinale

E. Ginger; S. O. & U. Adraka; B., O. & A. Ada; H. Adarak; G. Adhu; Bom. Adu; Mar. Ale, M. Inji; T. Inchi; Te. Allam; C. Sunti.

Chapter 47

Evolution of Indian Therapeutic System

Five thousand years ago, in the magnificent Himalayas, one of the greatest sages of India, Srila Vyasadeva wrote down the Vedas for the first time. This included a branch which is called **Ayurveda.** The word 'Ayur' means 'Life', while 'Veda' means 'Science'. Therefore, Ayurveda literally means the 'Science of Life'. It is not just a medicinal system, but also a way of life.

Ayurveda deals with the physical, as well as spiritual health. The medicinal form is governed by the Laws of Nature, which suggest that life is a combination of senses, mind, body and soul. According to the Science of Life, the structural aspect of every individual comprises five elements — earth, water, fire, air and space.

The **Unani system** of medicine was founded on the principles propounded by Galen, a Greek practitioner, in 5th century B.C. *Kitab-al-shifa*, the Magnum Opus of Abu Sina, an Arab philosopher and physicist, also known as Avicenna in English (A.D. 980 – 1037), played a role of great importance in the development of this system. In fact, today this style of medicine is not known as Galenic, as it was earlier called, but the Unani (Arabic name for Greek) system of medicine. It was later adapted and developed by the Arabs into an elaborate therapeutic system. It was introduced in India sometime around 10th century A.D.

This therapy is based on the Hippocratic Therapy of good health being equivalent to a perfect balance of the elements present, including the temperament of a person. Unani Medicine treats the patients with regard to the environment they are exposed to. The diagnosis is a mixture of modern pathology and traditional pulse reading technique. The remedy administered is that of diet control, herbal and animal based drugs, physiotherapy and surgery. Unani Medicine claims to cure neurotic as well as psychiatric problems.

Siddha—another type of therapeutic system is practised and restricted to a very small area in Tamil Nadu. Its origin can be traces back to over 3,000 years. It is more or less on the same level as Ayurveda. It has an identity of its own. This system comprises of the ancient medical treatises that are a compilation of valuable information on various herbs, drugs, diseases and the techniques to diagnose them. This system stresses on the therapeutic skills as pressure point massage that have proved to be effective in case of diabetes.

Ayurvedic Medicines are based on plants, animals extract and minerals both in single ingredient drugs and compound formulations, however,

Ayurveda does not rule out any substances from being used as a potential source of medicine.

Ayurvedic compound formulations are mainly divided into two groups:

1. Kasthausadhi (predominantly plant drugs), and
2. Rasausadhi (predominantly metals and minerals).

There are several categories of Kasthausadhi formulations such as Asavaristra, Avleha, Grafa Churena, Taila etc. and of Rasausadhis such as Bhasma, Pisti, Lauha, Kapibadkva, Rasayana etc.

The Ayurvedic drugs are derived from vegetable sources from the various parts of the plant like root, leaf, flower, fruit extrude or plant as a whole.

There are about 21 varieties of compound formulations in which some of the single drugs of animal origin (52 Nos). Mineral origin (55 Nos.) and plant origin (351 Nos.) are used. The details of the single drugs and other particulars can be had from the Ayurvedic Formulary of India, published by Govt. of India, Ministry of Health and Family Welfare.

Present Status of Ayurveda

India acquired independence from British rule in 1947 and become a Democratic Republic in 1950. Developments of Ayurveda in India after independence need to focus on various aspects:

1. Ayurvedic Education and Research

The integrated approach of Ayurvedic Education started by efforts of Leucas continued for about one more decade. The parallel Institutions started by All India Ayurvedic Congress were running concurrently. Apart from these two institutions of learning, one more institution working silently, without any kind of hindrances was, the Guru-Shishya Parampara. Based on experience of multifacetated pressure, it was decided to bring the Ayurvedic Education under the preview of universities in Independent India. By 1969 all the colleges imparting education in Ayurveda or other Indigenous system of medicine were affiliated to respective universities.

In 1970, **The Indian Medicine Central Council Act** which aims to standardise qualifications for Ayurveda and provide accredited institutions for its study and research was passed by the Parliament of India.

The **Central Council of Indian Medicine** is the statutory body constituted under The Indian Medicine Central Council Act, 1970 vide Gazette Notifaction Extraordinary Part (ii) Section 3(ii) dated 10.8.71. Since its establishment in 1971, **The Central Council of Indian Medicine** has been framing on and implementing various regulations including the Curricula and Syllabii in **Indian Systems of Medicine** viz. Ayurved, Siddha and Unani Tibb at Under-graduate and Post-graduate level.

Besides Graduate and Post-Graduate courses, different levels of training are being imparted for Para-medical staff, like Panchkarma Technicians, Ayurvedic Pharmacist etc. at different centers in India.

Now there are few institutions of national repute, which are conducting various programs in the field of Ayurveda, viz. Faculty of Ayurveda, Institute of Medical Sciences, Banaras Hindu University, Varanasi, Institute of Post Graduate Training & Research, Gujrat Ayurveda University, Jam Nagar, National Institute of Ayurveda, Jaipur & Rashtriya Ayurved Vidyapeetha, India.

The Ayurvedic medicines/drugs are becoming popular day-by-day and demand for its usage is increasing not only in the country but also worldwide. The inherent quality of Ayurvedic treatment of having negligible side/after effects, has made great potential for its production. A large number of medicinal plants, herbs, shrubs etc. are available in our country in the hilly/forest regions.

Govt. of India has set up a Board namely **Indian system of Medicine and Homoeoepathy (ISM & H)** in March,1995 and renamed as **Department of Ayurveda, Yoga and Naturopathy, Unani, Siddha and Homoeopathy (AYUSH)**, Ministry of Health and Family Welfare, Government of India, in November, 2003 with a view to providing focused attention to development of Education and Research in Ayurveda, Yoga and Naturopathy, Unani, Siddha and Homoeopathy systems. The Department continued to lay emphasis on upgradation of AYUSH educational standards, quality control and standardisation of drugs, improving the availability of medicinal plant material, research and development and awareness generation about the efficacy of the systems domestically and internationally.

Now all the Colleges of Indian Systems of Medicine are affiliated to various Universities in the country. These Colleges are following the minimum standards of education and Curricula and Syllabii, prescribed by the Central Council.

In India, over 100 colleges offer degrees in traditional Ayurvedic Medicine. The Indian government supports research and teaching in ayurveda through many channels at both the national and state levels, and helps institutionalise traditional medicine so that it can be studied in major towns and cities.

The state-sponsored **Central Council for Research in Ayurveda and Siddha (CCRAS)** is the premier institution for promotion of traditional medicine in India. The studies conducted by this institution encompass clinical, drug, literary, and family welfare research. To fight biopiracy and unethical patents, the Government of India, in 2001, set up the Traditional Knowledge Digital Library as repository of 1,200 formulations of various systems of Indian medicine, such as Ayurveda, Unani and Siddha. The library also has 50 traditional ayurveda books digitised and available online.

Standardisation of Ayurvedic and other traditional medicine, compound drugs is more complex than standardisation of single or combination pharmaceutical drugs. Government of India set up the **Ayurvedic Pharmacopoeia Committee (APC)** for laying down pharmacopoeial standards. So far pharmaceutical standards of 418 most widely used single crude Ayurvedic drugs have been laid down. First Volume of Pharmacopoeial Standards of 50 most commonly used Ayurvedic compound drugs has also been published in October, 2007. The science of standardisation of botanicals is constantly evolving and the pharmacopoeial monographs are accordingly revised from time to time.

The Ayurvedic Pharmacopoeia Committee is following international norms for pharmacopoeial monographs of single and compound Ayurvedic drugs. Scientific work for laying down pharmacopoeial standards for another 200 most commonly used Ayurvedic formulations as well as the work of preparation of pharmacopoeial standards for Ayurvedic plant based extracts has also been undertaken by the Ayurvedic Pharmacopoeia Committee in collaboration with laboratories of Department of AYUSH,

The 1st APC was constituted in 1962. Since then it is working continuously. The term of Committee remains for a period of 3 years from the date of its first meeting and the members hold office for that period.

To bring uniformity among the manufacturers and to follow the same formula of ingredients in the same proportion, two parts of Ayurvedic Formulary of India has been published by the Ayurvedic Pharmacopoeia Committee. The 1st Volume of Ayurvedic Pharmacopoeia of India (Formulations), contains 635 Formulations. Both parts are available in English and Hindi separately.

AFI Part I (1978) – 444 formulations

AFI Part II (2000) – 191 formulations

2. Patient Care Services

A number of Hospitals, Dispensaries run by Government, Local Administration provide treatment to the needy, employing Ayurvedic methods.

3. Manufacturing of Ayurvedic Medicine

In 1964, manufacturing of Ayurvedic Medicine was brought under the scope of Drugs and Cosmetics Act, through an amendment enacted by the parliament. As a result the government could exercise appropriated regulation over the manufacturing of Ayurvedic Medicine. This regulation helped the Industry of Ayurvedic Medicines to grow in a healthy environment.

The GMP (Good Manufacturing Practice) certification also played an important role to provide, quality standard as per the norms of World Health Organisation in the field of Ayurveda Industries. Recently Govt. of India has laid down separate GMP requirements for Ayurvedic manufactures and made it mandatory.

4. Cultivation of Medicinal Plants

Ayurveda advocated a harmonious interface of human beings with nature as it recognises him to be an integral part of the universe. Also, Ayurveda draws its therapeutic agents mainly from Plant Kingdom. Thus, the forests have been the conventional sources of Ayurvedic Medicines. However, under threatened ecological balance and dwindling forest resources, Ayurveda as a whole faces a major threat in near future.

So, more precise methods for propagation of Medicinal Plants should be devised through methodical research. Tropical Botanical Garden and Research Institute (TBGRI), and Centre for Indian Medical Heritage (ČIMH) promoted by Ayurvedic Trust are working in this direction besides many other agencies in the country.

Chapter 48

List of Drugs with their Common Name, Family, Distribution and Parts used

Name of drug	*Synonyms*	*Family*	*Distribution*	*Parts used*
Abies canadensis	Hemlock spruce	Pinaceae	North America	Bark
Abies nigra	Black spruce	Pinaceae	North America Canada	Amber resin
Abroma augusta	Olat kambal	Sterculiaceae	Bengal; Bihar; Sikkim	Leaves
Abroma radix	Olat kambal	Sterculiaceae	Bengal; Bihar; Sikkim	Root
Abrotanum	Southern wood	Compositae	Great Britain	Leaves & young shoots
Acalypha indica	Indian nettle	Euphorbiaceae	Throughout India	Whole plant
Achyranthes aspera	Prickly chaff flower	Amaranataceae	Throughout India	Whole plant excluding root
Aconitum napellus	Monk's hood	Ranunculaceae	Western Himalayas	Whole plant
Actaea spicata	Black shake-root	Ranunculaceae	Germany; Canada	Roots
Adonis vernalis	Pheasant's eye	Ranunculaceae	Northern Europe; Asia	Whole plant
Aegle folia	Bael	Rutaceae	India	Leaves
Aesculus hippocastanum	Horse chestnut	Sapindaceae	Europe; India; America	Ripe nut excluding outer shell
Aethusa cynapium	Garden hemlock	Umbelliferae	Europe; New England	Whole plant
Agaricus muscarius	Toad stool	Agaricaceae	Europe; Asia; America	Whole fungus except outer skin
Agnus castus	Chaste tree	Verbenaceae	Europe; France; Greece	Berries

Contd.

Name of drug	*Synonyms*	*Family*	*Distribution*	*Parts used*
Ailanthus glandulosus	Chinese sumach	Simarubaceae	Northern India	Stem-bark
Aletris farinosa	Star-grass	Liliaceae	Eastern United States	Rhizome
Allium cepa	Onion	Liliaceae	Cultivated in India	The red mature bulb
Allium sativum	Garlic	Liliaceae	Universally cultivated	The mature bulb
Aloe socotrina	Ghikumari; Mocha	Liliaceae	India; Africa; Sri Lanka	Inspissated juice of the leaves
Alstonia scholaris	Chatim; Dita bark	Apocynaceae	India; Sri Lanka; Burma	Bark
Anacardium orientale	Marking nut	Anacardiaceae	India	Resinous juice of seed
Andrographis paniculata	Kalmegh	Acanthaceae	Throughout India	Whole plant
Apocynum cannabinum	Indian hemp	Apocynaceae	U.S.A.; Canada	Roots
Aralia racemosa	American spikenard	Araliaceae	North America	Roots
Arnica montana	Leopard's bane	Compositae	Central Europe; Russia	Whole plant
Artemisia vulgaris	Nagadouna; Mugwort	Compositae	India; Europe; Canada	Roots
Arum triphyllum	Bog onion	Araceae	America; Canada	Roots
Asafoetida	Heeng; Devil's dung	Umbelliferae	India; Iran	Gum-resin
Asarum europaeum	European snake root	Aristolo-chiaceae	Throughout Europe	Whole plant
Asparagus officinalis	Common garden asparagus	Liliaceae	Europe	Young shoots
Avena sativa	Oat; jey	Gramineae	India	Seeds
Azadirachta indica	Nim; Margosa bark	Meliaceae	India; Burma	Fresh bark
Baptisia tinctoria	Wild indigo	Leguminosae	Southern New England; America	Bark of root
Belladonna	Deadly night shade	Solanaceae	Europe; Kashmir	Whole plant
Bellis perennis	Daisy	Compositae	Britain	Whole plant
Berberis vulgaris	Kashmal; Pipperidge	Berberidaceae	India; Europe; Asia	Bark of the root
Boerhaavia diffusa	Punarnava	Nyctaginaceae	India	Entire fresh herb with flowers
Bovista	Warted puff-ball	Lycoperdaceae	Europe; Asia minor	Ripe bovista (Fungus)
Bryonia alba	Wild hops	Cucurbitaceae	Middle & South Europe	Roots
Cactus grandiflorus	Night blooming cereus	Cactaceae	Tropical America	Flowering stems
Calendula officinalis	Garden marigold	Compositae	Cultivated in India	Fresh flowering tops and leaves

Contd.

Name of drug	*Synonyms*	*Family*	*Distribution*	*Parts used*
Calotropis gigentia	Madar; Akanda	Asclepiadaceae	India	Roots
Cannabis indica	Hashis	Cannabinaceae	Western Central Asia; India	Leaves
Cannabis sativa	Hemp; Gallow grass	Cannabinaceae	Western Central Asia; India	Flowering tops
Capsicum annum	Chilly	Solanaceae	India; South America	Ripe fruit
Carduus marianus	Blessed thistle	Compositae	Punjab; Himalayas	Seeds
Carica papaya	Melon tree; papaya	Caricaceae	Throughout India	Unripe fruits
Caulophyllum thalictroides	Blue cohosh	Berberidaceae	U.S.A.; Kentucky	Rhizome
Ceanothus americanus	New Jersey Tea	Rhamnaceae	Southern Canada; Texas	Leaves
Chamomilla	Bitter chamomile	Compositae	India; Asia; Europe	Whole plant
Chelidonium majus	Calandine	papaveraceae	Europe; Germany; France	Whole plant
Circuta virosa	Water hemlock	Umbelliferae	India	Roots
Cimicifuga racemosa	Black snake-root	Ranunculaceae	U.S.A.; Canada	Rhizome
Cinchona officinalis	Peruvian bark	Rubiaceae	India; Sikkim	Bark
Cinnamomum	Cinnamon	Lauraceae	India; Sri Lanka	Inner bark
Cocculus indicus	Indian cockle	Menispermaceae	India; Burma	Seeds
Coffea cruda	Coffee	Rubiaceae	India; Abyssinia	Seeds
Colchicum autumnale	Meadow saffron	Liliaceae	India; Europe	Bulb
Collinsonia canadensis	Stone-root	Labiatae	Canada; U.S.A.	Rhizome
Colocynthis	Bitter gourd	Cucurbitaceae	India; Ceylon; Japan	Pulp of the fruit
Conium maculatum	Poison hemlock	Umbelliferae	Asia; Europe; North Africa	Whole plant
Convallaria majalis	Lily of the valley	Liliaceae	Europe; Asia United States	Whole plant
Crataegus oxyacantha	Ban-sangli	Rosaceae	Asia; Europe	Berries
Crocus sativus	Saffron	Iridaceae	India; Europe; China	Dried stigma of flower
Croton tiglium	Purging nut	Euphorbiaceae	Bengal; Assam; Burma (Myanmar)	Oil from seeds
Cyclamen europoeum	Snow-bread	Primulaceae	Central & South Europe	Roots
Daphne indica	Spurge-laurel	Thymelaceae	West Indies; China	Bark of branches
Digitalis purpurea	Common fox-glove	Scrophulariaceae	India; Europe; England	Leaves of 2nd year growth
Dioscorea villosa	China root; Colic root	Dioscoriaceae	United States	Rhizomes
Drosera rotundifolia	Round leaved sundew	Droseraceae	Europe; North America	Whole plant

Contd.

Name of drug	*Synonyms*	*Family*	*Distribution*	*Parts used*
Dulcamara	Bitter-sweet	Solanaceae	Europe; Asia; Africa	Whole plant
Echinacea angustifolia	Black Sampson	Compositae	America; Central Europe	Whole plant
Equisetum hyemale	Scouring rush	Equisetaceae	U.S.A.	Whole plant
Eucalyptus globulus	Blue gum leaves	Myrtaceae	Universal	Fresh leaves
Eupatorium perfoliatum	Ague weed	Compositae	North America	Leaves & tops of flower
Euphrasia officinalis	Eye-bright	Scrophulariaceae	Europe; Asia	Whole plant
Ficus religiosa	Pipal; Ashwath	Moraceae	India	Tender leaves
Gelsemium sempervirens	Yellow jasmine	Logaminaceae	Virginia; Mexico	Rhizome
Geranium maculatum	Alum root	Geraniaceae	North America	Root
Gossypium herbaceum	Cotton plant	Malvaceae	Asia; Europe America	Bark of the root
Gratiola officinalis	Hedge hyssop	Scrofulariaceae	North America; Europe	Whole plant
Gymnema sylvestre	Mesasingi	Asclepiaricaceae	Central India	Leaves
Hamamelis virginica	Witch hazel	Hamameli-deaceae	U.S.A.; Canada	Bark of root and stem
Helleborus niger	Black hellebore	Ranunculaceae	Alpine regions	Rhizome
Holarrhena antidysenterica	Kurchi; Kura	Apocynaceae	Throughout India	Dried bark
Hydrastis canadensis	Golden seal	Ranunculaceae	Canada; U.S.A.	Rhizome
Hydrocotyle asiatica	Thick-leaved pennywort	Umbelliferae	Moist places of India	Whole plant
Hyoscyamus niger	Black henbane	Solanaceae	India; Europe; U.S.A.	Whole plant
Hypericum perforatum	St. John's wort	Hypericaceae	India; Asia; Europe	Whole plant
Ignatia amara	St. Ignatius' bean	Loganiaceae	Philippines Islands; China	The bean
Ipecacuanha	Ipecac	Rubiaceae	India; Brazil; America	Roots
Iris versicolor	Blue flag	Iridaceae	America; India; Europe	Rhizome
Jatropha curcas	Purging nut	Euphorbiaceae	Throughout India	Seeds
Janosia asoka	Ashok; Kankelia	Leguminosae	Evergreen forests of India	Bark
Justicia adhatoda	Adulsa; Vasaka	Acanthaceae	India	Leaves
Kalmia latifolia	Broad-leaved laurel	Ericaceae	North America	Leaves
Lachnanthes tinctoria	Spirit-weed	Haemodoraceae	North America	Whole plant
Lathyrus sativus	Chick-pea	Leguminosae	India; Southern Europe	Seeds
Laurocerasus	Cherry-laurel	Rosaceae	Persia; Turkey	Leaves

Contd.

Name of drug	*Synonyms*	*Family*	*Distribution*	*Parts used*
Ledum palustre	Wild rosemary	Ericaceae	Northern Europe; Asia	Whole plant
Lobelia inflata	Red Indian tobacco	Lobeliaceae	North America; Canada	Whole plant
Lycopodium clavatum	Club-moss	Lycopodiaceae	Bengal; Sikkim; Europe	The spores
Lycopus virginicus	Bugle-weed	Labiatae	North America	Whole plant
Melilotus alba	Sweet scented clover	Leguminosae	India; Europe; Mexico	Flowering tops
Menyanthes trifoliata	Buck-bean	Gentianaceae	America; Kashmir; Europe	The whole plant
Mezereum	Mezereon	Thymeliaceae	Europe	The bark
Millefolium	Yarrow	Compositae	Asia; North America; India	Whole plant
Myrica cerifera	Wax-myrtle	Myricaceae	Along the Atlantic coast	Bark of the root
Nux moschata	Nutmeg	Myristicaceae	East Indies; South America	Seeds
Nux vomica	Poison nut	Loganiaceae	Western Ghats; Himalayas	Seeds
Ocimum sanctum	Tulsi	Labiatae	India	Whole plant excluding root
Opium	Poppy	Papaveraceae	India	Gummy juice
Petroselinium sativum	Garden parsley	Umbelliferae	India; Europe	Whole plant
Physostigma venenosum	Calabar bean	Leguminosae	India; Brazil; Africa	Seeds
Phytolacca decandra	American night-shade	Phytolaccaeae	North America	Roots
Plantago major	Greater plantain	Plantaginaceae	India; Europe America	Whole plant
Podophyllum peltatum	May apple	Berberidaceae	United States	Rhizome
Psoralea corylifolia	Babchi; Bakuchi	Leguminosae	Throughout India	Seeds
Pulsatilla nigricans	Wind flower	Ranunculaceae	Europe; Russia; Asia	Whole plant
Ranunculus bulbosus	Buttercup	Ranunculaceae	Europe; United States	Whole plant
Ratanhia	Rhatany	Polygonaceae	Peru	Roots
Rauwolfia serpentina	Sarpagandha	Apocynaceae	India	Roots
Rhus toxicodendron	Poison-ivy; Poison oak	Anacardiaceae	Forests of United States	Leaves
Rhus venenata	Poison sumach	Anacardiaceae	Forests of United States	Leaves and stems
Robinia pseudocacia	Locust	Leguminosae	America	Bark of root & stem
Rumex crispus	Yellow dock	Polygonaceae	United States; Europe	Rhizome

Contd.

Name of drug	*Synonyms*	*Family*	*Distribution*	*Parts used*
Ruta graveolens	Bitter herb	Rutaceae	India; Western Asia	The whole plant
Sabadilla	Cevadilla seeds	Liliaceae	Mexico; West Indies	Seeds
Sabina	Savin	Coniferae	Europe; Asia; America	Stems and leaves
Salix nigra	Black-willow	Salicaceae	United States	Bark
Sambucus nigra	Elder	Caprifoliaceae	Britain; Japan; Europe	Leaves and flowers
Sanguinaria canadensis	Blood root	Papaveraceae	India; United States; Canada	Rhizome
Secale cornutum	Ergot of Rye	Hypocreaçeae	Found in fields on the rye plant	Whole fungus (Dried)
Senega	Seneca snake root	Polygalaceae	U.S.A.; Western New England	Dried roots
Staphysagria	Louse seeds	Ranunculaceae	Italy; Greek islands	Seeds
Stramonium	Thorn-apple	Solanaceae	India; North America	Whole plant
Sumbul	Sumbul root	Umbelliferae	Central Asia; Russia	Roots
Tabacum	Tobacco	Solanaceae	All over India	Leaves
Terminalia arjuna	Arjun	Combretaceae	Throughout India	Bark
Thuja occidentalis	American arbor-vitae	Cupressaceae	United States	Leaves and twigs
Tinospora cordyfolia	Gulancha	Menispermaceae	Throughout India	Stem
Tribulus terrestris	Gokhru	Zygophyllaceae	India (Kashmir)	Whole plant
Urtica urens	Dwarf nettle	Urticaceae	Great Britain; United States	Whole plant
Valeriana officinalis	Vaterian	Valerianaceae	India; Europe	Rhizome
Veratrum album	White hellebore	Liliaceae	Europe; Japan; Russia	Rhizome
Veratrum viride	American white hellebore	Liliaceae	North America	Rhizome
Verbascum thapsus	Common mullein	Scrophula-riaceae	India; Canada	Whole plant
Viburnum opulus	Cranberry high bush	Caprifoliaceae	Canada; U.S.A.; Europe	Bark
Viburnum prunifolium	Black-how	Caprifoliaceae	Central U.S.A.	Bark
Vinca minor	Lesser periwindle	Apocynaceae	India	Whole plant
Viola tricolor	Pansy	Violaceae	Cultivated in India	Whole plant
Viscum album	Mistletoe	Loranthaceae	India; Europe	Fresh leaves and berries
Withania somnifera	Aswagandha	Solanaceae	Throughout India	Roots

Drugs and their Abbreviations

Abies. c., Abies canadensis

Abies. n., Abies nigra

Abrom. ag., Abroma augusta

Abrot., Abrotanum

Absin., Absinthium

Acal. ind., Acalypha indica

Acet. ac., Acetic acid

Acon. nap., Aconitum napellus

Act. sp., Actaea spicata

Aesc. hip., Aesculus hippocastanum

Aesc. g., Aesculus glabra

Aeth. cy., Aethusa cynapium

Agar. m., Agaricus muscarius

Agn. cast., Agnus castus

Ail., Ailanthus glandulosa

Alet., Aletris farinosa

All. cepa., Allium cepa

All. sat., Allium sativum

Aloe. soc., Aloe socotrina

Alumn., Alumen

Alum., Alumina

Alum. met., Aluminium metallicum

Alum. sil., Aluminium silicata

Ambr., Ambra grisea

Am. ben., Ammonium benzoicum

Am. c., Ammonium carbonicum

Am. caust., Ammonium causticum

Am. m., Ammonium muriaticum

Amyl. n., Amyl. nitrosum

Anac., Anacardium orientale

Andro. pan., Andrographis paniculata

Anthr., Anthracinum

Anthra., Anthrakokali

Ant. ars., Antimonium arsenicosum

Ant. cr., Antimonium crudum

Ant. tart., Antimonium tartaricum

Apis. mel., Apis mellifica

Apoc. can., Apocynum cannabinum

Aral. rac., Aralia racemosa

Arg. met., Argentum metallicum

Arg. nit., Argentum nitricum

Arn. mon., Arnica montana

Ars. alb., Arsenicum album
Ars. iod., Arsenicum iodatum
Ars. s.f., Arsenicum sulphuratum flavum
Ars. s.r., Arsenicum sulphuratum rubrum
Art. vul., Artemisia vulgaris
Arum. tri., Arum triphyllum
Asaf., Asafoetida
Asar., Asarum europaeum
Aspar., Asparagus officinalis
Aur. met., Aurum metallicum
Aven. sat., Avena sativa
Azad. ind., Azadirachta indica
Bad., Badiaga
Bapt., Baptisia tinctoria
Bar. carb., Baryta carb
Bar. mur., Baryta muriatica
Bell., Belladonna
Bel. per., Bellis perennis
Benz. ac., Benzoic acid
Berb. vul., Berberis vulgaris
Blatta., Blatta orientalis
Boer. dif., Boerhaavia diffusa
Bor., Borax
Bov., Bovista
Brom., Bromium
Bry. alb., Bryonia alba
Bufo., Bufo rana
Cact., Cactus grandiflorus
Cal. ars., Calcarea arsenicosa
Cal. carb., Calcarea carbonica
Cal. fl., Calcarea fluorica
Cal. phos., Calcarea phosphorica
Calend., Calendula officinalis
Calot. gig., Calotropis gigentia
Camph., Camphora
Can. ind., Cannabis indica
Can. sat., Cannabis sativa
Canth., Cantharis
Caps., Capsicum
Carb. ac., Carbolic acid
Carbo. an., Carbo animalis.
Carbo. veg., Carbo vegetabilis
Card. mar., Carduus marianus.
Caul., Caulophyllum thalictroides
Caust., Causticum
Ceano. am., Ceanothus americanus
Cham., Chamomilla
Chel. maj., Chelidonium majus
Cic. vir., Cicuta virosa
Cimic., Cimicifuga racemosa
Cina., Cina
Clem., Clematis erecta
Cocc., Cocculus indicus
Coc. c., Coccus cacti
Coff., Coffea cruda
Colch., Colchicum autumnale
Coll., Collinsonia canadensis
Coloc., Colocynthis
Con., Conium maculatum
Crat. oxy., Crataegus oxyacantha
Croc., Crocus sativus
Crot. hor., Crotalus horridus
Crot. tig., Croton tiglium
Cup. ars., Cuprum aresenicosum
Cup. met., Cuprum metallicum
Cycl., Cyclamen europaeum
Dig., Digitalis purpurea
Dios., Dioscorea villosa
Dol., Dolichos pruriens
Dros., Drosera rotundifolia
Dulc., Dulcamara
Elaps., Elaps corallinus
Equis., Equisetum hyemale
Erig., Erigeron canadense

Eup. per., Eupatorium perfoliatum

Eup. pur., Eupatorium purpureum

Euphr., Euphrasia officinalis

Fer. met., Ferrum metallicum

Fer. phos., Ferrum phosphoricum

Ficus. rel., Ficus religiosa

Form., Formica rufa

Gels., Gelsemium sempervirens

Ger. mac., Geranium maculatum

Glon., Glonoinum

Graph., Graphites

Gymn. syl., Gymnema sylvestre

Ham., Hamamelis virginica

Hecla., Hecla lava

Hell., Helleborus niger

Helon., Helonias dioica

Hep. sul., Hepar sulphuris calcareum

Hol. andy., Holarrhena antidysenterica

Dydr., Hydrastis canadensis

Hydro. as., Hydrocotyle asiatica

Hyos., Hyoscyamus niger

Hyper., Hypericum perforatum

Ign., Ignatia amara

Iod., Iodum

Ipecac., Ipecacuanha

Iris., Iris versicolor

Jab., Jaborandi

J. ashoka., Jatropha ashoka

Just. ad., Justicia adhatoda

Kali bi., Kali bichromicum

Kali br., Kali bromatum

Kali carb., Kali carbonicum

Kali iod., Kali iodatum

Kali mur., Kali muriaticum

Kali phos., Kali phosphoricum

Kali. s., Kali sulphuricum

Kalm., Kalmia latifolia

Kreos., Kreosotum

Lac. c., Lac caninum

Lac. d., Lac. defloratum

Lach., Lachesis

Led., Ledum palustre

Lil. tig., Lilium tigrinum

Lob., Lobelia inflata

Lyco., Lycopodium clavatum

Lycpr., Lycopersicum esculentum

Lycps., Lycopus virginicus

Lyss., Lyssin

Mag. carb., Magnesia carbonica

Mag. mur., Magnesia muriatica

Mag. phos., Magnesia phosphorica

Med., Medorrhinum

Mel., Melilotus alba

Meph., Mephitis

Merc., Mercurius vivus

Merc. cor., Mercurius corrosivus

Merc. cy., Mercurius cyanatus

Merc. dul., Mercurius dulcis

Merc. i. f., Mercurius iodatus flavus

Merc. i. r., Mercurius iodatus ruber

Merc. sol., Mercurius solubilis

Mez., Mezereum

Mill., Millefolium

Murx., Murex

Mur. ac., Muriatic acid

Myric., Myrica serifera

Nat. carb., Natrum carbonicum

Nat. mur., Natrum muriaticum

Nat. phos., Natrum phosphoricum

Nat. sulph., Natrum sulphuricum

Nux. mos., Nux moschata

Nux. vom., Nux vomica

Oci. san., Ocimum sanctum

Op., Opium

Ox. ac., Oxalic acid
Petrol., Petroleum
Petros., Petroselinum sativum
Phos. ac., Phosphoric acid
Phos., Phosphorus
Phys., Physostigma
Phyto., Phytolacca decandra
Pic. ac., Picric acid
Plan., Plantago major
Plat., Platinum metallicum
Plb. met., Plumbum metallicum
Podo., Podophyllum peltatum
Psor. cor., Psoralea corylifolia
Puls., Pulsatilla nigricans
Pyrog., Pyrogenium
Ran. b., Ranunculus bulbosus
Rat., Ratanhia
Rauw. serp., Rauwolfia serpentina
Rhus. tox., Rhus toxicodendron
Rhus. v., Rhus venenata
Rob., Robinia pseudocacia
Ruta., Ruta graveolens
Sabad., Sabadilla
Sabal., Sabal serrulata
Sabin., Sabina
Samb., Sambucus nigra
Sang. c., Sanguinaria canadensis
Sanic., Sanicula aqua
Sars., Sarsaparilla
Sec. cor., Secale cornutum
Sel., Selenium
Seneg., Senega
Sep., Sepia
Sil., Silicea
Spig., Spigelia anthelmintica
Spong., Spongia tosta
Stan. met., Stannum metallicum
Staph., Staphysagria
Stram., Stramonium
Sulph., Sulphur
Symph., Symphytum officinale
Syz. jam., Syzygium jambolanum
Tab., Tabacum
Tarax., Taraxacum
Tarent., Tarentula hispanica
Tarent. c., Tarentula cubensis
Term. arj., Terminalia arjuna
Ther., Theridion
Thlaspi., Thlaspi bursa pastoris
Thuja., Thuja occidentalis
Trib. ter., Tribulus terrestis
Tril., Trillium pendulum
Tub., Tuberculinum
Urt. u., Urtica urens
Ust., Ustilago maydis
Uva., Uva ursi
Valer., Valeriana
Vario., Variolinum
Verat. alb., Veratrum album
Verat. vir., Veratrum viride
Vib., Viburnum opulus
Visc., Viscum album
With. som., Withania somnifera
Xan., Xanthoxylum fraxineum
Zinc., Zincum metallicum
Zing., Zingiber

Chapter 50

Contribution of Homoeopathic Stalwarts in the field of Pharmacy

Homoeopathic pharmacy was enriched time to time by different stalwarts for their contribution and experiments. A brief discussion is given below.

Dr Hahnemann (1755-1843): Master Hahnemann, in 1805, announced his new method of pharmacological process in the treatise, *'Fragmenta de Viribus Medicamentorum Positivis Sive in Sano Corpore Humano Observatis'* which included the first repertory of homoeopathic materia medica. Between 1811 and 1833 were published his *'Materia Medica Pura'* and *'Chronic Diseases'*.

Hahnemann was the first who introduced *'Centesimal scale'*, *'Fluxion potency'*, and *'50-millesimal scale'*.

Hahnemann also develops *'Multiple vial potency'*. In this method requires a new vial to be used for every stage of potentisation.

Dr William H Burt: Dr Burt introduced *'Straight potency'* (Conversion of trituration into liquid potency). As per Burt of London, 7x liquid potency can be prepared from its previous 6x trituration.

Burt advises using a small amount of alcohol for moistening the sugar of milk during trituration, as it will save the troubles of scrapping and stirring.

Dr Burt advises to avoid blue coloured (Colouring agent – Cobalt oxide, Cupric oxide) bottles for preserving drugs and potentised medicines as they have some dynamic affects which is injurious to drugs or potentised medicines.

Dr Burt was responsible for the actual proving of about 30 drugs. He works with crude doses as heroic proving. He proves Aesculus, Baptisia, Cactus grandiflorus, Caulophyllum, Collinsonia, Dioscorea, Hamamelis, Hydrastis, Iris vers, Leptandra, Phytolacca, Pulsatilla, Ustilago and Veratrum viride.

Burt's classic book, *'Physiological Materia Medica'* containing all that is known of the physiological action of our remedies; together with their characteristic indications and pharmacology. He classified drugs into two groups according to their action – Animal group (Cerebro-spinants) and Organic group (Ganglionics).

Albrecht von Haller (1708-1777): A well known physician, botanist, poet and novelist was the first known person, besides Hahnemann, who felt the need of testing medicines for their pure and peculiar effects in deranging the health of man, in order to learn what morbid state each medicine is capable of curing (F. N. to Sec. 108). Albrecht von Haller recommends the following in his 'Pharmacopoeia Helvetica,' Basel; Im Hof 1771, p.12. Haller describes

"Indeed, a medicine must first of all be assayed in a healthy body, without any foreign admixture. When the odour and taste of the medicine have been examined, a small dose of it must be taken, and attention must be paid to every change that occurs, to the pulse, the temperature, respiration and excretions. Then, having examined the symptoms encountered in the healthy person, one may proceed to trials in the body of a sick person".

Dr Johann Ernst Stapf (1788-1860): Stapf was the prover of thirty-two medicines. He was an indefatigable worker and was much esteemed by his fellow physicians for his extended knowledge.

It was reported that he used olfaction of the higher potencies to administer the remedies. He commenced his studies upon high potencies during the last of 1843 and published the results in June, 1844. In 1822 he became the editor of the, *"Archiv fur die homoeopathische Heilkunst"*, which was published at Leipzic, three times a year.

He proved the following medicines – Aconitum napellus, Ammonium carbonicum, Anacardium, Arnica montana, Arsenicum album, Asarum europaeum, Baryta carbonicum, Belladonna, Bryonia alba, Calcarea, Camphora, Cannabis sativa, Causticum, Chamomilla, Cinchona officinalis, Cina, Clematis erecta, Colocynthis, Digitalis purpurea, Dulcamara, Helleborus niger, Hepar sulphuris calcareum, Hyoscyamus niger, Ipecacuanha, Magnetis polus australis, Manganum aceticum, Mercurius solubilis, Moschus, Muriaticum acidum, Nitric acid, Nux vomica, Opium, Phosphorus, Phosphoricum acidum, Pulsatilla, Rhus toxicodendron, Ruta graveolens, Silicea, Spigelia anthelmia, Spongia tosta, Squilla maritima, Staphysagria, Veratrum album and Zincum metallicum.

He introduced a process to purify commercial lactose known as Stapf's process.

General Count Iseman von Korsakoff (1788-1853): He was impressed by Hahnemann's potentisation theory. He was the **real originator of high potencies**. He claimed that one single medicated globule when placed among many non-medicated globules communicate its medicinal power to the non-medicated globules. He claimed that all these globules had been medically activated and that their medicinal strength was almost equal to that of the original globule. He went on to do this with **13,500 unmedicated globules** and one single dry globule of **Sulphur 30**. He believed that the material division of the medicine ceased with the 6th potency.

He prepared high potency by dry grafting method.

Caspar Julius Jenichen (1787-1849): Jenichen of Wismar, Germany pursued the idea that further attenuation is not necessary for the potentisation of medicine, but *continuous succussion without dilution is sufficient*. He advocated that the degree of strength developed through potentisation was directly proportional to the number of strokes given. Thus he suggested that every ten strokes given would increase the dynamic strength of the medicine by one degree. He instructed to give only strokes without dilution to increase potency.

Dr Carl W Caspari (1798-1828): The first Homoeopathic Pharmacopoeia was written by Dr Carl W Caspari of Leipzig, Germany, in 1825. He published, 'Homoeopathisches Dispensatorium Fur Aerzte und Apotheker' thereby giving the first idea of homoeopathic pharmacopoeias for physicians and pharmacists. Dr Caspari was a member of Samuel Hahnemann's Provers Union and wrote the Homoeopathic Domestic Physician which included a chapter on Mesmerism.

Dr Constantine Hering (1800-1880): Dr Constantine Hering of Philadelphia was the first who introduced Decimal scale to potentise snake venoms. Now this scale is extensively used for the preparation of homoeopathic medicines as well as biochemic tissue salts.

Dr Hering described *five steps* involved in the drug proving in the preface of volume 1 of his Guiding Symptoms of Materia Medica. They are Probability, Confirmation, Corroboration, Verification and Characteristics.

Dr Vehsemeyer: Vehsemeyer of Berlin, in 1836, set forth the principles of Decimal scale, in a precise manner.

Dr Samuel Swan (1814-1893): Swan experimented with the concept of using *fractional part of potencies* for attenuation. He suggested that if one drop of tincture were used to make 1M potency, then 1/10th of a drop of the 1M would be used to make the 10M. This method had more to do with the dilution of the final potency, rather than the serial dilution of each potency along the way.

Bernhardt Fincke (1821-1906): He was an American physician and develops his own method of potentisation by a new machine named as '*Fincke Potentiser*'. He used to take 100 drops of drug substance in a glass jug. He allowed a stream of water to flow into it. For every drachm of water entering in and out of the vessel, he would count it as one potency. Thus 100 drachms of water entering and coming out of the vessel would raise the potency of the containing drug substance to 100. **He never believed the value of strokes**. He had paid importance only on the water with its exerting force on a medicinal substance in raising the potencies, and not on any strokes applied.

Dr Fincke proved many homoeopathic remedies like X-ray and others. The imponderable remedies proving credit goes to Dr Fincke. Saccharum lactis was also proved by Dr Fincke.

Thomas Skinner (1825-1906): Skinner was a high potency prescriber and he invented a machine for potentisation named '*Fluxion Centesimal Attenuator*' in 1878. It was first described in an article by Thomas Skinner in the Organon (Vol.1 P. 45). This device was designed to mount above a small sink in the office or home. The motive power was water pressure. The potencies are labeled 'FC' (*Fluxion Centesimal*) to differentiate them from Hahnemannian Centesimal potencies. Skinner's potencies were prepared by a process of *discontinuous fluxion* in contrast to the continuous fluxion of Swan and Fincke.

Carroll Dunham (1828-1877): Dunham introduced preparation of potentised homoeopathic medicines by machines. He used an abandoned oil mill for preparing potencies. He experimented with 125 strokes to raise one degree of the potency. His potencies were suffixed by letter 'D'.

Dr Willmar Schwabe (1839-1917): Dr Willmar Schwabe of Leipzig founded the Homoeopathic Central Pharmacy to manufacture and sell homoeopathic medicines in 1866. He created precise standards for homoeopathic pharmaceutical production which was published in 1872 as, '*Pharmacopoeia Homoeopathica Polyglotta*'.

He also introduced the semi manual and semi-mechanical trituration process.

Dr Pierre Schmidt (1894-1987): Dr Pierre Schmidt firstly coined the name 50-millesimal scale. He published an article entitled *"The Hidden Treasure of the Last Organon"*, in *"The British Homoeopathic Journal"* July October 1954. Another article was published by him in *"The Journal of the Institute of Homoeopathy"* December-January 1955-56. Potencies prepared under this method are named by Schmidt as *"Fifty Millesimal Potencies"* because of the fact that the material part of the medicine was said to be decreased by 50,000 times for each degree of dynamisation.

Dr P. N. Varma (1937-2018): Dr. P. N. Varma, the renowned homoeopathic scientist and the founder of Homoeopathic Pharmacopoeia Laboratory (HPL) in 1975 at Ghaziabad and of Central Council of Research in Homoeopahty (CCRH). The contribution of Dr P. N. Varma in establishing the '*Homoeopathic Pharmacopeia Laboratory*' was a trend-setter towards the statutory control of Homoeopathic medicines in the world of homoeopathy all over India and abroad.

He has authored many books on homoeopathy including the '*Encyclopedia of Homoeopathic Pharmacopoeias*', the first edition of which published in 1997. The latest four volume '*Encyclopedia of Homoeopathic Pharmacopoeia & Drug Index*' has been approved as a reference book for pharmacy by the Central Council of Homoeoapthy.

Dr P. N. Varma uses bioinformatics to give an explanation for homoeopathy. He took inspiration from the works of scientists of 'Kalyani University', who suggested gene expression as possible model of action in 'radiation protection' (protection from the hazardous effects of radiation) by homoeopathic medicine Ginseng 200 on biological models. Dr P. N. Varma says that the idea of individualistic medicine suggested by genomics is similar to '*constitutional medicine*' which homoeopathy has upheld for long. He uses immunology to explain that the self regulatory mechanisms of body, which is in turn controlled by genes, could be influenced by homoeopathic medicines. He replaces the word 'vital force' with a new terminology 'biological responses'. He says this concept requires more scientific work so that gene expression can be linked to homoeopathy.

Chapter 51

Pharmacovigilance (PV or PhV) (Drug Safety)

Word Meaning

The word Pharmacovigilance (Pv) is a mixture of Greek word "Pharmakon" which means *"medicinal substances"* and the Latin word "Vigilare" which means *"to keep watch"*. So Pharmacovigilance generally refers to continuous monitoring for unwanted effects and other – safety related aspects of marketed drugs.

Pharmacovigilance (Pv)
It is comprises of etymology

Pharmakon (Greek word)	Vigilare (Latin word)
↓	↓
Medicinal substances	To keep watch

Definition

1. Pharmacovigilance has been defined as: The science and activities relating to the **detection, assessment, understanding and prevention** of adverse effects or any other drug-related problem (WHO).
2. An umbrella term used to describe the processes for monitoring and evaluating ADRs.

   It is a key component of effective drug regulation systems, clinical practice and public health programs.
3. It is the study of the safety of marketed drugs examined under the practical conditions of clinical use in large communities.
4. It is the branch dealing with adverse drug reactions (ADRs), their recognition, and reporting.

Major aims of Pharmacovigilance

1. **Patient care**: To improve patient care and safety in relation to medicines, and all medical and para medical interventions.
2. **Public health:** To improve public health and safety in relation to the use of medicines.
3. **Risk benefit and assessment**: To contribute to the assessment of benefit, harm, effectiveness and risk of medicines.
4. **Communication:** To promote understanding, education and clinical training in pharmacovigilance and its effective communication to health professionals and the public.

Challenges in homoeopathic pharmacovigilance

- **Diversity of Remedies:** Homoeopathy encompasses a vast range of remedies derived from various sources. Tracking and monitoring the safety of such a diverse array of substances pose a challenge.

- **Diagnostic Complexity**: Homoeopathic treatments often rely on subjective symptoms for diagnosis. Distinguishing between the natural progression of a disease and potential adverse effects becomes challenging.
- **Quality Assurance**: Vigilant monitoring contributes to maintaining the
- **Standardisation**: Lack of standardised reporting systems and criteria for adverse events in homoeopathy hinders the establishment of a uniform pharmacovigilance framework.

Need of Pharmacovigilance in Homoeopathy

The core concerns of contemporary pharmacovigilance is the safety of modern medicines, traditional (herbal) medicines, vaccines, in some places, devices, substandard and falsified (SF) medical products. In addition to the above, reasons for Pharmacovigilance of homoeopathic drugs are:

1. **Misconceptions about the Homoeopathic drugs**: There are misconceptions regarding homoeopathic systems that these drugs are absolutely safe, can be taken for long time, they have only placebo effect, can be used in conjunction with other drugs etc. Such misconceptions are detrimental to the patients and the system. Pharmacovigilance can play a great role in resolving this notion.
2. **Adulterations and contaminations of Homoeopathic drugs**: Homoeopathic drugs have been found to be adulterated with heavy metals etc. There are spurious and misbranded drugs in the market. Different types of vehicles are used as per requirement like sugar of milk, globules, tablets, purified water, alcohol, glycerine, olive oil, almond oil etc. More over there is a practice of self preparation and dispensing of medicine by the physicians in their clinic or chambers. So there is a maximum chance of contamination of these vehicles while preparing or dispensing which can be a potential cause of ADE/ ADR.
3. **Malpractices**: Common malpractices are self medications, misuse of prescriptions, improper and indiscriminate use as 'over the counter' (OTC) drugs etc.
4. **Globalisation of AYUSH systems**: AYUSH systems are widely and thoroughly practiced in India since centuries irrespective of their use in other countries. Further many ASU&H drugs are manufactured for global use and they have moved beyond the traditional and cultural framework for which they were originally intended. Considering the growing use of ASU & H products globally; inclusion of traditional medicines in Pharmacovigilance system becomes important.
5. **Lack of safety profile of drug**: People round the globe are becoming conscious and more concerned about the safety of drugs they consume. Pharmacovigilance of homoeopathic drugs can help in creating a safety profile of each drug both generic and patent leading to their easy acceptability globally.
6. **Increased incidence of Objectionable Advertisements**: In recent times incidence of misleading and objectionable advertisements of homoeopathic drugs in print and electronic media are the global concern nowadays. Combination and patent medicines demanded to prevent diseases even incurable diseases. The drugs were marketed without clinical trials.

Milestones in the Evolution of Pharmacovigilance

- 1848: Fifteen-year-old Hannah Greener from the north of England died after receiving chloroform anaesthetic during a surgical procedure to remove an ingrown toenail. Chloroform had been brought into use in clinical practice the previous year, replacing ether, which caused more intense nausea and vomiting.
- 1937: Sulfanilamide elixir leads to the poisoning of more than one hundred people in the USA;
- 1938: The United States Congress passes the Federal, Drug and Cosmetic Act;
- 1955: Acetylsalicylic acid is confirmed as a cause of gastrointestinal diseases;
- 1961: An Australian doctor, William McBride, wrote a letter to the editor of "The Lancet" journal, in which he suggested a connection of congenital malformation (Phocomelia) of

babies born to women who took thalidomide during pregnancy. This alarming incidence initiated pharmacovigilance concept. In fact, he observed that the incidence of congenital malformations of babies (1.5%) had increased up to 20% in women who had taken thalidomide during pregnancy. At the same time, during a Pediatric Convention in Germany Dr. Lenz suggested a correlation between malformations and thalidomide and his suspect was published in a German Journal (Welt am Sonnatag).

- 1962: In USA, the amendment to Federal Food, drug & Cosmetic Act, requiring safety and efficacy data of drugs before premarketing submission, was approved. As a result of this amendment, the safety data have to include also teratogenicity test in three different animals.
- 1964: The UK launches the Yellow Card (YC) scheme for the spontaneous reporting of adverse drug reactions.
- 1965: In Europe, the disaster of thalidomide stimulated the development of a European legislation with the EC Directive 65/65. First European Pharmaceutical Directive.
- 1966: In 1966, a pilot study of Boston Collaborative Drug Surveillance Program started. It was the first group to conduct epidemiologic researches to quantify the potential adverse effects of drugs utilising in-hospital monitoring and had an essential role in the development and application of methods in drug epidemiology.
- 1968: The World Health Organization (WHO) established its first Collaborating Centre for International Drug Monitoring in 1968. This center later became the Uppsala Monitoring Centre (UMC), which played a pivotal role in promoting international collaboration in pharmacovigilance.
- 1970: In the 1970s, the United States Food and Drug Administration (FDA) implemented the Adverse Drug Reaction Reporting System (ADRRS), which required pharmaceutical companies to report any adverse reactions associated with their drugs. This system served as a model for other countries and remains an integral part of the modern pharmacovigilance system.
- 1978: In 1978 Uppsala Monitoring Centre (UMC) started in Sweden as the WHO collaborating centre for international drug monitoring. It operates the technical and scientific aspects of the WHO's worldwide pharmacovigilance network. Currently 136 countries are the full members of the WHO Programme for International Drug Monitoring.
- 1990: The International Conference on Harmonisation (ICH) issued guidelines for the structure and content of individual case safety reports (ICSRs). These guidelines standardised the way adverse event reports were submitted and managed.
- 1992: In 1992, the European Society of Pharmacovigilance (ESoP) was funded, turned into the International Society of Pharmacovigilance (IsoP). The aims of this society were to promote Pharmacovigilance, and enhance all aspects of the safe and proper use of medicines.
- 1995: The European Medicines Agency (EMA) was founded in 1995, and it is a decentralized body of the European Union (EU). One of its essential functions is the monitoring and assessment of the safety of drugs, and it has implemented several systems and programs to accomplish this goal.
- 1998: India joined the WHO ADR monitoring programme based in Uppsala, Sweden. This attempt was unsuccessful.
- 2000: In the early 2000s, the FDA and the European Medicines Agency (EMA) introduced the concept of a Risk Management Plan (RMP), which is a document that outlines the measures that pharmaceutical companies will take to ensure the safe use of their products.
- 2001: Eudra Vigilance database was created. It is the official European database for managing and analysing information on suspected adverse reactions to medicines which have been authorised for the market or being studied in European clinical trials.
- 2010: Europian Pharmacovigilance legislation passed.

- 2014: MHRA Good Pharmacovigilance Practice for medicines.
- 2017: The new EudraVigilance system is launched.

History of Pharmacovigilance in India

1983: In India awareness about the ADR was first started in October 1983 by organising a seminar under the auspices of *India Pharmacovigilance society* at Maulana Azad Medical College, New Delhi.

1986: A formal ADR monitoring system for India consisting of 12 regional centers, each covering a population of 50 million, was proposed.

1989: In 1989 ICMR sponsored the first project on ADR in India in the department of pharmacology Jawaharlal Nehru Medical College, Aligarh Muslim University, Aligarh.

1996: In India, clinical trials at the global standard level have started in1996.

1997: The first conference on ADR was organised in **January 1997** by the Department of Clinical Pharmacology, Seth GS Medical College and KEM Hospital, Mumbai.

1998: in 1998, India joined the WHO ADR monitoring programme based in Uppsala, Sweden. This attempt was unsuccessful.

1999: *Society of Pharmacovigilance India* (SoPI) was constituted and registered in 1999 as a dedicated platform for future discussions.

2005: *National Pharmacovigilance Programme* (NPP) established in **January 2005** was monitored by the *National Pharmacovigilance Advisory Committee* based in the Central Drugs Standard Control Organization (CDSCO), New Delhi. Two zonal centers – the South-West zonal center (located in the Department of Clinical Pharmacology, Seth GS Medical College and KEM Hospital, Mumbai) and the North-East zonal center (located in the Department of Pharmacology, All India Institute of Medical Sciences, New Delhi) – were to collate information from all over the country and send it to the Committee as well as to the Uppsala monitoring center in Sweden.

2006: First work related to the Adverse drug reaction (ADR) in AYUSH sector occurred in 2005 when Ibn Sina Academy of Medieval Medicine & Science (Aligarh), established a special cell namely *"Centre for safety & Rational Use of Indian Systems of Medicine"* in collaboration with WHO.

2007: After that Institute of Post Graduate Teaching & Research in Ayurveda (IPGT & RA), Jamnagar, conducted two days National workshop on 3rd and 4th December 2007.

2008: In 2008 Department of AYUSH, Ministry of Health and FW, Govt. of India, New Delhi, organised the first National Consultative Meet of *National Pharmacovigilance Programme* (NPP) for AYUSH drugs.

2010: *National Pharmacovigilance Programme* (NPP) was launched in 2010 under the command of *Central Drug Standard Control Organization* (CDSCO), by the Ministry of Health & Family Welfare, Government of India, New Delhi.

2011: *National Pharmacovigilance Programme* (NPP) was shifted from the *All India Institute of Medical Sciences* (AIIMS), New Delhi to the *Indian Pharmacopoeia Commission* (IPC), Ghaziabad, (U.P) as *National Coordinating Centre* (NCC) in April, 2011 by a Notification issued by the Ministry of Health & Family Welfare, Government of India, New Delhi, from where it is working since then. Following the conventional medicine, need of pharmacovigilance was also felt in herbal or traditional medicines. Consequently *National Pharmacovigilance Programme* (NPP) was established in various countries to collect, process, understand and report adverse events (AE) of the medicines including the herbal medicines. The *European Medicine Agency* (EMA) provided its rule for pharmacovigilance of herbal medicines and provided its reviews of various herbal medicines as per the available data.

2015: Indian Pharmacopoeia Commission – Pharmacovigilance Programme of India (IPC-PvPI) became the *National Coordinating Centre* (NCC) for *Materiovigilance Programme of India* (MvPI) from July in 2015.

2017: Indian Pharmacopoeia Commission, Pharmacovigilance Programme of India and National Coordinating Centre (IPC, NCC-PvPI) became a WHO Collaborating Centre for Pharmacovigilance in Public Health Programmes & Regulatory services from July, 2017.

2018: In March 2018 Ministry of AYUSH signed MoU with NCC-IPC subsequently National Pharmacovigilance Programme (NPP) for Ayurveda, Sidha, Unani & Homoeopathy was launched as Central sector schemes. It initiated its working with All India Institute of Ayurveda (AIIA), New Delhi, as the *National Pharmacovigilance Coordination Centre* (NPvCC).

Statistics

According to a report by the World Health Organization (WHO), adverse drug reactions (ADRs) are a significant cause of morbidity and mortality worldwide. The report states that ADRs are responsible for 7% of hospital admissions and are the 6th biggest cause of death in hospitals. In addition, the report estimates that up to 50% of ADRs are preventable. In comparison to the global average of 5%, India's ADR reporting rate is less than 1%.

In India, the Pharmacovigilance Programme of India (PvPI) has been established to monitor and evaluate the safety of medicines. According to the PvPI, there were 1,85,036 ADRs reported in India between 2010 and 2018. Of these, 7,541 ADRs were reported for homoeopathic medicines.

Framework of Pharmacovigilance (Homoeopathy)

Under the Ministry of AYUSH, Govt. of India, there are three tier Pharmacovigilance centres for homoeopathic system. They are as follows:

1. **National Pharmacovigilance Co-ordination Centre (NPvCC)**: It is a tertiary pharmacovigilance centre, acting as National Centre in the administrative structure of the program. Ministry of AYUSH, New Delhi has designated All India Institute of Ayurveda (AIIA), New Delhi as National Pharmacovigilance Coordination Centre (NPvCC).
2. **Intermediary Pharmacovigilance Centres (IPvCs)**: Secondary pharmacovigilance centres, acting as second level centres in the administrative structure of the program. All the national institutes (AYUSH) has been designated as IPvCs. For homoeopathy National Institute of Homoeopathy, Kolkata, West Bengal is the IPvC.

Note: The IPvC, Kolkata started functioning since 11.01.2018.

3. **Peripheral Pharmacovigilance Centres (PPvCs)**: Primary pharmacovigilance centres. They are relatively smaller ASU & H colleges or institutions including. These are the first contact ADR data collection units. They would be identified and coordinated by IPvCs in consultation with NPvCC. As we are discussing Pharmacovigilance in homoeopathy so here only Homoeopathic institutions designated as PPvCs all over India are given below. Each PPvC have been allotted with specific centre code (see page no. 597).

1. Central Research Institute for Homoeopathy, under CCRH, Noida, UP
2. National Homoeopathy Research institute in Mental Health, under CCRH Kottayam, Kerala.
3. Regional Research Institute for Homoeopathy, under CCRH, Gudivada.
4. Regional Research Institute for Homoeopathy, under CCRH, Guwahati.
5. Regional Research Institute for Homoeopathy, under CCRH, Kolkata.
6. Regional Research Institute for Homoeopathy, under CCRH, Mumbai.
7. Government Homoeopathic Medical College and Hospital, Bhopal.
8. Mahesh Bhattacharya Homoeopathic Medical College and Hospital, Howrah, West Bengal.
9. Sarada Krishna Homoeopathic Medical College, Kulasekharam, Kanyakumari, Tamil Nadu.
10. Father Muller Homoeopathic Medical College and Hospital University Road, Deralakatte, Mangaluru-575018.
11. Dr. Abhin Chandra Homoeopathic Medical College and Hospital, Unit-III, Kharvel Nagar, Bhubaneswar, 750001.

Pharmacovigilance is the science dedicated to reduce the risk of drug-related harms to the consumers. Looking into the conditions prevailing in the present scenario, it is high time to deliberate regarding the concerns over traditional and classical Ayurvedic, Siddha, Unani and Homoeopathy products and practices. Thus, the programme is initiated to collect, collate and analyse data to establish evidence for clinical safety of ASU & H

Centre Code	Name of the Peripheral Pharmacovigilance Centres (PPvCs)
001	Central Research Institute for Homoeopathy, under (CRI-H), Noida, U.P.
002	National Homoeopathy Research institute in Mental Health (NHRIMH), Kottayam, Kerala.
003	Regional Research Institute for Homoeopathy (RRI-H), Gudivada.
004	Regional Research Institute for Homoeopathy (RRI-H), Guwahati.
005	Regional Research Institute for Homoeopathy (RRI-H), Kolkata.
006	Regional Research Institute for Homoeopathy (RRI-H), Mumbai.
007	Government Homoeopathic Medical College and Hospital (GHMC & H), Bhopal.
008	Mahesh Bhattacharya Homoeopathic Medical College and Hospital (MBHMC & H), Howrah, West Bengal.
009	Sarada Krishna Homoeopathic Medical College (SKHMC), Kulasekharam, Kanyakumari, Tamil Nadu.
010	Father Muller Homoeopathic Medical College and Hospital (FMHMC & H), University Road, Deralakatte, Mangaluru-575018.
011	Dr. Abhin Chandra Homoeopathic Medical College and Hospital (ACHMC & H), Unit-III, Kharvel Nagar, Bhubaneswar, 750001.
012	Regional Research Institute for Homoeopathy (RRI-H), Imphal, Manipur.
013	Regional Research Institute for Homoeopathy (RRI-H), Agartaa, Tripura.
014	All India Institute of Medical Sciences, Raipur (AIMA, Raipur.
015	M.P.K. Homoeopathic Medical College, Jaipur (MPKHMC, Jaipur).
016	Clinical Research Unit for Homoeopathy, Port Blair (CRU-H), Port Blair.

drugs in a scientific manner for documenting clinical evidence of safety and to undertake surveillance of misleading advertisements of ASU & H drugs for regulatory actions.

The National Pharmacovigilance Co-ordination Centre (NPvCC) will undertake the pharmacovigilance activities under the guidance and technical support of Indian Pharmacopoeia Commission (WHO Collaborating Centre for Pharmacovigilance), Ghaziabad and Concerned programme officers at WHO Country Office India, NewDelhi. The National Pharmacovigilance Coordination Centre (NPvCC) in consultation with the Pharmacopoeial Commission of Indian Medicine and Homoeopathy (PCIM & H), if required, shall conduct the Causality Assessment of the signals received from the Intermediary Pharmacovigilance Centres (IPvCs) and intimate to the Ministry of AYUSH regarding confirmed ADRs and misleading advertisements to enable suitable action.

Ministry of Ayush, Govt of India

↓

Drug Policy Section, Ministry of Ayush

↓

National Pharmacovigilance Co-ordination Centre (NPvCC) (AIIA, New Delhi)

↓

Intermediary Pharmacovigilance Centres (IPvCs) (Homoeopathy) (NIH-Kolkata)

↓

Peripheral Pharmacovigilance Centres (PPvCs) (Homoeopathy) (16 centres all over India)

Terminologies/theories of Homoeopathy and ADR

Following terminologies and theories of Homoeopathy are closely related to ADR which should be clearly for expelling confusion and proper better understanding of pharmacovigilance.

1. **Homoeopathic literature and ADR**: The basic concept of pharmacovigilance of "making drug safe" is one of the factors that led to the discovery of homoeopathy by Hahnemann in 1796. In fact the toxicity or harm caused to the patient by the contemporary methods of treatment bent Hahnemann to leave medical practice and start translating books for his livelihood. In homoeopathy references of ADRs or similar phenomena are present in its literature years before the world community apprehended its threat in 1848. In later part of 18th century he warned the world community against the collateral damages by the applied drug during treatment.

   Hahnemann has denounced the administration of multifarious, compounds and haphazard administration of several substances at one time with unascertained efficacy as "very absurd which only lead to a blind and confused practice". He added that without the investigation (and unless their pure pathogenetic action on the healthy individual has previously been ascertained) all treatment of disease must continue to be not only a foolish, but even a criminal action, a dangerous attack upon human life. So since very beginning homoeopathy has tried to address the issue of safety of drug (Pharmacovigilance).

   Currently ADE/ADR is poorly reported or documented in homoeopathy. It may be either because of negligence on part of physician or non occurrence of ADR at all. A systematic review conducted on adverse effects of homoeopathic medicines concluded that anecdotal reports of adverse effects in homoeopathic publications were not well documented and mainly reported aggravation of current symptoms. Case reports in conventional medical journals pointed more to adverse effects of mislabeled 'homoeopathic products' than to true homoeopathic medicines.

2. **Drug proving and ADR**: Drug proving is a unique process of drug development in homoeopathy. Adverse drug reaction and Drug proving are closely related. In fact ADR or noxious effect of drug is the basis of drug development. Once the pathogenetic effect of the substance is known sub-molecular or ultra molecular doses of these substances are used in homoeopathic drug proving on healthy human being to produce symptoms and so generate new indications for clinical use of the homoeopathic medicine. In homoeopathy the disease producing power is the disease curing power in potentised form. In Organon of Medicine, the magnum opus in Homoeopathy, Hahnemann has referred ADR by different similar terminologies like *pernicious effect, noxious* and *poisonous character of substance* etc. and appreciated these past recorded ADRs as the first rudiments of the true, pure Materia medica.

3. **Homoeopathic Materia Medica and ADR**: Homoeopathic Materia Medica is a systemic record (available in the form of books and software's) of collection of symptoms of thousands of medicines. These symptoms are obtained by 'Drug Proving' conducted on basis of principles laid out in Organon by Dr. Hahnemann and 'Clinical Proving'. It contains proved symptoms, clinical symptoms etc. Proved symptoms as we have seen above has evolved from its pathogenetic power or so called ADR.

   In homoeopathic literatures numerous forms of correlations between remedies have been developed by stalwarts. According to Dr Gibson Miller, connection between drugs such as *complementary, inimical, antidote,* remedies that follow well have been classified. But as the Materia medica is expanding, the new remedies have no literature in remedy relationship. These relationship are practically important during prescribing. Does the violation of these relationships while prescribing cause any drug interaction that can be tested by recording of events for a long time for which reporting and documentation under pharmacovigilance will prove helpful.

4. **Homoeopathic Posology and ADR**: ADR is mainly caused by the immoderate doses of prescribed medicine. This was apprehended by Hahnemann in his early practice life. Hahnemann at the beginning of his practice used large doses of medicine like allopathic

system. He used large and repeated doses of Mercury for Lues venereal (1786). He prescribed *Verat alb* for bronchial asthma, 3 grains, every morning for 4 weeks and *Arnica montona* several grains of dysentery (1796). Due to unwanted aggravation and secondary effects he switched on to minimum doses, i.e. infinitesimal doses (1801). In higher potency (infinitesimal doses) the actual material of the drug is untraceable and that preparation exhibits the dynamic action in order to cure the patient. That is why the chance of ADR in high potency is minimum but long continued administration of mother tinctures and low potency medicines with immoderate doses which is prevalent now a day's may cause ADR like phenomena.

5. **Mode of Homoeopathic prescription and ADE/ADR**: Hahnemann clearly states about the application of single medicine at a time in Organon Sec. 272, 273, 274 and F.N. to Sec. 272.

Sec. 272: In no case is it requisite to administer more than one single, simple medicinal substance at one time.

Sec. 273: It was more consistent with nature and more rational to prescribe single, simple medicine at one time in a disease.

In contrary to that, prescriptions like polypharmacy, mixture of medicines, patent medicines, multiple biochemic tablets etc. given for long duration has become a fashion.

ADR will not occur at all cases of wrong prescription, but overdosing, administration of multiple drugs for long period, adulteration and contamination etc. always put threat for ADE/ADR in homoeopathy.

The flow of information in the system shall be handled confidentially. This also facilitates documentation of adverse drug reaction. It helps to develop system wise database of adverse drug reaction and improve the clinical safety of the drugs.

6. **Aggravation and ADR**: Aggravation is the intensification or worsening of the symptoms/condition of the patient after the administration of medicine. In homoeopathy, three types of aggravation are usually found. They are:

(i) **Homoeopathic aggravation**: Homoeopathic aggravation is the slight and apparent intensification (i.e. short and sharp aggravation) of the existing symptoms of the patient (which are similar to the applied medicine) after the application of a well-selected homoeopathic medicine, but the patient feels better inspite of the aggravation of the symptoms.

(ii) **Medicinal aggravation**: Medicinal aggravation can be defined as the appearance of new symptoms of the medicine in a patient after administration of wrongly selected medicine. In medicinal aggravation, many new symptoms appear in addition to the existing sufferings of the patient causing great distress to the patient.

(iii) **Disease aggravation**: Disease aggravation can be defined as the appearance of new symptoms belonging to the sphere of disease due to its natural tendency to progress. It indicates that the selected medicine is wrong and is not showing any impact on the disease condition. As a result, there will be progressive aggravation of the symptoms of the patient and the patient will feel worse both physically and mentally as well as the case will deteriorate in all respect as a whole.

Aggravation apparently looks similar to ADR but it is quite different. ADR is the unintended and noxious reaction of the drug which is not known earlier during different phases of medicinal/drug trial. But Aggravation of homoeopathic medicine is either expected or known. If at all beyond purview of aggravation it will be new symptoms of the drugs on that particular person that can be included in our Materia Medica after verification for future use.

Proceedings of National Pharmacovigilance Co-ordination Centre (NPvCC)

- **What to Report**: The programme for ASU &H drugs shall encourage reporting of
  (i) *all suspected drug related adverse events – seemingly insignificant or common adverse reactions.*
  (ii) *misleading advertisement of* ASU&H drugs.

The reporting should be done by using *Suspected Adverse Drug Reaction Reporting Form* for ASU & H drugs.

The reporting of these are important since they may highlight a widespread prescribing problem.

- **Who can Report**: Any health care professional can report suspected adverse drug events to the concerned PPvCs/IPvCs using *Suspected Adverse Reactions Reporting Form* for ASU & H Drugs.
- **Where to Report**: The reporting on prescribed format can be submitted to any Pharmacovigilance centre nearest to you or Email at NIH, Kolkata: ipvc.nih.kolkata@gmail.com or online at www.ayushsuraksha.com
- **What happens to the submitted Reports**: The information submitted shall be handled in confidentiality. Peripheral Pharmacovigilance Centres (PPvCs) shall forward the form to the respective Intermediary Pharmacovigilance Centres (IPvCs) who will carry out the causality analysis.

  This information shall be forwarded to the National Pharmacovigilance Co-ordination Centre (NPvCC). The data will be analysed and forwarded to the Ministry of AYUSH, Govt. of India.
- **Reporting backdrops**: The major weakness of the spontaneous reporting system by clinician is under-reporting. Overworked medical personnel do not always see reporting as a priority, especially if the symptoms are not serious. Even if the symptoms are serious, they may not be recognised as the possible effect of a particular drug.

Pharmacovigilance terms/definitions

Adverse Drug Events (ADEs): Any "untoward medical occurrence" that occurs alongside a drug that has not been conclusively attributed to the use of the drug itself. ADEs encompass side effects and laboratory results.

Serious Adverse Events (SAEs): Adverse drug events that are particularly serious, including those that are life-threatening, lead to congenital abnormalities, result in extended or unexpected inpatient hospitalisation or cause disability. Newly discovered SAEs for drugs on the market require expedited reporting by pharma companies to regulatory authorities.

Adverse Drug Reaction (ADR): WHO Technical Report No 498 (1972): A response which is noxious and unintended, and which occurs at doses normally used in humans for the prophylaxis, diagnosis, or therapy of disease, or for the modification of physiological function. "A response to a medicinal product which is noxious and unintended."

Suspected Adverse Drug Reactions: An adverse event that is suspected to be caused by a drug. If research confirms the correlation, it would become a confirmed adverse drug reaction.

Suspected Unexpected Serious Adverse Reactions (SUSARs): Adverse reactions that occur which do not line up with the adverse reactions currently outlined in the investigator brochure (before marketing) or product information including the SmPC and PIL (after marketing). Also called unexpected drug reactions.

Causality Assessment

Various causality terms are in use but the following are used most widely. Some, however, do not use all the terms, for instance many do not believe that a 'certain' classification is possible for a single report and other make no distinction between 'probable' and 'possible'. These definitions are however acceptable to Programme members who do use the terms. Where only 'possible' or 'unlikely' are used to describe reactions it must be understood that 'possible' include those reactions which are called by others 'probable' and 'certain', as well as 'possible'. Whilst 'conditional/unclassified' and 'unassessable/unclassifiable' are not causality terms, they describe the status of adverse reaction reports and therefore allow for practical communication about ADR issues.

1. **Certain**: A clinical event, including laboratory test abnormality, occurring in a plausible time relationship to drug administration, and which cannot be explained by concurrent disease or other drugs or chemicals. The response to withdrawal of the drug (de-challenge) should be clinically plausible. The event must be

definitive pharmacologically or phenomenologically, using a satisfactory re-challenge procedure if necessary.

2. **Probable/Likely:** A clinical event, including laboratory test abnormality, with a reasonable time sequence to administration of the drug, unlikely to be attributed to concurrent disease or other drugs or chemicals, and which follows a clinically reasonable response on withdrawal (de-challenge). Re-challenge information is not required to fulfil this definition.
3. **Possible**: A clinical event, including laboratory test abnormality, with a reasonable time sequence to administration of the drug, but which could also be explained by concurrent disease or other drugs or chemicals. Information on drug withdrawal may be lacking or unclear.
4. **Unlikely**: A clinical event, including laboratory test abnormality, with a temporal relationship to drug administration which makes a causal relationship improbable, and in which other drugs, chemicals or underlying disease provide plausible explanations.
5. **Conditional/Unclassified**: A clinical event, including laboratory test abnormality, reported as an adverse reaction, about which more data is essential for a proper assessment or the additional data are under examination.
6. **Un-assessable/Unclassifiable**: A report suggesting an adverse reaction, which cannot be judged because information is insufficient or contradictory, and which cannot be supplemented or verified

Reported Side Effects of some Homoeopathic Drugs

Aloe socotrina: Oxytocic and abortifacient effects of Vasicine and alkaloid derived from the plant. Adverse effects below 3x.

Andrographis paniculata: Induces sterility in males. Induces abortion.

Berberis vulgaris: Epistaxis, nausea, disruption of sex hormone synthesis. Immune suppressant. Should not be used in pregnancy.

Carduus marianus Insulin resistance. Allergic reaction to skin.

Chelidonium majus: Gastroenteritis, hepatotoxicity.

Chimaphilla umbellata: Reduces mineral absorption from gut on long term use.

Equisetum hymale: Loss of appetite, hypokalemia, loss of muscular control.

Gentiana lutea: Contains heavy metals in extract such as Zinc, Nickel, Chromium, Plumbum and Cadmium.

Grindelia robusta: May cause allergy in sensitive individual. Gastric irritation and diarrhoea. Should not be used during pregnancy.

Hamamelis verginica: Contains Safrole which is carcinogenic.

Holarrhena antidysenterica: Avoid in pregnancy, hypotension, insomnia and vertigo.

Hydrangea arborescens: It may cause allergy in sensitive patients due to Hydrangenol. Large dose may cause toxicity due to cynogenic glycoside.

Hydrastis canadensis: Should not be used in pregnancy. Contraindicated in pregnancy. In large dose causes ulceration. Diminish vitamin B absorption.

Lobelia inflata: Nausea, vomiting, dizziness and loss of uterine tone.

Panax ginseng: The histamine-liberating property would indicate caution for COPD patients.

Passiflora incarnata: Develops severe nausea, vomiting, drowsiness, prolonged QTc, and episodes of non-sustained ventricular tachycardia.

Rauwolfia serpentina: Tranquiliser, bradycardia, salivation, nausea hypogastric secretions, nasal congestion, diarrhoea, inhibition of menstruation, feminisation and impairment of sexual function in male.

Uva ursi: Musculopathy. Hydroquinone can be hepatotoxic

Viscum album: Large doses of Viscum proteins produce anaemia and haemorrhage in the liver and intestinal haemorrhage.

Misleading/Objectionable Advertisement regarding Homoeopathic Drugs

Surveillance on Misleading/Objectionable Advertisement of homoeopathic drugs through pharmacovigilance is an important step. Off and on we use to see advertisements in print and electronic media having false claim on different types of diseases and homoeopathy. Such advertisements exploit the people's belief on homoeopathy. Through this programme we can put a tap over misleading or objectionable advertisements and action can be taken as per provisions of the law. Ministry of AYUSH has been receiving written and online complaints of misleading advertisements of homoeopathic drugs. Such complaints are also registered in the GAMA (Grievances against Misleading Advertisements) portal maintained by the Department of Consumer Affairs (DoCA).

For enforcing Pharmacovigilance of ASU & H drugs multiple laws are available in India. Few important ones are given below:

1. The Drugs and Magic Remedies (Objectionable Advertisements) Act, 1954 and Rules 1955.
2. Drugs and Cosmetics act.1940 and Rules 1945.
3. The Food Safety and Standards Act, 2006.
4. The press council act 1978.
5. Cable Television Network Rules, 1994.
6. Code of Commercial Advertising on Doordarshan and All India Radio.
7. Electronics media monitoring centre (EMMC).
8. Norms of Journalist Conduct issued by the Press Council of India.
9. Code of Conduct of the News Broadcasters Association.
10. Emblems and Names (Prevention of Improper Use) Act, 1950.
11. Consumer Protection Act, 1986. 12. Etc.

Legal Provisions for ASU & H drugs:

1. **Drugs and Cosmetics act. 1940**
   - Section 3(a) & (h) chapter IVA from section 33B to 33O and first schedule pertain to ASU drugs.
   - Second schedule (4A) provides for quality standards of homoeopathic drugs.
2. **Drugs and Cosmetics rules. 1945**
   - Rules 151 to 170, schedules E (I), T, TA pertain to ASU drugs.
   - Rules 30AA, 67, 85(A to I), 106-A, schedule K, schedule M-I pertain to homoeopathy drugs.

The Drugs and Magic Remedies (Objectionable Advertisements) Act, 21 of 1954 and the Rules 1955 "Advertisement":

Section 3 of the Act says that no person shall take any part in the publication of any advertisement promoting a drug or leading to the use of a drug for the procurement of miscarriage in women or prevention of conception in women; the maintenance or improvement of the capacity of human being for sexual pleasure; and correction of menstrual disorders in women.

Section 3 further prohibits any advertisement promoting drugs for the diagnosis, cure, mitigation, treatment or prevention of any disease, disorder or condition specified in the Schedule. The schedule lists a number of diseases, disorders or conditions such as:

Appendicitis
Arteriosclerosis
Blindness
Blood poisoning
Bright's disease
Cancer
Cataract
Deafness
Diabetes
Diseases and disorders of brain
Diseases and disorders of optical system
Diseases and disorders of the uterus
Disorders of menstrual flow
Disorders of the nervous system
Disorders of the prostatic gland
Dropsy
Epilepsy
Female diseases (in general)
Fevers (in general)
Fits
Form and structure of the female breast

Gallstones, kidney & bladder stones

Gangrene

Glaucoma

Goitre

Heart diseases, syphilis, gonorrhoea, soft

High/Low blood pressure

Hydrocele Hysteria

Infantile paralysis

Insanity

Leprosy

Leucoderma

Lockjaw

Locomotor ataxia

Lupus

Nervous debility

Obesity

Paralysis

Plague

Pleurisy

Pneumonia

Rheumatism

Ruptures

Sexual impotence

Smallpox

Stature of persons

Sterility in women

Trachoma

Tuberculosis

Tumours

Typhoid fever

Ulcers of the gastro-intestinal tract

Venereal diseases, including chancre,

Venereal granuloma and lympho granuloma

Section 4 of the Act prohibits those advertisements relating to a drug if they contain any matter which directly or indirectly gives a false impression regarding the true character of the drug or makes a false claim for the drug or is otherwise false or misleading.

Section 5 of the Act prohibits advertisements of magic remedies for treatment of certain diseases and disorders.

Conclusions

Pharmacovigilance is a critical component of healthcare that ensures patient safety by identifying and managing the risks associated with the use of medicines. It is taught in different schools of pharmacy across the world, and students are provided with the knowledge and skills required to monitor and evaluate the safety and efficacy of medicines.

In homoeopathy, pharmacovigilance is equally important as it helps in assessing the safety and efficacy of homoeopathic medicines. Homoeopathic medicines are generally considered safe, but there have been instances where they have caused adverse effects. Therefore, it is essential to monitor and evaluate the safety and efficacy of homoeopathic medicines.

The establishment of Pharmacovigilance Programme of India (PvPI) is a significant step towards ensuring patient safety. It is essential to continue to monitor and evaluate the safety and efficacy of homoeopathic medicines to ensure patient safety.

Chapter 52

Artificial Intelligence (AI) in Homoeopathy

Definition

Artificial intelligence (AI), in its broadest sense, is intelligence exhibited by machines, particularly computer systems, as opposed to the natural intelligence of living beings.

Artificial intelligence is the general name of the technology for the development of machines, which are created entirely by artificial means and can exhibit behaviours and behaviours like human beings, without taking advantage of any living organism.

History of Artificial Intelligence

Artificial Intelligence is not a new word and not a new technology for researchers. This technology is much older than you would imagine. Even there are the myths of Mechanical men in Ancient Greek and Egyptian Myths. Following are some milestones in the history of AI which defines the journey from the AI generation to till date development.

1942: Alan Turing uses his Bombe device to crack the Enigma machine, allowing the Allies to decode German communications during World War II.

1943: The first work which is now recognized as AI was done by Warren McCulloch and Walter pits in 1943. They proposed a model of artificial neurons.

1949: Donald Hebb demonstrated an updating rule for modifying the connection strength between neurons. His rule is now called Hebbian learning.

1950: Alan Turing, an English mathematician proposes the "Turing Test" in his "*Computing Machinery and Intelligence*" to assess a machine's ability to exhibit intelligent behaviour similar to a human.

1955: An Allen Newell and Herbert A. Simon created the "*first artificial intelligence programme*" which was named as "*Logic Theorist*". This programme had proved 38 of 52 Mathematics theorems, and find new and more elegant proofs for some theorems.

1956: The word "*Artificial Intelligence*" first adopted by American Computer scientist John McCarthy at the Dartmouth Conference. For the first time, AI coined as an academic field. At that time high-level computer languages such as FORTRAN, LISP, or COBOL were invented. And the enthusiasm for AI was very high at that time.

1966: The researchers emphasised developing algorithms which can solve mathematical problems. Joseph Weizenbaum created the first chatbot in 1966, which was named as ELIZA.

1972: The first intelligent humanoid robot was built in Japan which was named as WABOT-1.

1978: Herbert Simon earned a Nobel Prize for his limited Rationality Theory, which is an important work on Artificial Intelligence.

1997: IBM Deep Blue beats world chess champion, Gary Kasparov, and became the first computer to beat a world chess champion.

2002: For the first time, AI entered the home in the form of Roomba, an autonomous robotic vacuum, revolutionising home cleaning. It uses sensors to navigate and avoid obstacles.

2006: AI came in the business world till the year 2006. Companies like Facebook, Twitter, and Netflix also started using AI.

2008: Apple introduces voice recognition features on the iPhone, marking the beginning of voice based AI interactions. The company integrates Siri as a virtual assistant a few years later.

2011: IBM's Watson wins on Jeopardy, demonstrating its ability to answer questions in natural language. Watson evolves into a versatile machine learning system.

2012: Google has launched an Android app feature "Google now", which was able to provide information to the user as a prediction.

2014: Amazon introduces Alexa, a virtual assistant that allows users to interact with devices using voice commands.

2017: Amper becomes the first AI music composer, collaborating with human musicians to create music.

2022: OpenAI – an artificial intelligence research company created ChatGPT, and launched the tool in November 2022 for automated conversations. It was founded by a group of entrepreneurs and researchers including Elon Musk and Sm Altman in 2015. OpenAI is backed by several investors, with microsoft being the most notable. ChatGPT uses *natural language processing* and deep learning to generate humanlike text, advancing AI-driven language capabilities.

2023: Gemini, formerly known as Bard, is a generative artificial intelligence chatbot developed by Google. It is Google's 'largest and most capable' AI that can process images, video, text, and even audio.

Now AI has developed to a remarkable level. The concept of Deep Learning, big data, and data science are now trending like a boom. Nowadays companies like Google, Facebook, IBM, and Amazon are working with AI and creating amasing devices. The future of Artificial Intelligence is inspiring and will come with high intelligence.

Role of AI in Homoeopathy

AI can potentially benefit homoeopathy in several ways by providing tools and techniques to enhance data analysis, diagnosis, treatment planning, quality control, patient education and research.

1. **Data analysis**: Homoeopathy relies on collecting and analysing large amounts of patient data to determine the most appropriate remedies for individual cases. AI can assist in analysing this data quickly and efficiently, identifying patterns and correlations that may not be immediately apparent to human practitioners. This can help in discovering new remedies, refining existing ones, and improving overall treatment outcomes.

2. **Diagnosis**: AI algorithms can analyse patient data, including symptoms, medical history, life style and genetic factors, to assist homoeopaths in making accurate diagnosis. This process, which traditionally relies on the practitioner's experience and intuition, can be significantly enhanced with AI's data-driven insights.

3. **Treatment planning**: AI can assist homoeopathic physician by suggesting most appropriate remedies and dosage for individual patients based on their unique characteristics. By analysing a vast database of remedies, historical treatment records, and patient outcomes, AI can identify patterns and trends that can guide the treatment process. This predictive capability can significantly improve the success rate of homoeopathic treatments, reducing trial and error and saving valuable time for both the practitioner and the patient.

4. **Quality control:** Homoeopathic remedies are prepared through a process called potentisation, which involves dilution and succussion. Ensuring the quality and consistency of remedies can be challenging. AI can assist in quality control by analysing manufacturing processes, monitoring parameters such as dilution ratios and succussion duration, and providing feedback to ensure that remedies are prepared accurately and consistently.

5. **Research and development:** AI can accelerate research and development in homoeopathy by automating certain aspects of the process. By analysing vast amounts of data from scientific literatures, clinical trials and experimental cases, AI can help researchers identify new remedies and treatment strategies. This could lead to the discovery of more effective and potent homoeopathic medicines, further expanding the scope and reach of this traditional system of medicine.

6. **Patient education:** AI can also play a crucial role in educating and empowering patients. AI-powered apps and platforms can provide patients with personalised health advice, help them track their symptoms and treatment progress, and even connect them with homoeopathic physician for online consultations. This can make homoeopathic treatment more accessible and convenient, especially for those living in remote areas or with limited access to healthcare services.

Note: While AI can provide valuable support to homoeopathic physicians, the fundamental principles and practice of homoeopathy should still be guided by the expertise and experience of trained professionals. AI should be seen as a tool to enhance and augment their capabilities rather than replace them.

Chapter 53

Abbreviations used in Homoeopathic Pharmacy

AAHP: American Association of Homoeopathic Pharmacists

AHPhA: American Homoeopathic Pharmaceutical Association

AHZ: Allgemeine Homoopathische Zeitung (Journal) – Heidelberg

AAS: Atomic Absorption Spectrophotometer

ADR: Adverse Drug Reaction

AFI: Ayurvedic Formulary of India

AIH: American Institute of Homoeopathy

APC: Ayurvedic Pharmacopoeia Committee

AYUSH: Ayurveda, Yoga & Naturopathy, Unani, Siddha and Homoeopathy

BAHM: British Association of Homoeopathic Manufacturers

BHP: British Homoeopathic Pharmacopoeia

BHS: British Homoeopathic Society

BIH: British Institute of Homoeopathy

BKTA: Bradykinin triacetate

B & T: Boericke and Tafel (Editors)

C: Centesimal potency

CCRAS: Central Council for Research in Ayurveda and Siddha

CCRH: Central Council for Research in Homoeopathy (India)

CCRIM and H: Central Council for Research in Indian Medicine and Homoeopathy

CH: Centesimal Potency prepared according to multiple vial potency (Hahnemannian) method

CIMH: Centre for Indian Medical Heritage

CK: Centesimal Potency prepared according to single vial potency (Korsakovian) method

CM: 100,000C

CRF: Case Report Form

D: Decimal scale as used in Germany, France and other European countries

D: Used at a time to denote the potencies prepared by Carroll Dunham

DL50: Dosalis Letalis, 50%

DMSO: Dimethyl Sulphoxide

DP: Drug Power

DSS: Decision Support System

DTAB: Drugs Technical Advisory Board

ED: Effective Dose

EIS: Executive Information System

ENA: Extra Neutral Alcohol

EP: Experimental Pharmacology

FC: Fluxion Centesimal potencies introduced by Dr Thomas Skinner

FDA: Foods and Drug Administration

FHP: French Homoeopathic Pharmacopoeia

GAP: Good Agricultural Practices

GCP: Good Clinical Practices

GHP: German Homoeopathic Pharmacopoeia

GHP: Good Harvesting Practices

GLC: Gas Liquid chromatography

GLP: Good Laboratory Practices

GMP: Good Manufacturing Practice

GNP: Gross National Product

GPS: Global Positioning System

HAB: Homoeopathiches Arzneibuch

HDP: Herbal Drug Preparations

HEPA filter: High efficiency Particulate Absorbing filter

HP: Homoeopathic Proving

HPC: Homoeopathic Pharmacopoeia Committee

HPUS: Homeopathic Pharmacopoeia of the United States

HPCUS: The Homoeopathic Pharmacopoeia Convention of the United States

HPI: Homoeopathic Pharmacopoeia of India

HPL: Homoeopathic Pharmacopoeia Laboratory

HPLC: High Pressure Liquid Chromatography

HPRS: Homoeopathic Pharmacopoeia of United States/Revision Service

HPTLC: High Performance Thin Layer Chromatography

HPT: Homoeopathic Pathogenetic Trials

HPUS: Homoeopathic Pharmacopoeia of United States

ICH: International Council for Harmonisation of Technical Requirements for Pharmaceuticals for Human Use

IHS: Indian Health Services

IM: Intramuscular

IMRP: Initial Medical Report Proforma

IP: Intraperitoneal

IPD: In-patient department

IPQC: In-process Quality Control

ISM&H: Indian system of Medicine and Homoeopathy

IV: Intravenous

KWC: Knowledge Work System

LD: Lethal Dose.

LM: 1/50 000 dilution

LSC: Liquid-Solid Chromatography

M: 1000C

MHRA: Medicines and Health care production Regulatory Agency

MIS: Management Information System

MM: 1,000,000C

MMM: 1,000,000,000C

NMR: Nuclear Magnetic Resonance

NTP: Normal temperature and Pressure

OAS: Office Automation System

OP: Over Proof

OPD: Outpatient department

OTC: Over the Counter.

PC: Paper Chromatography

PITNDPS: Prevention of Illicit Traffic in Narcotic Drugs and Psychotropic Substances

PSS: Physiological Salt Solutions

Q Potency: Quinquagintamillesimal potency/ 1/50 000 dilution

QSAR: Quantitative Structure Activity Relationships

RCT: Randomised Control Trial

R & D: Research & Development

RMP: Response Monitoring Proforma

Rx: Recipe, to take

SEC: Size Exclusion Chromatography

SEM: Scanning Electron Microscopy

SOPs: Standard Operating Practices

TBGRI: Tropical Botanical Garden and Research Institute

TLC: Thin Layer Chromatography

TPS: Transaction Processing System

TT: Tincture Trituration

UP: Under proof

UPLC: Ultra Performance Liquid Chromatography

USP: United States Pharmacopoeia

WHO: World Health Organisation

WPJ White Petroleum Jelly

X: To denote Decimal scale as used in Britain, Australia & India

XH: Decimal Potency prepared according to multiple vial potency (Hahnemannian) method

XK: Decimal Potency prepared according to single vial potency (Korsakovian) method.

Multiple Choice Questions (MCQ)

Pharmacy and Pharmacopoeia

- The word 'Pharmacopoeia' was originated from:

(a) French, (b) Latin, (c) German, (d) Greek.

Ans. (d)

- 'Pharmacopoeia' may be published by:

(a) Any medical or pharmaceutical society authorised by the Government

(b) The Government in charge of medical and family welfare

(c) Both

(d) Any pharmaceutical laboratory.

Ans. (c)

- First Homoeopathic Pharmacopoeia in the world:

(a) Homoeopathic Pharmacopoeia of India

(b) British Homoeopathic Pharmacopoeia

(c) German Homoeopathic Pharmacopoeia

(d) Homoeopathic Pharmacopoeia of United State.

Ans. (c)

- First Homoeopathic Pharmacopoeia published in:

(a) 1870, (b) 1865, (c) 1830, (d) 1825.

Ans. (d)

- First Homoeopathic Pharmacopoeia published by:

(a) Dr Hahnemann (b) Dr Boenninghausen

(c) Dr Carl W Caspari (d) Dr Kent

Ans. (c)

- First Homoeopathic Pharmacopoeia by Dr Carl W Caspari of Leipzig Germany in 1825:

(a) Homoeopathisches Dispensatorium Fur Aertze and Apotheker

(b) Homoeopathisches Arzneibuch

(c) Pharmacopie Homoeopathiaue Francaise

(d) None of them

Ans. (a)

- British Homoeopathic Pharmacopoeia published in:

(a) 1870, (b) 1845, (c) 1860, (d) 1825

Ans. (a)

- British Homoeopathic Pharmacopoeia published by:

(a) British Institute of Homoeopathy

(b) British Homoeopathic Society

(c) British Government, (d) None of these.

Ans. (b)

- Homoeopathic Pharmacopoeia of United State 1st edition published in:

(a) 1870, (b) 1897, (c) 1860, (d) 1825.

Ans. (b)

- Homoeopathic Pharmacopoeia of India 1st volume published in:

(a) 1825, (b) 1897, (c) 1895, (d) 1971.

Ans. (d)

- Homoeopathic Pharmacopoeia of India 2nd volume published in:

(a) 1971, (b) 1973, (c) 1974, (d) 1976.

Ans. (c)

- No. of monograph in Homoeopathic Pharmacopoeia of India 2nd volume:

(a) 200, (b) 100, (c) 250, (d) 150.

Ans. (b)

- Homoeopathic Pharmacopoeia of India 5th volume published in:

(a) 1986, (b) 1980, (c) 1998, (d) 1985.

Ans. (a)

- No. of monograph in Homoeopathic Pharmacopoeia of India 3rd volume:

(a) 105, (b) 115, (c) 125, (d) 135.

Ans. **(a)**

- Homoeopathic Pharmacopoeia of India 5th volume published in:

(a) 1980, (b) 1984, (c) 1986, (d) 1988.

Ans. **(c)**

- The Eighth Volume of HPI published by Government of India was in the year:

(a) 1998, (b) 2000, (c) 2002, (d) 2004.

Ans. **(b)**

- No. of monograph in Homoeopathic Pharmacopoeia of India 8th volume:

(a) 100, (b) 101, (c) 102, (d) 103.

Ans. **(b)**

- Homoeopathic Pharmacopoeia of India 9th volume published in:

(a) 2000, (b) 2005, (c) 2009, (d) 2007.

Ans. **(d)**

- Homoeopathic Pharmacopoeia of India 10th volume published in:

(a) 2013, (b) 2010, (c) 2015, (d) 2017.

Ans. **(a)**

- First Homoeopathic Pharmacopoeia published in India by:

(a) M Bhattacharya and Co's

(b) India Government

(c) Dr Mahendra Lal Sircar

(d) Rajedra Lal Datta

Ans. **(a)**

- First Homoeopathic Pharmacopoeia in India published by M Bhattacharya and Co's in:

(a) 1890, (b) 1891, (c) 1892, (d) 1895.

Ans. **(c)**

- First Homoeopathic Pharmacopoeia in India published by M Bhattacharya and Co's in 1892 called:

(a) Pharmaceutics Manual

(b) Pharmaceutics Literature

(c) Pharmaceutics Compendium

(d) Pharmaceutics Encyclopedia

Ans. **(a)**

- Encyclopedia of Homoeopathic Pharmacopoeia published in:

(a) 1990, (b) 1997, (c) 1999, (d) 2005.

Ans. **(b)**

- 'Encyclopedia of Homoeopathic Pharmacopoeia' in India edited by:

(a) Dr P N Verma (b) Dr P Sankaran

(c) Dr Jugole Kishore (d) Dr Diwan Harish Chand

Ans. **(a)**

- Chairman of the first "Homoeopathic Pharmacopoeia Committee" in 1962:

(a) Dr Jugole Kishore (b) Dr P Sankaran

(c) Dr B K Sarkar (d) Dr Diwan Harish Chand

Ans. **(c)**

- Who defines pharmacy as 'the art of preparing drugs for use and dispensing them as medicines':

(a) Dr Boenninghausen (b) Dr Willium Boericke

(c) Dr Clarke (d) Dr Farington

Ans. **(b)**

- Official pharmacy means:

(a) Preparation of the drugs according to the physician's prescription

(b) Preparation of the drugs according to the processes prescribed in Official Pharmacopoeias

(c) Preparation of the drugs according to Galenical pharmacy

(d) Preparation of the drugs according to Spagyric therapy

Ans. **(b)**

- Extemporous pharmacy means:

(a) Preparation of the drugs according to the physician's prescription

(b) Preparation of the drugs according to the processes prescribed in Official Pharmacopoeias

(c) Preparation of the drugs according to Galenical pharmacy

(d) Preparation of the drugs according to Spagyric therapy

Ans. (a)

Sources of Homoeopathic Drugs

- Medorrhinum is otherwise known as:

(a) Leuticum (b) Pestinum

(c) Aviaire (d) Glinicum

Ans. (d)

- Lachesis lanceolatus is otherwise known as:

(a) Crot hor (b) Elaps

(c) Toxicophis (d) Bothrops

Ans. (d)

- Theridion curassavicum is otherwise known as:

(a) Gray spider (b) Black widow spider

(c) Orange spider (d) Hairy Cuban spider

Ans. (c)

- Asgarea officinalis is otherwise known as:

(a) Sabadilla (b) Sabina

(c) Samb nigra (d) Sang can

Ans. (a)

- Moccassin snake is otherwise known as:

(a) Toxicophis (b) Bangarus

(c) Cenchris contortrix (d) Clotho arictans

Ans. (d)

- Serum anguillar ichthyotoxin is otherwise known as:

(a) Eel serum (b) Angustra vera

(c) Ichthyolum (d) Toxicophis

Ans. (a)

- Largest source of drug substances in homoeopathy is from:

(a) Animal kingdom (b) Plant Kingdom

(c) Mineral kingdom (d) Synthetic chemicals

Ans. (b)

- Which of these is used to prepare homoeopathic preparations?

(a) Plants (b) All of these

(c) Animals (d) Chemicals

Ans. (b)

- Homoeopathy uses preparations known as Nosodes. What are they?

(a) Disease extracts (b) Plant extracts

(c) Animal extracts (d) Extracts from minerals

Ans. (a)

- First Nosode introduced to Homoeopathy:

(a) Ambra grisea (b) Psorinum

(c) Variolinum (d) Syphilinum

Ans. (a)

- Who discovered the homoeopathic preparation 'Lachesis'?

(a) Dr C Hering (b) Dr J H Clarke

(c) Dr J T Kent (d) Dr Boenninghausen

Ans. (a)

- 'Aviare' is prepared from:

(a) TB of cattle (b) TB of bone tissue

(c) TB of chicken (d) TB of skin

Ans. (c)

- "Koumyss" is prepared from:

(a) Ass's milk (b) Cat's milk

(c) Curd (d) Milk cream

Ans. (a)

- Which among the following is a natural 'Imponderabilia' drug?

(a) Electricitas (b) Radium bromide

(c) Magnetis poli ambo (d) X-ray

Ans. (c)

- The drug which is not derived from Sarcode:

(a) Fel tauri (b) Thyroidinum

(c) Ustilago (d) Pituitrinum

Ans. (c)

- 'Cholesterinum' is a:

(a) Nosode (b) Sarcode

(c) Imponderabilia (d) Synthetic sources

Ans. (b)

- Thyroidinum is prepared from the healthy thyroid tissue of which animal:

(a) Man, (b) Sheep, (c) Pig, (d) Mice.

Ans. (b)

- Hering prepared Lyssin from the saliva of rabid dog by which method:

(a) Trituration of sugar of milk saturated with saliva

(b) Trituration of cane sugar saturated with saliva

(c) By potentisation using 1 drop of saliva and 99 drops of alcohol

(d) By potentisation using 2 drops of saliva and 98 drops of alcohol

Ans. (a)

- Only leaf of the plant is used for preparation of drug in case of:

(a) Aconitum nap (b) Pulsatilla nig

(c) Bryonia alba (d) Digitalis purpurea

Ans. (d)

- The following is not prepared from vegetable source:

(a) Sabina (b) Sabadilla

(c) Sepia (d) Staphysagria

Ans. (c)

- Coccus cacti belong to the class:

(a) Reptilia, (b) Insecta, (c) Asteroidea, (d) Pisces.

Ans. (b)

- Common name of Symphytum:

(a) Parsley (b) Comphrey

(c) Smilax (d) Quebracho

Ans. (b)

- Common name of Petroleum is:

(a) Coal oil

(b) Coal oil; Anthracite

(c) Coal oil; Anthracite; Black lead

(d) Coal oil; Anthracite; Black lead; Wood tar

Ans. (b)

- Common name of Arum triphyllum is:

(a) Indian pennywort (b) Indian turnip

(c) Indian liquorice (d) Indian cockle

Ans. (b)

- Common name of Actaea spicata is:

(a) Barberry (b) Bayberry

(c) Baneberry (d) Bearberry

Ans. (c)

- Common name of Vipera torva is:

(a) German viper (b) Cuban viper

(c) Yellow viper (d) Pit viper

Ans. (a)

- Purple cone-flower and Black Sampson are the common names of:

(a) Melilotus alba (b) Echinacea

(c) Eupat per (d) Cina

Ans. (b)

- "Blazing star" and Unicorn plant are the common names of:

(a) Hamam, (b) Hell, (c) Helonias, (d) Hyos.

Ans. (c)

- 'Lesser periwinkle' is the common name of:

(a) Ustilago (b) Xantho

(c) Uva ursi (d) Vinca minor

Ans. (d)

- 'Spanish fly' is the common name of:

(a) Causticum (b) Cantharis

(c) Terebinth (d) Tarantula cub

Ans. (b)

- Mephites is the poisonous secretion of the anal gland of which animal:

(a) Toad, (b) Wild lizard, (c) Wild cat, (d) Wild deer

Ans. (c)

- Glonoine is the drug prepared from

(a) Glycerine trichloride (b) Nitroglycerin

(c) Triglycerides (d) Benzene

Ans. (b)

- Chemical formula of Camphor is:

(a) $C_{10}H_{14}O$ (b) $C_{10}H_{16}O$
(c) $C_{10}H_{10}N_4O$ (d) $C_3H_5N_3O_9$

Ans. (b)

- The natural order of Podophyllum peltatum is

(a) Berberidaceae (b) Liliaceae
(c) Umbelliferae (d) Ranunculaceae

Ans. (a)

- Habitat of Acalypha indica is

(a) England, (b) America, (c) Germany, (d) India.

Ans. (d)

- Drugs which are prepared from the morbid product are called:

(a) Drugs, (b) Medicines, (c) Sarcodes, (d) Nosodes

Ans. (d)

- Medicine prepared from Indian bed bug:

(a) Cimex acanthia (b) Doryphora decemlineata
(c) Pulex irritans (d) Vespa crabro

Ans. (a)

- Medicine prepared from Cow's milk is:

(a) Lac felinum (b) Lac vaccinum
(c) Lac defloratum (d) Lac vaccinifloc

Ans. (b)

- Name the medicine prepared from Papal cross spider:

(a) Aranea diadema (b) Latrodectus hasselti
(c) Latrodectus katipo (d) Mygale lasiodora

Ans. (a)

- Tuberculinum was proved by:

(a) Heath (b) Fincke
(c) Fincke & Swan (d) Heath & Fincke

Ans. (c)

- Dr Hahnemann proved Ambra grisea in the year:

(a) 1827, (b) 1828, (c) 1832, (d) 1833.

Ans. (a)

- Brimstone is the common name of:

(a) Sulphur, (b) Silicea, (c) Alumina, (d) Calc ars.

Ans. (a)

- Plumbago is the common name of:

(a) Graphites (b) Plumb met
(c) Glonoine (d) Gun powder

Ans. (a)

- "Sal ammoniac" is the common name of:

(a) Amm carb (b) Amm mur
(c) Amm causticum (d) Ammon phos

Ans. (a)

- Complementary medicine of "Animal charcoal" is:

(a) Carbo veg, (b) Drosera, (c) Calc phos, (d) Phos.

Ans. (c)

- Chemical formula of Mag carb is:

(a) $MgCO_3$ (b) $MgCO_3.H_2O$
(c) $MgCO_3.2H_2O$ (d) $MgCO_3.3H_2O$

Ans. (d)

- Chemical formula of Hepar sulph is:

(a) Ca_2S, (b) $CaS.2H_2O$, (c) CaS_2, (d) CaS.

Ans. (d)

- Which among the following is prepared from mineral spring water?

(a) Sanic (b) Sanic; Wiesbaden
(c) Sanic; Wiesbaden; Skukum chuck
(d) Sanic; Wiesbaden; Skukum chuck; Selen

Ans. (c)

- Which among the following is a medicine prepared from Organic acid?

(a) Phos acid (b) Hydrocyanic acid
(c) Oxalic acid (d) All of the above

Ans. (c)

- Kreosotum is a:

(a) Inorganic compound (b) Organic compound
(c) Metal (d) Non metal

Ans. (b)

- What is the property common to the medicines Rheum and Rumex?

(a) Complimentary medicines
(b) Inimical medicines

(c) Proved by Hahnemann

(d) Both belong to the same family

Ans. (d)

- Choose the common names of medicines, Taraxacum, Senega and Ratanhia:

(a) Wild yam, Virgin's bower, Celandine

(b) Saw bread, Golden seal, Spurge olive

(c) Parsley, Lung wort, Mug wort

(d) Dandelion, Snake wort, Mapato

Ans. (d)

- American white hellebore is:

(a) Verat alb (b) Verat vir

(c) Hell (d) None of the above

Ans. (b)

- Kalmia, Ledum pal and Rhododendron belongs to the family:

(a) Ericaceae (b) Euphorbiaceae

(c) Labiatae (d) Melanthaceae

Ans. (a)

- Nux moschata belongs to the family:

(a) Melanthaceae (b) Myristicaceae

(c) Loganiaceae (d) Leguminosae

Ans. (b)

- Which of the following medicine does not belong to the Ranunculaceae family?

(a) Clematis erecta (b) Adonis vernalis

(c) Physostigma (d) Hydrastis can

Ans. (c)

- Name the medicines belonging to the family Lichens:

(a) Secale cor (b) Ustilago

(c) Lycopodium (d) Sticta

Ans. (d)

- Mercurialis perennis belongs to:

(a) Mineral kingdom (b) Euphorbiaceae

(c) Rubiaceae (d) Lichens

Ans. (b)

- Name one medicine belonging to Algae family:

(a) Ustilago (b) Sticta

(c) Usnea barbata (d) Fucus vesiculosis

Ans. (d)

- Ginseng belongs to the family:

(a) Araliaceae (b) Aristolochiaceae

(c) Araceae (d) Apocyanaceae

Ans. (a)

- Coca belongs to the family:

(a) Graminae (b) Linaenae

(c) Smilaceae (d) Thymelaceae

Ans. (b)

- Name the medicine coming under Polygalaceae:

(a) Rheum (b) Rumex

(c) Senega (d) All of the above

Ans. (c)

- What is not a Sarcode:

(a) Thyroidinum (b) Fel tauri

(c) Pituitrin (d) Ustilago

Ans. (d)

Collection of drug Substances

- Which plants are more effective and possess more medicinal virtue?

(a) Plants cultivated in botanical gardens

(b) Plants cultivated in home

(c) Wild plants (d) All

Ans. (c)

- Barks of resinous trees are collected during:

(a) Early Summer (b) Early Winter

(c) Early Autumn (d) Early Spring

Ans. (d)

- Resins are collected in which season:

(a) Early Summer (b) Early Winter

(c) Early in autumn (d) Time of development of leaves and blossoms

Ans. (d)

Vehicles

- Sugar of milk is chemically:

(a) Sucrose, (b) Maltose, (c) Lactose, (d) Fructose.

Ans. (c)

- Placebo is:

(a) Medicated substance (b) Unmedicated substance

(c) Poisonous substance (d) None of these

Ans. (b)

- Placebo may be prescribed in the form of:

(a) Phytum, (b) Rubrum, (c) Lactopen,

(d) Nihilinum, (e) All of these

Ans. (e)

- 'Placebo is the second best remedy without which no good homoeopathist could not practice medicine'-stated by:

(a) Hahnemann (b) H A Roberts

(c) Stuart Close (d) Carroll Dunham

Ans. (c)

- Placebo is discussed in 6th edition of Organon in the aphorism:

(a) 270, (b) 272, (c) 280, (d) 281.

Ans. (d)

- Placebo has been pointed out as something of an unmedicinal nature by Hahnemann in 5th edition of Organon:

(a) 91, (b) 140, (c) 260.

Ans. (a)

- Administration of something of an unmedicinal character is mentioned in Sec.:

(a) 91, (b) FN 96, (c) 90, (d) 91 and FN to 96.

Ans. (d)

- The percentage of alcohol in Proof Spirit is:

(a) 95%, (b) 88%, (c) 66%, (d) 57.1%.

Ans. (d)

- Stapf's process is done to detect purity of:

(a) Purified water (b) Alcohol

(c) Lactose (d) Olive oil

Ans. (a)

- Quantity of absolute alcohol required for Stapf's process?

(a) 450 ml (b) 1 litre

(c) 2 litre (d) 500 ml

Ans. (c)

- Ethyl alcohol is:

(a) Monohydric (b) Dihydric

(c) Trihydric (d) Tetrahydric

Ans. (a)

- The sizes of globule vary from:

(a) 5 to 80 (b) 8 to 80

(c) 8 to 90 (d) 10 to 80

Ans. (d)

- Which of the following is false?

(a) Sp. Gr. of Olive oil is 0.813-0.890

(b) Sp. Gr. of Glycerine is 1.255-1.266

(c) Sp. Gr. of Dilute alcohol is 0.913-0.916

(d) Sp. Gr. of Absolute alcohol is -0.7935

Ans (a)

- Specific Gravity of Olive oil at 20°C is:

(a) 0.813-0.890 (b) 1.255-1.266

(c) 0.913-0.916 (d) 0.910-0.913

Ans (d)

- Mention the vehicle by which you can prepare liniment:

(a) Purified water (b) Alcohol

(c) Glycerin (d) Olive oil

Ans. (d)

- Tablets are prepared from:

(a) Sugar of milk (b) Glucose

(c) Fructose (d) Sucrose

Ans. (a)

Different Scales of Preparation of Drugs

- Dr. Hearing introduced:

(a) Decimal scale (b) Centesimal scale

(c) 50-Millesimal scale (d) None of the above

Ans. (a)

- Decimal scale was introduced by:

(a) Dr. C. Hering (b) Hahnemann
(c) Hartlaub (d) None

Ans. **(a)**

- Ratio of drug substance and vehicle in Decimal Scale:

(a) 1:9, (b) 1:99, (c) 1:999, (d) 1:4999.

Ans. **(a)**

- Ratio of drug substance and vehicle in Centesimal Scale:

(a) 1:9, (b) 1:99, (c) 1:999, (d) 1:4999.

Ans. **(b)**

- Ratio of drug substance and vehicle in 50-Millesimal Scale:

(a) 1:9, (b) 1:99, (c) 1:999, (d) 1:4999.

Ans. **(d)**

- The term 'New dynamisation method' mentioned by Hahnemann in Organon of Medicine in:

(a) Sec. 136 (b) Sec. 138
(c) FN 1 to Sec. 132 (d) Sec. 161

Ans. **(c)**

- The term 'Renewed dynamisation' mentioned by Hahnemann in Organon of Medicine in:

(a) Sec. 136 (b) Sec. 138
(c) FN 1 to Sec. 132 (d) Sec. 161

Ans. **(d)**

- An article 'My experience about Hahnemann's 50-Millesimal scale potency' was written by:

(a) Hahnemann (b) Charles Pahud
(c) William Boericke (d) Pierre Schmidt

Ans. **(b)**

- For 1st 50-Millesimal scale potency ……….. potency of Trituration is needed:

(a) 8X, (b) 4X, (c) 3C, (d) 4C.

Ans. **(c)**

- The drug strength of 1st '50-Millesimal potency' is

(a) $\frac{1}{5} \times \frac{1}{10^8}$, (b) $\frac{1}{50} \times \frac{1}{10^8}$, (c) $\frac{1}{5} \times \frac{1}{10^{10}}$, (d) $\frac{1}{50} \times \frac{1}{10^{10}}$.

Ans. **(c)**

- Hahnemann has recommended potencies in Sec. 270, 6th edition:

(a) $\frac{0}{1}$ to $\frac{0}{30}$ only (b) $\frac{0}{1}$ to $\frac{0}{20}$ only
(c) $\frac{0}{1}$ to $\frac{0}{40}$ only (d) $\frac{0}{1}$ to $\frac{0}{60}$ only

Ans. **(a)**

- The treatment in '50-Millesimal scale' must be started with potency from the:

(a) Higher degrees of dynamisation
(b) Mild degrees of dynamisation
(c) Lowest degrees of dynamisation
(d) Moderate degrees of dynamisation

Ans. **(c)**

- Q-potency is the term used to designate:

(a) Centesimal potency (b) 50-Millesimal potency
(c) Decimal potency (d) None of these

Ans. **(b)**

- The flame '50-Millesimal scale' was given by:

(a) Hahnemann (b) Pierre Schmidt
(c) Kent (d) Hering

Ans. **(b)**

- Who gave the name 50-Millesimal to the New dynamisation method?

(a) Horace (b) Gellert (c) Boenninghausen
(d) Pierre schmidt (e) William Boericke.

Ans. **(d)**

- 50-Millesimal scale is described in which edition of Organon of Medicine?

(a) 4th edition (b) 5th edition
(c) 6th edition (d) None of these

Ans. **(c)**

- 50-Millesimal scale of preparation is mentioned in aphorism in 6th edition

(a) 270, (b) 268, (c) 269, (d) 253.

Ans. **(a)**

- In case of 50-Millesimal potency, the method of repetition of doses in chronic diseases:

(a) Once a day or once every alternate day
(b) Once every 2, 3, 4 or 6 hours

(c) Every hour or oftener

Ans. (a)

- In 50-Millesimal scale the crude substance is reduced to what level by trituration:

(a) 5c (b) 10c (c) 6c (d) 3c

Ans. (c)

- The drug strength of the mother tincture in 50-Millesimal scale is:

(a) $\frac{1}{6}\times\frac{1}{10^6}$, (b) $\frac{1}{5}\times\frac{1}{10^8}$, (c) $\frac{1}{8}\times\frac{1}{10^8}$, (d) None of these.

Ans. (b)

Methods of Preparing Homoeopathic Drugs (Old Method)

- Dr. Hahnemann has given idea about the preparation of medicine in Sec.:

(a) 22 - 27 (b) 264 - 271
(c) 146 - 161 (d) None of these

Ans. (b)

- Drug power of mother tincture in class I:

(a) $\frac{1}{2}$, (b) $\frac{1}{6}$, (c) $\frac{1}{10}$, (d) $\frac{1}{100}$.

Ans. (a)

- Drug power of mother tincture in class II:

(a) $\frac{1}{2}$, (b) $\frac{1}{6}$, (c) $\frac{1}{10}$, (d) $\frac{1}{100}$.

Ans. (a)

- Drug power of mother tincture in class III:

(a) $\frac{1}{2}$, (b) $\frac{1}{6}$, (c) $\frac{1}{10}$, (d) $\frac{1}{100}$.

Ans. (b)

- Drug power of mother tincture in class IV:

(a) $\frac{1}{2}$, (b) $\frac{1}{6}$, (c) $\frac{1}{10}$, (d) $\frac{1}{100}$.

Ans. (c)

- Drug power of mother tincture in class V(A):

(a) $\frac{1}{2}$, (b) $\frac{1}{6}$, (c) $\frac{1}{10}$, (d) $\frac{1}{100}$.

Ans. (c)

- Drug power of mother tincture in class V(B):

(a) $\frac{1}{2}$, (b) $\frac{1}{6}$, (c) $\frac{1}{10}$, (d) $\frac{1}{100}$.

Ans. (d)

- Drug power of mother tincture in class VI(A):

(a) $\frac{1}{2}$, (b) $\frac{1}{6}$, (c) $\frac{1}{10}$, (d) $\frac{1}{100}$.

Ans. (c)

- Drug power of mother tincture in class VI(B):

(a) $\frac{1}{2}$, (b) $\frac{1}{6}$, (c) $\frac{1}{10}$, (d) $\frac{1}{100}$.

Ans. (d)

- Drug power of mother tincture in class VII:

(a) $\frac{1}{2}$, (b) $\frac{1}{6}$, (c) $\frac{1}{10}$, (d) $\frac{1}{100}$.

Ans. (c)

- Ratio of drug substance and alcohol for preparation of mother tincture in Class I:

(a) 1:2 (b) 3:2 (c) 3:4 (d) 1:1

Ans. (d)

- Ratio of drug substance and alcohol for preparation of mother tincture in Class II:

(a) 1:2 (b) 3:2 (c) 3:4 (d) 1:1

Ans. (b)

- Ratio of drug substance and alcohol for preparation of mother tincture in Class III:

(a) 1:2 (b) 3:2 (c) 3:4 (d) 1:1

Ans. (a)

- Ratio of drug substance and alcohol for preparation of mother tincture in Class IV:

(a) 1:2 (b) 3:2 (c) 1:5 (d) 1:1

Ans. (c)

- Ratio of drug substance and purified water for preparation of mother solution in Class V(A):

(a) 1:3 (b) 3:2 (c) 1:5 (d) 1:9

Ans. (d)

- Ratio of drug substance and purified water for preparation of mother solution in Class V(B):

(a) 1:9 (b) 1:99 (c) 1:5 (d) 1:1

Ans. (b)

- Ratio of drug substance and alcohol for preparation of mother solution in Class VI(A):

(a) 1:5 (b) 3:2 (c) 1:9 (d) 1:99

Ans. (c)

- Ratio of drug substance and alcohol for preparation of mother solution in Class VI(B):

(a) 1:5 (b) 3:2 (c) 1:9 (d) 1:99

Ans. (c)

- Mother tincture prepared from most juicy plants under:

(a) Class I, (b) Class II, (c) Class III, (d) Class IV.

Ans. **(a)**

- Mother tincture prepared from medium juicy plants under:

(a) Class I, (b) Class II, (c) Class III, (d) Class IV.

Ans. **(b)**

- Mother tincture prepared from least juicy plants under:

(a) Class I, (b) Class II, (c) Class III, (d) Class IV.

Ans. **(c)**

- Mother tincture prepared from dried vegetables and animal substance under:

(a) Class I, (b) Class II, (c) Class III, (d) Class IV.

Ans. **(d)**

- Mother solution prepared in aqueous solution under:

(a) Class V(A) & V(B) (b) Class VI(A) & VI(B)
(c) Class VII (d) Class VIII

Ans. (a)

- Mother solution prepared in alcoholic solution under:

(a) Class V(A) & V(B) (b) Class VI(A) & VI(B)
(c) Class VII (d) Class VIII

Ans. **(b)**

- Trituration from dry, insoluble medicinal substances done under:

(a) Class VII (b) Class VIII (c) Class IX

Ans. **(a)**

- Trituration from liquid, insoluble medicinal substances done under:

(a) Class VII (b) Class VIII (c) Class IX

Ans. **(b)**

- Trituration from fresh vegetable and animal substances done under:

(a) Class VII (b) Class VIII (c) Class IX

Ans. **(c)**

- Drug prepared under Class I:

(a) Acon nap (b) Euphresia
(c) Nux vomica (d) Acid phos

Ans. **(a)**

- Drug prepared under Class II:

(a) Symphytum (b) Euphresia
(c) Thuja occ (d) All of them

Ans. **(d)**

- Drug prepared under Class III:

(a) Symph (b) Arn mont
(c) Thuja occ (d) Acid nitric

Ans. **(b)**

- Drug prepared under Class IV:

(a) Nux vom (b) Viscum album
(c) Mez (d) Phos

Ans. **(a)**

- Drug prepared under Class V(A):

(a) Bryo alba (b) Acid phos
(c) Lyco (d) Dulc

Ans. **(b)**

- Drug prepared under Class V(B):

(a) Bryo alba (b) Caust
(c) Lyco (d) Dulc

Ans. **(b)**

- Drug prepared under Class VI(A):

(a) Glon (b) Aloe soc
(c) Berb vulg (d) Digit

Ans. **(a)**

- Drug prepared under Class VI(B):

(a) Bell, (b) Ign, (c) Colch, (d) Ars alb.

Ans. **(d)**

- Drug prepared under Class VII:

(a) Bell, (b) Ign, (c) Colch, (d) Opium.

Ans. **(d)**

- Drug prepared under Class VIII:

(a) Acid fluoric, (b) Lach, (c) Podo, (d) Anac or

Ans. **(b)**

- Drug prepared under Class IX:

(a) Ammon carb (b) Caust

(c) Medo (d) Hydrast can

Ans. (c)

- A Mother tincture is:

(a) An alcoholic solution (b) Alcoholic extract

(c) Dilution of the drug (d) Aqua alcoholic extract

Ans. (b)

- An example for drug prepared from Class VI (A) of old method of mother tincture preparation:

(a) Guaiacum (b) Iodum

(c) Graphitis (d) Anacardium

Ans. (a)

- Thuja occ is prepared according to old method under class:

(a) Class I, (b) Class II, (c) Class III, (d) Class IV.

Ans. (c)

- Anacardium orientale is prepared according to old method under class:

(a) Class IV (b) Class IX

(c) Class VII (d) Both Class IV and IX

Ans. (d)

- Pulsatilla is prepared according to old method under class:

(a) Class I, (b) Class II, (c) Class III, (d) Class IV.

Ans. (c)

- Lachesis is prepared according to old method under class:

(a) Class IV (b) Class VII

(c) Class VIII (d) Class IX

Ans. (c)

- Snake venom can be preserved in deep-freeze being kept in:

(a) Glycerine (b) Vaseline

(c) Rosemary oil (d) Sesame oil

Ans. (a)

- Type of drug prepared under Class IX of Old method is:

(a) Fresh vegetables and animals, (b) Insoluble solids, (c) Insoluble liquids, (d) Minerals.

Ans. (a)

- Hepar sulph is prepared by mixing Calcium carbonate and Sulphur in the ratio:

(a) 1:3 (b) 1:2 (c) 2:1 (d) 1:1

Ans. (d)

Methods of Preparing Homoeopathic Drugs (New Method)

- Maceration of mucilaginous substance is done for:

(a) 7 to 14 days (b) 3 to 6 days

(c) 15 to 30 days (d) 2 to 4 days

Ans. (c)

- The following is not a process included under old method:

(a) Extraction (b) Maceration

(c) Trituration (d) Solution

Ans. (b)

- Drug power of Moschus by new method of preparation is:

(a) $\frac{1}{10}$, (b) $\frac{1}{2}$, (c) $\frac{1}{5}$, (d) $\frac{1}{20}$.

Ans. (d)

- Drug power of medicine in new method of preparation is:

(a) $\frac{1}{10}$, (b) $\frac{1}{20}$, (c) $\frac{1}{30}$, (d) $\frac{1}{100}$.

Ans. (a

- Gummy substances prepared by method of:

(a) Percolation (b) Solution

(c) Polarimeter (d) Maceration

Ans. (d

Potentisation

- In homoeopathy, a process which brings about a quantitative reduction in the drug substance but qualitative increase in its medicinal or therapeutic property is known:

(a) Ionisation (b) Potentisation

(c) Succussion (d) Dilution

Ans. (b)

- Potentisation helps:

(a) To explore the dynamic curative properties of the drug.
(b) To minimise the drug effects of material doses.
(c) To explore the uncommon peculiarities characteristic of the natural substances or drugs during proving.
(d) All of them

Ans. (d)

- How many process of Potentisation?

(a) Two, (b) Three, (c) Four, (d) Five.

Ans. (a)

- How many scales are uses for Succussion?

(a) Two, (b) Three, (c) Four, (d) Five.

Ans. (b)

- How many scales are uses for Trituration?

(a) Two, (b) Three, (c) Four, (d) Five.

Ans. (a)

- Where Hahnemann described the process of preparing medicine by Trituration?

(a) Materia Medica Pura
(b) Chronic Diseases Vol.-I
(c) Chronic Diseases Vol.-II
(d) Medicine of Experience

Ans. (b)

- How long you will have to triturate to get one potency?

(a) 10 minutes (b) 20 minutes
(c) 60 minutes (d) 90 minutes

Ans. (c)

- Succussion is a method of Potentisation of:

(a) Soluble drug substances
(b) Solid drug substances
(c) Insoluble drug substances
(d) All of the above

Ans. (a)

- The process by which the latent curative properties of drugs are brought into activity is called as:

(a) Dynamisation (b) Potentisation
(c) None of above (d) Both

Ans. (d)

- The drugs which are insoluble in alcohol or water become soluble by the process of:

(a) Succussion (b) Trituration
(c) Both (d) None of above

Ans. (b)

- The insoluble substances are triturated first to:

(a) 1x potency (b) 3x potency
(c) 7x potency (d) 4x potency

Ans. (b)

- The new method of dynamisation of drugs is known as:

(a) Potentisation (b) Medicamentanum positives
(c) Medicamentanum an globuli (d) None of these

Ans. (c)

- In homoeopathy, a process which brings about a quantitative reduction in the drug substance but a qualitative increase in its medicinal or therapeutic property is known as:

(a) Potentisation (b) Succussion
(c) Ionisation (d) Dilution

Ans. (a)

- Fluxion potency is a peculiar process when medicines prepared by trituration are converted into potency by succussion. What are the levels at which it is carried out?

(a) 30 to 200 (b) 2X to 4C
(c) 6X to 8X (d) 12X to 14X

Ans. (c)

- Dynamisation theory was introduced in which edition of Organon:

(a) 1st edition (b) 2nd edition (c) 3rd edition
(d) 4th edition (e) 5th edition

Ans. (e)

- The process in which the dynamic curative powers of the crude drug substance are activated by means of friction:

(a) Vehicle (b) Dilution
(c) Potentisation (d) Solution

Ans. (c)

- The dynamic power of a medicine to influence the vitality of a living organism in conditions of health and disease:

(a) Potency (b) Dilution
(c) Potentisation (d) Solution

Ans. (a)

- The potency of homoeopathic medicines derived by displacement is known as:

(a) Decimal potency (b) Centesimal potency
(c) 50-Millesimal potency (d) Fluxion potency

Ans. (d)

- Regarding the number of strokes in succussion process A.H.P. and G.H.P. still advocates:

(a) 2 strokes (b) 6 strokes
(c) 10 strokes (d) 8 strokes

Ans. (c)

- From which triturated potency the drug is converted to liquid potency:

(a) 4x (b) 6x (c) 8x (d) 12x

Ans. (b)

- Which of the following is a high potency preparation used in homoeopathy?

(a) 6c (b) 6M (c) 6x (d) 30c

Ans. (b)

- Fluxion potency is a peculiar process when medicines prepared by Trituration are converted into potency by succussion. What are the levels at which it is carried out:

(a) 30 to 200 (b) 2x to 4c
(c) 6x to 8x (d) 12x to 14x

Ans. (c)

External Application

- What is the route of administration of external application?

(a) Rubbing (b) Local application
(c) Both (d) None of these

Ans. (c)

- In external application, the method which does not contain any medicament:

(a) Fomentation (b) Plasters
(c) Both (d) None of above

Ans. (a)

- In which aphorism of 'Organon of Medicine' sixth edition mentioned about external application:

(a) 170-180, (b) 144-152, (c) 281-284, (d) 284-285

Ans. (d)

- For preparing 'Ointment' 1 part of required mother tincture is mixed with 9 parts of:

(a) Purified water (b) White petroleum jelly
(c) Olive oil (d) Glycerine

Ans. (b)

- Ointment prepared by mixing mother tincture and white petroleum jelly in the ratio of:

(a) 1:9 (b) 1:4 (c) 1:10 (d) 1:5

Ans. (a)

- For preparing 'Liniment' 1 part of required mother tincture is mixed with 9 parts of:

(a) Purified water (b) White petroleum jelly
(c) Olive oil (d) Glycerine

Ans. (c)

- For preparing 'Glycerole' 1 part of required mother tincture is mixed with 9 parts of:

(a) Purified water (b) White petroleum jelly
(c) Olive oil (d) Glycerine

Ans. (c)

- For preparing 'Lotion' 1 part of required mother tincture is mixed with 9 parts of:

(a) Purified water (b) White petroleum jelly
(c) Olive oil (d) Glycerine

Ans. (a)

- To make uniform colour of external application (Lotions) which is mixed with?

(a) Mother tincture with purified water
(b) Mother tincture with alcohol
(c) Mother tincture with olive oil

(d) Mother tincture with glycerine

Ans. (a)

Various constituents in plant substances

- The alkaloid of Belladonna:

(a) Quinine (b) Colchicine
(c) Brucine (d) Atropine

Ans. (d)

- The alkaloid of Acon nap:

(a) Aconitine (b) Ergotine
(c) Hydrastine (d) Piperine

Ans. (a)

- The alkaloid of Cinchona officinalis:

(a) Quinine (b) Emitine
(c) Cocaine (d) Atropine

Ans. (a)

- The alkaloid of Ipecacuanha:

(a) Nicotine (b) Emitine
(c) Cocaine (d) Ipecine

Ans. (b)

- The alkaloid of Nux vomica:

(a) Caffeine (b) Quinine
(c) Strychnine (d) Morphine

Ans. (c)

- Morphine is the alkaloid of:

(a) Nux vomica (b) Tabacum
(c) Opium (d) Cannabis indica

Ans. (c)

- Which of the following is the glycoside present in Cinchona?

(a) Quinidine (b) Isoquinoline
(c) Cinchonine (d) Quinovin

Ans. (d)

Drug Proving

- The quality of an ideal prover:

(a) Sick, (b) Emotional, (c) Idle, (d) Trustworthy.

Ans. (d)

- Qualities of prover are described in Sec.:

(a) 72 (b) 80 (c) 126 (d) 288

Ans. (c)

- Aphorism which deals with best prover:

(a) 144 (b) 145 (c) 141 (d) 148

Ans. (c)

- The word used by Dr. Trinks in his Annals to describe the proving of person:

(a) Hg (b) Lg (c) Ng (d) Gn (e) Bg

Ans. (c)

- In proving medicines are given to healthy persons in:

(a) Large doses (b) Moderate doses
(c) Minute doses (d) Single minute doses

Ans. (c)

- Proving of narcotic medicines are mentioned in Sec.:

(a) 108 (b) 113 (c) 119 (d) 128

Ans. (b)

- Medicine for proving should be given in simple unadulterated form-this statement is given in Sec.:

(a) 123 (b) 118 (c) 115 (d) 116

Ans. (a)

- Which among the following is not required for apprehending the picture of disease?

(a) Freedom from prejudice (b) Sound senses
(c) Attention in observing and fidelity in tracing the picture of the disease
(d) Rational explanation

Ans. (d)

- Medicine to be proved has to be taken:

(a) At night (b) Empty stomach
(c) Each dose after taking food
(d) Morning and night

Ans. (b)

- During proving of the narcotics we observe the:

(a) Primary action (b) Secondary action

(c) Alternating action (d) All of these

Ans. (b)

- Drug proving on healthy a person's was thought of for the first time by:

(a) Hippocrates (b) Paracelsus
(c) Hahnemann (d) Albrecht Von Haller

Ans. (d)

- Best prover:

(a) Medical students (b) Physician
(c) Oversensitive patient (d) Childern

Ans. (b)

- In which of the below that nothing can be accurately observed during proving?

(a) When large doses taken
(b) When moderate doses taken
(c) When small doses taken
(d) When minute doses taken

Ans. (a)

- The subject on whom a drug is proved is called:

(a) Prover (b) Ideal prover
(c) Best prover (d) All of them

Ans. (a)

- Ideal prover should be:

(a) Healthy and intelligent
(b) Delicate, sensitive and irritable
(c) Trustworthy and lover of truth
(d) All of the above

Ans. (d)

- For what we cannot prove the drug on animal?

(a) Subjective and mental symptoms cannot be studied.
(b) Animal cannot give the finer and finest modalities
(c) The effect of the same drug is different from those of human beings
(d) All of the above

Ans. (d)

- The medicine must be tested on:

(a) Male (b) Female
(c) Male and Female (d) Animal

Ans. (c)

- Alternating actions which are produced by some medicines should be:

(a) No need to note down (b) Noted
(c) No hard and fast rule (d) None of these

Ans. (b)

- The recording of drug will be more accurate and complete if the prover is:

(a) Literate (b) Illiterate
(c) Physician himself (d) All of them

Ans. (c)

- Medicine to be proven must be:

(a) Perfectly well known
(b) Purity must be assured
(c) Genuineness must be assured
(d) All of above

Ans. (d)

- Diet during proving should be purely:

(a) Nutritious (b) Green vegetables
(c) Salads (d) Wine brandy coffee

Ans. (a)

- During the drug proving the mental condition of prover should be

(a) Avoid the over-exertion of mind and body
(b) No urgent business
(c) Devote himself to careful self observation
(d) All of the above

Ans. (d)

- What will happen if we prove the medicine in sick person?

(a) The symptoms of disease and the symptoms of the proven medicine mixed together
(b) If the medicine to be proved similar to the case the patient may cure
(c) Both (d) None of these

Ans. (c)

- Why potentised medicine should be employed in proving?

(a) Crude medicinal substance do not exhibit their full medicinal power
(b) By potentisation the latest curative power of drugs are developed
(c) Potentisation brings medicines to act on dynamic plane
(d) All of the above

Ans. **(d)**

- The proving must be done on:

(a) Animals (b) Human being (c) Both
(d) None of the above (e) Physician

Ans. **(b)**

- During the time of proving the prover should avoid taking:

(a) Medicinal things (b) Nutritious diet
(c) Stimulants like coffee, wine (d) Specious diet

Ans. **(a), (c), (d)**

- We must prove the drug in:

(a) Dilutions (b) Massive doses
(c) Both (d) None of the above

Ans. **(c)**

- The medicine must be tested on both male and female in order also to reveal the alterations of the health they produce in the sexual sphere in Sec.:

(a) 122 (b) 124 (c) 127 (d) 132

Ans. **(c)**

- Proving of drugs on healthy individuals is not easy as (Homoeopathy, the science of Therapeutics by C. Dunaham):

(a) The doses by which the corresponding varieties of symptoms are produced, differ widely in different drugs
(b) The susceptibility of different provers to the same drug is different
(c) The susceptibility of provers to different preparations of the same drug is very various and apparently capricious.
(d) All of the above

Ans. **(d)**

- Albrecht Von Haller says about human proving in:

(a) British Homoeopathic journal
(b) Pharmacopoeia Helvetica
(c) Friend of Health (d) None of these

Ans. **(b)**

Posology and Homoeopathic Posology

- 'The study of doses' is called the:

(a) Potency (b) Potentisation
(c) Posology (d) Pharmacology

Ans. **(c)**

- Posology is related with:

(a) Potency (b) Dose (c) Both (d) None

Ans. **(c)**

- In which aphorism Dr. Hahnemann has given idea about the homoeopathic posology?

(a) 105-145, (b) 146-154, (c) 245-258, (d) 262-263

Ans. **(c)**

- To employ the proper dose a physician has to see the:

(a) Susceptibility of the patient
(b) Seat, nature and intensity of the disease
(c) Stage, duration of disease
(d) All of the above

Ans. **(d)**

- Homoeopathic dose includes:

(a) Potency (b) Quantity (c) Form
(d) Number of administration (e) All of them

Ans. **(e)**

- Too large dose of homoeopathic medicine is:

(a) Injurious (b) Beneficial
(c) Ineffective (d) None of these

Ans. **(a)**

- 'The dose is appropriate which will be proportionate to the degree of susceptibility of the patient'-stated by:

(a) Hahnemann (b) Stuart Close
(c) Fincke (d) H A Roberts

Ans. (b)

- "Poison is everything and nothing is without poison, the dose makes it a poison or a remedy" declared by:

(a) Hahnemann (b) Asclepiades (c) Paracelsus
(d) Rademacher and Hahnemann both

Ans. (c)

- Logic and advantages of diluting, plussing and dividing the dose:

(a) Greatly stimulates the vital force and smoothly overpowers the artificial disease
(b) To avoid unwanted aggravations in very sensitive patients
(c) For best result succussion and plussed dose
(d) Unchanged and unmodified dose produces an aggravation
(e) All of them

Ans. (e)

- Monopharmacy means:

(a) Application of only single, simple medicine to a patient at a time
(b) Application of two medicines at a time
(c) Application of multiple medicines at a time
(d) None of these

Ans. (a)

- Polypharmacy means:

(a) Application of only single, simple medicine to a patient at a time
(b) Application of many medicines or the mixture of many medicines to a patient at a time
(c) Application of two medicines at a time
(d) None of these

Ans. (b)

- 'The same potency is not repeated on more than two occasions'-commented by:

(a) Hahnemann (b) Stuart Close
(c) J T Kent (d) H A Roberts

Ans. (c)

- Selection of potency depends upon:

(a) Susceptibility (b) Patient
(c) Nature of remedy (d) All of them

Ans. (d)

- Acute diseases with lowered vitality:

(a) Requires higher potency
(b) Requires medium potency
(c) Requires low potency and in repeated doses
(d) None of these

Ans. (c)

- Diseases in dynamic pathology require:

(a) Higher potency (b) Medium potency
(c) Lower potency (d) None of these

Ans. (a)

- Diseases in organic pathology require:

(a) Higher potency (b) Medium potency
(c) Lower potency (d) None of these

Ans. (c)

- Minimum dose means:

(a) Selection of similar potency to that of natural disease
(b) The potency which can cure a natural disease
(c) The potency which can kill a patient
(d) The dose which enough to excited the vital force.

Ans. (d)

- The most suitable degree of minuteness for sure and gentle effect can be found out by:

(a) Experience and experiment
(b) Experiment and research
(c) Pure experimentation, careful observation of sensitiveness of the patient and accurate experience
(d) Proper case taking and miasmatic diagnosis

Ans. (c)

- Homoeopathicity is:

(a) Pathology of disease (b) Potentisation
(c) Relationship between drug and patient

(d) Individualisation

Ans. (c)

- 'The decisive amount is always a minimum, an infinitesimal' is stated by:

(a) Fincke (b) Maupertuis

(c) Hahnemann (d) Hippocrates

Ans. (a)

- Homoeopathic medicines are used in:

(a) Physiological doses (b) Toxic doses

(c) Material doses (d) Dynamic doses

Ans. (d)

- Peripheral symptoms appear as a result of comparatively:

(a) Smaller doses (b) Large doses

(c) Minute doses (d) None of above

Ans. (a)

- 'Arsenic album' in a smaller dose develops:

(a) Specific dynamic symptoms

(b) Generic dynamic symptoms

(c) Both (d) None of above

Ans. (b)

- Selection of potency depends upon the:

(a) Susceptibility of the patient

(b) Nature of the disease

(c) Nature of the medicine (d) All of them

Ans. (d)

- If the susceptibility of a patient is more what potency should be given?

(a) High (b) Low

(c) Moderate (d) Mother tincture

Ans. (a)

- Sensitive persons of nervous, sanguine and choleric temperament needs:

(a) Higher potency (b) Lower potency

(c) Moderate potency (d) Mother tincture

Ans. (a)

- Acute diseases respond well to:

(a) Higher potencies (b) Lower potencies

(c) Moderate potencies (d) Mother tincture

Ans. (a)

- In case of mental diseases needs:

(a) Higher potencies (b) Lower potencies

(c) Moderate potencies (d) Mother tincture

Ans. (a)

- Where the gross pathological changes taken place, very much effective in:

(a) Higher potencies (b) Lower potencies

(c) Moderate potencies (d) Mother tincture

Ans. (b)

- Disease characterised by diminished vital reaction requires:

(a) Higher potency (b) Lower potency

(c) Moderate potency (d) Mother tincture

Ans. (b)

- Oversensitive persons require

(a) Higher potencies (b) Lower potency

(c) Moderate potency (d) Either of the above

Ans. (c)

- In case of extreme idiosyncrasy, preferred potency is:

(a) Lower (b) Medium

(c) Higher (d) No specificity

Ans. (b)

- More the susceptibility, potency will be:

(a) Higher (b) Lower

(c) Either of two (d) No change

Ans. (a)

- Higher potencies are adapted to:

(a) Sanguine temperament (b) Robust persons

(c) Both (d) None of above

Ans. (a)

- Lower potencies are adapted to:

(a) Nervous temperament

(b) Phlegmatic individuals

(c) Both (d) None of above

Ans. (b)

- Susceptibility and potency are:

(a) Directly proportional to each other
(b) Inversely proportional to each other
(c) Not related (d) None of the above

Ans. (a)

- Criteria for selection of potency are:

(a) Seat of disease (b) Duration of action of drug
(c) Sensations (d) Totality

Ans. (a)

- Law of Simplex means:

(a) Similar medicine (b) Single medicine
(c) Simple medicine (d) Single medicine in simple form

Ans. (b)

- It is wrong to attempt complex means when simple means suffice. This statement is given in Sec.:

(a) 274 (b) 273 (c) 68 (d) 234

Ans. (a)

- If polypharmacy is continued for a prolonged period it may produce:

(a) Chronic disease (b) Complex disease
(c) Contagious disease (d) Drug disease

Ans. (d)

- Repetition of doses are called as:

(a) Pharmaconomy (b) Pharmacology
(c) Pharmacopollaxy

Ans. (c)

- According to aphorism 247 'Organon of Medicine', in acute diseases medicine can be repeated at:

(a) Every 24, 8, 6 hourly
(b) Every 24, 12, 8, 4 hourly
(c) Every 24, 8, 6, 4 hourly
(d) Every 24, 12, 8 hourly

Ans. (b)

- The frequency of repetition of medicines in acute diseases depends on the:

(a) Nature of disease (b) Intensity of disease
(c) Duration of disease (d) Course of disease

Ans. (b)

Prescription Writing

- The word prescription was originated from:

(a) French (b) Latin (c) German (d) Greek

Ans. (b)

- The prescription consists of:

(a) Two parts (b) Three parts
(c) Four parts (d) Five parts

Ans. (c)

- The 'Superscription' part of prescription includes:

(a) Name of the patient (b) Age and sex
(c) Address (d) All of them

Ans. (d)

- The 'Inscription' part of prescription includes:

(a) Name of the remedy, its potency, its quantity
(b) Name of the vehicle
(c) Quantity of vehicle (d) All of them

Ans. (d)

- The 'Subscription' part of prescription includes:

(a) Directions to the pharmacist how he is to dispense the remedy
(b) Name of the vehicle
(c) Quantity of vehicle (d) All of them

Ans. (a)

- The 'Signature' part of prescription includes:

(a) Directions to the patient
(b) Signature of the physician
(c) Registration no and date (d) All of them

Ans. (d)

- Most important part of the prescription:

(a) Superscription (b) Inscription
(c) Subscription (d) Signature

Ans. (b)

- Rx stands for the........ word 'Recipe':

(a) Greek (b) Latin (c) German (d) None

Ans. (b)

- Q L or Quantum libet means:

(a) As much as required
(b) As much as you please
(c) As much as one can repeat (d) None of these

Ans. (a)

- 'P.C' is the abbreviated word in prescription writing for

(a) Placebo (b) As prescribed
(c) After food (d) Before food

Ans. (c)

Drug Administration

- The subject dealing with the routes of administration of medicines is termed as:

(a) Pharmacopallaxy (b) Pharmacology
(c) Pharmacognosy (d) Pharmaconomy

Ans. (d)

- Route of administration of medicine is mentioned in 5th edition of Organon under:

(a) § 264-265 (b) § 272-274
(c) § 288-292 (d) None of them

Ans. (c)

- Route of administration of medicine is mentioned in 6th edition of Organon under:

(a) § 264-265 (b) § 272-274
(c) § 284-285 (d) None of them

Ans. (c)

- What is the route of administration of external application?

(a) Rubbing (b) Local application
(c) Both (d) None of these

Ans. (c)

- The ideal route of administration of homoeopathic medicine is:

(a) Mouth (b) Skin (c) Injection (d) Inhalation

Ans. (a)

- Pharmaconomy stands for:

(a) Identification of drug
(b) Route of administration of drug
(c) Deals with different aspect of drugs
(d) Role of drug in the body

Ans. (b)

Drug – Medicine – Remedy

- Genuine medicine denotes:

(a) Adulterated (b) Unadulterated
(c) None of these

Ans. (b)

- Mercury's vegetable analogue is:

(a) Podo (b) Mez (c) Sil (d) Phyto

Ans. (a)

- Acute complementary medicine of Calc phos is:

(a) Psor (b) Bacil (c) Syphil (d) Medo

Ans. (b)

- Chronic complementary medicine of Bryonia is:

(a) Rhus tox (b) Calc carb (c) Medo (d) Nat mur

Ans. (d)

- Acute complementary medicine of Sepia is:

(a) Nux vom (b) Sulph (c) Puls (d) Lach

Ans. (a)

- One among the following is an inimical medicine of Allium cepa:

(a) Allium sat (b) Aloe soc (c) Squilla (d) Sars

Ans. (d)

- Complementary medicine of Camphor:

(a) Kali nit (b) Canth (c) Coffea
(d) All of the above

Ans. (b)

- Complementary medicine of Carbo animalis:

(a) Calc carb (b) Kali carb
(c) Mag carb (d) Calc phos

Ans. (d)

- Name the medicine, which is not an inimical to Sepia:

(a) Bryo alba (b) Lach (c) Puls (d) Sabad

Ans. (d)

- This medicine is complementary to Carbo veg in stitches in the heart:

(a) Kali carb (b) Drosera

(c) Phos (d) All of the above

Ans. (a)

- All are complementary except:

(a) Ignatia – Nat. mur (b) Merc. – Sil

(c) Bell – Calc. (d) Apis mel – Nat. mur

Ans. (b)

General knowledge of Legislastion in relation to Homoeopathic Pharmacy

- Chapter III of the Central Council of Homeopathy Act deals with:

(a) Recognition of medical qualifications

(b) Central register (c) Miscellaneous

(d) Number of seats allocated in Central Council in each state.

Ans. (a)

Model Questions

Pharmacy and Pharmacopoeia

1. Define Pharmacopoeia and discuss various Homoeopathic Pharmacopoeias. Discuss the necessity of Pharmacopoeia.
2. What is Pharmacopoeia? Write down different Pharmacopoeia in detail.
3. Short questions: (a) First Homoeopathic Pharmacopoeia of USA was published in which year and by whom? (b) When was first edition of AHP published and by whom? (c) BHP was published in which year and by whom? (d) How many volumes of Homoeopathic Pharmacopoeia of India (HPI)? Which is the year of publication of first vol. of HPI and give number of monographs?
4. What is Pharmacy? What are the different branches of Homoeopathic Pharmacy? Write down the sources of Homoeopathic Pharmacy in detail. Name the two specialties of Homoeopathic Pharmacy.
5. Write the history and development of Homoeopathic pharmacy. Write down the difference between Pharmacy and Pharmacopoeia.
6. Give two branches of Pharmacy proper. What is Pharmacomania and Pharmacophobia?
7. Write the scope of homoeopathic pharmacy in relation to National Economy. Discuss the relation of homoeopathic pharmacy with Materia Medica.
8. Who is a pharmacist? Write any three essential qualities of an ideal pharmacist.

Sources of Homoeopathic Drugs

1. What do you understand by the drugs? What are the different sources from which drugs are collected? Illustrate your sources with a few examples. How the following specimens are collected and preserved for preparing homoeopathic medicines: (a) Substances (b) Whole plants.
2. What are the sources of homoeopathic drugs. Discuss in detail about the sources of drugs from vegetable and animal kingdom with two examples. What is imponderabilia?
3. From what sources we get the following drugs and state which of them are polychrest remedies of our Materia Medica? Sulphur, Sepia, Bryonia, Lycopodium, Phosphorus, Glonoine, Dulcamara, Psorinum, Thyroidinum.
4. Write an essay about the sources of homoeopathic drugs with two examples.
5. Short questions: (a) Name the two medicines prepared from bulb of fruit. (b) Name the two medicines prepared from diseased products of plants. (c) Name the two medicines prepared from diseased product of animal. (d) Name the medicines prepared from energy of full moon and sun rays. (e) Name two examples of medicines prepared from dried root. (f) Name two medicines prepared from flowers. (g) Name two medicines prepared from secretion of glands.
6. Write short Notes on: (a) Nosodes, (b) Imponderabilia, (c) Sarcodes, (d) Tautopathic drugs.

Collection of drug Substances

1. Write briefly about the collection of plants for the preparation of drugs.
2. What are the general and specific rules for collecting of vegetable drug substances?
3. What are the general and specific rules for collecting of animal drug substances?

4. Short questions: (a) Flowers are collected in which weather and when? (b) Leaves are collected in which season and when? (c) When the roots of annuals and biennials are collected? (d) Whole plants are collected in which season and when?
5. Discuss the method of collection of Nosodes and Sarcodes for preparing medicines.
6. How to procure and preserve herbs from which mother tinctures are prepared?

Homoeopathic Pharmaceutical Instruments and Appliances

1. Mention ten pharmaceutical instruments or appliances, their uses and cleansing methods. What are the uses of mortar and pestle in a homoeopathic laboratory? What all types of containers are used for the preservation of mother tinctures and dilutions?
2. What are the types of spatula? What are the uses of funnel and chopping board?
3. Short questions: (a) What is the types and uses of hydrometer? What are the uses of thermometer and Water bath?
4. What are the uses of spatula? What all materials are used for the – manufacture of spatula? Draw and level different parts of water bath when in operation. Write a brief note on water bath.
5. Draw and level different parts of Percolator in operation.

Cleansing of Utensils

1. How will you cleanse the utensils, corks and phials for a homoeopathic pharmacy? And what kind of phials should be used for homoeopathic medicines? What is contamination?
2. How to clean wooden instruments? How to clean knife?

General Laboratory and Laboratory Methods

1. What is Chromatography? Mention three basic types of Chromatography.
2. How can you differentiate the process of decantation from that of filtration? Why the former process is necessary before the latter?
3. Write short notes on: (a) Distillation. (b) Sedimentation. (c) Crystallisation.
4. How to determine the moisture content of a drug?

Brief Study of Standardisation of Drugs

1. Define standardisation. Write down different methods of drug standardisation for vegetable and animal kingdom. What are the parameters to standardise mother tinctures, mother solutions and attenuations in brief.
2. What are the standards of finished preparations?

Vehicles

1. How sugar of milk is prepared for Homoeopathic purposes and what are Homoeopathic globules made of?
2. Name the different vehicles used in homoeopathic pharmacy. Describe about the preparation, properties and uses of sugar of milk.
3. How can you prepare dilute alcohol and for what purpose it is generally used?
4. What are the impurities generally found in alcohol and how to remove them? What do you understand by drug-strength and strength by volume of spirit?
5. What is vehicle? Classify them. How can you prepare Purified water on small scale? What are the common impurities present in Purified water with the tests to detect them?
6. Define vehicle. Classify the vehicles used in homoeopathy. Write in detail about Sugar of Milk. Name of the process for the purification of Sugar to Milk.
7. What are the common characters of an ideal vehicle? Describe the process of preparation of ethanol from molasses. What are the common impurities present in alcohol and how to detect them?

8. Which raw material is used for the preparation of globules? How will you prepare globules? Write about the medication of globules. How will you determine the size of globules? What are the uses of globules?
9. How can you prepare ethyl alcohol from starchy materials? Mention three disadvantage of ethyl alcohol as a vehicle.
10. Name the liquid vehicles. Write in detail about Glycerine. Describe the uses of Glycerine in homoeopathic pharmacy.
11. Write four examples for semi-solid vehicles. Write two synonyms of Vaseline. What are the common vehicles used for preparing ointments. Write waxes in detail.
12. Write any three important features of cones.
13. Write briefly: (a) Stapf's process (b) 60° O P ethanol (c) Proof spirit (d) Metrology.
14. Write short notes on: (a) Preparation of Sugar of Milk (b) Globules (c) Purified water (d) Rectified spirit.
15. How globules are medicated and why in some cases the globules do not stand medication?
16. What is the chemical formula of Glycerine and give its molecular wt.? Name two varieties of petroleum jelly.
17. Short questions: (a) Name the two solid vehicles. (b) Name two types of alcohol. (c) Give the chemical formula and molecular wt. of Sugar of Milk.
18. What is Placebo? Is Placebo and Sac lac are same? In what circumstances placebo is being prescribed? 'Placebo is the second best remedy'– give your opinion.
19. What is Biochemic tablet? How it is prepared? Describe its mode of administration in acute and chronic diseases. 'Biochemic powder (trituration) are more powerful in action than tablets' – if so, why? if not, why not?
20. Write short notes on: (a) Placebo (b) Sac lac (c) Liquid vehicles (d) Dispensing alcohol.
21. Is it possible to convert Rectified Spirit into Absolute alcohol? If so, describe the methods of its preparation in short.

Different Scales of Preparation of Drugs

1. What is meant Decimal and Centesimal scales? What is the relation between Decimal and Centesimal potencies? What are the usual designations of the two scales of attenuations?
2. Who coined the term 50-Millesimal scale? What is the principle of 50-Millesimal scale?
3. Discuss the merits of 50-Millesimal scale of potency over Centesimal scale. Describe the preparation of 0/2 in LM scale from one liquid drug substance.
4. Who introduced 50-Millesimal scale and in which edition of Organon of Medicine?
5. Mention the scale generally used in Biochemic System. Name its inventor. How tissue salts are triturated under the scale?
6. What are the ratio and symbol of Decimal and Centesimal scale? What is the ratio and symbol of 50-Millesimal scale?
7. What important scale of Potentisation has been discarded by the new official Homoeopathic Pharmacopoeia? How is the 1st potency represented according to this Pharmacopoeia?
8. Write the inventor and the principle of Centesimal scale of preparation of drugs.

Methods of Preparing Homoeopathic Drugs (Old Method)

1. Write down the old method of preparation of mother tincture in detail.
2. Write down the difference between old method and new method of preparation of drugs.
3. What is mother tincture and what is meant by the drug power of a mother tincture? Are Allopathic and Homoeopathic tinctures the same? If not, how do they differ? Give the drug strength of the followings: Aresenicum album, Nux vomica, Phosphorus.
4. Short questions: (a) What is the ratio and drug power of Class I and II? (b) What is the ratio of drug power of Class II A? (c) What is the ratio and drug power of 6A and 6B?

5. Describe the preparation of mother tincture according to Class I and Class II with examples.

Methods of Preparing Homoeopathic Drugs (New Method)

1. Discuss in detail about the modern method of preparation of mother tinctures from vegetable sources. Indicate their superiority of the mother tinctures produced by older methods. What are the two methods of preparation of mother tincture according to new method?
2. Define Maceration, what are the substances taken for Maceration? Write the conditions and process of Maceration. What are the difference between Maceration and Percolation?
3. Write short notes on: (a) Maceration, (b) Filtration, (c) Percolation, (d) Magma.
4. Write the modern methods of preparation of mother tincture. Define Percolation and explain in detail.

Potentisation

1. Write down the origin and evolution of the theory of dynamisation. What are the different scales of trituration and succussion? What is the process of potentisation?
2. What is potentisation? What is the process of potentisation with scales? Describe the process of preparation of 1st LM potency.
3. How knowledge of potency is utilised in the selection of remedy? What is natural potentisation?
4. Define drug dynamisation. What are the different methods of potentisation? Write them in detail. In succussion how many scales are used?
5. What is fluxion potency? What is the starting point of jumping and fluxion potency? How do you differentiate between potency and dilution?
6. What is trituration? What are the requirements necessary for trituration? Why do we triturate drugs? How are triturations converted in fluid potencies?
7. What is drug strength? Justify why Homoeopathic medicines are potencies and not dilutions.
8. Mention what type of remedies would you expect other than in liquid state at least up to the 6x potency and why? Give examples.

External Application

1. Explain why Hahnemann was against the external application of medicine.
2. What are the disadvantages of external application? Name the two vehicles used as base for external application.
3. State the method of preparation of three external applications with examples.
4. What are opodeldocs. Write its preparation and its uses. Define olfaction.
5. Discuss the different external applications, their scope and limitation in Homoeopathic system.
6. What is the scope of external application in homoeopathy? Describe the uses of any four external applications and their method of application. Name the various oils used in the preparation of external applications. Write about olive oil.
7. Write short notes on: (a) Ointment (b) Poultices (c) Lotion (d) Bath.
8. Discuss Hahnemann's views regarding external applications.
9. Write short notes on: (a) Fomentations (b) Cerates (c) Poultices.

Preservation of Drugs and Potentised Medicines

1. Describe the general rules to be taken in preservation of drugs and potentised medicines.
2. What precaution is to be observed in keeping Homoeopathic medicines?
3. How will you preserve the drug substances?
4. Short questions:
   (a) How to preserve Carbo vegetable and Camphor?

(b) How to preserve Nitric acid and Picric acid?

(c) For storing Fluoric acid, which bottles are used and which coloured bottles are not used?

5. Mention the names of the substances for which glass-stoppered bottles are used.

Pharmacology

1. Define Pharmacology. What are the two branches of Pharmacology?
2. Write short notes on: (a) Pharmacopoeia (b) Pharmacodynamics (c) Posology (d) Pharmacognosy.

Drug action

1. Define drug action. Discuss general principles of drug action. What is Physiological action?
2. Classify drugs according to drug action.

Various Constituents in Plant Substances

1. Mention various constituents in plant substances with one example for each.
2. What is an alkaloid? Name few alkaloids.
3. Write short notes on: (a) Synonym (b) Common name (c) Glycoside (d) Alkaloids.
4. Write the alkaloids of Nux vomica.
5. Define the active principles (Resinoids) with examples. What are tannins?

The Technique of Drug Proving

1. Discuss the history and evolution of Homoeopathic drug proving.
2. Define drug proving. Write down the main instructions of drug proving as given by Hahnemann.
3. Mention the essential qualities of ideal prover. Who is best prover and why? What precautionary measure is to be taken by the prover during drug proving? Why drugs are not proved on lower groups of animals?
4. What is drug proving? Whom do you select for provers? What special advantage one may have when a physician prove drugs on himself?
5. Mention the criteria's for selection of a substance for proving. How can we know the disease curing power of drugs? Which substance can be taken for proving? Write with reasons why the dose and repetitions of a drug is necessary during its proving. Can a drug be proved on disease persons? Justify your statement.
6. What are the objectives of drug proving? Whom you will select as an ideal prover? Give your reasons. Under what circumstances sequential appearance of symptoms can be observed in proving? Write the advantages and disadvantages of proving on animals. Symptoms of which action of drugs are recorded in proving?
7. Site the merits of drug proving on healthy human being. Write the merits when the first dose is sufficient enough to produce the symptoms on the prover. Write the Hahnemannian instruction regarding the diet and regimen during drug proving.
8. Describe the technique Homoeopathic drug proving.
9. Answer in a few lines: (i) Clinical proving (ii) Idisyncratic prover, (iii) Day book (iv) Diet of a prover, (v) Best prover.
10. Discuss the methods of preparation and doses of drug substances for proving. What precautions to be taken during drug proving?

Posology and Homoeopathic posology

1. What do you mean by posology? Mention the factors responsible for the selection of dose. Describe Hahnemannian posology with reference.
2. Write as essay on selection of potency.
3. State briefly the different factors to be considered during the selection of potency.
4. "The greater the susceptibility, higher the potency"-Explain.

5. State how the knowledge of susceptiblilty helps for potency selection.
6. How 'selection of potency' depends upon the 'susceptibility of the patient?
7. What are the relations between dose and susceptibility?
8. Why is the minimum dose in homoeopathy? Discuss favourable conditions for the action of homoeopathic dose. What are the disadvantages of large doses in homoeopathy?
9. "Only one, single, simple medicine should be given to the patient at one time"- Elucidate.
10. What is monopharmacy? Describe it with the remarks of Hahnemann in favour of it in Organon of Medicine.
11. What are the reasons for applying only single, simple medicinal substance at a time? What are the disadvantages of polypharmacy?
12. Write an essay on Homoeopathic Posology – Types of potency and its selection, Types of doses.
13. Define Monopharmacy and give reasons for following it in Homoeopathy.

Prescription Writing

1. Define Prescription. What are the parts of a prescription? Describe the importance of a prescription. What are the norms and forms of an ideal prescription?
2. Write in detail about the different parts of an ideal prescription. What are the criteria to be followed, so as to make an ideal prescription? What are the advantages of writing prescription?
3. Describe the importance of the legal part of a prescription. Write an ideal prescription for a girl aged 12 years suffering from headache and describe different parts of that prescription.
4. Describe in detail the process of prescription of sugar of milk. What is the importance of signature?
5. Justify why prescription writing is compulsory of a physician. Write a prescription for a lady who is suffering from leucorrhoea. What are the merits and demerits of writing prescription?
6. What is prescription? As a medical man, how will you write a prescription for a boy who is suffering from acute tonsillitis?
7. What are the contents of inscription? Name the two parts of prescription writing. Write a model prescription and explain its parts. What are the contents of signature (parts of prescription writing)?
8. How will you write out a prescription giving complete instruction to the pharmacist as also to the patient?
9. Write about prescription, components, mode of writing and validity.

Drug Administration

1. Discuss briefly the different routes for administration of homoeopathic drugs.
2. What are the principles of drug administration?

Drug – Medicine – Remedy

1. What do you understand by the drugs? What are the different types of drugs? What is genuine medicine? What is the difference between Drug and Medicine?
2. What is remedy? Give examples. What is polychrest remedy? Give examples. What is Similimum?
3. What is Relationship of Remedies? Discuss in details the Complementary and Antidotal relations with examples.

Scope of Homoeopathic Pharmacy in relation to Materia Medica, National Economy and Organon of Medicine

1. How the knowledge of Pharmacy helps to increase the knowledge of Materia Medica?
2. Write the scope Homoeopathic Pharmacy in relation to Materia Medica Organon of Medicine and National Economy.

3. Write an essay about scope of Homoeopathic Pharmacy in relation to Materia Medica.

General Knowledge of Legislastion in Relation to Homoeopathic Pharmacy

1. Write an essay about the legislation in relation with homoeopathic pharmacy.
2. What are the conditions for grant of homoeopathic manufacturing license?
3. Write down the character, moral and responsibilities of homoeopathic practitioner to their patient.
4. Write short notes on: (a) Dangerous Drugs Act (b) Drugs and cosmetic Act (c) Pharmacy Act (d) Labelling and Packing of homoeopathic medicines.

Glossary

Adverse Event: Any untoward medical occurrence that may present during treatment with a pharmaceutical product, but which does not necessarily have a causal relationship with this treatment.

Adverse Drug Reaction (ADR): A response which is noxious and unintended, and which occurs at doses normally used in humans for the prophylaxis, diagnosis, or therapy of disease, or for the modification of physiological function (WHO, 1972). An adverse drug reaction, contrary to an adverse event, is characterised by the suspicion of a causal relationship between the drug and the occurrence, i.e. judged as being at least possibly related to treatment by the reporting or a reviewing health professional.

In homoeopathic drug-provings a conventional ADR will not occur, because there are no toxicologic effects of the proving substances, since they usually are administered in high dilutions.

Adverse Proving Symptom: An adverse Proving Symptom is defined as a symptom, which is likely to be caused by the administration of the proving substance and adversely affects the well being of a volunteer, disturbs the normal daily routine and may require the withdrawal of the volunteer from the homoeopathic drug-proving. It will be recorded on the Adverse Event Form, attached to the Case Report Form (CRF) of each volunteer. Therefore be any unfavourable and unattended sign, symptom, or disease temporally associated with the administration of a proving substance, whether or not related to it.

Aldehyde: It is a class of organic compound formed by the oxidation of the primary alcohols e.g., Acetyldehyde etc.

Allersode: It is the term used to describe homoeopathic dilutions of antigens, i.e. substances that, under suitable conditions, can induce the formation of antibodies. Antigens include toxins, ferments, precipitinogens, agglutinogens, opsonogens, lysogens, venins, agglutinins, complements, opsonins, amboceptors precipitins and most native proteins.

American Association of Homoeopathic Pharmacists (AAHP): A nonprofit organisation established in 1923 that represents the interests of homoeopathic drug manufacturers, distributors, and and individual pharmacists. In December 2001, the AAHP Web site stated that, AAHP had "24 corporate and 16 individual members representing over 70% of the homoeopathic community."

Anhydrous: It is defined as a substance that is completely free from water is known as anhydrous.

Arndt-Schulz Law: An obsolete law stating that weak stimuli excite physiologic activity, moderately strong ones favor it, strong ones retard it, and very strong ones arrest it. Also called Amdt's Law, it was proposed by Rudolph Arndt (1835-1900), a German psychiatrist.

Atom: The smallest particle of an element which can enter into a chemical combination. It is composed of subatomic particles (protons, neutrons, electrons) whose number and arrangement characterise the element.

Avogadro's Hypothesis: Under the same conditions of pressure and temperature equal volumes of all gases contain equal number of molecules.

Avogadro's Number. The number of molecules in a gram molecular weight of a substance, approximately 6.023×10^{23}. (A mole is the number of grams of a substance equal to its molecular weight).

Back Potency: Two to three potencies prior to the frequently used potencies are called back potency. Examples: For 30CH potency, the back potencies would be 29CH, 28CH or 27CH potency.

Basophil: A type of leucocytes that remain coated with IgE (Immunoglobulin E), a protein antibody.

Bioassay: Estimation of the potency of an active principle in a unit quantity of preparation or defect and using biological methods is known as 'Biological assay or Bioassay'

Blister Pack: It is a term for several types of pre-formed plastic packaging used for small consumer goods. Blister packs are commonly used as unit-dose packaging for pharmaceutical tablets, capsules or lozenges. Blister packs can provide barrier protection for shelf life requirements, and a degree of tamper resistance. Blister packs are the new age method of dispensing Homoeopathic Medicines, in which medicated globules are dispensed.

Capillary Analysis: Is a simple method of standardisation given elaborately in the German Homoeopathic Pharmacopoeia, used to estimate the approximate alcohol content and other constituents in crude drugs, tinctures and even very low potencies.

Chemical Symbol: An abbreviation for the complete/full name of an element or compound/any other chemical substance is known as chemical symbol.

Classical Homoeopathy: Use of a single remedy prescribed according to the individual's presentation and history.

Clinical Pharmacology: It is that branch of science that deals with the evaluation of the drug in clinical setting is known as clinical pharmacology.

Clinical Trial: A systematic study on pharmaceutical products in human subjects (including patients and other volunteers) in order to discover or verify the effects of and/or identify any adverse reaction to investigational products, and/or to study the absorption, distribution, metabolism and excretion of the products with the objective of ascertaining their efficacy and safety.

Combination Remedy: A mixture containing more than one Homoeopathic Medicine.

Complex Homoeopathy: More than one remedy used concurrently.

Compound: A substance whose molecules consists of unlike atoms and whose constituents cannot be separated by physical means.

Concordant Remedies: The drugs whose actions are similar, but are of dissimilar origin to another are said to be concordant and they follow each other well.

Examples of concordant remedies are China and Calcarea, Pulsatilla and Sepia, Nitric acid and Thuja, Belladonna and Mercurius, Ignatia and Zinc.

Condense: It means to make or become dense.

Condensation: A process that is used for making or being dense something is known as condensation.

Control Group: The comparison group in drug-trials not being given the studied drug.

Day Book: It is a book given to the prover to write symptoms, when they are fresh in their memory, in chronological order.

Diskets: Diskets are tablets made up of cane sugar. Its porosity is less than that of tablets. Nowadays diskets available in varying sizes are used as vehicles to dispense the homoeopathic medicines.

Dosage Form: The pharmaceutical form in which a product is presented for therapeutic administration, e.g. tablet, cream.

Double-Blind Placebo Clinical Trials: Refers to experiments in which neither the experimenter nor the subjects know whether a specific treatment was prescribed or a placebo (a "fake" medicine that looks and tastes like a Homoeopathic Medicine).

Dyscrasia: An abnormal or physiologically unbalanced state of the body

Electromagnetic Field: An electric or magnetic field or a combination of the two, as in an electromagnetic wave.

Electromagnetic Wave: A travelling disturbance in space produced by the acceleration of an electric charge, comprising an electric field and a magnetic field at right angles to each other, both moving at the same velocity in a direction normal to the plane of the two fields.

Elutriation: Mixing of rough insoluble substances like chalk etc. in water so that, the finer light powdery portion of the substances may be poured off after the coarser particles have settled in the bottom. It is done sometimes merely to wash away such impurities as gravel etc.

Energy Medicine: The theme of energy permeates many areas of health care, from acupuncture to homoeopathy, as well as many systems of bodywork and movement therapy, and increasingly mainstream medicine (MRI scans for example).

Excipient; Any component of a finished dosage form other than an active ingredient.

Gene: A discrete unit (that is each small part) of DNA bound to a protein and arranged linearly in the thread-like structure known as chromosome.

Gene Therapy: To replace the defective genes by healthy ones.

Generic Medicine: A medicine that, in comparison to a registered medicine: (a) has the same quantitative composition of therapeutically active substances, being substances of similar quality to those used in the registered medicine; and (b) has the same pharmaceutical form; and (c) is bioequivalent; and (d) has the same safety and efficacy properties.

Healthy Volunteer: The volunteer has to be healthy in the sense of being free from important physical or psychic symptoms and does not consider himself to need medical treatment. The investigator too —after having taken the case history and done clinical examination—does not see an indication for medical treatment.

High Potency Remedies: Remedies of a 100°C potency or higher.

Homotoxicology: A system developed by German homoeopath Hans Heinrich Reckeweg, who claimed that symptoms are the result of the body's attempt to use "homotoxons" to detoxify the body. Reckeweg developed many homoeopathic mixtures said to enhance "homotoxon" production. He also claimed that his remedies activate a "greater defence system" that can neutralise and excrete homotoxins.

Hormesis: The concept, based on the (obsolete) Arndt-Schulz Law—that concentrations of potentially toxic substances below the amount that cause inhibition (toxicity) will cause stimulation. (It is well-known that substances can have different effects at different concentrations, but they do not follow the general pattern proposed by homoeopathy advocates.)

Ideal Prover: The physician himself is the ideal prover.

Investigational Product: A proving substance (drug), prepared according to a Homoeopathic Pharmacopoeia or a placebo/blank administered or used as a reference in HDP.

Isodes: Sometimes called detoxodes, are homoeopathic dilutions of botanical, zoological or chemical substances, including drugs and excipients, that have been ingested or otherwise absorbed by the body and are believed to have produced a disease or disorder.

Magma: The thick residue of the soft doughy mass (molten mass) resulting from the expression of the floid part of certain substances (pounded fresh plant).

Master Prover (or Project Director): The Master Prover is the chief person responsible for the entire proving project from start to end.

Menstrum: It is a liquid which is capable of penetrating the tissues of plant or animal substances and capable to dissolve the active principles.

Merc: It is the inert, fibrous and insoluble material remaining after expression of the juice from drug material or after maceration or percolation.

Molding Vehicle: The vehicle which can be moulded into a particular shape and size. They are usually solid and semi-solid vehicles, e.g., globules, tablets, pilules, cones.

Molecule: The smallest particle of an element or compound that is capable of existing separately without loss of any original chemical properties.

Molecular Biology: That part of biology which attempts to interpret biological events in terms physico-chemical properties of molecules in cells.

Monograph: The general plan of Pharmacopoeias is to lay down the direction for the selection and preparation of drugs, that are thoroughly adapted to the purpose of homoeopathic prescribing. These directions and specifications for each drug are called 'Monographs'.

Mother Solution: It is the drug pharmaceutically prepared from the drug substance of mineral and chemical source as the strongest alcoholic, or aqueous solvent by the process dissolving in alcohol or purified water or exposing as the case may be.

Mother Substance: It is the drug pharmaceutically prepared from the drug substance of any source insoluble in liquid vehicle as the strongest solid solvent by the process of trituration with sugar of milk.

Mother Tincture: It is the drug pharmaceutically prepared from the drug substance of vegetable and animal kingdom, using strong alcohol as a vehicle (solvent) by the process of immersion, maceration and percolation.

Over-the-counter (OTC) Drugs: Medicines which are available for purchase from a shop, pharmacy etc. without a prescription(i.e. non prescription medicines).

pH: It is defined as the hydrogen ion concentration mole/litre.

Plussing: Extension of a dose by adding water to the remedy solution and succussing further.

Principal Investigator (In Homoeopathic Literature also referred to as: Master Prover; Coordinator; Director of Proving): Is responsible for the conduct and organisation of the Homoeopathic Drug-Proving following GCP Guidelines, e.g., contact with Independent Ethical Commission and the report of severe adverse events, storing of study documents.

Proprietary Name: The registered trademark of the therapeutic goods or the unique name assigned to the goods by the sponsor and appearing on the label.

Protocol: A document that describes the objective(s), design, methodology, statistical considerations, and organisation of a trial. The protocol usually also gives the background and rationale for the trial, but these could be provided in other protocol referenced documents.

Throughout the ICH, GCP Guideline the term protocol refers to protocol and protocol amendments.

Q-Potency: Q-potency is the term used to designate 50-Millesimal potency.

Quantum Theory: The theory that the emission or absorption of energy by atoms or molecules is not continuous but occurs in discrete amounts, each amount (energy-packet) being called a quantum.

Schedule J: It is the Objectionable Advertisement Act. According to this Act, there are certain incurable diseases which should not be proclaimed to be cure.

Schedule M: It is the Factory rule which guides about the requirement for pharmacy laboratory.

Serial Dilution: Serial dilution means that each dilution is prepared from the dilution immediately preceded it.

Sifting: It is a process of separating finer portions of comminuted drugs from the coarser particles by the use of a sieve. This is determining particle size.

Supervisor (Proving Doctor): A person responsible for the direct contact with the volunteer(s). He reviews the diaries (journals) together with each volunteer in order to clarify and if necessary amend the symptoms.

Tablets: Tablets are unit forms of solid medicinal substances with or without suitable diluents prepared from sugar of milk by the process of compressing or moulding.

Tautopathic, Tautopathically: Using the 'same' substance potentised as a remedy (rather than a 'similar' substance).

Therapeutic: Pertaining to the healing art, concerned with remedies for diseases.

Topical: Applied to a certain area of the skin for a localised effect.

Toxicology: The science which treats of poisons, their effects, antidotes and recognition.

Transdermal: Applied to the skin for a systemic effect by the diffusion or continuous absorption of the active ingredient through the skin.

Ultramolecular Potency: Homoeopathic product which is so dilute that the original substance is absent.

Unicist: One who adheres to the principle of single remedy/single dose.

Volunteer (In homoeopathic literature also referred to Prover): Person who takes the proving substance and reports any symptoms that occur by keeping a diary and direct contact with the investigator.

Wash: During preparation of alcohol, when percentage reaches up to 12-15%, it kills the enzyme present in yeast. This 12-15% alcoholic solution is called wash.

Whey: During preparation of sugar of milk, the solution remaining after removal of fat and protein is called whey.

Index

A

B

C

D